# *OSCE in*
# Clinical Surgery

# *OSCE in*
# Clinical Surgery


**Himanshu Prasad**
MBBS DNB (General Surgery) MCh Pursuing
Senior Resident (Academic)
Department of Neurosurgery
All India Institute of Medical Sciences
Jodhpur, Rajasthan, India
Ex-Senior Resident (Nonacademic)
Department of Neurosurgery
All India Institute of Medical Sciences
New Delhi, India
*Email: himanshuprasad1@gmail.com*

***Co-Authors***

**Neha Kalwadia**
MBBS DNB (General Surgery) MCh Pursuing
Senior Resident
Department of Plastic and
Reconstructive Surgery
Medical College and Hospital
Kolkata, West Bengal, India
*Email: nkalwadia@gmail.com*

**Shubham Jain**
MBBS MS (General Surgery)
Assistant Professor
Department of General Surgery
ESI Medical College
Alwar, Rajasthan, India
Ex-Senior Resident
Department of General Surgery
SMS Medical College,
Jaipur, Rajasthan, India
*Email: shubham.jain12101994@gmail.com*

**Manali Jain**
MBBS MS MCh Pursuing
Senior Resident
Department of Urology
All India Institute of Medical Sciences
Jodhpur, Rajasthan, India
*Email: manalijain281996@gmail.com*


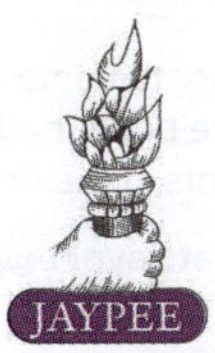



**JAYPEE BROTHERS MEDICAL PUBLISHERS**
*The Health Sciences Publisher*
**New Delhi | London**

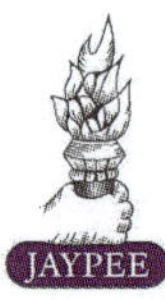

**Jaypee Brothers Medical Publishers (P) Ltd**

**Headquarters**
EMCA House, 23/23-B
Ansari Road, Daryaganj
New Delhi 110 002, India
Landline: +91-11-23272143, +91-11-23272703
+91-11-23282021, +91-11-23245672
e-mail: jaypee@jaypeebrothers.com

**Corporate Office**
4838/24, Ansari Road, Daryaganj
New Delhi 110 002, India
Phone: +91-11-43574357
Fax: +91-11-43574314
e-mail: jaypee@jaypeebrothers.com

**Overseas Office**
JP Medical Ltd.
83, Victoria Street, London
SW1H 0HW (UK)
Phone: +44-20 3170 8910
e-mail: info@jpmedpub.com

**EU GPSR** Authorised Representative
Logos Europe, 9 rue Nicolas Poussin
17000, La Rochelle, France
Phone: +33 (0) 6 67 93 73 78
e-mail: contact@logoseurope.eu

Website: www.jaypeebrothers.com
Website: www.jaypeedigital.com



**Inquiries for bulk sales may be solicited at:** jaypee@jaypeebrothers.com

***OCSE in Clinical Surgery***

*First Edition:* **2025**

*Reprint:* **2026**

ISBN: 978-93-5696-841-7

*Printed at: Samrat Offset Pvt. Ltd.*

**Dedicated to**

*My parents and family*
*for their immense love and support.*

# Contributors

**Aakansha Vashistha**
Assistant Professor
Department of Plastic Surgery
Sawai Man Singh Medical College
Jaipur, Rajasthan, India

**Ashish Jain**
Assistant Professor
Department of Community Medicine
RNT Medical College
Udaipur, Rajasthan, India

**Kajal Salvi**
Junior Resident
Department of Obstetrics and Gynecology
Government Medical College
Nagpur, Maharashtra, India

**Kaavya Agarwal** MBA
IILM University
Gurugram, Haryana, India

**Preeti Joon**
Senior Resident
Department of Pediatric Neurology
All India Institute of Medical Sciences
Jodhpur, Rajasthan, India

**Rajat Singhal**
Senior Resident
Department of Interventional Radiology
Christian Medical College
Vellore, Tamil Nadu, India

**Saurav Sharma**
Senior Resident
Department of Pediatric Oncology
All India Institute of Medical Sciences
New Delhi, India

**Shrikrishna Parab**
Senior Resident
Department of Plastic Surgery
Vardhman Mahavir Medical College
New Delhi, India

**Venkatesh Gadapaga**
Assistant Professor
Department of General Surgery
RVM Institute of Medical Sciences and Research Center
Hyderabad, Telangana, India

# Preface

Surgery is the expertise of human anatomical knowledge and applied surgical skills to remove or repair the body part. A surgical practical examination is a subjective clinical assessment of the postgraduate student.

This *OSCE in Clinical Surgery* is dedicated to DNB General Surgery final exam-going students and post-MS General Surgery candidates who are going to take the DNB final exit examination for a comprehensive understanding of the objective structured clinical examination (OSCE) pattern, which is an integral part of the DNB surgery broad specialty exit examination.

We tried to design the questions and answers, including a variety of clinical scenarios and clinical pictures from the standard reference books, to introduce the students with the OSCE pattern of examination so that they can prepare accordingly, it is not meant to cover the whole syllabus.

We heartily welcome all your insightful suggestions and criticism for the enhancement and refinement of our knowledge.

**Himanshu Prasad**

# Acknowledgments

As a surgeon will tell you, the training and practice with surgical acumen take dedication and hard work.

I would like to thank my surgical mentors for their inspiration and guidance.

I would especially like to thank the co-authors for using their expertise to assist me in bring all of the chapters together as a book.

I convey my sincere thanks to Shri Jitendar P Vij (Group Chairman), Mr Ankit Vij (Managing Director) of M/s Jaypee Brothers Medical Publishers (P) Ltd, New Delhi, India, and their team for their efforts and suggestions for helping me to present my idea and its execution in the form of the book.

It is my prayer and hope that this book will be an invaluable tool in OSCE examination preparation for general surgery.

# Acknowledgements

# Contents

## SECTION 1: Basic Principles



## SECTION 2: General Pediatrics

## SECTION 3: Preoperative Care



## SECTION 4: Trauma



## SECTION 5: Elective Orthopedics



## SECTION 6: Skin, Plastic and Reconstructive



## SECTION 7: Head and Neck

## SECTION 8: Endocrine and Breast



## SECTION 9: Cardiothoracic



## SECTION 10: Vascular



## SECTION 11: Abdominal



## SECTION 12: Genitourinary

## SECTION 13: Transplantation



## SECTION 14: Miscellaneous



## SECTION 15: Revision Spotter

1

SECTION

# Basic Principles

CHAPTER

# 1 Metabolic Response to Injury

## QUESTIONS

**Q1. Answer the following:**

a. Define term milieu interieur and term given by
b. Define homeostasis word and term coined by
c. "There is a circumstance attending accidental injury which does not belong to the disease, namely that the injury done, has in all cases a tendency to produce both the deposition and means of cure" statement given by
d. Biochemist who divided metabolic response to injury in humans into "ebb" and "flow" phase

**Q2. Hypermetabolism and increased nitrogen excretion are closely related to the magnitude of the initial injury and show a graded response.**

1. The following graphs showing the above mentioned thing—define a and b
2. Enumerate the proinflammatory cytokines produced in first 24 hours which act directly on hypothalamus to cause pyrexia.
3. Enumerate two characteristics of CARS.
4. Classical pathway of the stress response consist of
5. Effect of GH in metabolic response to injury

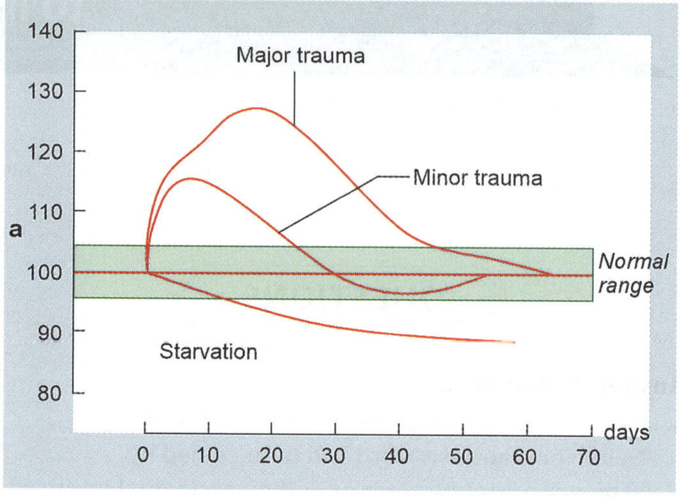


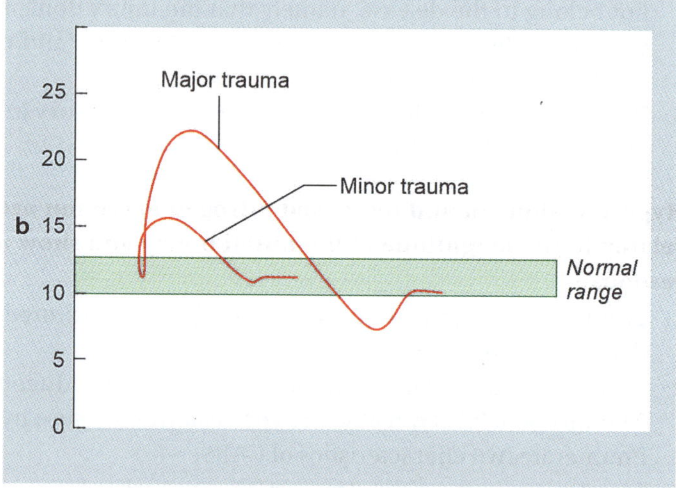


*Source:* Bailey and Love, 28th edition, page 2.

**Q3. Answer the following:**

a. Name two endogenous cytokinin antagonist
b. Th2 type counter inflammatory response regulated by
c. What includes specialized proresolving mediator (SPM)?
d. Hepatic acute phase promoted by

**Q4. Answer the following:**

a. Define systemic inflammatory response syndrome (SIRS)
b. SIRS is initially driven by which cytokines
c. SIRS is followed rapidly by increased plasma levels of
d. If SIRS prolonged or excessive may evolve into

**Q5. Regarding Ebb phase answer the following:**

a. Characterized by
b. Physiological role

**Q6. Figure showing the major catabolic and anabolic signaling pathways involved in skeletal muscle homeostasis.**

What is A, B, and C in given figure?

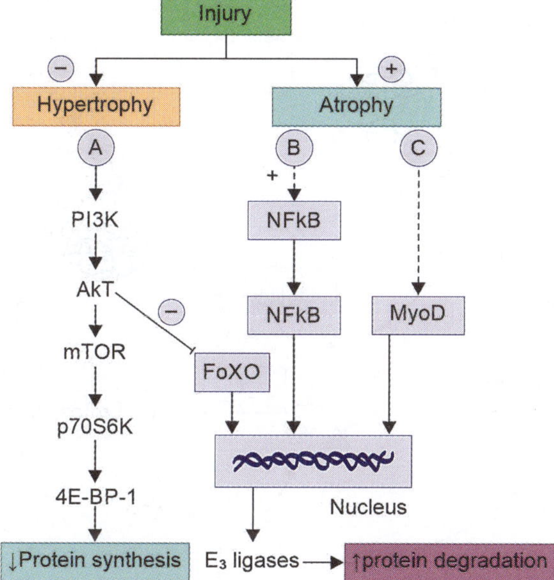


**Q7. Answer the following:**

a. Name the amino acid in given figure
b. The predominant mechanism involved in skeletal muscle wasting is

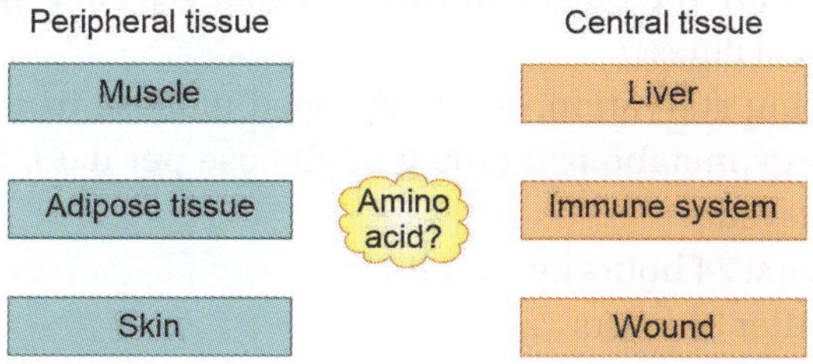


**Q8. Answer the following:**

a. Effect on albumin TER following major injury/sepsis
b. Why acute phase protein response (APPR) represents double edge sword?

c. The hepatic acute phase response represents are prioritization of body protein metabolism toward the liver and is characterized by
d. Autocannibalism, resulting in continuing how much urinary nitrogen loss.

**Q9. The intercellular effector mechanisms involved in degrading myofibrillar protein into free amino acids.**

What is A and B?

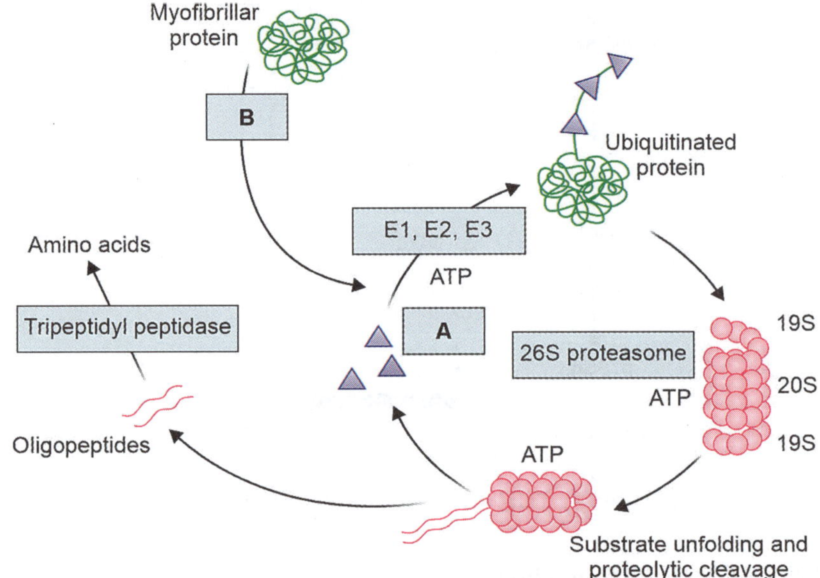


*Source:* Bailey and Love, 28th edition, page 6.

**Q10. Answer the following:**

a. What are the body composition changes after major surgery or critical illness?
b. During starvation, the body need glucose to sustain cerebral energy metabolism (100 g of glucose per day). Mention this is achieved:
   - First 24 hours by ............
   - After 24 hours ...........
c. According to modern guidelines on fasting prior (before surgery) to GA or spinal anesthesia allow intake of clear fluids up to how much hours
d. What are the advantages of carbohydrate drink at this time of preop?

**Q11. Figure showing changes in body weight that occur in serious sepsis, after uncomplicated surgery and in total starvation.**

What A, B, and C depict in graph?

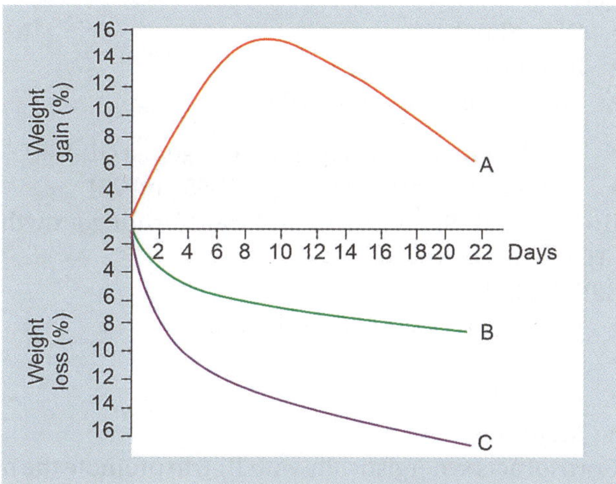


*Source:* Bailey and Love, 28th edition, page 8.

## ANSWERS

**Ans. 1** a. • *Term milieu interieur:* Claude Bernard

• *Terms means:* Body systems act to maintain internal constancy.

b. *Homeostasis:* Physiological process which maintains most of the steady states of the organism' (Walter Cannon); i.e., complex homeostatic responses involving the brain, nerves, heart, lungs, kidneys, and spleen work to maintain body constancy.

c. John Hunter

d. Sir David Cuthbertson (1930)

**Ans. 2** 1. a. Resting metabolic rate (%)

b. Nitrogen excretion (gN/day)

2. IL-1, tumor necrosis factor alpha (TNF-$\alpha$), IL-6, and IL-8

3. *Two characteristics:*

i. Results in immunosuppression

ii. An increased susceptibility to opportunistic (nosocomial) infection

4. *Consist of:*

- Afferent nociceptive neurons
- The spinal cord

- Thalamus
- Hypothalamus
- Pituitary

5. *Effect:*
   - Direct lipolytic
   - Insulin antagonizing
   - Proinflammatory properties

**Ans. 3** a. • Interleukin-1 (IL-1) receptor antagonist (IL-IRa)
- TNF-soluble receptors (TNF-sR-55 and 75)

b. IL-4, IL-5, IL-9, and IL-13 and transforming growth factor beta (TGF-β)

c. SPM Includes:
- Essential fatty acid-derived lipoxins
- Resolvins
- Protectins
- Maresins

d. Cortisol acts synergistically with IL-6 to promote the hepatic acute phase response

**Ans. 4** a. Systemic inflammatory response syndrome (SIRS) is an exaggerated defense response of the body to a noxious stressor (infection, trauma, surgery, acute inflammation, ischemia or reperfusion, or malignancy, to name a few) to localize and then eliminate the endogenous or exogenous source of the insult

Systemic inflammatory response syndrome following major injury:

b. Is driven initially by proinflammatory cytokines (e.g., IL-1, IL-6, and TNF-α).

c. Is followed rapidly by increased plasma levels of cytokine antagonists and soluble receptors (e.g., IL-1Ra and TNF-sR).

d. If prolonged or excessive may evolve into a counter inflammatory response syndrome.

**Ans. 5** a. *Characterize by:*
- Tissue edema (from vasodilatation and increased capillary leakage)
- Increased basal metabolic rate (hypermetabolism)
- Increased cardiac output
- Raised body temperature
- Leukocytosis
- Increased oxygen consumption
- Increased gluconeogenesis

b. To conserve both circulating volume and energy stores for recovery and repair.

**Ans. 6** a. Insulin-like growth factor-1 (IGF-1)
b. TNF-α
c. Myostatin

**Ans. 7** a. Branched chain amino acids. Ala—alanine; Gin—glutamine
b. ATP-dependent ubiquitin-proteasome pathway (lysosomal cathepsins and the calcium-calpain pathway play facilitatory and accessory roles.)

**Ans. 8** a. Increased threefold (following major injury/sepsis)
b. *Reason:* Proteins important for recovery and repair, but only at the expense of valuable lean tissue and energy reserves.
c. The hepatic acute phase response represents are prioritization of body protein metabolism toward the liver and is characterized by:
- *Positive reactants (e.g., CRP):* Plasma concentration ↑
- *Negative reactants (e.g., albumin):* Plasma concentration ↓

d. 10–20 gN/day (equivalent to 500 g of wet weight lean tissue)

**Ans. 9** A. Ubiquitin
B. Caspases, cathepsins, and calpain

**Ans. 10** a.
- Catabolism leads to a ↓ in fat mass and skeletal muscle mass.
- Body weight may paradoxically ↑ because of expansion of extracellular fluid space.

b.
- By mobilizing glycogen stores
- There after by hepatic gluconeogenesis from amino acids, glycerol, and lactate

c. 2 hours
d. Reduces perioperative anxiety and thirst and ↓ postoperative insulin resistance.

**Ans. 11** A. Sepsis and multiorgan failure
B. Uncomplicated major surgery
C. Starvation

# 2 CHAPTER

# Shock and Blood Transfusion

## QUESTIONS

**Q1. Answer the following:**

a. Define shock.
b. What is ischemic reperfusion syndrome?
c. Classify shock.
d. What is distributive shock and enumerate some example?
e. Define endocrine shock and enumerate causes.

**Q2. Answer the following:**

a. What is the effect on mixed venous saturation on distributive shock?
b. What is effect on systemic vascular resistance on distributive shock?
c. What is effect of cardiac output on distributive shock?

**Q3. Answer the following:**

a. Enumerate features of mild, moderate, and severe shock.
b. BP fall after how much of % circulatory volume loss.
c. What is the effect of distributive shock in capillary refill?
d. What is the last sign of shock?

**Q4. Answer the following:**

a. Define multiple organ failure.
b. How will you manage multiple organ failure?
c. Percentage of mortality in multiple organ failure
d. Effect of organ failure on:
    - Lungs
    - Kidney
    - Clotting
    - Cardiac

**Q5. Define:**

a. Responders
b. Transient responders
c. Nonresponders

**Q6. Answer the following:**

a. Vasopressor agent of choice in distributive shock and cardiogenic shock
b. The minimum standard and additional modalities for monitoring of the patient in shock
c. What is the normal central venous pressure (CVP) response, how will you measure and interpretate it?
d. What is the best measure of organ perfusion and the best monitor of the adequacy of shock therapy?

**Q7. Answer the following:**

a. The only clinical indicators of perfusion of the gastrointestinal tract and muscular beds are
b. Patients with a base deficit over ............ have a much higher morbidity and mortality than those with no metabolic acidosis.
c. Name new methods for monitoring regional tissue perfusion and oxygenation are

**Q8. Mixed venous oxygen saturation (MVOS)**

a. Define
b. Measured by
c. What is the normal value?
d. <50% suggestive of
e. >70% suggestive of
f. Effect of sepsis on MVOS

**Q9. Answer the following:**

a. Laser Doppler flowmetry used to monitor which organ
b. Near-infrared spectroscopy used to monitor which organ
c. Sublingual capnometry used to monitor which organ
d. Tissue oxygen electrode used to monitor which organ

**Q10. Answer the following:**

a. Define occult hypoperfusion.
b. How is it manifested?
c. Effect of occult hypoperfusion on mortality
d. What are global perfusion end points and traditional endpoints in context to improvement in mortality and morbidity in high-risk surgical patients?

**Q11. What is % of blood loss in:**

a. Class 1 hemorrhagic shock
b. Class 2 hemorrhagic shock
c. Class 3 hemorrhagic shock
d. Class 4 hemorrhagic shock

**Q12. Answer the following:**

a. How much blood one can donate at a time and max of how much time in a year?
b. Each unit of blood tested for
c. What is the benefit of leukodepleted blood donation?

**Q13. Answer the following:**

a. Packed cells are stored in
b. Fresh frozen plasma (FFP) stored at and its shelf life
c. What is cryoprecipitate and its use?
d. How are platelets stored?
e. What are the factors contained in prothrombin complex concentrates?

**Q14. Answer the following:**

a. Write three indication for blood transfusion.
b. What is the level of Hb probably will benefit from transfusion?

**Q15. Enumerate the complications from:**

a. Single transfusion
b. From massive transfusion

## ANSWERS

**Ans. 1** a. Shock is a systemic state of low tissue perfusion that is inadequate for normal cellular respiration with insufficient delivery of oxygen and glucose, cells switch from aerobic to anaerobic metabolism. If perfusion is not restored, cell death ensues.

b. Systemic hypoperfusion leads to → cellular and organ damage which leads to → tissue hypoxia and local activation of inflammation.

- Once normal circulation is restored to these tissues further injury occurs.
- The acid and potassium lead to direct myocardial depression, vascular dilatation, and further hypotension; this activates leukocytes then cellular and humoral elements activated by the hypoxia (complement, neutrophils, and microvascular thrombi), overwhelm the local anti-inflammatory response and are pushed back into the systemic circulation, where they cause injury to distant organs such as the lungs and the kidneys. This leads to acute lung injury, acute renal injury, cerebral oedema, multiple organ failure, and death.

- Reperfusion injury can currently only be attenuated by reducing the extent and duration of tissue hypoperfusion.

c. *Classification of shock:*
   - Hemorrhagic/hypovolemic shock
   - Cardiogenic shock
   - Obstructive shock
   - Distributive shock
   - Endocrine shock

d. Inadequate organ perfusion is accompanied by vascular dilatation with hypotension, low systemic vascular resistance, inadequate afterload, and a resulting abnormally high cardiac output.

e. Combination of hypovolemic, cardiogenic or distributive shock. Causes of endocrine shock include hypothyroidism and hyperthyroidism and adrenal insufficiency.

**Ans. 2** a. High
b. Low
c. High

**Ans. 3** a. Clinical features of shock

| | ***Compensated*** | ***Uncompensated*** | |
|---|---|---|---|
| | ***Mild*** | ***Moderate*** | ***Severe*** |
| Lactic acidosis | + | ++ | +++ |
| Urine output | Normal | Reduced | Anuric |
| Conscious level | Mild anxiety | Drowsy | Comatose |
| Respiratory rate | ↑ | ↓ | Labored |
| Pulse rate | ↑ | ↑ | ↑ |
| Blood pressure | Normal | Mild hypotension | Severe hypotension |

b. 30–40% of circulating volume has been lost.
c. Capillary refill will be brisk, despite profound shock.
d. Hypotension

**Ans. 4** a. ≥2 failed organ systems
b. Support of organ systems, with ventilation, cardiovascular support, and hemofiltration/dialysis until there is recovery of organ function.
c. 60%
d. 
   - *Lungs:* Acute respiratory distress syndrome (ARDS)
   - *Kidney:* Acute renal insufficiency
   - *Liver:* Liver failure and coagulopathy
   - *Cardiac:* Cardiovascular failure

**Ans. 5** a. There is a good and sustained improvement in blood pressure in response to a bolus transfusion.

b. There is an improvement in the blood pressure but this is not sustained. The rate of hemorrhage is less than the rate of volume administration.

c. There is no improvement in the blood pressure to a bolus transfusion. The rate of hemorrhage is greater than the rate of volume administration.

**Ans. 6** a. • *Distributive shock:* Phenylephrine and noradrenaline

• *Cardiogenic shock:* Dobutamine is the agent of choice.

b.

| ***Monitoring for patients in shock*** | |
|---|---|
| *Minimum additional modalities:* | *Additional modalities:* |
| • ECG | • Central venous pressure |
| • Pulse oximetry | • Invasive blood pressure |
| • Blood pressure | • Cardiac output |
| • Urine output | • Base deficit and serum lactate |

c. There is no "normal" CVP for a patient in shock, some patients may require a CVP of 5 $cmH_2O$, whereas some may require a CVP of 15 $cmH_2O$ or higher. Further, ventricular compliance can change from minute to minute in the shocked state, and CVP is a poor refection of end diastolic volume (preload).

Central venous pressure measurements should be assessed dynamically as the response to a fluid challenge. A fluid bolus (250–500 mL) is infused rapidly over 5–10 minutes. The normal CVP response is a rise of 2–5 $cmH_2O$, which gradually drifts back to the original level over 10–20 minutes. Patients with no change in their CVP are empty and require further fluid resuscitation. Patients with a large, sustained rise in CVP have high preload and an element of cardiac insufficiency or volume overload.

d. Urine output

**Ans. 7** a. Lactic acidosis (lactate and base deficit) and the mixed venous oxygen saturation

b. >6 mmol/L

c. • Muscle tissue oxygen probes

• Near-infrared spectroscopy

• Sublingual capnometry

**Ans. 8** a. MVOS - Percentage saturation of $O_2$ returning to the heart from the body is a measure of the $O_2$ delivery and extraction by the tissues.

b. Accurate measurement is via analysis of blood drawn from a long central line placed in the right atrium.
c. 50–70%.
d. Hypovolemic or cardiogenic shock
e. Sepsis and some other forms of distributive shock
f. Disordered utilization of oxygen at the cellular level and AV shunting of blood at the microvascular level. Therefore, less $O_2$ oxygen is presented to the cells, and those cells cannot utilize what little oxygen is presented. Thus, venous blood has a higher oxygen concentration than normal.

**Ans. 9** a. Gut
b. Brain and Muscle
c. Gut
d. Muscle

**Ans. 10** a. The state of normal vital signs and continued underperfusion
b. Persistent lactic acidosis and low mixed venous oxygen saturation
c. Patients with occult hypoperfusion for >12 hours have two to three times the mortality of patients with a limited duration of shock
d. • Base deficit
• Lactate
• Mixed venous oxygen saturation

**Ans. 11** a. <15%
b. 15–30%
c. 30–40%
d. >40%

**Ans. 12** a. Up to 450 mL
b. • Hepatitis B
• Hepatitis C
• Human immunodeficiency virus (HIV) 1 and HIV-2
• Syphilis
c. Donations are leukodepleted as a precaution against variant Creutzfeldt-Jakob disease (this may also reduce the immunogenicity of the transfusion).

**Ans. 13** a. SAGM (saline-adenine-glucose-mannitol) solution to increase shelf life to 5 weeks at 2–6°C.
b. –40°C to –50°C with a 2 years shelf life (first-line therapy in the treatment of coagulopathic hemorrhage)
c. Supernatant precipitate of FFP and is rich in fibrinogen, factor VIII, and XIII. It is stored at –30°C with a 2 years shelf life. It is given in low-fibrinogen states or factor VIII deficiency.

d. On a special agitator at 20–24°C and have a shelf life of only 5 days.
e. Highly purified concentrates prepared from pooled plasma. They contain factors II, IX and X. Factor VII may be included or produced separately.
*Indication:* Emergency reversal of anticoagulant (warfarin) therapy in uncontrolled hemorrhage

**Ans. 14** a.
- Acute blood loss (to replace circulating volume and maintain oxygen delivery)
- Perioperative anemia (to ensure adequate oxygen delivery during the perioperative phase)
- Symptomatic chronic anemia, without hemorrhage or impending surgery

b. <6 g/dL

**Ans. 15** a. Complications from a single transfusion include:
- Incompatibility hemolytic transfusion reaction
- Febrile transfusion reaction
- Allergic reaction
- Infection:
  - Bacterial infection (usually due to faulty storage)
  - Hepatitis
  - HIV
  - Malaria
- Air embolism
- Thrombophlebitis
- Transfusion-related acute lung injury (usually from FFP)

b. Complications from massive transfusion include:
- Coagulopathy
- Hypocalcemia
- Hyperkalemia
- Hypokalemia
- Hypothermia

# CHAPTER 3

# Wound Healing and Tissue Repair

## QUESTIONS

**Q1. Answer the following:**

a. What are the stages of wound healing?
b. What is described as the immediate phase occurring before inflammation?
c. What is the role of alpha granules in hemostasis?
d. Write functions of thrombin in hemostasis.

**Q2. Answer the following:**

a. Enumerate reactions take place in early inflammatory phase and late inflammatory phase.
b. Arrange these in sequence dolor, calor, rubor, and tumor (NEET SS 2022).
c. Enumerate the changes that take place in proliferation phase of wound healing.
d. Enumerate the changes that take place in remodeling phase of wound healing.

**Q3. Answer the following:**

a. What is predominant collagen seen in remodeling phase of wound healing?
b. What is the ratio of type I and type III in remodeling phase of wound healing?
c. Maximal tensile strength is to be achieved by how much time post injury (NEET SS 2022).

**Q4. Identify the stages of bone healing (a), (b), (c), and (d).**

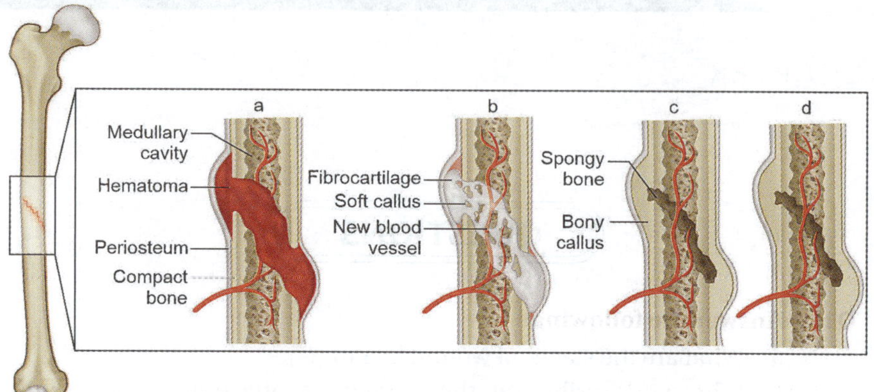


*Source:* Bailey and Love, 28th edition, page 26.

**Q5. Answer the following:**

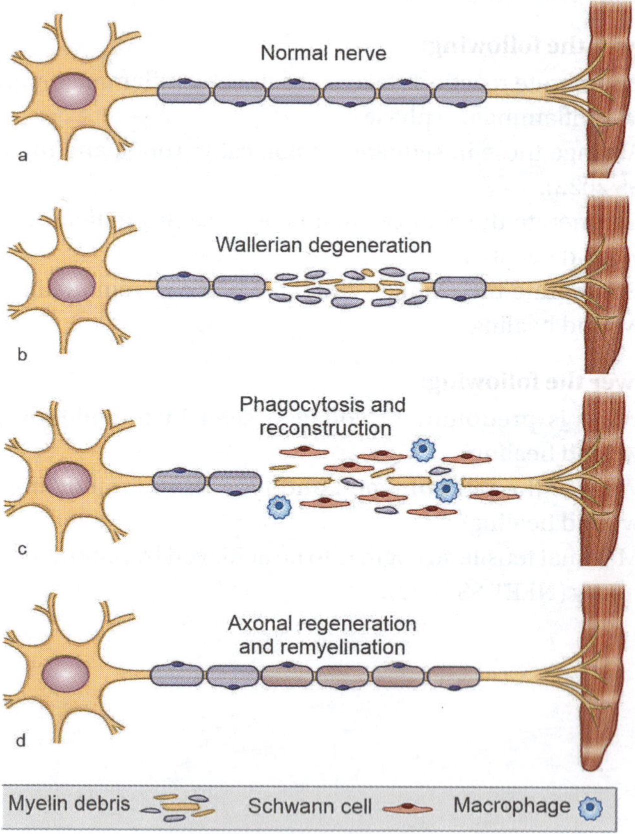


*Source:* Bailey and Love, 28th Edition, page 27.

a. What is depicted in this image?
b. Band of Büngner formed by and what is the role of it?
c. Which of the following stage in above image showing Wallerian degeneration and band of Büngner?
d. Define Wallerian degeneration.

**Q6. Answer the following:**

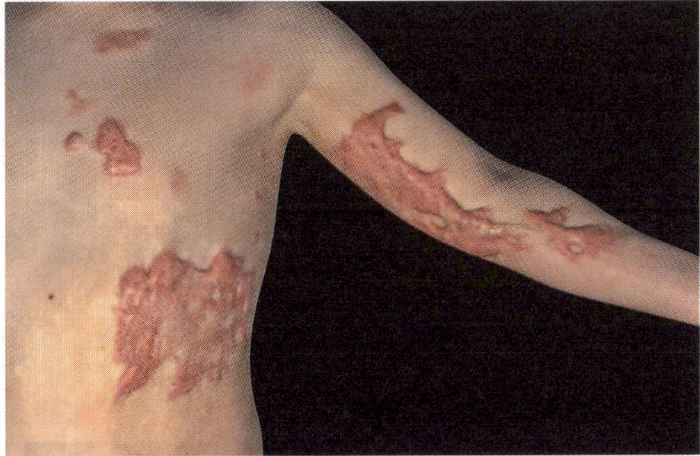

*Source:* Bailey and Love, 28th edition, page 28.

a. Enumerate two differences between keloid and hypertrophic scar.
b. Identify the scar in image.

**Q7. Identify the wound class according to us center for disease and control surgical wound classification.**

a. Open cardiac massage.
b. Open, fresh, accidental wounds.
c. Incision in which acute, nonpurulent inflammation is encountered.
d. Hernia repair.

**Q8. Answer the following:**

a. What is tetanus prone wound and high-risk tetanus prone wounds?
b. Postexposure management for treatment prone wounds in children 8 years old.

**Q9. Answer the following:**

a. Medical grade larvae used in biological debridement.
b. Give an example of enzymatic debridement.
c. Explain autolytic debridement.

**Q10. Answer the following:**

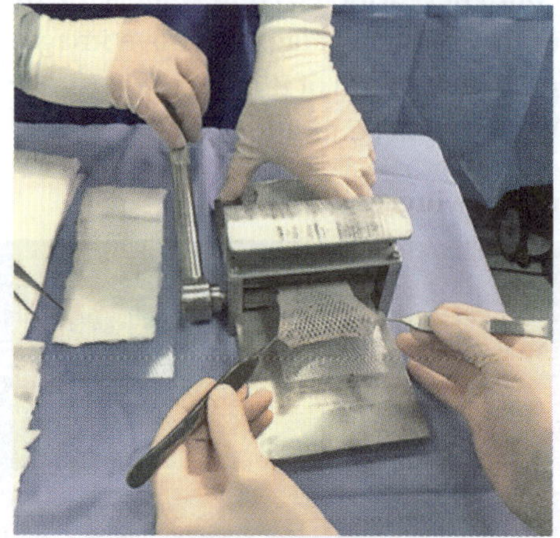

*Source:* Bailey and Love, 28th edition, page 30.

a. Explain the procedure depicted in image.
b. Give one difference between graft and flap.

**Q11. Answer the following:**

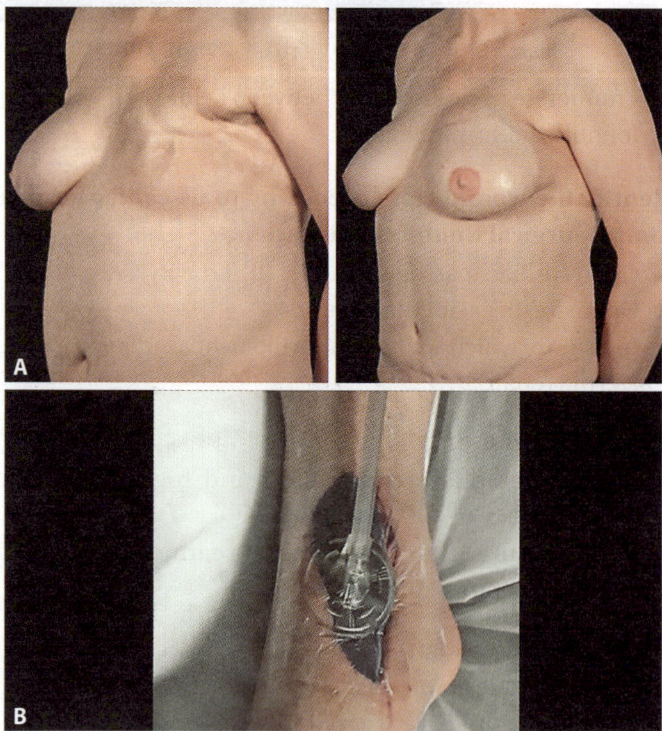


*Source:* Bailey and Love, 28th edition, page 31.

a. Which flap used in above image A?
b. Image B showing which type of therapy and how it helps wound healing?

## Q12. Answer the following:

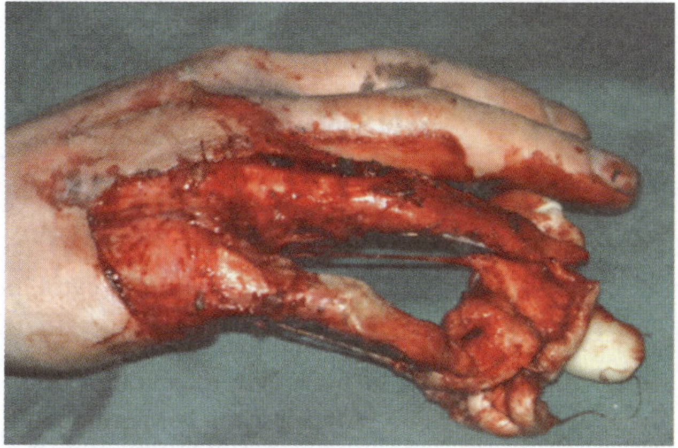

*Source:* Bailey and Love, 28th edition, page 33.

a. Identify the type of injury.
b. Explain the above type of injury.
c. What is morel Lavallee lesion?
d. Which dye used for to delineating viable and nonviable tissue in degloving injury?

## Q13. Answer the following:

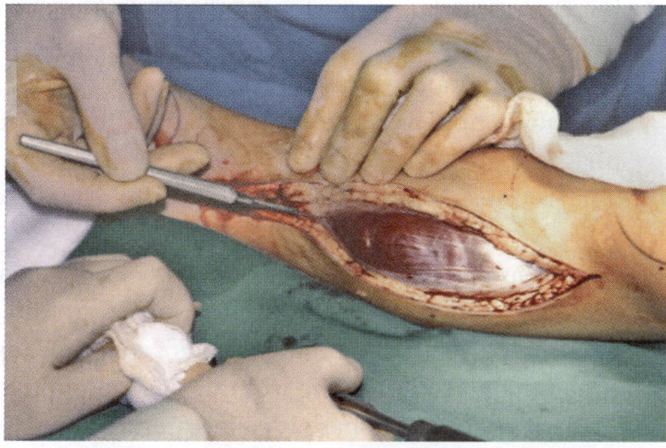

*Source:* Bailey and Love, 28th edition, page 34.

a. Characteristics of acute compartment syndrome of lower limb.
b. Which procedure depicted in above image?
c. What incisions to be given for above procedures?

**Q14. According to UIS national injury advisory panel staging of pressure injuries answer the following:**

a. Description of stage 3.
b. Description of stage 2.
c. Enumerate bed sore preventive scores.

## ANSWERS

**Ans. 1** a. Inflammation, proliferation and remodeling

b. Hemostasis

c. It contain hundreds of proteins, including cytokines and GF [transforming growth factor beta (TGF-β), platelet-derived growth factor (PDGF), fibroblast growth factor (FGF), EDGF, and vascular endothelial growth factor (VEGF)].

These aid in the chemotaxis, extracellular matrix deposition, epithelialization, and angiogenesis.

d. Production of fibrin, which aids in stabilizing the platelet plug and creates a scaffold for cell infiltration

**Ans. 2** a. *Early inflammatory phase (days 1–2):*

- Platelet activation causes an influx of inflammatory cells led by PMNL, platelets, and the local injured tissue also release vasoactive amines such as histamine and serotonin, which increase vascular permeability, thereby aiding infiltration of inflammatory cells
- Early inflammatory phase (days 2–3)
- Monocyte appear in wound and differentiate into macrophages

b. Rubor (redness), tumor (swelling), calor (heat), and dolor (pain)

c. It starts around day 3 and lasts for 2–4 weeks. It consists mainly of fibroblast activity with the production of ground substance (glycosaminoglycans and proteoglycans), collagen, angiogenesis, and reepithelialization of the wound. The wound tissue formed in the early part of this phase is called granulation tissue. It has a pink and granular appearance.

d. Begins 2–3 weeks after injury and lasts for a year or more. This phase is characterized by maturation of collagen.

**Ans. 3** a. Type I collagen is the predominant collagen seen in the remodeling phase of wound healing
b. 4:1
c. 12 weeks postinjury

**Ans. 4** a. Hematoma formation and inflammation
b. Soft callus
c. Hard callus formation from osteoblasts forming woven bone
d. Remodeling proceeds with osteoclasts and osteoblasts facilitating the conversion of woven bone into lamellar bone

**Ans. 5** a. Degeneration and regeneration after peripheral nerve injury
b. SCs proliferate and migrate alone to the basal lamina to form bands of Büngner, which guide the axon to reinnervate toward the corresponding target
c. Stage B
d. When normal nerves suffer a physical injury, the portion of the lesion site and its distal stump undergo destruction and break down to produce myelin debris. This degenerative process is called Wallerian degeneration.

**Ans. 6** a.

| *Hypertrophic scars* | *Keloid scars* |
|---|---|
| Hypertrophic scars do not extend beyond the boundary of the original incision or wound. They are more common in areas of increased tension, wounds crossing tension lines, deep dermal burns and wounds left to heal by secondary intention (longer than 3 weeks) | Keloid scars extend beyond the boundaries of the original incision or wound, do not spontaneously regress and are difficult to treat. The etiology is unknown but genetic predisposition is implicated. They often occur as a result of relatively minor trauma and mainly in those with darker skin pigmentation |

b. Multiple keloid scars

**Ans. 7** a. Class III contaminated
b. Class III contaminated
c. Class III contaminated
d. Class I clean

**Ans. 8** a.

| *Tetanus-prone wounds* | *High-risk tetanus-prone wounds* |
|---|---|
| • Puncture-type injuries in a contaminated environment<br>• Bites<br>• Compound fractures<br>• Containing foreign bodies<br>• Wounds or burns with systemic sepsis | Any tetanus-prone wound with:<br>• Heavy contamination, e.g., soil or manure<br>• Wound requiring surgery with >6-hour delay<br>• Extensive devitalized tissue |

b. Children aged 5–10 years

| Who have received an adequate priming course but no pre-school booster | Who not received an adequate priming course | For high risk tetanus prone: |
|---|---|---|
| Immediate reinforcement dose of vaccine | Immediate reinforcement dose of vaccine | • Immediate reinforcing dose of vaccine<br>• One dose of human tetanus immunoglobulin 2 in a different site |

**Ans. 9** a. Larvae of *Lucilia sericata* (release proteolytic and antimicrobial substances to remove necrotic tissue)

b. Collagenase or papain—urea

c. Using dressings such as hydrocolloids or transparent films to retain moisture and allow wound enzymes to selectively liquefy nonviable tissue

**Ans. 10** a. Meshing a split-thickness skin graft

b.

| *Graft* | *Flap* |
|---|---|
| No inherent blood supply and is dependent on a well-vascularized recipient site for survival and wound healing. Split-thickness skin grafts consist of the epidermis and a small portion of dermis whereas full-thickness skin grafts consist of the epidermis and the majority of the dermis | Contains tissue with its intrinsic blood supply that is transferred from one part of the body (donor) to another (recipient). The blood supply of the flap therefore does not rely on the recipient site like a skin graft. A free fap contains tissue with its vascular pedicle that is surgically detached and transferred from its original location to a distant recipient site |

**Ans. 11** a. Left mastectomy and delayed left breast reconstruction with a deep inferior epigastric artery perforator free fap and nipple reconstruction

b. Negative-pressure wound therapy for a lower limb wound

**Ans. 12** a. Degloving injury of the right little and ring fingers

b. Avulsion of skin + subcutaneous fat from the underlying fascia + muscle/bone

c. *Morel Lavallee lesion:* Disruption of perforating vascular and lymphatic vessels may result in a characteristic hemolymphatic collection between the fascial planes.

d. Indocyanine green

**Ans. 13** a. Increased interstitial pressure within a closed osteofascial compartment, which results in microvascular compromise. It is a surgical emergency as delayed treatment may lead to irreversible muscle ischemia and significant long-term morbidity.

b. Fasciotomy of the leg pressure ≤30 mm Hg between the diastolic pressure and intracranial pressure (ICP)

c. A medial longitudinal incision 1–2 cm posterior to the medial border of the tibia decompresses the superficial and deep posterior compartments. A lateral longitudinal incision 2 cm lateral to the anterior tibial border decompresses the peroneal and anterior compartments.

**Ans. 14** a. Full-thickness skin loss

b. Partial-thickness skin loss with exposed dermis

c. Scores:
- Braden scale
- Waterlow score
- Norton risk assessment scale

CHAPTER

# 4 Tissue Engineering and Regenerative Therapies

## QUESTIONS

**Q1. Define with one example.**

a. Totipotent
b. Pluripotent
c. Multipotent
d. Unipotent

**Q2. Answer the following:**

a. What are stem cells?
b. Enumerate types of stem cells.

**Q3. Answer the following:**

a. What are somatic stem cells?
b. Enumerate types of somatic stem cells (SSC).

**Q4. Answer the following:**

a. Mesenchymal stem cells morphologically resembles.
b. What are the sources of mesenchymal stem cells?
c. Mesenchymal stem cells isolated from
d. Uses of mesenchymal stem cells.

**Q5. Answer the following:**

a. Who discovered induced pluripotent stem cells?
b. Enumerate property of induced pluripotent stem cells.
c. Write one disadvantage of induced pluripotent stem cells.

**Q6. Answer the following:**

a. What are the sources of natural and artificial scaffolds?
b. Role of scaffold in tissue engineering

**Q7. Answer the following:**

a. Enumerate challenges to tissue engineering.
b. Enumerate safety concern in tissue engineering.

**Q8. Answer the following:**

a. Embryonic stem cells are obtained after how many days of fertilization.

b. Yamanaka factors includes which genes?

c. What lineages can be produced by placenta?

d. Skeletal stem cells are which type of cell lineage.

## ANSWERS

**Ans. 1** a. to d.

| *Term* | *Definition* | *Examples* |
|---|---|---|
| Totipotent | Ability to form all differentiated cells in the embryo and extraembryonic tissue (e.g., placenta) | Zygote, morula |
| Pluripotent | Ability to form all lineages of the body but not extraembryonic tissue (e.g., placenta) | Embryonic stem cells (ESCs)—derived from the blastocyst inner cell mass |
| Multipotent | Adult stem cells that can form multiple cells in a particular cell lineage | Skeletal stem cells (SSCs) |
| Unipotent | Cells from one cell type | Osteocytes and chondrocytes |

**Ans. 2** a. Stem cells undifferentiated or nonspecialized cells through cell division to renew themselves indefinitely.

b. *Classification:*
- Embryonic stem cell—early embryo
- Fetal stem cell-tissue from the fetus
- Adult or somatic stem cell
- Induced pluripotent stem cells—derived from reprogramming adult specialized cells

**Ans. 3** a. Capacity to differentiate into a limited number of specialize cells types: They are multipotent, e.g., replace senescent or damage cells in the blood and gut mucosa

b. *Types of SSC:*
- Hematopoietic stem cells—treatment for hematological malignancy
- Mesenchymal stem cells for tissue engineering
- Endothelial progenitor cells/stromal cells
- Neural stem cells

**Ans. 4** a. Fibroblast
b. Bone marrow, adipose tissue, and umbilical cord
c. Iliac crest, aspiration, and liposuction
d. burns treatment, repair of cartilage defects

**Ans. 5** a. Shinya Yamanaka
b. *Retroviral or lentiviral transfection to introduce factors:*
- Pluripotent
- Autologous
- No rejection

c. By using retro virus genomic integration of virus may lead to activation of oncogenes.

**Ans. 6** a. Natural—intact human tissue and artificial—implantable biomaterials
b. *Requirement of scaffold of used in tissue engineering:*
- Provide structural support for cells
- Allow cells to attach, migrate and proliferate
- Enable oxygen, nutrients and regulatory factors access to all cells
- Deliver signals to promote cell migration and proliferation
- Biocompatible non immunogenic and ideally biodegradable

**Ans. 7** a. *Challenges to tissue engineering:*
- Delivery of oxygen
- Delivery of nutrients
- Flat tissue grow easily
- Tubular structure and organs difficult to grow

b. *Safety concerns:*
- Malignant transformation
- Infection
- Graft rejections
- Need for immunosuppressive therapy

**Ans. 8** a. 5 Days
b. Genes - OCT 3/4, $SOX_2$ and either Kruppel-like factor and C-MYC (together designated the OSKM reprogramming factors) or NANOG and LIN28
c. Unipotency, multipotency, totipotency but not pluripotency
d. Multipotency

CHAPTER

# 5 Surgical Infection

## QUESTIONS

**Q1. Answer the following:**

a. *Staphylococcus aureus* is found in the nasopharynx of up to how much percentage of the population?

b. Which organism responsible for pseudomembranous colitis?

c. What rapid testing available for *Clostridium difficile* (*C. difficile*)?

d. Recommended empirical treatment available for *C. difficile.*

e. Which is the principal organism that acts in synergy with aerobic gram-negative bacilli to cause surgical site infections (SSIs)?

**Q2. Answer the following:**

a. What is endogenous and exogenous source of infection?

b. Enumerate risk factors for increased risk of wound infection.

**Q3. Answer the following:**

a. What is decisive period and its interval?

b. What is HAI (hospital-acquired infection)?

c. Define major SSI.

**Q4. Answer the following:**

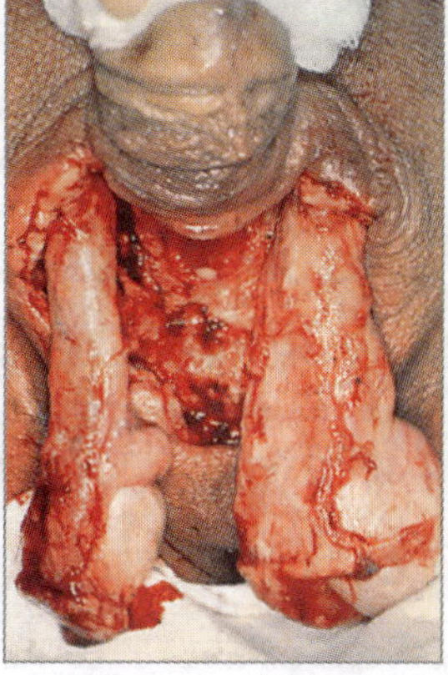

*Source:* Bailey and Love, 28th edition, page 58.

a. Identify the image presentation.
b. Enumerate the operative points to be consider during management of necrotizing fasciitis.
c. What is Meleney's synergistic gangrene?

**Q5. Enumerate the universal precautions have been drawn by CDC in USA and largely adopted by UK.**

**Q6. Define:**

a. SIRS
b. Sepsis
c. Severe sepsis or sepsis syndrome

**Q7. Answer the following:**

a. What is sepsis bundle?
b. Explain Sepsis Six.
c. What are the components of Sepsis Six?

**Q8. Answer the following:**

a. What are the infection rate with antibiotic prophylaxis in clean type of surgery?
b. What are the infection rates without antibiotic prophylaxis in dirty (pus or perforation, or incision through an abscess) type of surgery?

**Q9. Name the procedure depicted in image and when it to be done.**

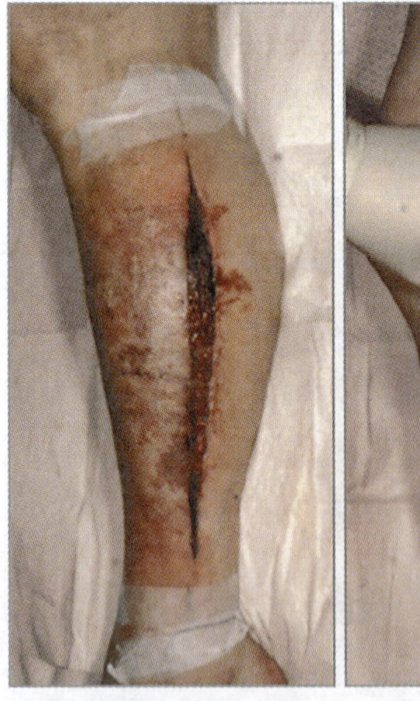
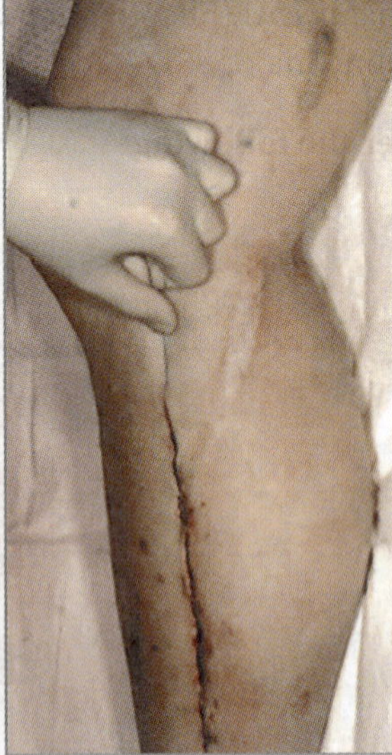

*Source:* Bailey and Love, 28th edition, page 63.

**Q10. Enumerate three principles for use of antibiotics therapy in SSI.**

**Q11. Answer the following:**

a. Use of narrow spectrum antibiotics.
b. Use of broad spectrum antibiotics.

## ANSWERS

**Ans. 1** a. *Staphylococcus aureus* (nasopharynx of up to 15% of the population)

b. *Clostridium difficile* is the cause of pseudomembranous colitis, in which destruction of the normal colonic bacterial fora by antibiotic therapy allows an overgrowth of the normal gut commensal *C. difficile* to pathological levels

c. Rapid testing for *C. difficile* is now available in the form of testing either *C. difficile* glutamate dehydrogenase (GDH) antigen or *C. difficile* toxin A/B. The *C. difficile* GDH Ag rapid test qualitatively detects for the presence of *C. difficile* GDH antigen in feces. On the other hand, the *C. difficile* toxin A/B rapid test qualitatively detects for the presence of *C. difficile* toxins A and B in feces. These rapid tests apply lateral flow immunochromatography and are for professional in vitro diagnostic use. Results are usually returned from this rapid testing in >30 minutes.

d. Empirical treatment with metronidazole or vancomycin is recommended while awaiting results.

e. Bacteroides fragilis is the principal organism that acts in synergy with aerobic gram-negative bacilli to cause SSIs, including intra-abdominal abscesses after colorectal or gynecological surgery. They are sensitive to the imidazoles (e.g., metronidazole) and some cephalosporins (e.g., cefotaxime)

**Ans. 2** a.

| ***Endogenous*** | ***Exogenous*** |
|---|---|
| Present in or on the host, e.g., SSSI following contamination of the wound from a perforated appendix | Acquired from a source outside the body, such as the operating theatre (inadequate air filtration, poor antisepsis) or the ward (e.g., poor handwashing compliance). The cause of hospital-acquired infection (HAI) |

b.
- Malnutrition (obesity and weight loss)
- Metabolic disease (diabetes, uremia, and jaundice)
- Immunosuppression [cancer, acquired immunodeficiency syndrome (AIDS), steroids, chemotherapy, and radiotherapy]

- Colonization and translocation in the gastrointestinal tract
- Poor perfusion (systemic shock or local ischemia)
- Foreign body material
- Poor surgical technique (devitalized tissue, dead space, and hematoma)

**Ans. 3** a. • *Decisive period:* Interval before bacterial growth becomes established enough to cause an infection after a breach in the tissues, whether caused by trauma or by surgery.
- Interval 4-hour

b. Infection acquired from the environment or the staff following surgery or admission to hospital

c. A wound that either discharges significant quantities of pus spontaneously or needs a secondary procedure to drain it. The patient may have systemic signs such as tachycardia, pyrexia, and increase WBC.

**Ans. 4** a. Fournier's gangrene

b. The finger test can be used in the diagnosis of patients who present with suspected necrotizing fasciitis. The area of suspected involvement is first infiltrated with local anesthesia. A 2-cm incision is made in the skin down to the deep fascia. Lack of bleeding is a sign of necrotizing fasciitis. On some occasions, a dishwater-colored fluid is noticed seeping from the wound. A gentle, probing maneuver with the index finger covered by a sterile glove is then performed at the level of the deep fascia. If the tissues dissect with minimal resistance, the finger test is positive. Tissue biopsies are then sent for frozen section analysis.

c. Abdominal wall infections are known as Meleney's synergistic gangrene and scrotal infections as Fournier's gangrene

**Ans. 5** Universal precautions have been drawn up by CDC in the USA and largely adopted by the NHS in the UK. In summary, these are:

- Use of a full face mask ideally, or protective spectacles.
- Use of fully waterproof, disposable gowns and drapes, particularly during seroconversion.
- Boots to be worn, not clogs, to avoid injury from dropped sharps.
- Double gloving needed (A larger size on the inside is more comfortable)
- Allow only essential personnel in theatre.
- Avoid unnecessary movement in theatre.
- Respect is required for sharps, with passage in a kidney dish.
- Slow meticulous operative technique is needed with minimized bleeding.

**Ans. 6** a. SIRS is presence of two out of three of the following:
- Hyperthermia (>38°C) or hypothermia (<36°C)
- Tachycardia (>90/min, no β-blockers) or tachypnea (>20/min)
- White cell count >12 × 109/L or <4 × 109/L

b. Sepsis is SIRS + documented source of infection

c. *Evidence of failure of one or more organs:* Respiratory (acute respiratory distress syndrome), cardiovascular (septic shock follows compromise of cardiac function and fall in peripheral vascular resistance), renal (usually acute tubular necrosis), hepatic, blood coagulation systems, or central nervous system

**Ans. 7** a. Combination of evidence-based objectives that must be completed within 6 hours for patients presenting with severe sepsis, septic shock, and/or lactate >4 mmol/L.

b. The Sepsis Six is the name given to a bundle of medical therapies designed to reduce mortality in patients with sepsis. Drawn from international guidelines that emerged from the Surviving Sepsis Campaign, the Sepsis Six was developed by the UK's Sepsis Trust.

c. The components of the Sepsis Six are:
- Give three to patients: (1) Intravenous fluid challenge, (2) intravenous antibiotics, and (3) oxygen and monitor urine output
- Take three from patients: (4) Blood cultures, (5) full blood count, and (6) lactate.

**Ans. 8** Surgical site infection rates relating to wound contamination with and without using antibiotic prophylaxis

| *Type of surgery* | *Infection rate with prophylaxis (%)* | *Infection rate without prophylaxis (%)* |
|---|---|---|
| Clean (no viscus opened) | 1–2 | 1–2 |
| Clean-contaminated (viscus opened, minimal spillage) | 3 | 6–9 |
| Contaminated (open viscus with spillage or inflammatory disease) | 6 | 13–20 |
| Dirty (pus or perforation, or incision through an abscess) | 7 | 40 |

**Ans. 9**
- Delayed primary closure of a fasciotomy wound after 3–5 days
- Delayed primary or secondary closure can be undertaken when the wound is clean and granulating. Gross-infected wounds may be left to heal by secondary intention, particularly where there is a loss of skin cover and healthy granulation tissue develops.

**Ans. 10** Principles for the use of antibiotic therapy:

- Antibiotics do not replace surgical drainage of infection.
- Only spreading infections or signs of systemic infection justify the use of antibiotics.
- Whenever possible, the organism and sensitivity should be determined.

**Ans. 11** a. To treat a known sensitive infection; for example, MRSA (which may be isolated from pus) is usually sensitive to vancomycin or teicoplanin, but not flucloxacillin.

b. Combinations of broad-spectrum antibiotics can be used when the organism is not known or when it is suspected that several bacteria, acting in synergy, may be responsible for the infection.

# 6

# Tropical Infections and Infestations

CHAPTER

## QUESTIONS

**Q1. Answer the following:**

a. What are the diagnostic pointers for infection with *Entamoeba histolytica*?

b. How will you treat amoebiasis?

**Q2. Answer the following:**

a. What is Loeffler's syndrome?

b. What is pathogenesis of ascariasis?

**Q3. Answer the following:**

a. What is depicted in the given image?

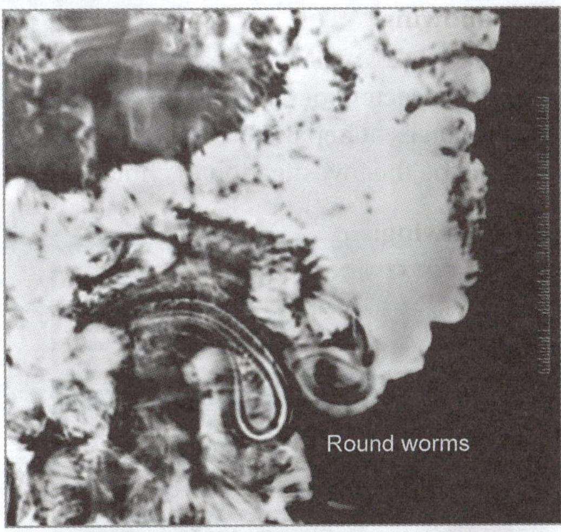


*Source:* Bailey and Love, 28th edition, page 70.

b. How will you diagnose and manage the condition shown in part A?

**Q4. Answer the following:**

a. Explain diagnosis and pathogenesis of cholangiohepatitis.
b. How will you manage asiatic cholangiohepatitis?

**Q5. Answer the following:**

a. Identify the condition depicted in the given image.

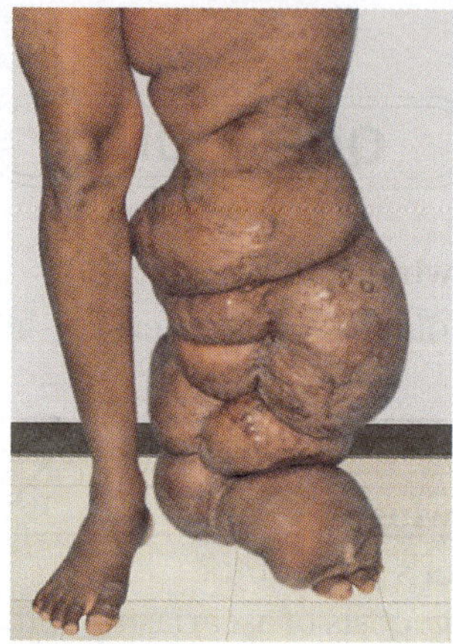

*Source:* Bailey and Love, 28th edition, page 73.

b. How will you manage the condition shown in part A?

**Q6. Answer the following:**

a. What is the cause of hydatid disease?
b. Explain the characteristics of cyst.
c. Explain the stages of hepatic hydatid cyst.
d. What should be the investigation of choice for hydatid cyst?

**Q7. Answer the following:**

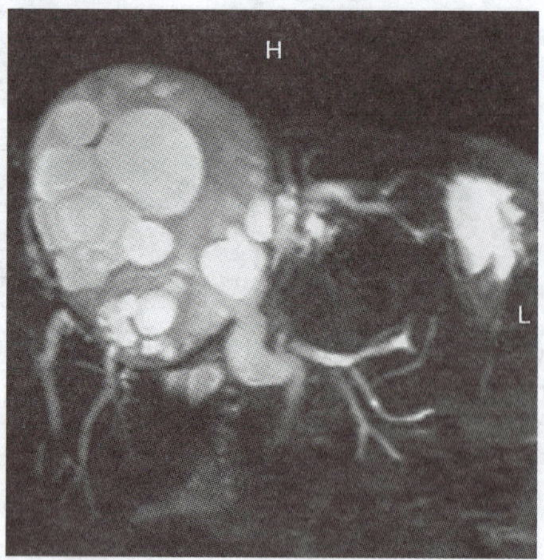


*Source:* Bailey and Love, 28th edition, page 75.

a. Identify the mode of imaging and diagnosis of given image.
b. What is surgical treatment of the same?

**Q8.**

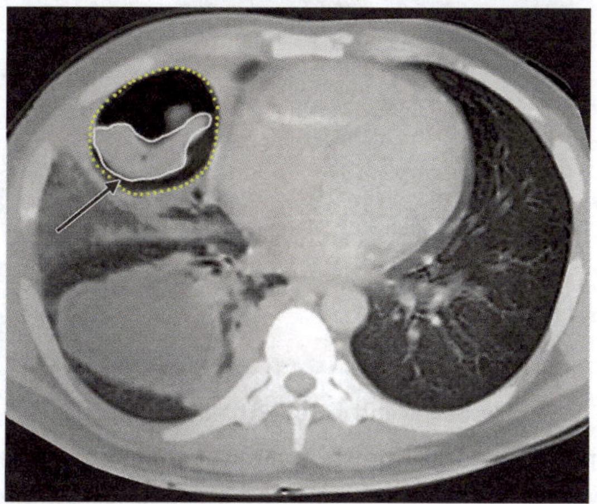

*Source:* Bailey and Love, 28th edition, page 77.

**While on a high-altitude trip a young mountaineer complained of sudden shortness of breath, cough, and copious expectoration consisting of clear fluid and flaky material. At first, it is thought to be due to pulmonary edema, which is ruled out later. On the basis of computed tomography (CT) finding, kindly make diagnosis.**

**Q9. Answer the following:**

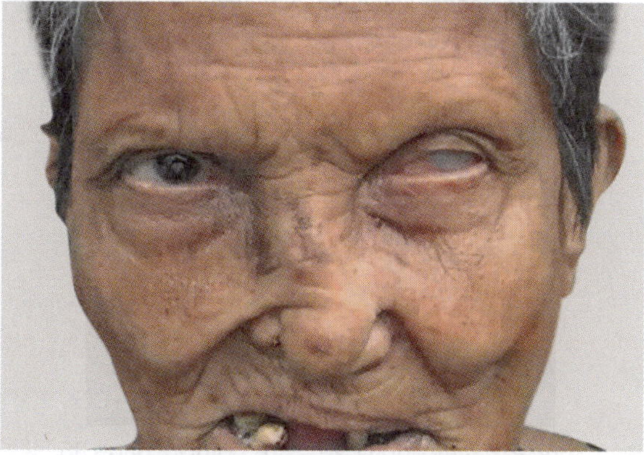

*Source:* Bailey and Love, 28th edition, page 79.

a. Identify the condition shown in given image.
b. What are the diagnosis points for the same?
c. How will manage the condition given in Part A?

## Q10. Answer the following:

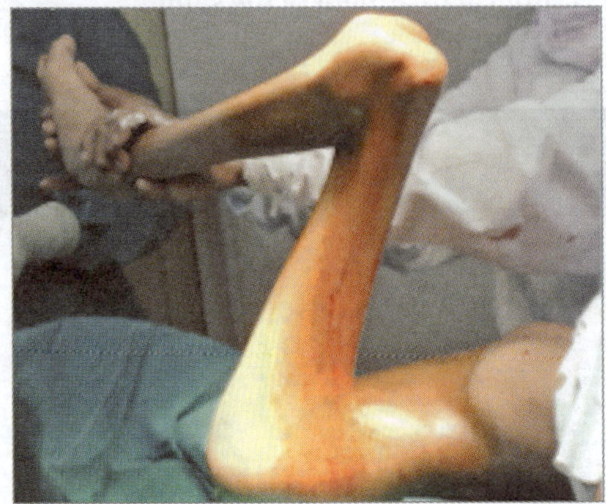

*Source:* Bailey and Love, 28th edition, page 85.

a. Identify the condition shown in the given image.
b. How will you differentiate the shown condition in Part A with Guillain-Barre syndrome (GBS)?
c. What is the pathogenesis of mycetoma?

## Q11. Answer the following:

a. What is pathology of tropical chronic pancreatitis?
b. How will you diagnose it?
c. What is the treatment strategy for same?
d. Identify the image and associated pathology.

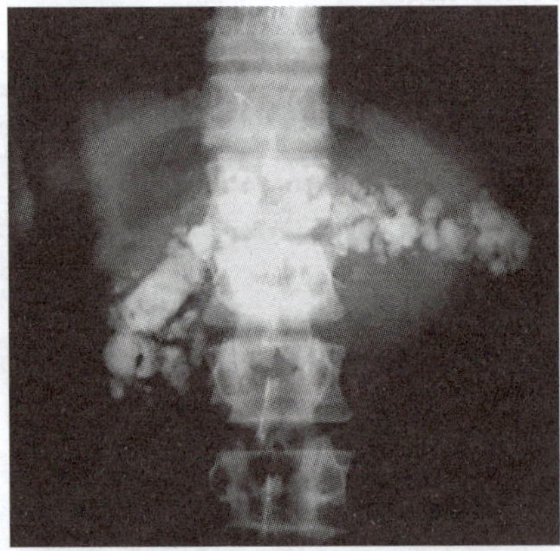

*Source:* Bailey and Love, 28th edition, page 86.

**Q12. Answer the following:**

a. What is shown in the given Figure A?

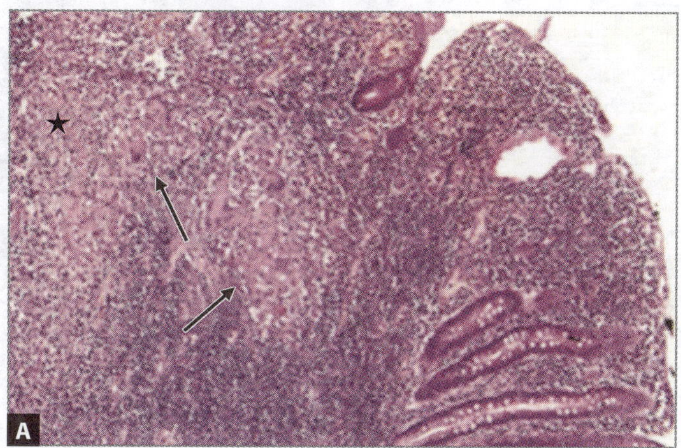

*Source:* Bailey and Love, 28th edition, page 88.

b. What is shown in the Figure B?

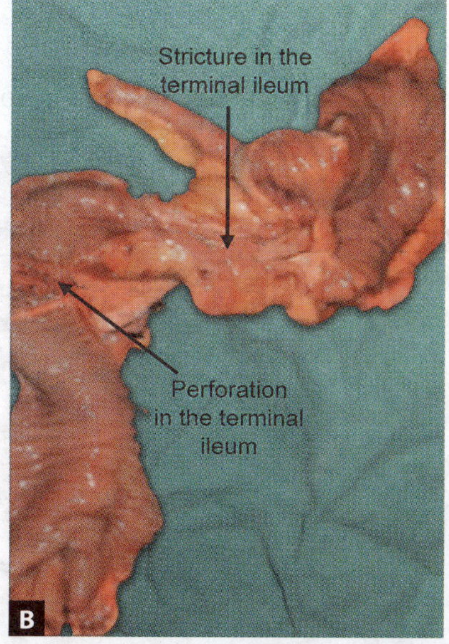


*Source:* Bailey and Love, 28th edition, page 89.

c. How will you investigate the condition given in Part B?

## Q13. Answer the following:

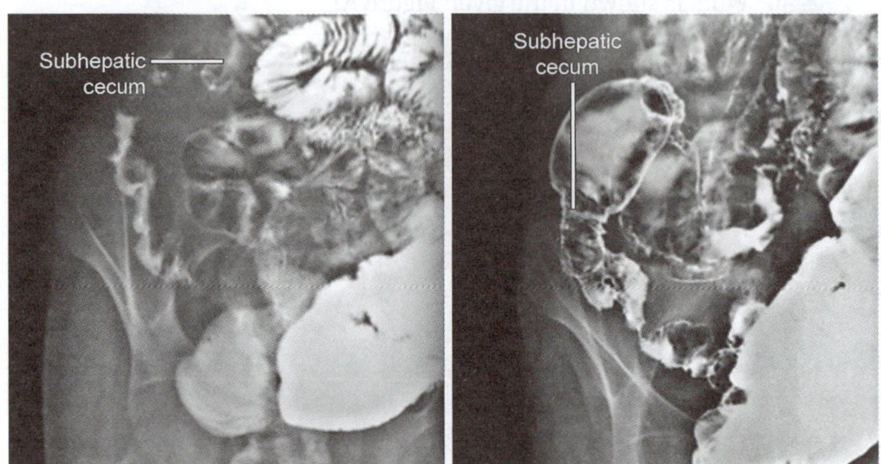


*Source:* Bailey and Love, 28th edition, page 90.

a. What is shown in the given scan?
b. How will you treat this condition?

## Q14. Answer the following:

a. Identify the condition depicted in given histology.

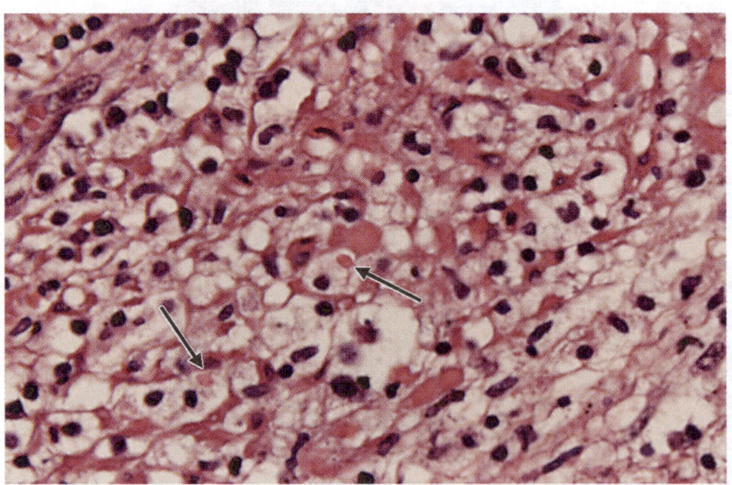

*Source:* Bailey and Love, 28th edition, page 90.

b. How will you treat the given condition?

## ANSWERS

**Ans. 1** a. Diagnostic pointers
- Diarrhea—bloody mucoid (endemic area)
- Upper abdominal pain, fever, cough, and malaise
- Chronic cases—a mass in the right iliac fossa may be an ameboma
- Sigmoidoscopy shows typical ulcers—biopsy and scrapes may be diagnostic
- Serological tests
- Intraoperative cholangiography (IOC), ultrasonography (USG), and computed tomography (CT).

b. Treatment
- Medical management—metronidazole and tinidazole
- Large abscesses—aspiration or pigtail catheter drainage is combined with drug treatment.
- Surgical—for complications, such as rupture into the pleural, peritoneal, or pericardial cavities.
- Acute toxic megacolon and severe hemorrhage are intestinal complications.
- *Treated with intensive supportive therapy followed by resection and exteriorization:* Subtotal colectomy with terminal ileostomy and closure of the rectal stump.
- Suspected case of amoeba in a colonic mass, cancer should be excluded by appropriate imaging and biopsy.

**Ans. 2** a. *In ascariasis:* The larval stage in the lungs causes pulmonary symptoms—dry cough, chest pain, dyspnea, and fever—referred to as Loeffer's syndrome.

b. *Ascariasis:* Pathogenesis
- Intestinal nematode affecting humans
- Humid atmosphere and poor sanitary conditions, hence, is seen in the tropics and resource-poor countries.
- Larvae cause pulmonary symptoms; adult worms cause gastrointestinal, biliary, and pancreatic symptoms.
- Distal ileal obstruction is due to a bolus of worms; ascending cholangitis and obstructive jaundice are due to infestation of the common bile duct.

- Acute pancreatitis occurs when a worm is lodged in the pancreatic duct.
- Perforation of the small bowel is rare.

**Ans. 3** a. Barium meal and follow-through showing roundworms in the course of the small bowel with barium seen inside the worms.

b. Diagnosis and management
   - Barium meal and follow-through will show worms scattered in the small bowel.
   - USG may show worms in the common bile duct (CBD) and pancreatic duct.
   - Plain abdominal radiograph and contrast CT scan will show the worms as tubular or curvilinear structures.
   - Medical management—anthelmintics is the first even in obstruction.
   - Surgery is a last resort for acute abdomen—various options are available.

**Ans. 4** a. *Asiatic cholangiohepatitis:* Pathogenesis and diagnosis
   - Occurs in far eastern tropical zones
   - The causative parasite is Clonorchis sinensis, opisthorchis, or fasciola.
   - Produces bile duct hyperplasia, intrahepatic duct dilatation, and stones.
   - Increases the risk of cholangiocarcinoma.
   - May remain dormant for many years.
   - When active, there are biliary tract symptoms in a generally unwell patient.
   - Stool examination for eggs or worms is diagnostic.
   - Ultrasonography of the hepatobiliary system and endoscopic retrograde cholangiopancreatography (ERCP) is also diagnostic.

b. Treatment
   - Medical treatment can be curative in the early stages.
   - Surgical treatment is cholecystectomy, exploration of the CBD, and some form of biliary-enteric bypass.
   - *Prevention:* Consider offering hepatobiliary USG as a screening procedure to recently arrived migrants from endemic areas.

**Ans. 5** a. Left lower limb filariasis—elephantiasis

b. Medical treatment—diethylcarbamazine (DEC) is very effective in the early stages before the gross deformities of elephantiasis have developed. Early stages of limb swelling, intermittent pneumatic compression helps treatment has to be repeated over a prolonged period.

**Ans. 6** a. Echinococcus granulosus, commonly called the dog tapeworm.

b. The cyst is characterized by three layers:

1. Outer pericyst, which is derived from compressed host organ tissues;
2. Intermediate hyaline ectocyst, which is noninfective; and
3. Inner endocyst, which is the germinal membrane and contains viable parasites that can separate, forming daughter cysts.

Colder climates caused by Echinococcus multilocularis, in which the cyst spreads from the outset by actual invasion rather than expansion.

c.

| | |
|---|---|
| CL (cystic lesion) | Unilocular anechoic cystic lesion without internal echoes or septations |
| CE (cystic echinococcosis) 1 | Uniformly anechoic cyst with fine internal echoes that represent protoscolices after rupture of a vesicle, called "hydatid sand" |
| CE 2 | Cyst with internal septation representing the walls of the daughter cyst described as multivesicular, honeycomb, cartwheel or rosette formation |
| CE 3 (transitional stage) | *Description of daughter cyst:*<br>• *3A:* Daughter cysts with detached laminated membrane<br>• *3B:* Daughter cysts inside a solid matrix |
| CE 4 | Daughter cysts can no longer be seen (inactive/degenerative) mixture of hypoechoic and hyperechoic features—like a bag of wool |
| CE 5 | Calcification of the wall; either partial or complete (inactive/degenerative) |

*Source:* Bailey and Love, 28th edition, page 74.

d. USG and CT scan.

**Ans. 7** a. MRCP showing a large hepatic hydatid cyst with daughter cysts communicating with the CBD, causing obstruction and dilatation of the entire biliary tree.

b. Surgical treatment—Minimal access therapy is best summarized by the mnemonic puncture, aspiration, injection, and respiration (PAIR). This is done after adequate drug treatment with albendazole, although praziquantel has also been used.

**Ans. 8** CT scan showing the "water lily" sign (arrow).

**Ans. 9** a. *Frontal view of the face showing eye changes in leprosy:* Paralysis of orbicularis oculi and loss of eyebrows.

b. *Leprosy:* Diagnosis

- Typical clinical features and awareness of the disease should help to make a diagnosis

- The face has an aged look, with collapse of the nasal bridge and ocular changes
- Thickened peripheral nerves, patches of anesthetic skin, claw hands, foot drop, and trophic ulcers are characteristic.
- Microbiological examination of the acid-fast bacillus and typical histology on skin biopsy are confirmator.

c. *Leprosy:* Treatment
- Multiple-drug therapy × 1 year.
- Team approach
- Surgical reconstruction requires the expertise of a hand surgeon, orthopedic surgeon, and plastic surgeon.
- Education of the patient and general public should be the keystone in prevention.

**Ans. 10** a. Patient with polio showing marked wasting of the left upper arm muscles with flexion contractures of the left knee and hip; there is equinus deformity of the foot.

b. The disease targets the anterior horn cells, causing lower motor neuron paralysis. Muscles of the lower limb are affected twice as frequently as those of the upper limb. Fortunately, only 1–2% of sufferers develop paralytic symptoms, but when they do occur, the disability causes much misery. When a patient develops fever with muscle weakness:
- GBS needs to be excluded.
- The latter has sensory symptoms and signs.
- Cerebrospinal fluid (CSF) fluid analysis should help to differentiate the two conditions.

c. *Mycetoma:* Pathogenesis
- Mostly occurs in the "mycetoma belt"
- There are two types—eumycetoma and actinomycetoma
- Caused by fungi or bacteria entering through a site of trauma, which may not be apparent; hence the foot is most commonly affected.
- Produces a chronic, specific, granulomatous, progressive, and destructive inflammatory lesion.
- Results in tissue destruction, deformity, disability, and sometimes death.

**Ans. 11** a. *Pathology of tropical chronic pancreatitis:*
- Almost exclusively occurs in resource-poor countries and is due to malnutrition; alcohol is not a cause.
- Cassava ingestion is regarded as an etiological factor because of its high content of cyanide compounds.

- Dilatation of pancreatic ducts with large intraductal stones.
- Fibrosis of the pancreas as a whole.
- A high incidence of pancreatic cancer in those affected by the disease.

b. *Diagnosis of tropical chronic pancreatitis:*
- The usual sufferer is a type 1 diabetic under 40 years of age.
- Serum amylase may be elevated in an acute exacerbation.
- Plain radiograph shows stones along the pancreatic duct.
- Ultrasonography and CT scan of the pancreas confirm the diagnosis.
- ERCP should be used as an investigation only when combined with a therapeutic procedure.

c. Treatment of tropical chronic pancreatitis
- Mainly medical—pain relief, insulin for diabetes, and pancreatic supplements for malnutrition.
- Surgery is reserved for intractable pain when all other methods have been exhausted.
- Operations are side-to-side pancreaticojejunostomy; resection in extreme cases.

d. Plain radiograph of the abdomen showing large stones along the main pancreatic duct typical of tropical chronic pancreatitis.

**Ans. 12** a. Histology of ileocecal tuberculosis showing epithelioid cell granuloma.

b. *Emergency limited ileocolic resection:* Specimen showing a tuberculous stricture in the terminal ileum and perforation of a transverse ulcer just proximal to the stricture.

c. *Intestinal tuberculosis:* Investigations
- Raised inflammatory markers, anemia, and positive sputum culture
- Interferon gamma (IFN-γ) release assays for subclinical infection.
- Ultrasonography of the abdomen may show localized areas of ascites.
- Chest radiograph shows pulmonary infiltration.
- Barium meal and follow-through shows multiple small bowel strictures particularly in the ileum, with a subhepatic cecum.
- If symptoms warrant, the genitourinary tract is also investigated.

**Ans. 13** a. Series of a barium meal and follow-through showing strictures in the ileum, with the cecum pulled up into a subhepatic position. Intestinal tuberculosis

b. *Tuberculosis:* Treatment
   - Patients should ideally be under the combined care of a physician and surgeon.
   - Vigorous supportive and full-drug treatment are mandatory in all cases.
   - Symptomatic strictures are treated by the appropriate resection, e.g., local ileocolic resection or strictureplasty or resection as an elective procedure once the disease is completely under control.
   - Acute intestinal obstruction from distal ileal stricture is treated by thorough resuscitation followed by resection with ileostomy or primary anastomosis.
   - One-stage resection and anastomosis can rarely be considered if the patient's general condition permits.
   - Perforation is treated by appropriate local resection and anastomosis or ileostomy if the condition of the patient is very poor; this is later followed by restoration of bowel continuity after the patient has fully recovered with antitubercular chemotherapy.

**Ans. 14** a. Histology of enteric perforation of the small intestine showing erythrophagocytosis (arrows) with predominantly histiocytic proliferation.

b. Treatment of bowel perforation from typhoid:
   - Intensive care unit (ICU) care
   - Resuscitate and give intravenous (IV) antibiotics
   - Laparotomy
   - Perforation (terminal ileum)
   - Exteriorization
   - Close the peritoneum and leave the wound open for secondary closure.

# CHAPTER 7 Basic Surgical Skills

## QUESTIONS

**Q1. Answer the following:**

a. What are the objectives of correct surgical positioning?

b. What are the points to consider prepositioning planning?

**Q2. Answer the following:**

a. What is rose position?

b. What is Trendelenburg position?

c. What is reverse Trendelenburg position?

**Q3. Identify the position shown in image.**

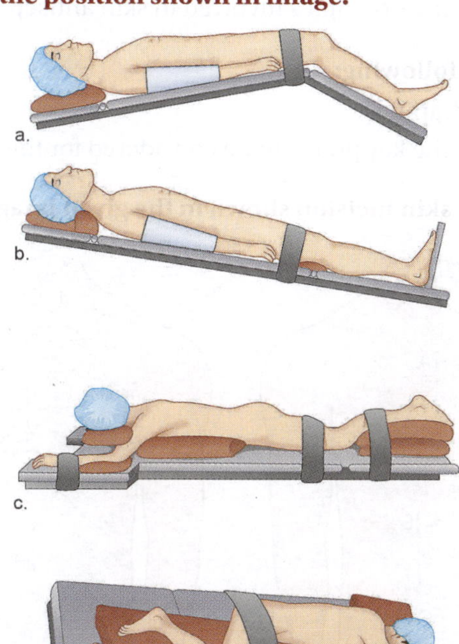


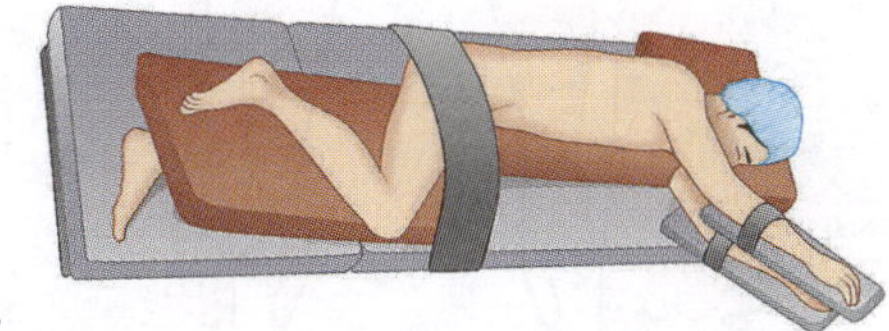


*Source:* Bailey and Love, 28th edition, pages 95 and 96.

**Q4. What are potential complications specific to supine positioning?**

**Q5. Answer the following:**

a. How will you give prone position?
b. When is this position used?
c. What are the key points to be considered in prone positioning?
d. What are the potential complications for the same?

**Q6. Answer the following:**

a. What are the key points to be considered in lateral positioning?
b. What are the potential complications for the same?

**Q7. Answer the following:**

a. What are the key points to be considered in lithotomy positioning?
b. What are the potential complications for the same?
c. What is Lloyd-Davies position?

**Q8. Answer the following:**

a. What is ideal timing of hair removal from surgical site?
b. What are the principles involved in skin antisepsis?

**Q9. Answer the following:**

a. What is draping?
b. What are the key points to be considered for the same?

**Q10. Identify the skin incision shown in the given image.**

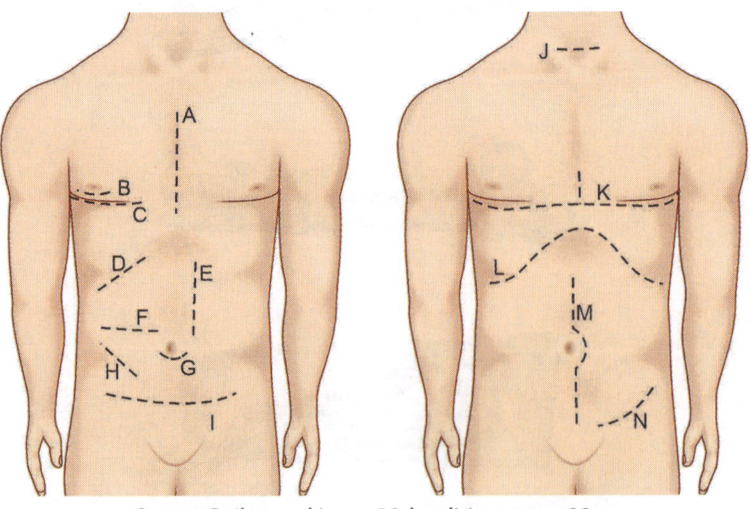


*Source:* Bailey and Love, 28th edition, page 98.

**Q11. Enumerate one use of these surgical blade.**

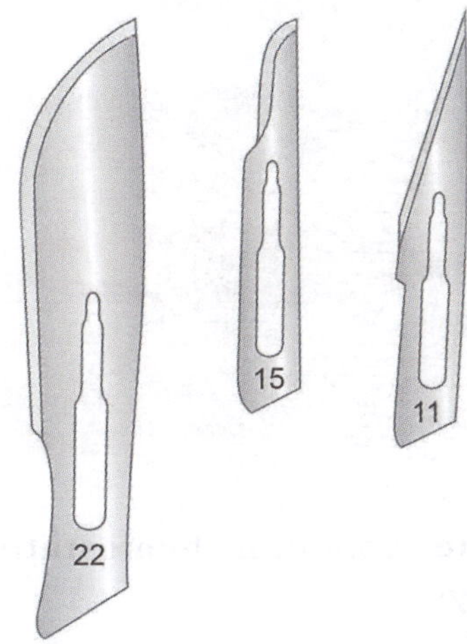


*Source:* Bailey and Love, 28th edition, page 98.

**Q12. Answer the following:**

a. What is maximum flow rate and maximum pressure of $CO_2$ insufflation in creating pneumoperitoneum for laparoscopic surgery (Iniss 2023 Nov)?
b. What is Palmer's point?
c. How will you confirm intraperitoneal placement of Veress needle?

**Q13. Answer the following:**

a. What is absorption rate and tensile strength of silk suture?
b. What is absorption rate and tensile strength of polyglactin suture (vicryl)?
c. What is absorption rate and tensile strength of polydioxanone (PDS) suture?
d. What is absorption rate and tensile strength of polyglycaprone suture (monocryl)?

**Q14. Name the suture technique shown in given figures.**

a.

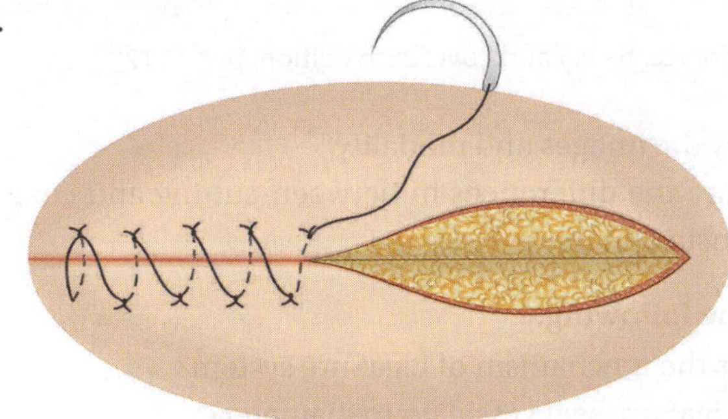

b.

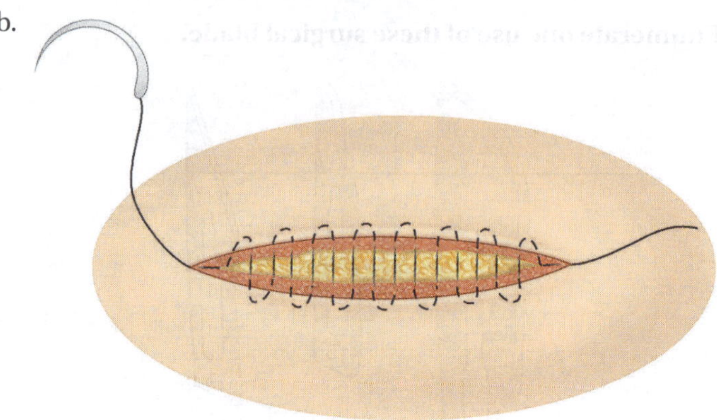

**Q15. What are the common hemostatic technique used intraoperatively?**

**Q16. Answer the following:**

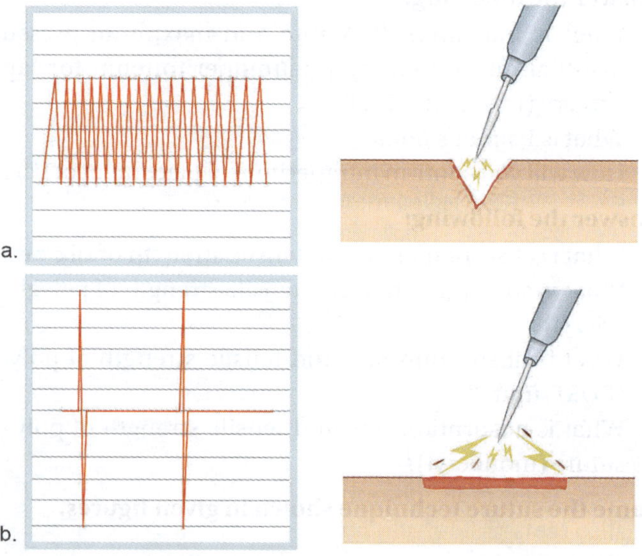


*Source:* Bailey and Love, 28th edition, page 112.

a. Identify the images and modality
b. What are the differences in between cutting and coagulation of tissue using diathermy?

**Q17. Answer the following:**

a. What is the mechanism of LigaSure system?
b. Does LigaSure seal vessel up to diameter?

**Q18. Answer the following:**

a. What is harmonic scalpel?

b. What is the mechanism of action (MOA)?

**Q19. Answer the following:**

a. What is the use of Thunderbeat STM?

b. What is current role of drain placement in gastrointestinal (GI) surgery?

**Q20. Answer the following:**

a. What are the indications for placement of the nasogastric tube?

b. What are the contraindications of nasogastric tube?

c. What are the complications associated with nasogastric tube?

**Q21. Name the type of drain used in a, b, and c?**

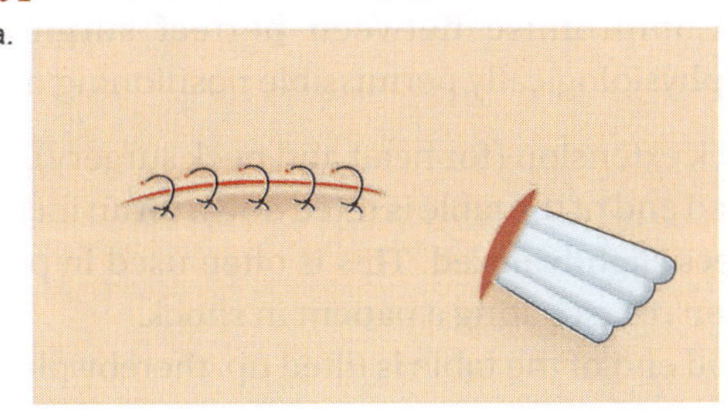


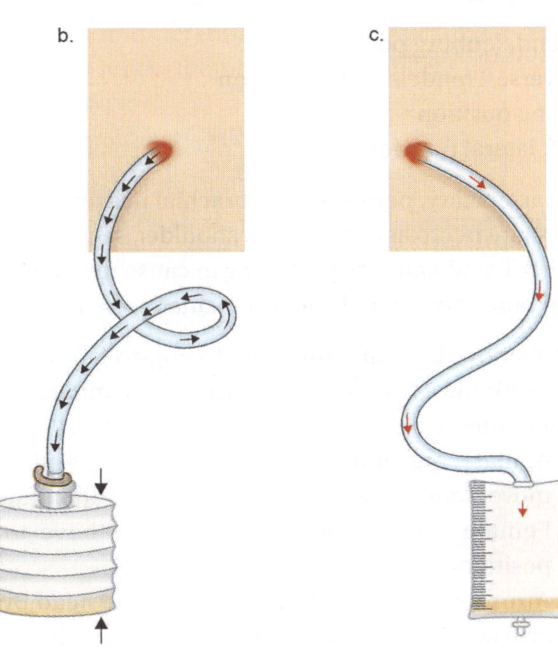

## ANSWERS

**Ans. 1** a. Objectives of correct surgical positioning:
1. Safe anesthesia and surgery
2. Reduce adverse physiological insults
3. Optimize exposure and ergonomics
4. Maintain patient's dignity by avoiding unnecessary exposure

b. Prepositioning planning
1. Final checks of the operating table and accessories.
2. Optimum positioning of laparoscopic stacks, electrosurgical unit, surgical ancillaries, and nursing trolley.
3. Passive diathermy leads and underbody heating blankets placed appropriately
4. Age, body habitus, and joint mobility to be considered.
5. Compromise between perfect surgical positioning and physiologically permissible positioning needs to be reached.

**Ans. 2** a. Neck extension (for head and neck surgery).

b. Head end of the table is tilted down on an incline with the patient's knees slightly flexed. This is often used in pelvic procedures and when resuscitating a patient in shock.

c. Head end of the table is tilted up, thereby placing the head higher than the feet.

**Ans. 3** a. Trendelenburg position

b. Reverse Trendelenburg position

c. Prone position

d. Left lateral position

**Ans. 4**
1. Ulnar, axillary, peroneal, and brachial neuropraxia.
2. Pressure necrosis of the heels, shoulder, sacral region, and scalp.
3. Steep Trendelenburg position can cause respiratory compromise and raise intracranial and intraocular pressure.

**Ans. 5** a. Intubation done first followed by log-rolled onto the operating bed with the assistance of at least four members of the team.

b. Spinal surgery

c.
1. Axillary and lateral chest rolls are essential to aid in the movement of the chest, abdomen, and diaphragm.
2. Female breasts and male genitalia have to be carefully positioned.
3. Arms may be placed by the side of the head by reversing the arm boards with care taken to avoid shoulder dislocation.

4. Toes should be elevated of the bed by placing pads under the shins.
5. Specially designed pillows with a hollow to accommodate the face and endotracheal tube, while gently supporting the forehead and chin, are also used.

d. Potential complications
- Brachial plexus injury (BPI) and shoulder dislocation.
- Facial trauma, including blindness secondary to vascular congestion of the eye.
- Pressure necrosis (i.e., breasts, external genitalia, and pressure-bearing bony prominences).
- Displacement of the endotracheal tube (ET).

**Ans. 6** a. For lateral positioning
1. The lower leg is slightly flexed at the knee, a pillow is placed between both the legs, and the upper leg is flexed in a more exaggerated position.
2. The arms are usually placed in stirrups.
3. Maintaining cervical alignment of the head is very important.

b. Potential complications
1. Respiratory complications secondary to preferential ventilation of one lung over the other and accidental endobronchial migration of the tube.
2. Traction injury of the brachial plexus injury and ulnar nerve injury.
3. Corneal abrasions and ocular trauma.

**Ans. 7** a. Lithotomy positioning
1. Bilateral lower limb are simultaneously placed in the stirrups.
2. The fingers should not extend past the edge of the table (as they can be crushed or even amputated accidentally).
3. The legs should not be externally rotated or unduly abducted.
4. Sequential compression devices may be useful to prevent venous stasis, especially in major operations.

b. Potential complications
1. Venous and arterial insufficiency (long procedures can lead to limb ischemia and compartment syndrome, besides having a higher chance of deep vein thrombosis (DVT).
2. Digital amputation
3. Damage to the sciatic nerve (due to hyperflexion).
4. Saphenous and peroneal neuropraxia when legs are placed in the stirrups.

c. Lithotomy—Positioned supine and legs flexed at the hip and knee and placed in stirrups (position the hips are flexed to 90°).

Lloyd-Davies position—modification of the lithotomy position with hips minimally flexed to around 15° with a 30° head-down tilt.

**Ans. 8** a. On the operating table after a dose of prophylactic antibiotic is given.

b. The principles involved in skin antisepsis are as follows:
1. Alcohol-based antiseptic solution (WHO recommends the use of chlorhexidine alcohol)
2. Extensions of the main incision, additional incisions, and drain placement have to be factored in when planning the preparation of the surgical site.
3. Cotton-tipped swab can be used to clean the umbilicus.
4. For dirty wounds, it is advisable to start from an area of lower bacterial contamination and move toward a region with greater contamination (clean procedures, starting from the area where skin incision is likely to be made and working toward the periphery is advised).
5. Using concentric circles, horizontal, or vertical lines do not make a difference in preventing surgical site infection (SSI).
6. Allow the antiseptic solution to dry and to avoid dripping of the solution onto the diathermy electrodes or pooling under the patient.

**Ans. 9** a. Process of forming a sterile perimeter around the operating site using disposable or reusable sterile sheets. Drape sheet form a fluid-resistant barrier; they are antistatic, fame resistant, lint free, and although waterproof, are porous enough to prevent heat build-up.

b. Key points
1. Stand an arm's length away from the OT table and spread the drapes with arms extended.
2. Avoid reaching across the operating table to drape.
3. Avoid sharp towel clips as that pierce the drapes and contaminate
4. If breach in sterile technique, then redo the process.
5. Customized drapes for nondisposable equipment such as laparoscopic cords, ultrasonic devices, image intensifiers, and light handles.
6. The routine use of transparent adhesive skin drapes (with or without antibiotic impregnation) over the surgical site cannot be recommended based on the available literature.

**Ans. 10** a. Sternotomy;
b. Periareolar;
c. Inframammary;
d. Subcostal;
e. Paramedian;
f. Transverse;
g. Periumbilical;
h. McBurney's;
i. Pfannenstiel;
j. Kocher's incision for thyroidectomy;
k. Clamshell thoracotomy;
l. Chevron incision;
m. Midline incision;
n. Inguinal incision.

**Ans. 11** 1. 22—For abdominal incisions;
2. 15—For arteriotomy and abscess drainage; and
3. 11—For minor surgical procedures.

**Ans. 12** a. 1-4 liters per minute and increased to a maximum pressure of 15 mm Hg and with a maximum flow rate of 20 L/min.
b. Palmer's point—3 cm below the left costal margin, in the midclavicular plane is the location (for Veress needle insertion).
c. Using a combination of the following techniques:
1. The hanging drop method (drop of water is placed in the hub of the needle; on elevating the abdominal wall the resultant loss of intra-abdominal pressure (IAP) would result in the drop emptying into the abdominal cavity.
2. Free flow of saline into the peritoneal cavity and no return of bowel content or blood on aspiration.
3. Abdominal pressure reading of less than 10 mm Hg.

**Ans. 13**

| *Suture* | *Absorption rate* | *Tensile strength* |
|---|---|---|
| a. Silk (Fibrous encapsulation in body at 2–3 weeks) | Absorbed slowly over 1–2 years | Loses 20% when wet; 80–100% lost by 6 months (Because of tissue reactions and unpredictability, silk is increasingly not recommended.) |
| b. Polyglactin suture (vicryl) | Hydrolysis minimal until 5–6 weeks. Complete absorption 60–90 days | Approximately 60% remains at 2 weeks. Approximately 30% remains at 3 weeks<br>*Raw material:* Copolymer of lactide and glycolide in a ratio of 90:10, coated with polyglactin and calcium stearate |

*Contd...*

*Contd...*

| Suture | Absorption rate | Tensile strength |
|---|---|---|
| c. PDS | Hydrolysis minimal at 90 days. Complete absorption at 180 days | Approximately 70% remains at 2 weeks. Approximately 50% remains at 4 weeks. Approximately 14% remains at 8 weeks |
| d. Poliglecaprone suture (Monocryl) | 90–120 days | 21 days maximum |

**Ans. 14** a. Continuous suture technique.
b. Subcuticular suture technique

**Ans. 15**

| *Common hemostatic technique used intraoperatively.* | | |
|---|---|---|
| ***Mechanical*** | ***Thermal*** | ***Chemical or topical hemostatic agents*** |
| • Digital pressure<br>• Ligatures<br>• Hemostatic clamps and ligating clips<br>• Vascular stapling devices<br>• Wound packing<br>• Bone wax<br>• Image-guided embolization | • Electrosurgery<br>• Cryosurgery<br>• Argon beam coagulation<br>• Vessel sealing devices | • *Physical:* Absorbable collagen, gelatin, and oxidized cellulose<br>• *Biological:* Topical thrombin, fibrin sealant, and tranexamic acid |

**Ans. 16** a. (a) Cutting; and (b) coagulation (tissue using monopolar diathermy).

b.

| Cutting | Coagulation |
|---|---|
| ↓Voltage current | ↑Voltage current |
| Continuous (current on 100% of time) | Interrupted (current flows 6% of the time and off for the remaining 94%) |
| Energy concentrated over a small area | Large area |
| Tissue is heated rapidly and to a higher temperature, causing vaporization of tissue, and thereby resulting in "cutting" tissue | Allows the tissue to cool slightly, so tissue heating is slower than with cutting mode. Its dehydration effect (loss of cellular fluid and protein denaturation), resulting in coagulation of tissue. Dehydration is not as effective as vaporization for cutting tissue but is ideal for hemostasis. Bleeding is stopped by a combination of the distortion of the walls of the blood vessel, coagulation of the plasma proteins, and stimulation of the clotting cascade |

*Contd...*

*Contd...*

| *Cutting* | *Coagulation* |
|---|---|
| Minimal lateral spread and collateral damage | Extensive lateral spread |
| Cutting divides tissue by generating sparks, which arc to the tissue; this is most efficient when the tip is held just above the tissue | Similar to cutting and works best when held just above the tissue, with no contact or minimal contact with tissue |
| *Uses:* Clean cut of tissue<br>To be used to dissect and divide tissue and not just to make skin incisions | *Uses:* Coagulation and achieving hemostasis |

**Ans. 17** a. Advanced bipolar technology that uses the body's collagen and elastin to both seal and divide, it reduce instrument handling when dissecting, ligating, and grasping—a valuable asset particularly during laparoscopic surgery. The feedback-sensing technology incorporated in the instrument is designed to manage the energy delivery in a precise manner and results in automatic discontinuation of energy once the seal is complete, thus removing any concern that the surgeon has to use guesswork as to when the seal is complete.

b. Up to 7 mm diameter, with an average seal time of 2–4 seconds.

**Ans. 18** a. Uses ultrasound technology to cut tissues while simultaneously sealing them. It utilizes a hand-held ultrasound transducer and scalpel that is controlled by a hand switch or foot pedal.

b. MOA—The scalpel vibrates in the 20,000–50,000 Hz range and cuts through tissues, effecting hemostasis by sealing vessels and tissues by means of protein denaturation caused by vibration rather than heat. Provides cutting precision, even through thickened scar tissue, and visibility is enhanced because less smoke is created by this system during use, compared with routine electrosurgery.

**Ans. 19** a. Simultaneously, using ultrasonic vibration and bipolar diathermy (Combined both modalities in a single device), this device can seal and divide arteries and veins up to 7 mm in diameter in a shorter amount of time with no smoke or mist.

b. Current role of drain placement in GI surgery:

| *Avoid routine drain placement following:* | *Consider routine drain placement following:* | *Selective use of drains following:* |
|---|---|---|
| • Colonic surgery<br>• Small bowel resections<br>• Hepatic resections<br>• Cholecystectomy | • Esophageal surgery<br>• Major pancreatic resection | • Rectal surgery<br>• Gastric resections |

**Ans. 20** a. Indications for placement of the nasogastric tube:

| *Drainage purposes* | *Feeding purposes* |
|---|---|
| • Postoperative paralytic ileus (Conservative management)<br>• Bowel obstruction (adhesional or partial) (conservative management)<br>• Decompression of the stomach before an emergency operation<br>• Prophylactically, when postoperative ileus is anticipated following extensive bowel handling | • Following procedures in the upper aerodigestive tract (nasogastric or nasoenteral)<br>• In patient with motor neurone disease (MND) or stroke |

b. Contraindications:

- Base of skull fracture as this may result in cranial injury.
- Esophageal stricture or recent esophageal surgery (unless under vision).

c. Complications

1. Upper airway damage—pressure necrosis of the nasal allowing to the placement of an oversized tube or following prolonged placement.
2. Reflux esophagitis
3. Pulmonary aspiration due to impaired function of the lower gastroesophageal sphincter.
4. Inadvertent placement into the lungs
5. Bleeding and perforation (traumatic placement)

**Ans. 21** a. Corrugated drain open drainage of a wound.

b. Closed suction drain (vacuum-assisted drainage system)

c. A closed, nonsuction drain (used to drain the abdominal cavity)

CHAPTER 8

# Diagnostic Imaging

## QUESTIONS

**Q1. What are the simple systems for checking radiographs?**

**Q2. What are the band classification of typical doses of ionizing radiation from common imaging procedure?**

**Q3. Answer the following:**

a. Identify the imaging modality and possible diagnosis of the given image.

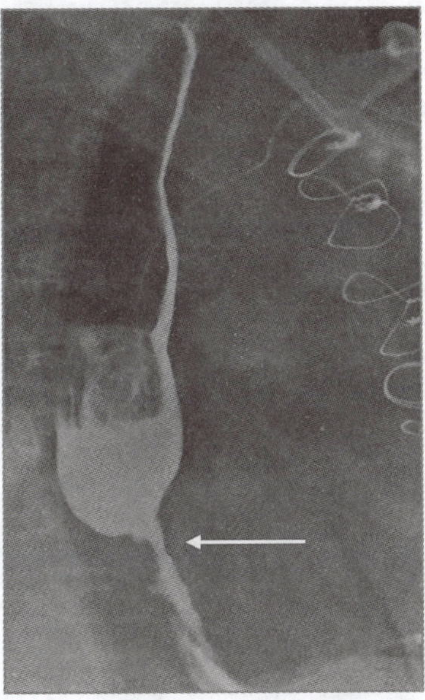

*Source:* Bailey and Love, 28th edition, page 120.

b. Identify the imaging modality and possible diagnosis of the given image.

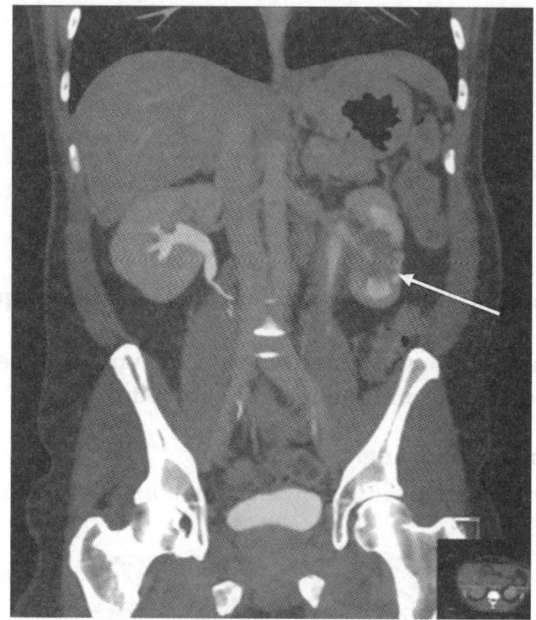

*Source:* Bailey and Love, 28th edition, page 121.

c. Identify the imaging modality and possible diagnosis of the given image.

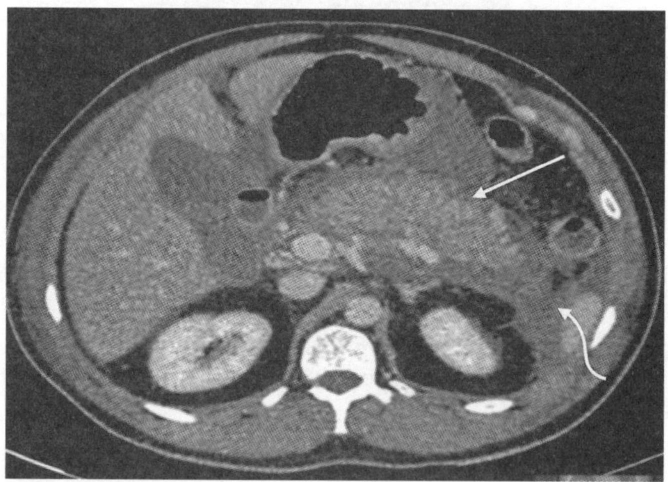

*Source:* Bailey and Love, 28th edition, page 123.

**Q4. Answer the following:**

a. Identify the imaging modality and possible diagnosis of the given image.

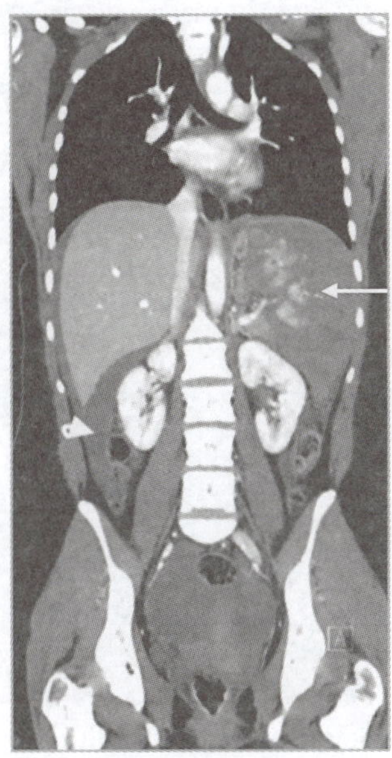

*Source:* Bailey and Love, 28th edition, page 135.

b. Identify the imaging modality and possible diagnosis of the given image.

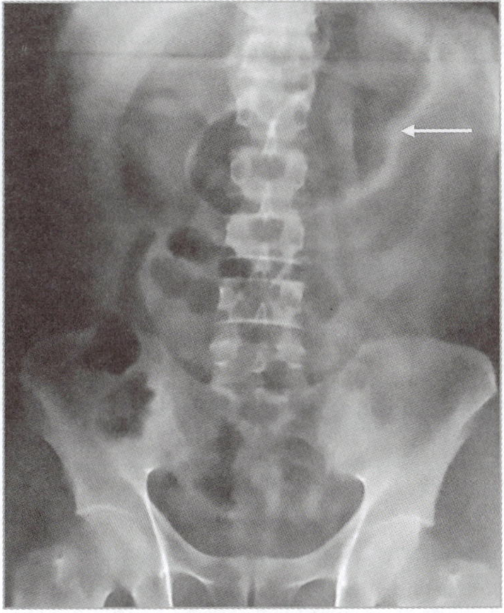

*Source:* Bailey and Love, 28th edition, page 137.

c. Identify the imaging modality and possible diagnosis of the given image.

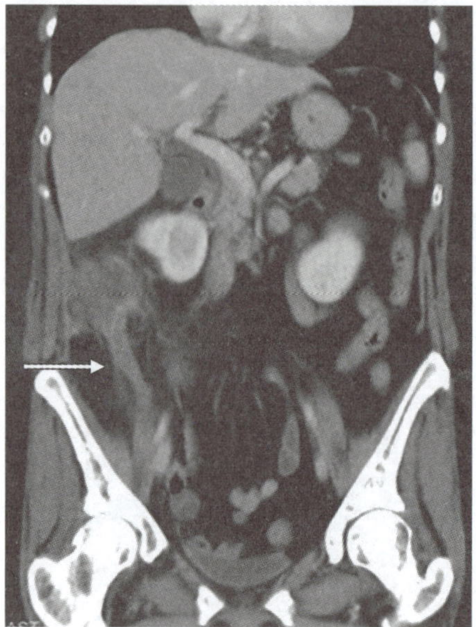

*Source:* Bailey and Love, 28th edition, page 138.

**Q5. Answer the following:**

a. Identify the imaging modality and possible diagnosis of the given image.

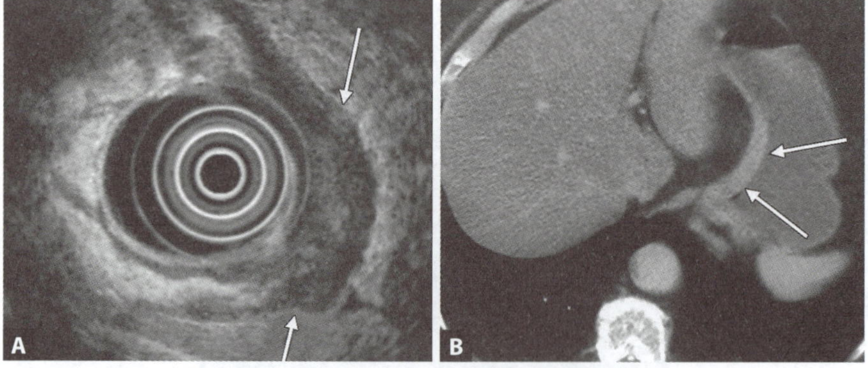


*Source:* Bailey and Love, 28th edition, page 141.

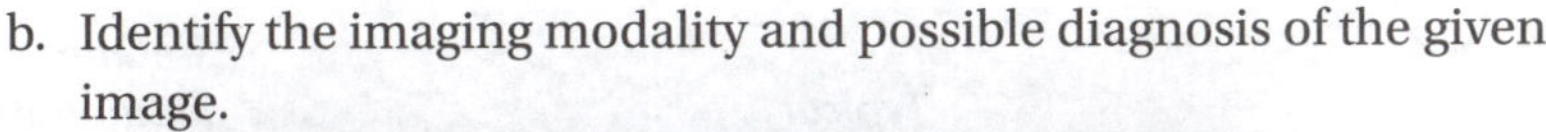


b. Identify the imaging modality and possible diagnosis of the given image.

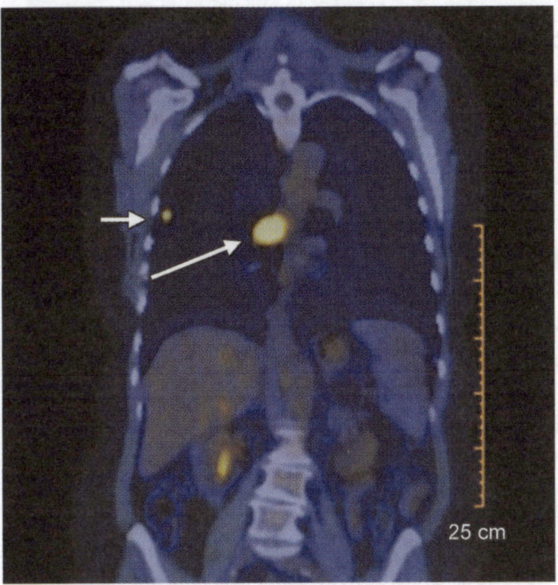


*Source:* Bailey and Love, 28th edition, page 142.

## ANSWERS

**Ans. 1**

- A simple system for checking radiographs.
- *Label:* Name of patient
- *Site:* Date of examination
- Side (check marker)
  - What part is the film centered on?
  - Does the film cover the whole area required?
  - Is there more than one view?
- *Quality:* Is the penetration appropriate?
- *Compare:* How have the appearances changed from previous images?
- Conclude
  - Is the diagnosis clear?
  - Is further imaging needed?

**Ans. 2**

| *Symbol* | *Typical effective dose (mSv)* | *Examples* | *Lifetime additional risk of cancer induction/ examination* |
|---|---|---|---|
| None | 0 | US; MRI | 0 |
| ☢ | <1 | CXR; XR limb, pelvis, lumbar spine; mammography | <1:20,000 |
| ☢☢ | 1–5 | IVU; NM (e.g., bone); CT head and neck | 1:20,000–1:4,000 |
| ☢☢☢ | 5.1–10 | CT KUB; NM (e.g., cardiac) | 1:4,000–1:2,000 |
| ☢☢☢☢ | >10 | Extensive CT studies, some NM studies (e.g., some PET/CT) | >1:2,000 |

(CXR: chest X-ray; CT: computed tomography; PET: positron emission tomography; IVU: intravenous urography; KUB: kidneys, ureters, bladder; US: ultrasound; MRI: magnetic resonance imaging)

*Source:* Bailey and Love, 28th edition, page 119.

**Ans. 3**

a. Barium swallow examination showing a malignant stricture (arrow) due to an esophageal carcinoma.

b. Coronal maximum intensity projection image from a computed tomography intravenous urogram shows a transitional cell carcinoma in the left renal pelvis (arrow) with normal excretion of contrast on the right.

c. Axial computed tomography scan of a patient with acute pancreatitis demonstrates a swollen edematous pancreas (arrow) with extensive peripancreatic free fluid (curly arrow).

**Ans. 4**

a. Coronal computed tomography image of the body shows a grade V splenic injury ("shattered spleen"; arrow) with vascular injury at the hilum and free fluid around the spleen and liver (arrowhead).

b. Plain abdominal radiograph showing an abnormal appearance to the gastric wall, which is very clearly visualized owing to the presence of gas both inside the lumen and outside the lumen (arrow). This is Rigler's sign of hollow organ perforation, in this case due to a duodenal ulcer.

c. Acute appendicitis. Contrast-enhanced computed tomography scan reconstructed in the coronal plane demonstrates a thickened appendix in the right iliac fossa (arrow) with inflammatory changes in the surrounding fat and reactive thickening of the cecal pole.

**Ans. 5** a. (A) Endoscopic ultrasound in gastric cancer. The hypoechoic tumor (arrows) is infiltrating the layered structure of the gastric wall and extending out beyond the serosa. (B) Computed tomography scan demonstrates thickening and enhancement of the gastric wall in the same area (arrows). The stomach is distended with water to provide low-density contrast.

b. Positron emission tomography shows fluorodeoxyglucose uptake in a carcinoma of the lung (short arrow) and mediastinal lymph nodes (long arrow).

CHAPTER 9

# Gastrointestinal Endoscopy

## QUESTIONS

**Q1. Answer the following:**

a. How will you disinfect endoscopes?

b. Enumerate risk of endoscopy.

**Q2. What is the incidence of bacteremia in following procedures?**

a. Rectal digital examination

b. Dental extraction

c. Colonoscopy

d. ERCP

e. Esophageal dilatation/prosthesis

**Q3. Name low-risk and high-risk conditions associated with risk of thromboembolic events according to underlying condition.**

**Q4. According to British Society of Gastroenterology and European Society of Endoscopy 2021 guidelines for the management of endoscopy in patients with antiplatelets or anticoagulant therapy. Kindly give management for following:**

a. Low-risk procedure

b. High-risk procedure

**Q5. Identify the condition and treatment of the following images:**

a. Image A

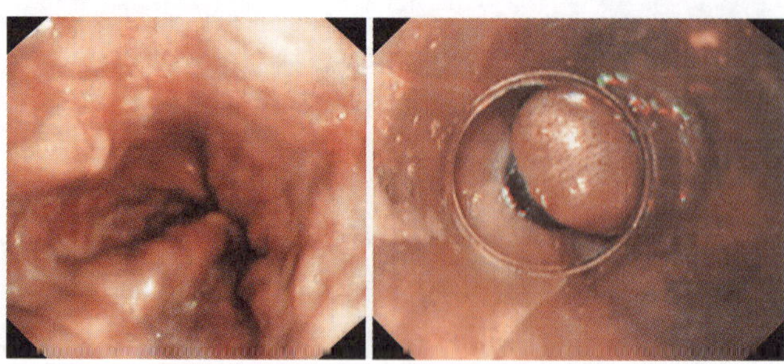

b. Image B

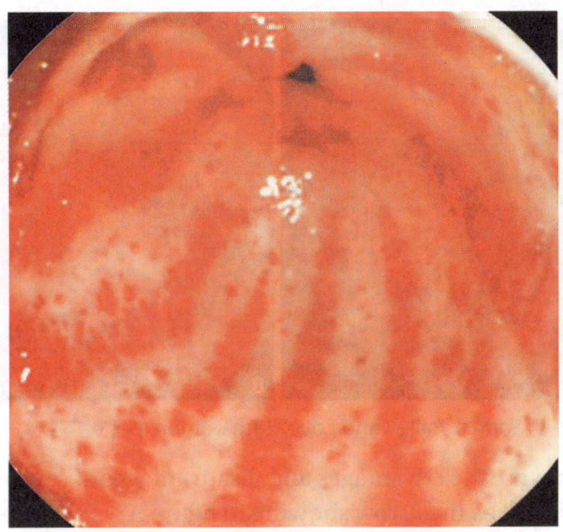

c. Image C

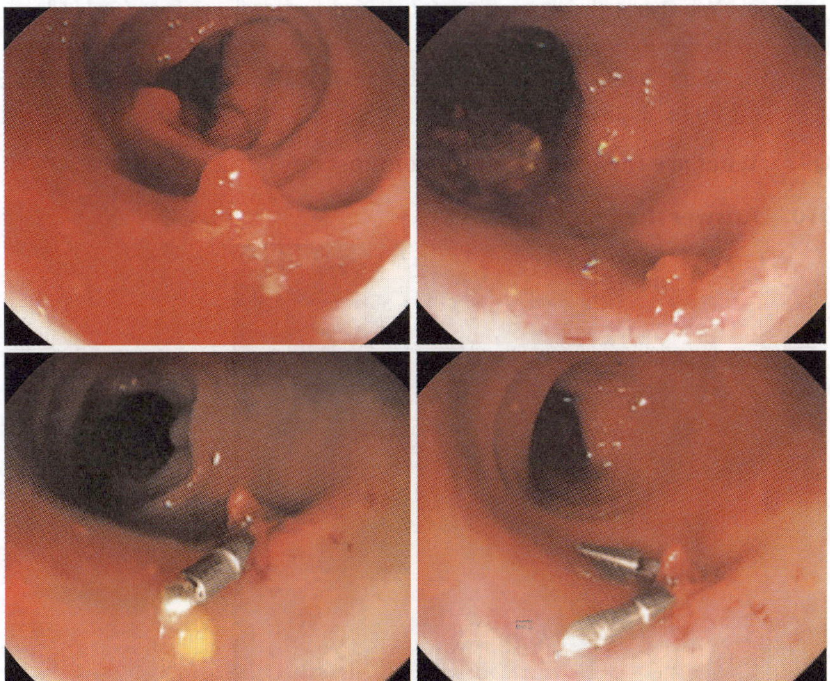

*Source for images A to C:* Bailey and Love, 28th edition, page 149.

**Q6. What are the symptoms of esophageal perforation?**

**Q7. Answer the following:**

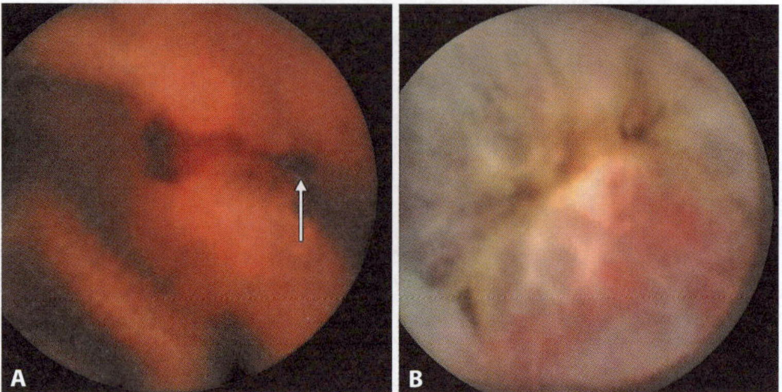


*Source:* Bailey and Love, 28th edition, page 154.

a. What are the advantages and disadvantages of capsule endoscopy?
b. What does the arrow showing in figure A?
c. Identify the condition seen in figure B.

**Q8. Answer the following:**

a. What are the current established indications for single/double balloon endoscopy?
b. What are the risk factors for post ERCP pancreatitis (NEET SS 2022, 2023)?

**Q9. What are the indications of colonoscopy?**

**Q10. Answer the following:**

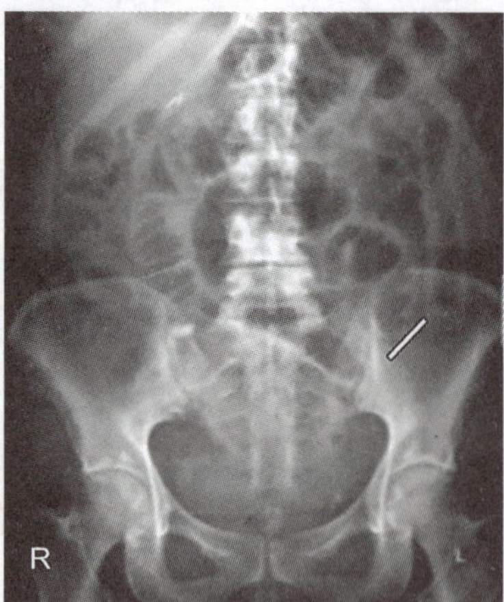


*Source:* Bailey and Love, 28th edition, page 160.

a. Identify the condition in the given image.
b. What are the indications for endoscopic ultrasound?

# ANSWERS

**Ans. 1** a. *Disinfection of endoscopes*

1. All channels must be brushed and irrigated throughout the disinfection process.
2. All instruments and accessories should be traceable to each use, patient, and cleaning cycle.
3. All staff should be trained and protected (particularly if glutaraldehyde is used in view of its immune-sensitizing properties).
4. Regular monitoring of disinfectant power and microbiological contamination should be performed.

b. *The risks of endoscopy*

1. Sedation-related cardiorespiratory complications.
2. Damage to dentition
3. Aspiration
4. Perforation or hemorrhage after endoscopic dilatation/ therapeutic endoscopic ultrasound (EUS).
5. Perforation, infection, and aspiration after percutaneous endoscopic gastrostomy insertion.
6. Perforation or hemorrhage after flexible sigmoidoscopy/ colonoscopy with polypectomy.
7. Pancreatitis, cholangitis, perforation, or bleeding, after endoscopic retrograde cholangiopancreatography.

**Ans. 2** a. 4%

b. 30–60%

c. 2–4%

d. ▪ ERCP (no duct occlusion)—6%
 ▪ ERCP (duct occluded)—11%

e. Esophageal varices band ligation—6%

**Ans. 3**

| *High risk* | *Low risk* |
|---|---|
| • Atrial fibrillation with valvular heart disease<br>• Mechanical mitral valve<br>• Mechanical valve and previous thromboembolic event | • Deep vein thrombosis<br>• Uncomplicated atrial fibrillation<br>• Bioprosthetic valve<br>• Mechanical aortic valve low |

**Ans. 4.**

a.

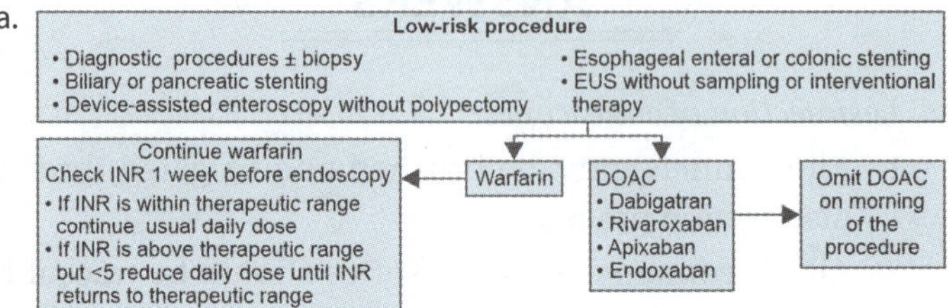


(EUS: endoscopic ultrasound; DOAC: Direct oral anticoagulants; INR: international normalized ratio)

*Source:* Bailey and Love, 28th edition, page 148.

b.

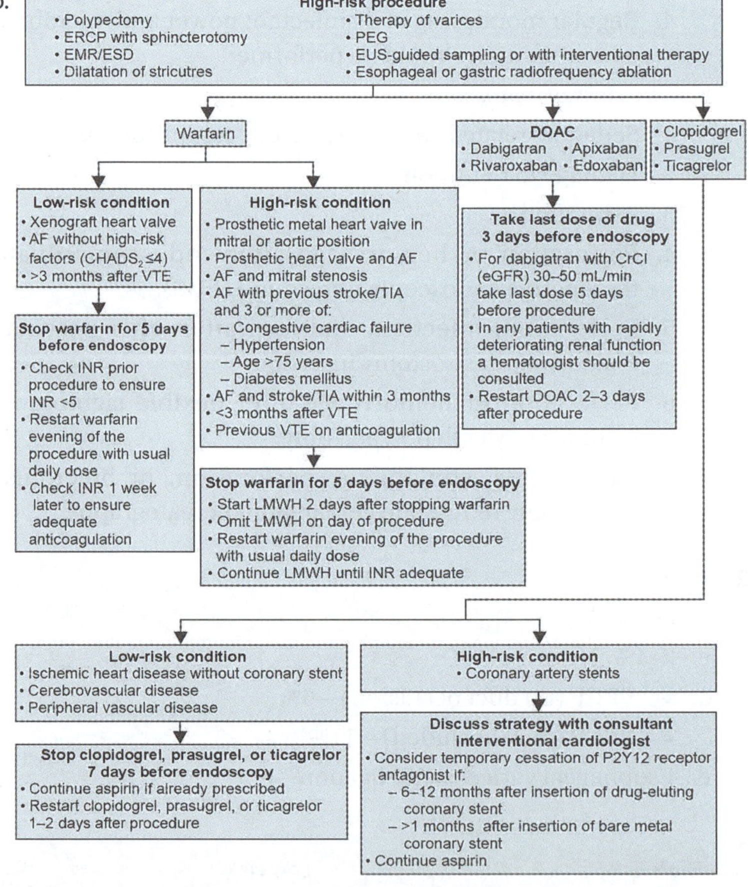


(AF: atrial fibrillation; ERCP: Endoscopic retrograde cholangiopancreatography; EMR: endoscopic mucosal resection; ESD: endoscopic submucosal dissection; EUS: endoscopic ultrasound; DOAC: direct oral anticoagulants; INR: international normalized ratio; PEG: percutaneous endoscopic gastrostomy; LMWH: low-molecular-weight heparin; TIA: transient ischemic attack; VTE: venous thromboembolism)

*Source:* Bailey and Love, 28th edition, page 148.

**Ans. 5** a. Grade 2 esophageal varices (treated by band ligation).

b. Gastric antral vascular ectasia (treated with argon plasma coagulation).

c. A gastric ulcer with active bleeding (treated with adrenaline injection to achieve hemostasis, two hemoclips are then applied to prevent rebleeding).

**Ans. 6.** *Symptoms of endoscopic esophageal perforation.*

1. Neck/chest pain
2. Increasing tachycardia
3. Dysphagia/drooling saliva
4. Hypotension
5. Abdominal pain
6. Surgical emphysema

**Ans. 7** a.

| *Advantage* | *Disadvantage* |
|---|---|
| • Able to visualize the entire small bowel, preferable for patients<br>• No sedation<br>• Painless | • No biopsies<br>• Not controllable and no accurate localization<br>• Variable transit incomplete studies owing to battery life.<br>• Not suitable for patients with strictures.<br>• Large capsule to swallow. |

b. Angioectasias

c. Crohn's disease (small bowel)

**Ans. 8** a.
- Bleeding from the gastrointestinal bleeding (GIT) of obscure cause.
- Iron deficiency anemia with normal colonoscopy and gastroscopy.
- Visualization of and therapeutic intervention for abnormalities seen on traditional small bowel imaging/capsule endoscopy.

b. Risk factors for postendoscopic retrograde cholangiopancreatography (ERCP) pancreatitis.

| *Definite* | *Possible* |
|---|---|
| 1. Suspected sphincter of Oddi dysfunction (SOD)<br>2. Young age<br>3. Normal bilirubin<br>4. Prior ERCP-related pancreatitis<br>5. Difficult cannulation<br>6. Pancreatic duct contrast injection<br>7. Pancreatic sphincterotomy<br>8. Balloon dilatation of biliary sphincter | 1. Female sex<br>2. Low volume of ERCPs performed<br>3. Absent common bile duct (CBD) stone |

**Ans. 9** Indications for colonoscopy:

1. Rectal bleeding [unexplained after proctoscopy/sigmoidoscopy]
2. Abdominal pain related to bowel actions
3. Iron deficiency anemia [combined with esophago-gastro duodenoscopy (OGD)]
4. Right iliac fossa mass if imaging suggestive of colonic origin
5. Unexplained alteration in bowel habit
6. Chronic diarrhea (>6 weeks) after sigmoidoscopy/rectal biopsy and negative celiac serology
7. Follow-up of colorectal cancer (CRC) and polyps
8. Screening of patients with a family history of CRC
9. Assessment/removal of a lesion seen on radiological examination
10. Assessment of ulcerative colitis/Crohn's extent and activity
11. Surveillance of inflammatory bowel disease
12. Surveillance in patients with acromegaly or following ureterosigmoidostomy

**Ans. 10** a. Malignant colonic obstruction relieved by insertion of a self-expanding metal stent (palliated or temporarily relief).

b.

| *Diagnostic* | *Therapeutic* |
|---|---|
| • Staging of esophageal/gastric malignancy staging of hepatobiliary malignancy<br>• Diagnosis of choledochol microlithiasis | • Biopsy of paraesophageal lymph nodes<br>• Biopsy of submucosal upper gastrointestinal lesions<br>• Biopsy of pancreaticobiliary mass<br>• Biopsy of portal lymphadenopathy biopsy of left adrenal and left liver masses<br>• Transgastric drainage of pancreatic pseudocyst<br>• Celiac plexus block |

CHAPTER

# 10 Principles of Minimal Access Surgery

## QUESTIONS

**Q1. Answer the following:**

a. Who performed the first experimental laparoscopic procedure?

b. Who performed the first thoracoscopy?

**Q2. Expand the following:**

a. NOTES

b. HALS

c. SILS

**Q3. Answer the following:**

a. What are the advantages of minimal access surgery?

b. What are the limitations of minimal access surgery?

**Q4. Identify the images a, b, and c.**

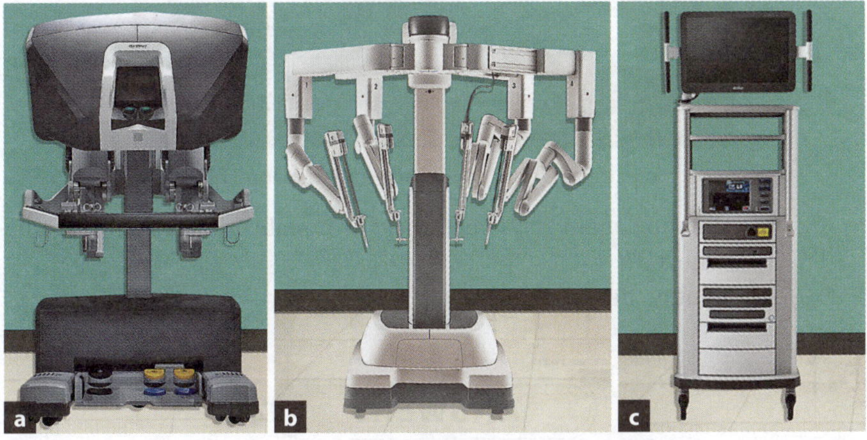


*Source:* Bailey and Love, 28th edition, page 166.

**Q5. Identify the system in the given image.**

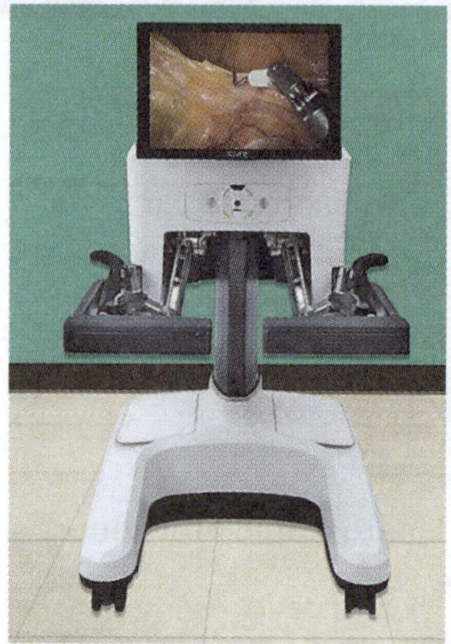

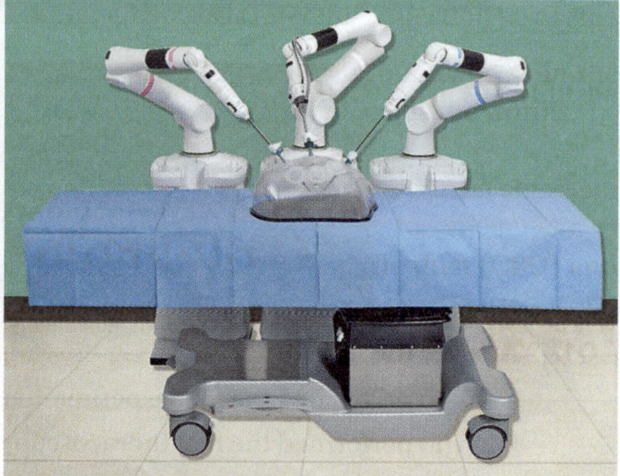

*Source:* Bailey and Love, 28th edition, page 168.

**Q6. Answer the following:**

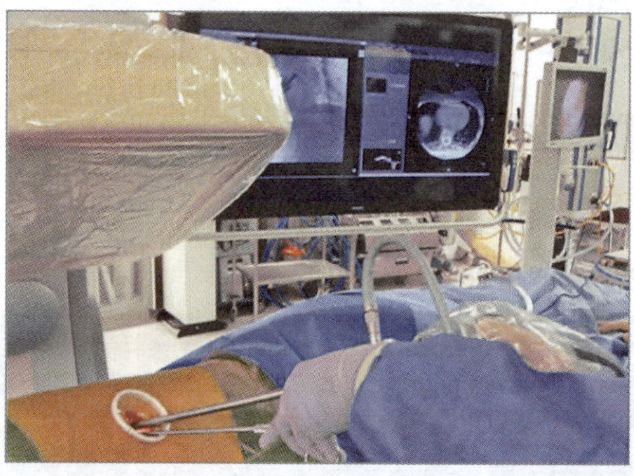

*Source:* Bailey and Love, 28th edition, page 175.

a. After how many days does port site nonabsorbable suture can be removed?
b. Identify the given image

## ANSWERS

**Ans. 1** a. Kelling in 1901
b. Jacobaeus

**Ans. 2** a. Natural orifice translumenal endoscopic surgery (NOTES)
b. Hand-assisted laparoscopic surgery
c. Single-incision laparoscopic surgery

**Ans. 3** a. Advantages of minimal access surgery
- Decrease in wound size
- Reduction in wound infection, dehiscence, bleeding, herniation, and nerve entrapment
- Decrease in wound pain
- Improved mobility
- Decreased wound trauma
- Decreased heat loss
- Improved visualization

b. Limitations of minimal access surgery
- Lack of 3D vision
- Loss of tactile feedback
- Hemostasis
- Extraction of large specimens
- Learning curve and increased operative time
- Cost
- Reliance on new technologies

**Ans. 4** *The da Vinci Xi system:*
a. Surgeon console
b. Da Vinci Xi robot
c. Vision cart

**Ans. 5** The Versius robotic system

**Ans. 6** a. Nonabsorbable sutures or skin staples have been used, they can be removed from the port sites after 7–10 days.
b. Image-guided video-assisted thoracoscopic surgery with the use of a navigationally placed fiducial marker to guide tumor resection.

# CHAPTER 11 Tissue and Molecular Diagnosis

## QUESTIONS

**Q1. Answer the following:**

a. Enumerate the reasons for analysis of tissue.

b. What are the common types of tissue samples?

**Q2. Identify the specimen a, b, and c, and possible diagnosis.**

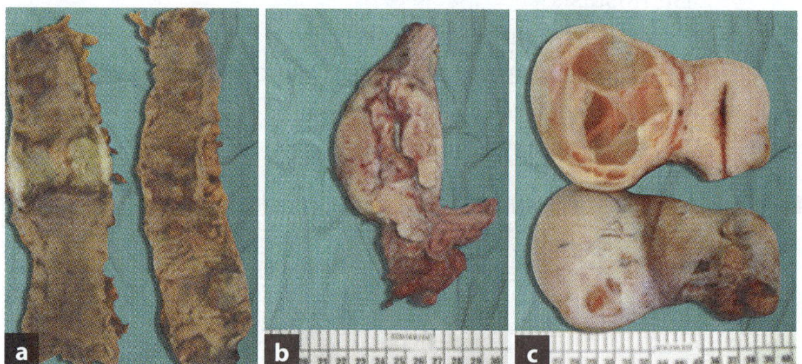

*Source:* Bailey and Love, 28th edition, page 180.

**Q3. What is the sequence of events in histological processing?**

**Q4. Identify the specimen along with associated histology.**

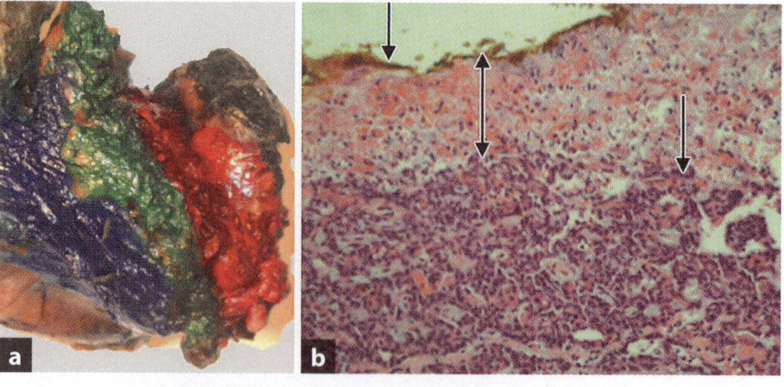

*Source:* Bailey and Love, 28th edition, page 181.

**Q5. Identify the image a, b, and c.**

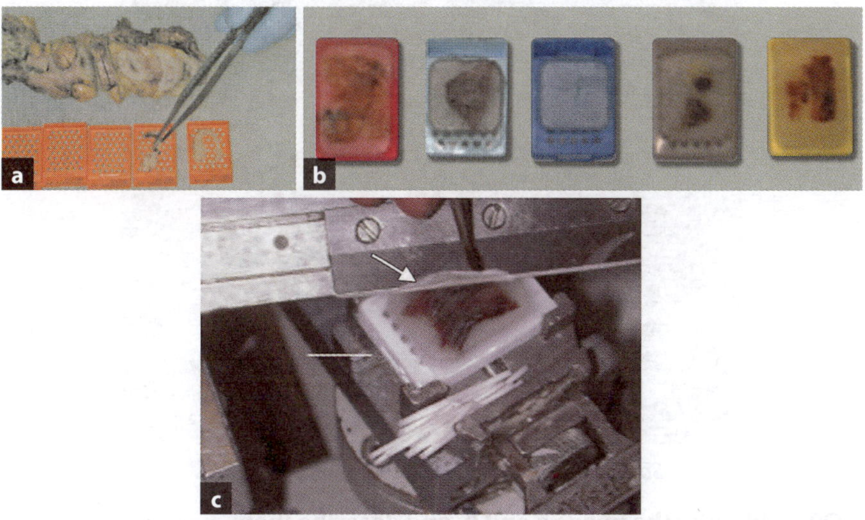

*Source:* Bailey and Love, 28th edition, page 181.

**Q6. What are the advantages and disadvantages of frozen section?**

**Q7. Answer the following:**

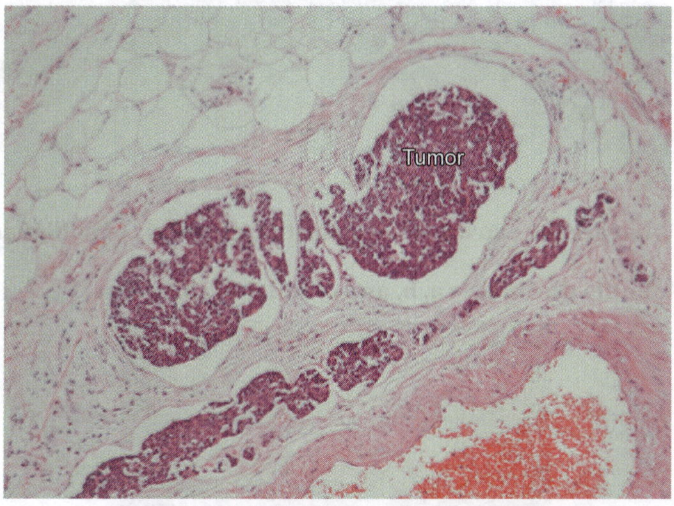


*Source:* Bailey and Love, 28th edition, page 183.

a. What are the microscopic features of malignancy?

b. Which step is shown in the figure?

**Q8. Identify the image and describe it.**

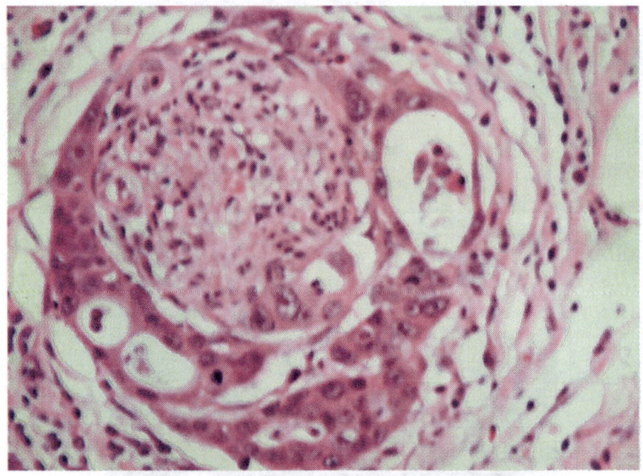

*Source:* Bailey and Love, 28th edition, page 183.

**Q9. Identify the image a and b, and describe them.**

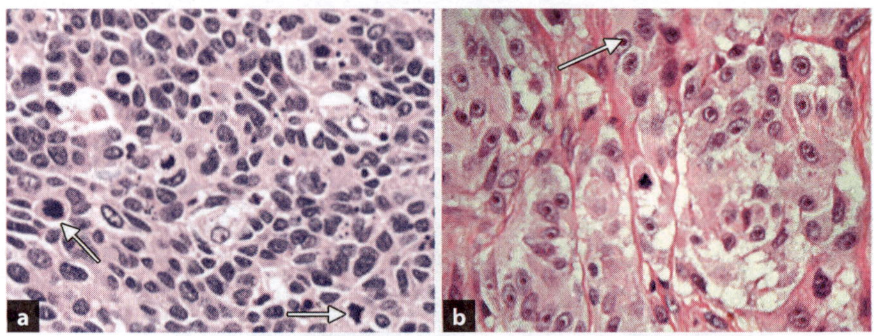


*Source:* Bailey and Love, 28th edition, page 184.

**Q10. What are the causes of false positive diagnosis of malignancy?**

**Q11. Identify the images a, b, and c, and describe them.**

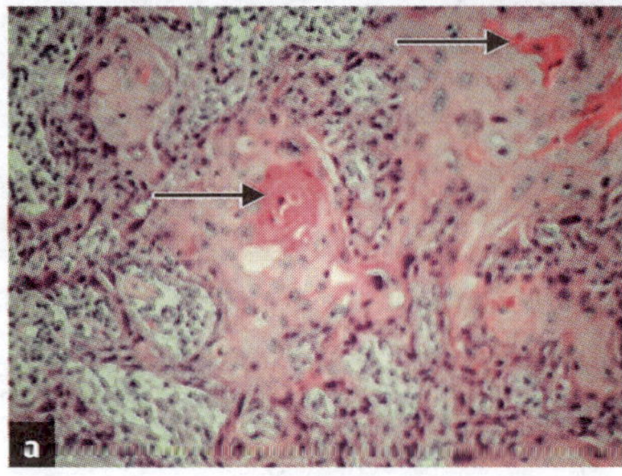

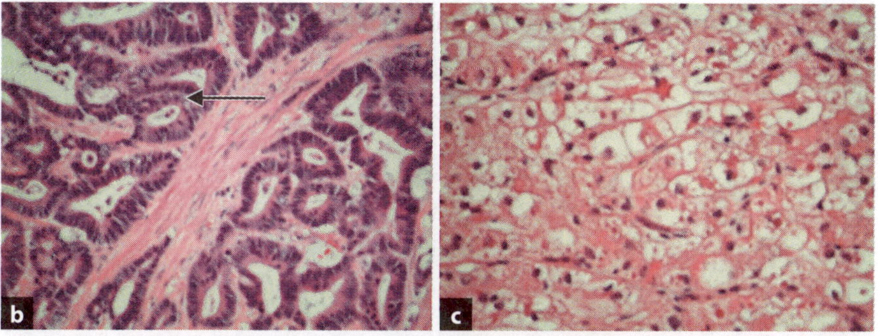

*Source:* Bailey and Love, 28th edition, page 185.

**Q12. Identify the images a and b, and describe them.**

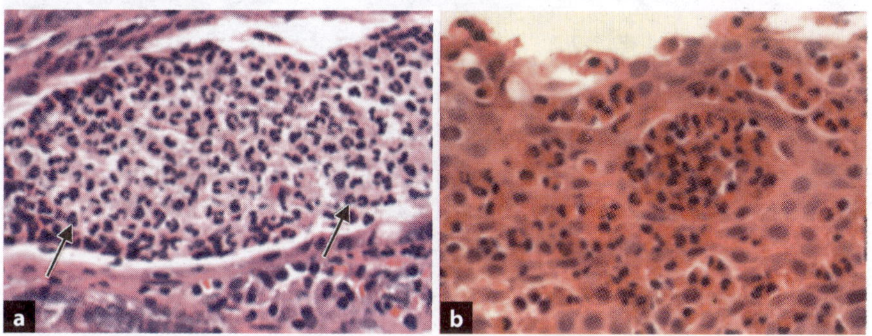

*Source:* Bailey and Love, 28th edition, page 186.

**Q13. Identify the given images and describe them.**

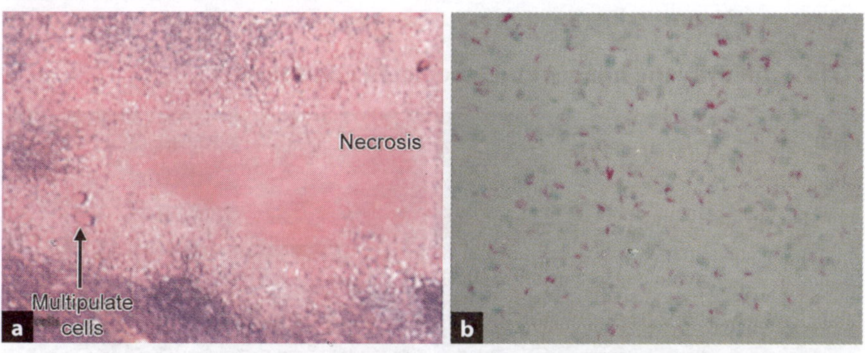


*Source:* Bailey and Love, 28th edition, page 186.

**Q14. Name four special stains and their uses in tissue assessment.**

**Q15. Identify the stains used in images a and b.**

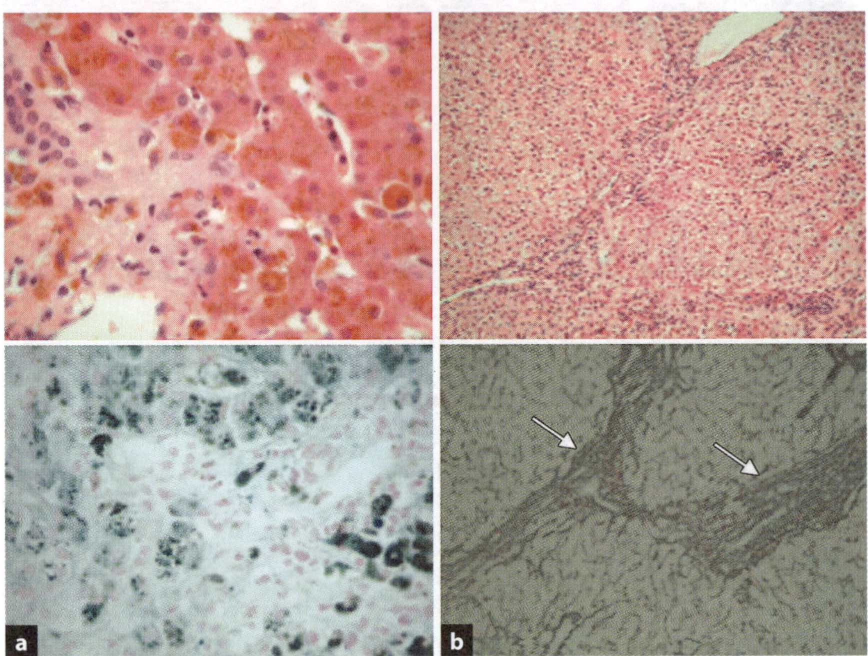


*Source:* Bailey and Love, 28th edition, page 189.

**Q16. Name immunological stains used for:**

- Epithelial
- Vascular
- Myoid
- Lung
- GIST
- Neuroendocrine tumor

**Q17. Identify the images and associated condition.**

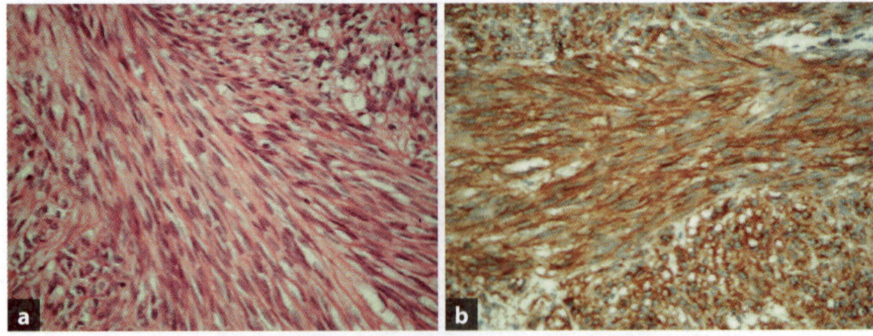


*Source:* Bailey and Love, 28th edition, page 190.

**Q18. Enumerate the uses of immunohistochemistry.**

**Q19. Answer the following:**

a. What is next generation sequencing (NGS)?
b. Write two examples of proto oncogenes and tumor suppressor genes.

**Q20. Answer the following:**

a. What are the indicators for molecular analysis of tumor tissue?
b. Enumerate various methods for detection for molecular changes.

**Q21. Answer the following:**

a. Name some tumor types that respond to immune checkpoint inhibitor drugs.
b. MSI is regulated by which genes.
c. What are the tests for MSI and mismatch repair gene?
d. What is clinicopathological correlation between MSI-H CRC?

**Q22. What are the molecular analysis in colorectal carcinoma?**

**Q23. Answer the following:**

a. Name two tumor associated with anaplastic lymphoma kinase (ALK) fusion.
b. Name one tumor associated with fibroblast growth factor receptor (FGFR) fusion.
c. Name one tumor associated with neurotrophic tyrosine receptor kinase (NTRK) fusion.

## ANSWERS

**Ans. 1** a. Reasons for analysis of tissue

*Diagnosis*
- Confirmation/rejection of a clinical diagnosis
- Additional diagnoses
- Classification of neoplasia
- Classification of non-neoplastic disease

*Staging of malignancy*

*Prognosis*

*Management*
- Selection of therapy
- Assessment of response to treatment

*Cancer screening programs and related programs*
- Cervical, bowel, breast, inflammatory bowel disease, and Barrett's esophagus

*Clinical trial support*

*Audit*

b. Common types of tissue sample

*Histology*

- Formalin—fixed tissue
  - Biopsy
    - Punch (e.g., skin)
    - Mucosal (e.g., oral, bronchial, gastrointestinal)
    - Core needle biopsy (e.g., liver)
    - Curatting (e.g., prostate, endometrium)
    - Excisional biopsy
  - Resection
- Fresh tissues
  - Frozen section for diagnosis
  - Tissue banking
  - Research purpose
  - For some special stains, requires fresh tissue

*Cytology*

- Cervical
- Brushing, washing, and scraping
- Fine—needle aspiration
- Sputum
- Fluids (pleural fluid, ascitic fluid)

**Ans. 2** a. Specimen of colon—familial adenomatous polyposis

b. Specimen of esophagogastrectomy
Content—distal esophageal tumor after opening.

c. Uterus and cystic lesion

**Ans. 3** *Histological processing:* Sequence of events

- Receipt of specimen
- Macroscopic (gross) description
- Sampling of specimen (unless small enough to submit in its entirety)
- Specimen or samples placed in cassette(s)
- Production of paraffin wax block(s).
- Cutting of 5-μm sections with microtome
- Sections placed on glass slides
- Sections stained with H&E
- Histopathologist examines slides, taking clinical and macroscopic findings into account
- Further studies on tissue, if necessary.
- Entry of report onto computer system.

**Ans. 4** a. Specimen—pancreatoduodenectomy specimen (posterior view)

b. Yellow ink (thick arrow)

Tumor (thin arrow) lies close to the surface.

Double-headed arrow—Measure the distance between the tumor and a surface or a resection margin.

**Ans. 5** a. Tissue sample from specimen in a cassette for processing.

b. Paraffin wax blocks. Cassettes of different colors allow the organization of samples and specimens into groups, e.g., according to specialty or degree of urgency.

c. Thick arrow—Cut from a paraffin wax block

Thin arrow—Cut from a microtome.

**Ans. 6**

| ***Advantages*** | ***Disadvantages*** |
|---|---|
| Quick diagnosis | • Poorer quality sections<br>• Potential reduction in accuracy and precision of histological diagnosis<br>• Labor intensive<br>• Disruptive<br>• Infection risk<br>• Small sample required<br>• Some tissue types are difficult to process |

**Ans. 7** a. *Microscopic features of malignancy*

- Metastasis
- Invasion
  - Of surrounding tissue
  - Vascular (intraluminal tumor and/or tumor in blood vessel wall)
  - Perineural
- Architectural abnormalities
- Necrosis
- Numerous mitotic figures
- Atypical mitotic figures
- Nuclear abnormalities
  - Pleomorphism
  - Enlargement
  - Hyperchromicity
  - Chromatin clumping
- Nucleolar enlargement and multiplicity

b. Step shown—Vascular invasion

**Ans. 8** Perineural invasion (adenocarcinoma)

**Ans. 9** a. Neuroendocrine cancer (nuclear pleomorphism and variation in nuclear size).

Arrows suggestive of mitotic figures.

b. Malignant melanoma
Arrows suggestive of nuclear pleomorphism and prominent nucleoli.

**Ans. 10** *Causes of false-positive diagnoses of malignancy*

- Interchanged samples
- Contamination
- Interpretative error
- Treatment-induced change, e.g., radiotherapy
- Ulceration

**Ans. 11** a. Squamous cell carcinoma (well-differentiated)
Arrows—Foci of keratinization.

b. Adenocarcinoma (well-differentiated)
Arrows—Gland formation.

c. Clear cell carcinoma (metastatic)—composed of sheets of cells with clear cytoplasm (most likely renal origin)

**Ans. 12** a. Inflammatory process (acute) characterized by numerous neutrophils.

b. Esophageal mucosa infiltrated by numerous eosinophils with bright red cytoplasm, many of which are forming clusters most likely eosinophilic esophagitis.

**Ans. 13** a. Granuloma with necrosis
Symptoms of (S/o) tuberculosis (TB) (multinucleate giant cells of Langhans).

b. Ziehl–Neelsen (ZN) stain shows pink acid-fast rod-shaped bacilli, S/o mycobacterial infection.

**Ans. 14** *Common special stains*

- *Periodic acid–Schiff (PAS):* Glycogen, fungi
- *D-PAS:* mucin
- *Perl's prussian blue:* Iron
- *Reticulin:* Reticulin fibers, fibrosis
- *van Gieson:* Collagen
- *Congo red:* Amyloid
- *Ziehl–Neelsen:* Mycobacteria

**Ans. 15** a. a. Brown pigment (biopsy).
b. Perl's stain (iron)

b. a. Liver biopsy stained with hematoxylin and eosin (severity of fibrosis cannot be determined). +
b. Reticulin stain [S/o fibrous bridges (arrows)]

**Ans. 16**

| *Some immunohistochemical stains used for tumors* | | |
|---|---|---|
| ***Cell type/site of origin*** | ***Site of origin/cell type*** | ***Prognosis and treatment*** |
| • *Epithelial (carcinoma):* Cytokeratins<br>• *Lymphoid (lymphoma):* CD45, CD3 (T cells), CD20 (B cells)<br>• *Melanocytic (melanoma):* S100, HMB45, Melan A<br>• *Neuroendocrine:* Synaptophysin, chromogranin<br>• *Vascular:* CD31<br>• *Myoid:* Desmin, actin | • *Prostate:* Prostate-specific antigen (PSA)<br>• *Lung:* Thyroid transcription factor-1 (TTF-1)<br>• *Thyroid:* Thyroglobulin<br>• *Colorectum:* Cytokeratin 20 (CK20), CDX2<br>• *Liver:* Hepatocyte-specific antigen (HSA)<br>• *Gastrointestinal stromal tumor (GIST):* CD117, DOG-1 | • *Breast carcinoma and gastric carcinoma:* HER-2<br>• *Neuroendocrine tumors:* Ki67 proliferation index<br>• Screening for mutations<br>• *Colorectal carcinoma:* Mismatch repair proteins (MLH1, MSH2, MSH6, and PMS2) |

**Ans. 17** a. Metastatic tumor composed of spindle cells—gastrointestinal stromal tumor (GIST).

b. Positive immunohistochemical (IHC) CD117 supportive diagnosis of GIST.

**Ans. 18** *Uses of Immunohistochemistry (IHC)*

- Cell type
- Neoplasia
  - Direction of differentiation/phenotype
  - Determination of anatomical site of origin
  - Confirmation of neoplasia
  - Grading
  - Selection of treatment
  - Detection of/screening for mutations
  - Prognosis
- Microorganisms—detection
- Other
  - Amyloid
  - Immunoglobulins
  - Complement

**Ans. 19** a. NGS—Performs massively parallel sequencing, allowing simultaneous examination of millions of fragments of DNA for molecular alterations, applicable to formalin-fixed tissue, allows evaluation of many DNA regions in a single assay and displays increased analytical sensitivity (i.e., the ability to detect low-frequency alleles) compared with Sanger sequencing or conventional PCR. Widely clinically used targeted NGS panels can identify multiple known mutations and other variants in 20–500 genes of interest in a single test.

b. Genes

| *(Proto-) oncogenes* | *Tumor suppressor genes* |
|---|---|
| • *KRAS*<br>• *BRAF*<br>• *EGFR*<br>• *BCL2* | • *TP53*<br>• *BRCA1/2* |

**Ans. 20** a. *Indications for molecular analysis of tumor tissue*

- Diagnosis and classification
- Selection of therapy
- Prognosis
- Staging
- Monitoring disease burden
- Screening for germline mutations
- Confirmation of neoplasia (e.g., clonality)

b. *Detection methods for main molecular changes*

- *Point mutations and small insertions and deletions:* NGS, PCR
- *Fusions:* Fluorescence in situ hybridization (FISH), NGS, PCR
- *Amplifications:* FISH, NGS
- *Tumor mutation burden:* NGS
- Immunohistochemistry may be a very useful initial test, and is often sufficient.

**Ans. 21** a. *Tumor types that may respond to immune checkpoint inhibitor drugs*

- Breast carcinoma
- Urothelial carcinoma
- Non-small cell lung cancer
- Small cell lung cancer
- Hepatocellular carcinoma
- Malignant melanoma

b to d.

Microsatellite instability and mismatch repair genes

Microsatellite instability (MSI)

*Regulated by four main genes:*

1. MLH1
2. PMS2
3. MSH2
4. MSH6.

Genetic changes responsible for MSI

1. Sporadic hypermethylation of MLH1 (more common; 85%)
2. Germline mutation, i.e., Lynch syndrome (less common)

Microsatellite unstable (MSI-H) tumors

- 15% of colorectal carcinoma (CRC)
- 30% of endometrial carcinoma

*Tests*

a. Immunohistochemistry
    - Recommended for all newly diagnosed CRCs
    - The preferred initial test in most centers
b. PCR-based microsatellite testing
c. NGS

*Clinicopathological correlation:* MSI-H CRC

- Typically right sided
- More likely to have mucinous element histologically
- Likely to have BRAF V600E mutation

*Clinical value*

- Phenotypic classification, e.g., medullary CRC is typically MSI-H
- Prognosis, e.g., MSI-H better prognosis overall
- Selection of drug therapy, e.g., MSI-H CRC responds better to ICIs and has no response to 5-fluorouracil.
- Screening for germline mutation, i.e., Lynch syndrome

**Ans. 22** *Molecular analysis in colorectal carcinoma*

Mismatch repair gene abnormalities

- Multiple considerations

KRAS or NRAS mutation

- Predicts resistance to epidermal growth factor receptor (EGFR) inhibitors

Tumor mutation burden

- Predicts response to immune checkpoint inhibitors (ICI) therapy

BRAF V600E mutation

- Poor prognosis in metastatic CRC
- Predictive of response to therapy

NTRK fusion

- Uncommon (<1% CRC)
- Usually MSI-H
- Poor prognosis
- *Specific therapy available:* Tyrosine kinase inhibitors

**Ans. 23** a. Nonsmall cell lung carcinoma, renal cell carcinoma

b. Bladder carcinoma

c. Colorectal cancer (CRC)

# CHAPTER 12 Principles of Oncology

## QUESTIONS

**Q1. Answer the following:**

Name the scientist

a. Who pointed out importance of chromosomal abnormalities in cancer cells in 1914?

b. Who demonstrated deoxyribonucleic acid (DNA) was a genetic material within chromosome in 1940?

c. In which year Watson and Crick described the structure of DNA?

**Q2. What are the features of malignant transformation given by Hanahan and Weinberg?**

**Q3. Answer the following:**

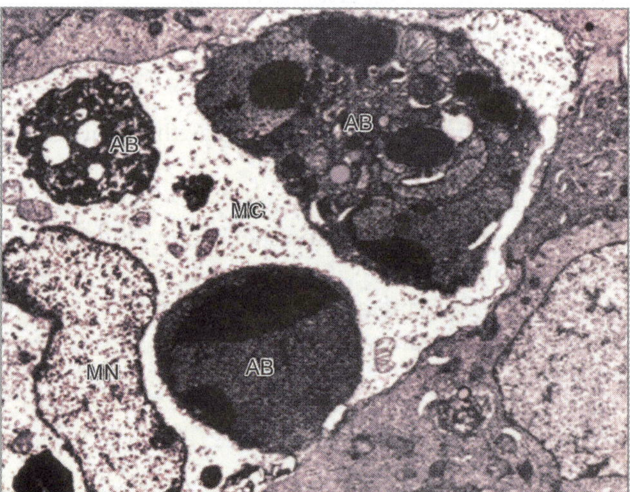


*Source:* Bailey and Love, 28th edition, page 199.

a. What is shown in the given image?

b. What is apoptosis?

c. What is EMT?

**Q4. Answer the following:**

a. Who proposed possible role of the immune system in eliminating nascent cancers in 1909?
b. Who gave the Seed soil hypothesis?
c. Warburg effect.

**Q5. Answer the following:**

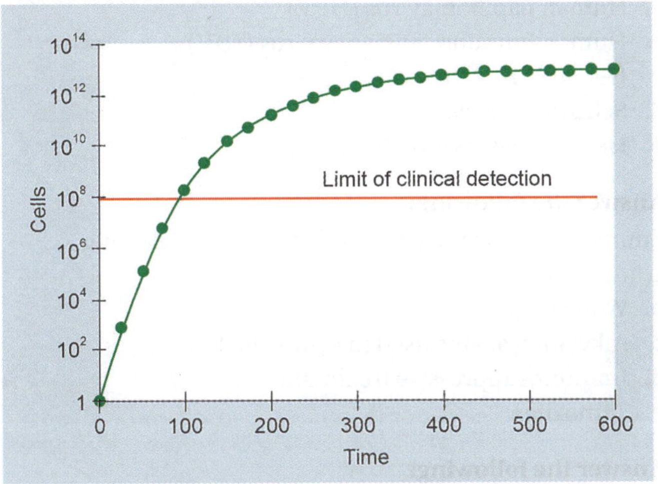


*Source:* Bailey and Love, 28th edition, page 201.

a. Identify the given graph.
b. What does it describe?

**Q6. Name the genes associated with the following conditions:**

a. Familial adenomatous polyposis (FAP)
b. Hereditary nonpolyposis colorectal cancer (HNPCC1), Lynch syndrome 1
c. HNPCC2
d. Peutz-Jeghers syndrome
e. Cowden syndrome
f. Multiple endocrine neoplasia (MEN) type 1
g. MEN type 2A
h. MEN type 2B
i. Li-Fraumeni
j. Familial cutaneous malignant melanoma

**Q7. Answer the following:**

a. Name three recessive inherited syndrome.
b. Name three inherited syndrome which require active surveillance in order to prevent or making early diagnosis.

**Q8. Answer the following:**

Enumerate the cancer associated with the following:

a. Tobacco
b. Alcohol
c. Ultraviolet (UV) exposure
d. Ionizing radiation

**Q9. Answer the following:**

Enumerate the cancer associated with the following:

a. Human papillomavirus (HPV)
b. Human immunodeficiency virus (HIV)
c. Hepatitis B
d. Schistosomiasis
e. Helicobacter pylori (*H. pylori*)

**Q10. Answer the following:**

Enumerate the cancer associated with the following:

a. Asbestos
b. Wood dust
c. Alkylating agents used in cytotoxic therapy
d. Immunosuppressive treatment
e. Tamoxifen

**Q11. Answer the following:**

Enumerate the cancer associated with the following:

a. Aflatoxins
b. Obesity/lack of physical exercise

**Q12. What are the criteria screening based on Wilson-Jungar criteria for screening program?**

**Q13. Answer the following:**

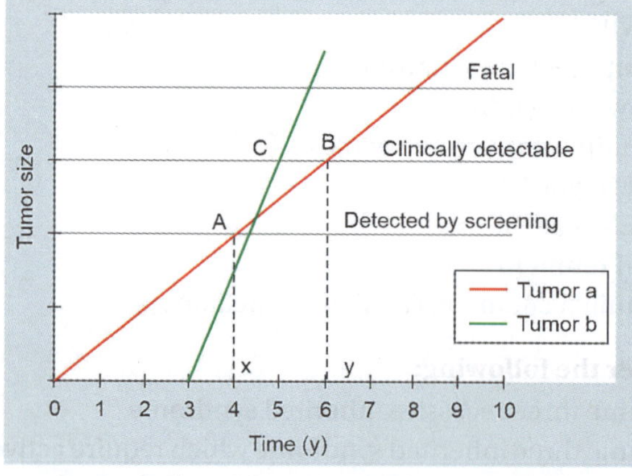


*Source:* Dailey and Love, 20th edition, page 205.

a. What does a, b, and c signifies in the given graph?
b. What does Gleason system grade used for?
c. What does Tx depict in staging of colorectal cancer?
d. What does T4 depict in staging of colorectal cancer?
e. What depicts nodal staging of colorectal cancer?

**Q14. What are the advantages and disadvantages of multidisciplinary team?**

**Q15. Answer the following:**

a. Name two drugs that act as spindle poisons.
b. Name a bioreductive drug which act as a DNA cross linking, preferentially active at sites of low oxygen tension.
c. Name two motor inhibitors and there mode of action and tumor sensitive to drug.

**Q16. Answer the following:**

a. Name two mitogen-activated protein kinase (MEK) inhibitors and there mode of action and tumor sensitive to drug.
b. Name two RAF inhibitors and there mode of action and tumor sensitive to drug.
c. Name one phosphoinositide 3-kinase (PI3K) inhibitors and there mode of action and tumor sensitive to drug

**Q17. Name Histone deacetylase (HDAC) inhibitors and there mode of action and tumor sensitive to drug.**

**Q18. Name three oncological emergencies and their treatment.**

## ANSWERS

**Ans. 1** a. Theodor Boveri
b. Oswald Avery
c. 1953

**Ans. 2** *Features of malignant transformation*

- Establish an autonomous lineage
- Resist signals that inhibit growth
- Sustain proliferative signaling
- Obtain replicative immortality
- Evade apoptosis
- Acquire angiogenic competence
- Acquire ability to invade, disseminate, and implant

- Evocation of inflammation
- Evade detection/elimination
- Loss of specialist cell function
- Develop ability to change energy metabolism

**Ans. 3** a. Electron micrograph of apoptotic bodies (AB) engulfed by a macrophage. Macrophage nucleus (MN) and macrophage cytoplasm (MC).

b. Apoptosis, taken from the Greek for "leaf fall", is a form of programmed cell death that occurs as the direct result of internal cellular events instructing the cell to die. Unlike necrosis, which is a form of traumatic cell death resulting from acute cellular injury, apoptosis is an orderly and internally driven process.

c. Epithelial cells behave as if they were mesenchymal cells and the process is termed epithelial-mesenchymal transition (EMT). EMT is a crucial step in malignant transformation and many of the genes and proteins implicated in the formation of cancer control processes are involved in EMT, e.g., Src, *RAS*, integrins, Wnt/β-catenin, Notch.

**Ans. 4** a. Paul Ehrlich

b. Stephen Paget

c. Warburg effect—Cancer cells can alter their metabolism even when oxygen is abundant; they break down glucose but do not, as normal cells would do, send the resulting pyruvate to the mitochondria for conversion, in an oxygen-dependent process, to carbon dioxide. This is the phenomenon of aerobic glycolysis, or the Warburg effect, and leads to the production of lactate.

**Ans. 5** a. Gompertzian curve

b. Gompertzian curve—(Growth of a typical tumor) In its early stages, growth is exponential but, as the tumor grows, the growth rate slows. This decrease in growth rate probably arises because of difficulties with nutrition and oxygenation. The tumor cells are in competition: Not only with the tissues of the host, but also with each other.

**Ans. 6** a. *APC* gene

b. DNA mismatch repair genes (*MLH1; MSH2; MSH6*)

c. DNA mismatch repair genes (*MLH1; MSH2; MSH6*)

d. *STK11*

e. *PTEN*

f. Menin

g. *RET*

h. *RET*

i. *P53*
j. *CDNK2A; CDK4*

**Ans. 7** a. 1. Xeroderma pigmentosum
2. Ataxia-telangiectasia
3. Bloom syndrome

b. 1. Cowden syndrome
2. Ataxia-telangiectasia
3. Bloom syndrome

**Ans. 8** a. Lung cancer, head and neck cancer, bladder cancer
b. Head and neck cancer, esophageal cancer, hepatocellular carcinoma
c. Melanoma, nonmelanoma, skin cancer
d. Leukemia, breast cancer, lymphoma, thyroid cancer

**Ans. 9** a. Cervical cancer, penile cancer, head and neck cancer
b. Kaposi's sarcoma, Lymphomas, germ cell tumors, anal cancer
c. Hepatocellular carcinoma
d. Bladder cancer
e. Stomach cancer

**Ans. 10** a. Mesothelioma
b. Paranasal sinus cancers
c. Leukemia lymphoma lung cancer
d. Kaposi's sarcoma
e. Endometrial cancer

**Ans. 11** a. Hepatocellular carcinoma
b. Breast endometrium kidney colon esophagus

**Ans. 12** Criteria for screening (based on Wilson–Junger criteria for a screening program)

| *The disease:* | *The test:* | *The program:* |
|---|---|---|
| • Recognizable early stage<br>• Treatment at early stage more effective than at later stage<br>• Sufficiently common to warrant screening | • Sensitive and specific<br>• Acceptable to the screened population<br>• Safe<br>• Inexpensive | • Adequate diagnostic facilities for those with a positive test<br>• High-quality treatment for screen-detected disease to minimize morbidity and mortality<br>• Screening repeated at intervals if disease of insidious onset<br>• Benefit must outweigh physical and psychological harm |

**Ans. 13** a. Illustration of lead time and length bias.
Tumor "a" is a steadily growing tumor; its progress is uninfluenced by any treatment.

a indicates the time at which the tumor would be diagnosed in a screening program,

b indicates the time at which the tumor would be diagnosed clinically, i.e., in the absence of any screening program.

If the date of diagnosis is used as the start time for measuring survival, then, in the absence of any effect from treatment, the screening program will, artefactually, add to the survival time.

The amount of "increased" survival is equal to y–x years, in this example just over 2 years. This artefactual inflation of survival time is referred to as lead time bias.

Tumor b is a rapidly growing tumor; again its progress is uninfluenced by treatment. It grows so rapidly that, in the interval between two screening tests, it can cross both the threshold for detectability by screening and that of clinical detectability (at point C).

It will continue to progress rapidly after diagnosis and the measured survival time will be short.

Length time bias—Phenomenon, whereby those tumors that are "missed" by the screening program are associated with decreased survival.

b. Gleason system grade used for Staging of colorectal cancer.

c to e. Answer given in table below:

| | | |
|---|---|---|
| • TX, Primary tumor cannot be assessed<br>• T0, No evidence of primary tumor<br>• Tis, Carcinoma in situ or intramucosal carcinoma<br>• T1, Tumor invades submucosa<br>• T2, Tumor invades muscularis propria<br>• T3, The tumor has grown through the muscularis propria and into the subserosa, which is a thin layer of connective tissue beneath the outer layer of some parts of the large intestine, or it has grown into tissues surrounding the colon or rectum.<br>• T4, Tumor directly invades beyond bowel<br>a. The tumor has grown into the surface of the visceral peritoneum<br>b. The tumor has grown into or has attached to other organs or structures | • NX, Regional lymph nodes cannot be assessed<br>• N0, No metastases in regional nodes<br>• N1a, Metastases in 1 regional lymph node<br>• N1b, Metastases in 2 or 3 regional lymph nodes<br>• N1c, There are nodules made up of tumor cells found in the structures near the colon that do not appear to be lymph nodes<br>• N2a, Metastases in 4–6 regional lymph nodes<br>• N2a, Metastases in ≥7 regional lymph nodes<br>• MX, Not possible to assess the presence of distant metastases | • M0, No distant metastases<br>• M1a, The cancer has spread to one other part of the body beyond the colon or rectum<br>• M1b, The cancer has spread to >1 part of the body other than the colon or rectum<br>• M1c, The cancer has spread to the peritoneal surface |

**Ans. 14**

| *Advantages* | *Disadvantages* |
|---|---|
| • Open debate concerning management of complex patients with many specialists<br>• Decision making is open, transparent, and explicit<br>• Team members educate each other<br>• A useful educational experience for trainees and students<br>• Performance can be monitored by managers | • Less confident and less articulate members of the team may not be able to express their views, even though their views may be extremely important.<br>• May become a rubber-stamping exercise in which the class solutions implied by guidelines are applied to disparate individuals.<br>• Decisions are made in the absence of patients and their carers.<br>• Clinicians are able to avoid having to take responsibility for their decisions and their actions—"corporate responsibility."<br>• Time-consuming and resource intensive: takes multiple busy clinicians away from clinical practice for hours at a time. |

**Ans. 15** a. Vincristine
Vinblastine

b. Mitomycin C

c. Temsirolimus
Everolimus
*Mode of action*
- Inhibit mTOR, a key component in the PI3K/AKT/mTOR pathway

*Tumor sensitive to drug*
- Neuroendocrine tumors
- Renal cancer

**Ans. 16** a. Trametinib
Selumetinib
Mechanism of action (MOA) inhibit the MAPK pathway
*Sensitive to:* Neurofibroma, melanoma

b. Dabrafenib Vemurafenib
MOA Inhibit the MAPK pathway
Sensitive to melanoma

c. Idelalisib
MOA Inhibit mTOR, a key component in the PI3K/AKT/mTOR pathway
Sensitive to renal cancer, neuroendocrine tumor

**Ans. 17** 1. Panobinostat
2. Vorinostat
3. Entinostat

MOA

Acetylation of histones is associated with increased transcription of genes; inhibiting deacetylation can decrease expression of mutated or dysregulated genes.

*Sensitive to:*

- Cutaneous T-cell lymphoma (Panobinostat, Vorinostat)
- Melanoma (Entinostat)

**Ans. 18** There are a limited number of true emergencies in oncology. Those that require immediate recognition and management are:

- *Cord compression:* Rapid diagnosis and management to relieve pressure on the spinal cord is essential to obtain the best results for patients. Ideally, treatment should be instituted when cord compression is threatened rather than when it has already occurred. Management is likely to include steroids and either neurosurgery or radiotherapy.
- *Neutropenic sepsis:* Rapid diagnosis and antibiotic therapy are essential. There is a strong inverse relationship between the time taken to start antibiotics and the chance of patient survival.
- Immune side effects including hypophysitis, adrenal failure, and insulin-dependent diabetes.

# 13 CHAPTER Surgical Audit and Research

## QUESTIONS

**Q1. Answer the following:**

a. What is clinical audit (NEET SS)?
b. What are essential steps to establish audit cycle?

**Q2. Answer the following:**

a. Who is producer of below database?
   - PubMed
   - PubMed central
b. Name two data base which have subscription availability only.
c. What is coverage of Cochrane collaboration and library?

**Q3. Answer the following:**

a. Which is the first randomized controlled trial (RCT) undertaken by West Midlands Research Collaborative (WMRC)?
b. What are the questions to answer before undertaking research?

**Q4. Enumerate different types of study (NEET SS).**

**Q5. Answer the following:**

a. What is type I and II error (NEET SS)?
b. Expand SUNRISE trial.

**Q6. Answer the following:**

a. What are the key features of research integrity?
b. What is mean, mode, median, and range (INI SS 2023 Nov)?

**Q7. Answer the following:**

a. What test used for [NEET SS 2022]?
   - Numerical and normally distributed data
   - Numerical but not normally distributed
   - Categorical data
b. What is significance of confidence interval (CI)?
c. What is the meaning of $p = 0.05$?

**Q8. Answer the following:**

a. Expand consort (NEET SS).
b. What is the consort checklist for authors?
c. Expand Prisma (NEET SS).

**Q9. What is IMRAD (DNB THEORY 2022)?**

## ANSWERS

**Ans. 1** a. Clinical audit is a process used by clinicians who seek to improve patient care. The process involves comparing aspects of care (structure, process, and outcome) against explicit criteria and defined standards.

b. Audits are formal processes that require a structure.
The following steps are essential to establish an audit cycle:
- Define the audit question in a multidisciplinary team.
- Identify the body of evidence and current standards.
- Design the audit to measure performance against agreed standards based on strong evidence. Seek appropriate advice (local audit department in the UK) and ensure institutions have agreed to undertake the audit.
- Measure over an agreed interval.
- Analyze results and compare performance against agreed standards.
- Undertake gap analysis:
  - If all standards are reached, reaudit after an agreed interval.
  - If there is a need for improvement, identify possible interventions such as training, and agree with the involved parties.
- Reaudit

**Ans. 2** a.
- US National Library of Medicine (NLM)
- US National Institutes of Health (NIH) free digital archive

b. CINAHL AND EMBASE

c. Preparing, updating, and promoting the accessibility of Cochrane Reviews published online in The Cochrane Library

**Ans. 3** a. The first RCT undertaken by the WMRC (West Midlands Research Collaborative) was the ROSSINI trial, which explored the clinical effectiveness of a simple wound-edge protection device in reducing wound infections after abdominal surgery.

b. Questions to answer before undertaking research:
   - Why study?
   - Answer a useful question
   - Practical
   - Possible available time and with the available resources
   - Benefit from collaboration to increase numbers or make best use of high-technology equipment
   - Findings are expected
   - Research governance requirements
   - Ethical issues
   - Impact

**Ans. 4**
- Observational—evaluation of condition or treatment in a defined population retrospective: Analysis of past events prospective: contemporaneous collection of data
- Case control—series of patients with a particular disease or condition compared with matched control patients
- Cross-sectional—measurements made on a single occasion, not looking at the whole population but selecting a small similar group and expanding results
- Longitudinal—measurements taken over a period of time, not looking at the whole population but selecting a small similar group and expanding results
- Experimental—two or more treatments are compared. Allocation to treatment groups is under the control of the researcher
- Randomized—two or more randomly allocated treatments
- Randomized includes a control group with standard controlled treatment

**Ans. 5** a.
   - *Type I error:* Benefit is perceived when really there is none (false positive).
   - *Type II error:* Benefit is missed when it was there to be found (false negative).

b. *SUNRISE:* Single Use Negative pRessure dressing for Reduction In Surgical site infection following Emergency laparotomy

**Ans. 6** a. *Features:*
   - Honesty
   - Accountability and transparency
   - Professional courtesy and fairness
   - Good stewardship

b.

| *Mean:* The result of dividing the total by the number of observations (the average) | *Median:* The middle value with equal numbers of observations above and below—used for numerical or ranked data | *Mode:* The value with the highest frequency observed—used for nominal data collection | *Range:* The largest to the smallest value |
|---|---|---|---|

**Ans. 7** a.

| Numerical and normally distributed (e.g., blood pressure)—use an unpaired t-test to compare two groups or a paired t-test to assess whether a variable has changed between two-time points | Numerical but not normally distributed (e.g., tumor size)—use a Mann–Whitney U-test to compare two groups or a Wilcoxon signed rank test to assess whether a variable has increased/stayed the same/decreased between two-time points | Categorical (e.g., admitted or not admitted to an intensive care unit)—a chi-squared test can be used to compare two groups |
|---|---|---|

b. *Confidence intervals* are the best guide to the possible range in which the true differences are likely to lie. A CI that includes zero usually implies a lack of statistical significance.

c. $p = 0.05$ means that there is only a 1:20 chance that the differences between the variables would have happened by chance when in fact there is no real difference.

**Ans. 8** a. Consolidated standards of reporting trials

b. CONSORT checklist for authors.

- Title—identify as randomized trial
- Abstract—structured format
- Introduction—prospectively defined hypotheses, clinical objective
- *Methods:*
    - Protocol
    - Assignment
    - Masking (blinding)
- *Results:* Participant flow and follow-up, analysis
- *Comment:*
    - Specific interpretation of study
    - Sources of bias
    - External validity
    - General interpretation

c. Preferred Reporting Items for Systematic Reviews and Meta-Analyses

**Ans. 9**
- IMRAD
- *IMRAD form:* Introduction, methods, results, and discussion
  - *Introduction:* Short and brief background of the study should be presented and then the aims of the trial or audit outlined.
  - *Methods:* The methodology and study design should be given in detail. It is important to identify potential biases. New techniques or investigations should be detailed in full; if they are common practice or have been described elsewhere, this should be referenced instead of described.
  - *Results:* Results are almost always best shown diagrammatically using tables and figures. Results shown in the form of a diagram need not then be duplicated in the text.
  - *Discussion:* It is important not to repeat the introduction or reiterate the results in this section. The study should be interpreted intelligently and any suggestions for future studies or changes in management should be made. It is prudent not to indulge in fights of fantasy or wild imagination about future possibilities; most journal editors will delete these. Recently, a standard format for the discussion section has been promoted, and journals such as the BMJ are keen that authors use it.
  - *References:* This section should include all relevant papers recording previous studies on the subject in question. The reference section does not usually have to be exhaustive, but should include up-to-date articles. Remember to present the references in the style of the journal of submission.

CHAPTER

# 14 Ethics and Law in Surgical Practice

## QUESTIONS

**Q1. Answer the following:**

a. What are the information disclosed during a formal and tangible discussion to establish valid consent for treatment?

b. What are the features of valid consent for adult?

**Q2. Answer the following:**

a. How incapacity established in patient?

b. What is doctrine of double effect?

## ANSWERS

**Ans. 1** a. Disclosed during a formal and tangible discussion, must include:

- The condition and the reasons why it warrants surgery.
- The type of surgery proposed and how it might correct the condition.
- The anticipated prognosis and expected side effects of the proposed surgery
- The unexpected hazards of the proposed surgery
- Any alternative and potentially successful treatments other than the proposed surgery
- The consequences of no treatment at all

b. For consent to be valid, adult patients must:

- Have capacity to give it—be able to understand, remember, and deliberate over the information disclosed to them about treatment choices, and to communicate those choices.
- Not be coerced into decisions that reflect the preferences of others rather than themselves.
- Have been given sufficient information for these choices to be based on an accurate understanding of reasons for and against proceeding with specific treatments.

**Ans. 2** a. Incapacity in England and Wales is established (in those aged 16 years and over) by a two-stage test. First, the functional test for incapacity is employed—is the person unable to make the relevant decision? If they are able to make the decision, the presumption of capacity endures. If they are unable to make the decision, then the second (diagnostic) stage must be employed—is there an impairment or disturbance of the mind or the brain? If so, the two stages in combination result in a conclusion of incapacity.

b. Doctrine of double effect is set of ethical criteria which Christian philosophers have advocated foe evaluating the permissibility of acting when ones otherwise.

CHAPTER

# 15 Human Factors, Patient Safety, and Quality Improvement

## QUESTIONS

**Q1. What are the principles proposed by porter that support value-based approach to healthcare?**

**Q2. What are the factors that contribute to patient safety incidents?**

**Q3. What are the safety checklist to be considered?**

a. Before induction of anesthesia.
b. Before skin incision.
c. Before patient leaves operating room.

**Q4. Answer the following:**

a. What are the information to be provided before seeking consent for surgery?
b. What are the common medication errors?

**Q5. What is coal face errors and what are the well-recognized and potential errors?**

**Q6. Answer the following:**

a. What are the failures in operative technique?
b. Draw the pyramid showing hierarchy of competence.

**Q7. Answer the following:**

a. What are never events?
b. What are the benefits of measuring clinical outcomes as a part of a quality improvement cycle?
c. What are the four stages of high value quality improvement or clinical audit activity?

**Q8. Answer the following:**

a. What are clinical outcome measures and clinical audit?
b. Name three pioneers of quality improvement and their quotes on data.

**Q9. Answer the following:**

a. What are seven stages to be consider when undertaking improvement?

b. Enumerate examples of tools used in quality improvement.

**Q10. What are seven types of waste in healthcare and possible solutions?**

**Q11. Answer the following:**

a. What is Six Sigma?

b. Expand DMAIC.

**Q12. Identify the mode of imaging with associated condition in image A and B.**

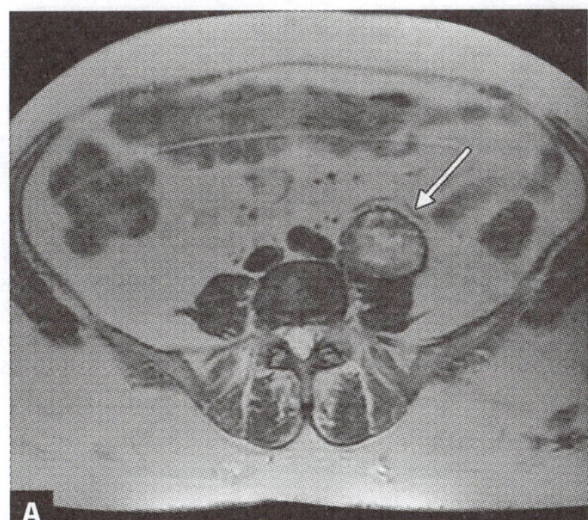


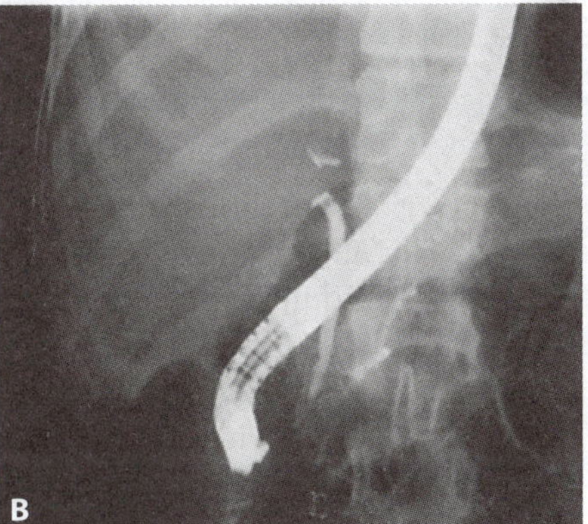


## ANSWERS

**Ans. 1** Porter proposed six principles that support a value-based approach to healthcare:

1. Organize care around medical conditions—care should be based upon the medical needs of a community.
2. Measure outcomes and costs for every patient.
3. Align reimbursement with value—to support better outcomes and more efficient care.
4. Systems integration—organize treatment around matching patient, treatment, and location.
5. Geography of care provide centers of excellence for complex care.
6. Information technology provides integration of the healthcare system.

**Ans. 2** *Factors that contribute to patient safety incidents:*

- *Human factors:*
  - Inadequate patient assessment; delays or errors in diagnosis
  - Failure to use or interpret appropriate tests
  - Error in performance of an operation, treatment, or test
  - Inadequate monitoring or follow-up of treatment
  - Deficiencies in training or experience
  - Fatigue, overwork, and time pressures
  - Personal or psychological factors (e.g., depression or drug abuse)
  - Patient or working environment variation
  - Lack of recognition of the dangers of medical errors
- *System failures*:
  - Poor communication between healthcare providers
  - Inadequate staffing levels
  - Disconnected reporting systems or over-reliance on automated systems
  - Lack of coordination at handovers
  - Drug similarities
  - Environment design, infrastructure
  - Equipment failure owing to lack of parts or skilled operators
  - Cost-cutting measures by hospitals
  - Poor governance structures and inadequate systems to report and review patient safety incidents
- *Medical complexity*:
  - Advanced and new technologies
  - Potent drugs, their side effects and interactions
  - Working environments—intensive care and operating theatre

**Ans. 3** a. *Before induction of anesthesia:*

  - Has the patient confirmed his/her identity, site, procedure, and consent?
  - Is the site marked?
  - Is the anesthesia machine and medication applicable check complete?
  - Is the pulse oximeter on the patient and functioning?
  - Does the patient have a:
    - Known allergy?
    - Difficult airway or aspiration risk?
    - Risk of >500 mL blood loss (7 mL/kg in children)?

b. *Before skin incision:*

  - Confirm all team members have introduced themselves by name and role.

- Confirm the patient's name, procedure, and where the incision will be made.
- Has antibiotic prophylaxis been given within the last 60 minutes?
- Anticipated critical events:
  - *To surgeon:*
    - What are the critical or nonroutine steps?
    - How long will the case take?
    - What is the anticipated blood loss?
  - *To anesthetist:* Are there any patient-specific concerns?
  - *To nursing team:*
    - Has sterility (including indicator results) been confirmed?
    - Are there equipment issues or any concerns?
  - Is essential imaging displayed?

c. *Before patient leaves operating room:*
- Nurse verbally confirms:
  - The name of the procedure
  - Completion of instrument, sponge, and needle counts
  - Specimen labeling (read specimen labels aloud, including patient name)
  - Whether there are any equipment problems to be addressed.
- To surgeon, anesthetist, and nurse:
  - What are the key concerns for recovery and management of this patient?
  - Revised

**Ans. 4** a. Information to be provided when seeking consent for surgery.
- The condition and the reasons why it warrants surgery.
- The type of surgery proposed and how it might correct the condition.
- The anticipated prognosis and expected side effects of the proposed surgery.
- The unexpected hazards of the proposed surgery.
- Any alternative and potentially successful treatments other than the proposed surgery.
- The consequences of no treatment at all.

b. Common medication errors include:
- Poor assessment or inadequate knowledge of patients and their clinical conditions;
- Inadequate knowledge of the medications;
- Dosage calculation errors;
- Illegible handwriting;
- Confusion regarding the name or the mixing up medications.

**Ans. 5**
- Errors where patients identify the surgeon as being responsible for a defined episode of care.
- Cuschieri and others have described coal-face errors as those that can potentially be committed by surgeons during the care of their patients and include:
  - Diagnostic and management errors
  - Resuscitation errors
  - Prophylaxis errors
  - Prescription/parenteral administration errors
  - Situation awareness, identification and teamwork errors
  - Technical and operative errors

**Ans. 6** a. Failures in operative technique include:
- Cognitive errors of judgement, such as late conversion of a difficult laparoscopic procedure into an open one;
- Procedural, when the steps of an operation are not followed or are omitted;
- Executional, when, for example, too much force is used, which may result in damage that may or may not have consequences;
- Misinterpretation of anatomy/pathology, which is compounded by minimal access surgery with the limitations of a two-dimensional image;
- Misuse of instrumentation, such as with energized dissection modalities (e.g., diathermy)
- Missed iatrogenic injury either at the time of surgery or diagnosed late.

b.

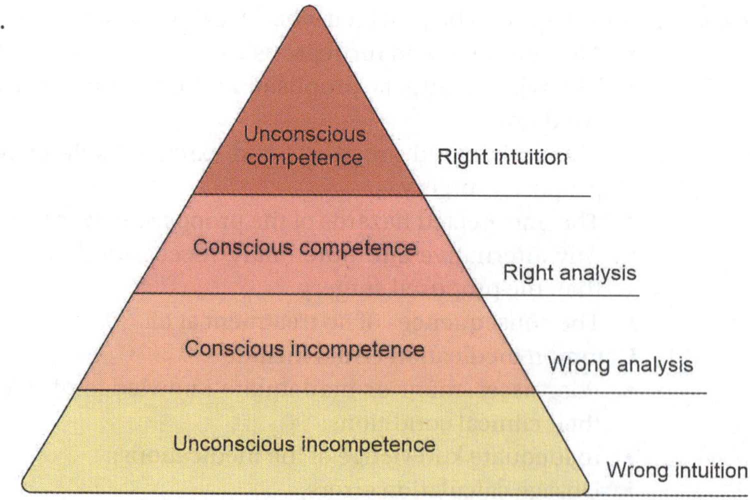

**Ans. 7** a. Incidents can be defined as events that could have or did result in unintended and/or unnecessary serious harm. One subset of serious incidents is a never or serious reportable event. These events are considered to be wholly preventable; for example, a retained abdominal swab or instrument, where guidance providing strong systemic protective barriers should have been implemented, namely checklists. Each "never event" type has the potential to cause serious harm to the patient or even death.

b. Measuring clinical outcomes as part of a quality improvement cycle can help to:

- Improve the quality of clinical care, with shorter hospital stays, better outcomes and fewer complications, reduced readmissions, and greater patient satisfaction.
- Inform the development of national clinical audits, including driving participation, data completeness, and accuracy.
- Support shared decision making and empowerment of patients, including their treatment options and choice of provider.
- Improve the oversight and management of clinicians, their teams and practices, thus reassuring patients that their clinical care is being actively monitored and improved.
- Help medical specialty associations to become increasingly transparent and patient focused.
- Support team and individual quality improvement, including providing information for appraisal and revalidation.
- Learn from, spread, and celebrate best practice.

c. Four stages of high value quality improvement or clinical audit activity:

1. Preparation and planning
2. Measurement of performance
3. Implementation of change
4. Sustainment and evaluation of the improvement

**Ans. 8** a. Clinical outcome measures refer specifically to outcomes of healthcare interventions, whether they are to do with diagnosis, treatment, or care received by service users. Ideally, they should be outcomes that are important to patients rather than to the healthcare provider (PROM—patient-reported outcome measure), and there should be evidence that they reflect the quality of the interventions and their effect.

Outcome measures are what are commonly used in clinical audit when outcomes achieved are compared with evidence-based standards of clinical care.

b. 1. *William Edwards Deming (1900–1993):*
   - American engineer, statistician, author, and management consultant. Pioneered the PDSA (plan–do–study–act) cycle
   - "In God we trust, all others bring data."

   2. *Peter Ferdinand Drucker (1909–2005):*
   - Austrian-born American management consultant and educator
   - "What gets measured gets improved."

   3. *Donald Berwick (B. 1946):*
   - American pediatrician. Former President and Chief Executive Officer of the Institute for Healthcare Improvement
   - Sequence of reactions that challenge data: "The data are wrong." "The data are right but it's not a problem." "The data are right; it is a problem but not my problem." "I accept the burden of improvement."
   - Process

**Ans. 9** a. Healthcare Improvement Scotland identifies seven stages when undertaking improvement:

1. Discovering is about defining the aims and vision; understanding what the problem is and what data are available.
2. Exploring is about defining the present state and visualizing the future state.
3. Designing is about defining how to move from the present state to the future state and identifying the priorities.
4. Refining is about testing change, learning from the data, and identifying the benefits.
5. Introducing is about managing communications and building the will and culture to change.
6. Spreading is about showing the improvements, telling the story, and disseminating the message.
7. Closing is about capturing and sustaining the learning.

b. Examples of tools used in quality improvement.

- *Organizational:*
  - Root cause analysis
  - Benefits realization planning
  - Demand and capacity planning

- Process mapping
- Value stream mapping
- Kanban and 5 'S'
- *Graphical:*
  - Driver diagrams
  - Fishbone cause and effect
  - Diagrams
  - Spaghetti diagrams
  - Box, frequency, and scatter Plots
  - Pareto charts
  - Run charts
  - Statistical process control charts

**Ans. 10** Seven types of waste in healthcare and possible solutions:

1. *Overproduction:*
   - *Example:* Ordering unnecessary preoperative tests
   - *Solution:* Implementation of evidence-based preassessment pathways
2. *Inventory:*
   - *Example:* Storing excessive medication or supplies in ward storage with a risk of them going out of date.
   - *Solution:* Alphabetically ordered medication cupboards with small amounts of commonly used drugs in conjunction with an efficient replenishment system.
3. *Waiting:*
   - *Example:* Patients waiting long periods to come to theatre.
   - *Solution:* Staggered admission times aligned to operating theatre schedule.
4. *Waste of transportation:*
   - *Example:* Using trolleys to bring ambulatory day patients to the operating theatre.
   - *Solution:* Better design of the admissions process to enable patients to walk to theatre.
5. *Waste of overprocessing:*
   - *Example:* Using computed tomography scans to assess children with possible appendicitis.
   - *Solution:* Consider whether ultrasound could be used instead.
6. *Defect:*
   - *Example:* Patients arriving for surgery with incomplete or inappropriate preoperative paperwork.
   - *Solution:* More robust checking systems before patients come to theatre.

7. *Motion:*
   - *Example:* Frequent searching in theatres and the anesthetic room to find necessary drugs and equipment.
   - *Solution:* An efficient theatre layout, common to all operating theatres in the hospital, where everything needed is easily available with minimal movement and always in the same place.

**Ans. 11** a. Six Sigma refers to another business performance methodology that has been adopted for use in healthcare. The fundamental objective of the Six Sigma methodology is the implementation of a measurement-based strategy that focuses on process improvement and especially on reducing unnecessary variation.

b. One of its submethodologies is DMAIC (Defne, Measure, Analyze, Improve, and Control), which is an improvement system for existing processes that fall below specification and require incremental improvement.

**Ans. 12**

- *Image A:* Axial magnetic resonance images demonstrating a well-defined abdominal mass with whorled stripes in a fluid-filled central cavity (arrows). This 60-year-old woman had had an abdominal hysterectomy 10 years previously and presented with pyrexia and flank pain. The cause was due to the late presentation of a retained surgical swab.
- *Image B:* Endoscopic retrograde cholangiopancreatography radiograph showing an iatrogenic bile duct injury.

# CHAPTER 16 Global Health and Surgery

## QUESTIONS

**Q1. Answer the following:**

a. What is four dimensions for access for surgery?
b. What is the geographical access?

**Q2. Answer the following:**

a. What are considered essential staffing at district hospital?
b. What are the core indicators to monitor the realization of universal access to safe, affordable surgical, and anesthesia care?

**Q3. What are the core packages for strengthening emergency and essential surgical care and anesthesia?**

## ANSWERS

**Ans. 1** a. Timeliness, capacity, safety, and affordability
b. Geographical access is the ability of a patient to reach a surgical facility within 2 hours, which is the crucial time for life-threatening hemorrhage. Capacity denotes that the facility has the required infrastructure and workforce and is able to perform safe surgery.

**Ans. 2** a. A surgeon, anesthetist and obstetrician (SAO) at the district hospital are considered essential staffing.
b. *Core indicators:* Monitor the realization of universal access to safe, affordable surgical, and anesthesia care.

**Ans. 3** Core packages for strengthening emergency and essential surgical care and anesthesia.

| *Emergency procedures packages include:* | *Planned care packages can include:* |
|---|---|
| • Basic trauma package (e.g., fracture treatment, trauma laparotomy, and debridement)<br>• Basic obstetric package (e.g., caesarean section)<br>• Basic emergency general surgical package (e.g., laparotomy and incision and drainage) | • General surgical package (e.g., hernia repair and bowel resection)<br>• Obstetric and gynecological package (e.g., hysterectomy)<br>• Specialist surgical package (e.g., cataract, clubfoot correction)<br>• Palliative surgical package (e.g., diversion colostomy and analgesics) |

2

SECTION

# General Pediatrics

# 17 CHAPTER Pediatric Surgery

## QUESTIONS

**Q1. Answer the following:**

a. Enumerate four examples of difference between infants and older children.
b. What are their implications?

**Q2. Answer the following:**

a. How to calculate maintenance fluid requirement in pediatric age group?
b. How to calculate systolic blood pressure (SBP) in pediatric age group?
c. How to calculate circulating blood volume?

**Q3. What are the preoperative fasting instruction for pediatric patients:**

a. Clear fluid
b. Breast milk
c. Solids

**Q4. Answer the following:**

a. What is Amyand's hernia?
b. What is Litter's hernia?
c. Incidence of inguinal hernia in infants and its risk factor.

**Q5. Answer the following:**

a. Testicular descent usually completed by
b. When to schedule orchidopexy in undescended testis (UDT)?
c. What is Denis brown pouch?
d. Explain fowler Stephans orchidopexy and its indication.

**Q6. Answer the following:**

a. Identify the image depicted.
b. What is depicted in single arrow and double arrow?

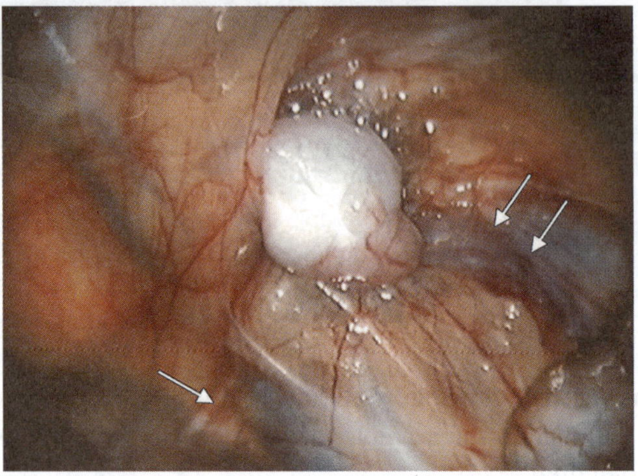

*Source:* Bailey and Love, 28th edition, page 258.

**Q7. Answer the following:**

a. Identify the clinical image and Doppler USG suggestive.
b. Surgery to be done at what time from onset of symptoms improves outcome.

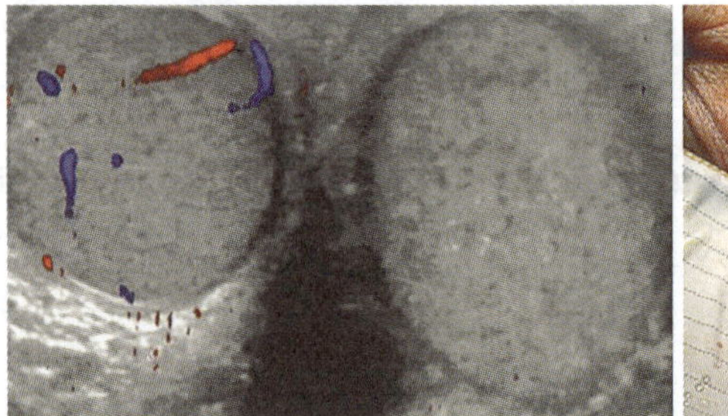
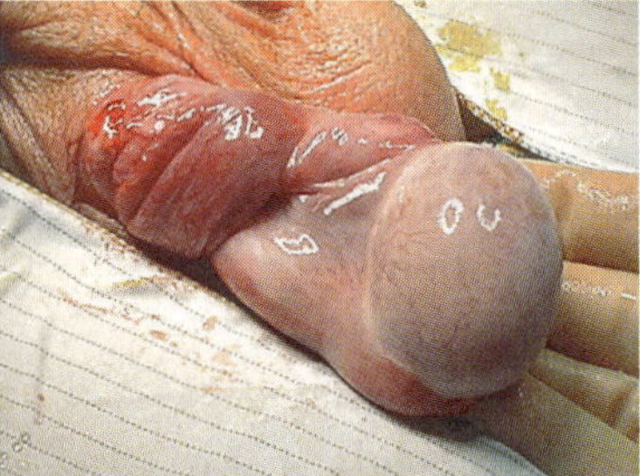

*Source:* Bailey and Love, 28th edition, page 258.

**Q8. Answer the following:**

a. Name three organisms involved in epididymo-orchitis seen after puberty in sexually active male and what are the presenting symptoms?
b. What is Prehn's sign?

**Q9. Answer the following:**

a. Olive tumor seen in
b. Explain Ramstedt's pyloromyotomy and used in

**Q10. Answer the following:**

a. Enumerate A, B, C.
b. Which of the following becomes median umbilical cord?

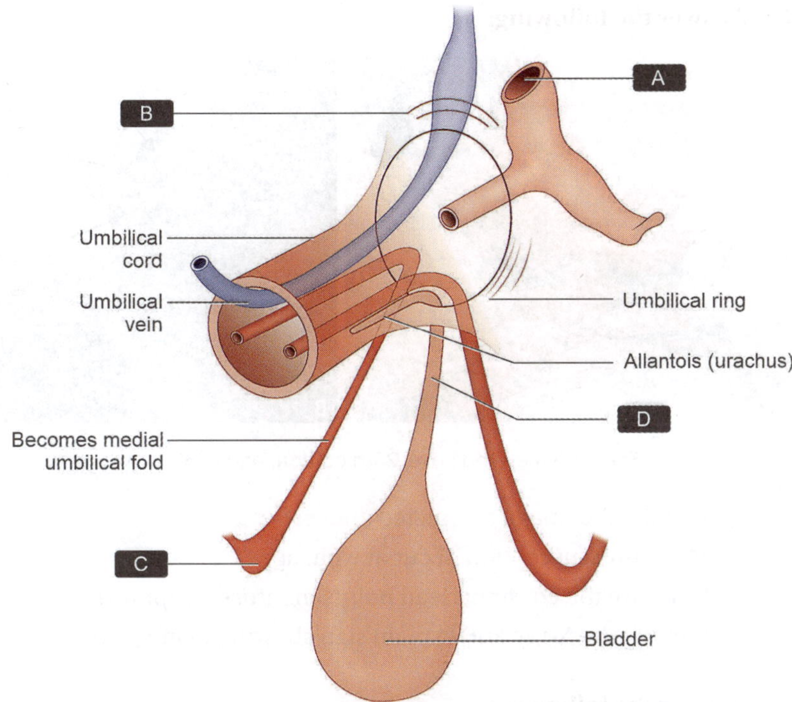


*Source:* Bailey and Love, 28th edition, page 259.

**Q11. Answer the following:**

a. What is depicted in image?

b. What type of alkalosis seen in infantile hypertrophic pyloric stenosis (IHPS)?

c. How do you manage alkalosis in IHPS?

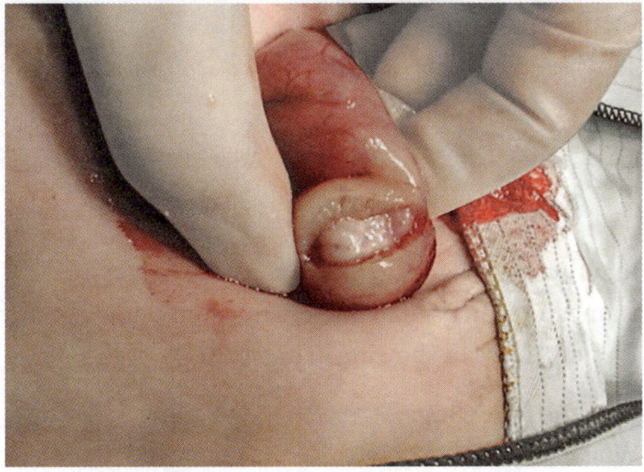

*Source:* Bailey and Love, 28th edition, page 260.

## Q12. Answer the following:

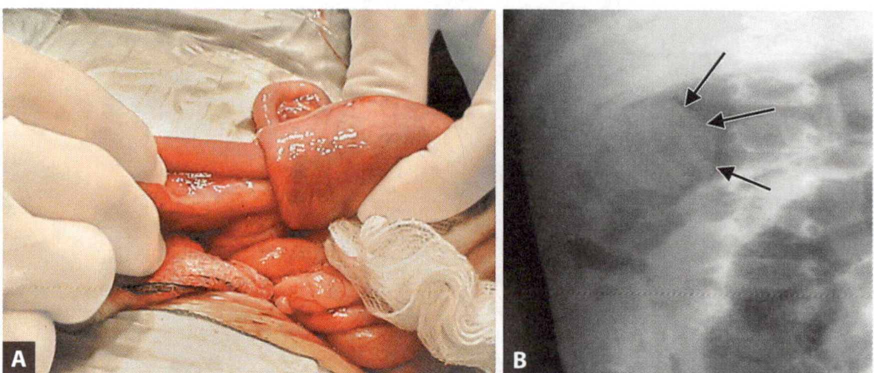


*Source:* Bailey and Love, 28th edition, page 260.

a. Identify the image a depicted above.
b. Most intussusception occur at what age
c. What are the common lead points in intussusception?
d. Identify the X-ray and explain sign showing in image B.

## Q13. Answer the following:

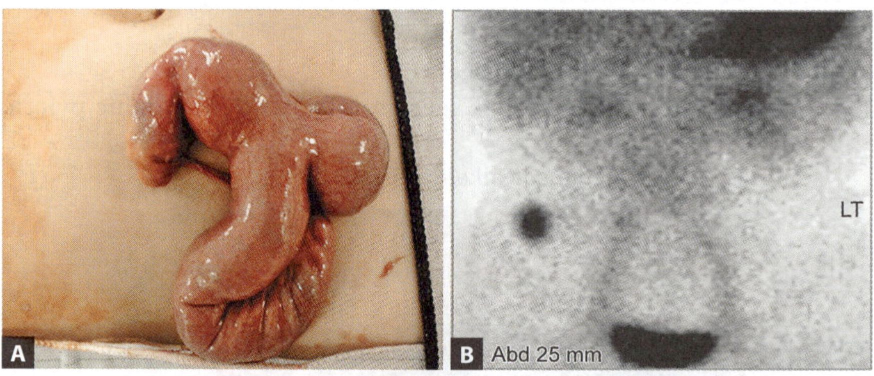


*Source:* Bailey and Love, 28th edition, page 261.

a. Identify the image A.
b. Name the scan used to demonstrate the ectopic gastric mucosa.
c. Identify the scan showing in image B.

## Q14. Answer the following:

a. What is neuroblastoma?
b. Nephroblastoma.

## ANSWERS

**Ans. 1** a. *Infants:*

- Wide abdomen
- Broad costal margin and a shallow pelvis
- Liver edge comes below the costal margin, and the bladder is partly intra-abdominal
- Ribs are more horizontal and are flexible
- Umbilicus is relatively low lying

b. *Implications:*

- *Incisions*: Transverse supraumbilical incisions have better access than vertical midline incisions.
- Abdominal trauma (including surgical incisions) can easily damage the liver or bladder
- Ventilation requires more diaphragmatic movement than in adults due to geometry of the ribs.
- Stoma in the lower abdomen of an infant sited carefully for its bag as it may interfere with the umbilicus.

**Ans. 2** a. Maintenance fluid requirement

| ***Weight*** | ***Daily requirement of fluid mL/kg/day*** | ***mL/kg/HR*** |
|---|---|---|
| Neonate | 120–150 | 5 |
| First 10 kg | 100 | 4 |
| Second 10 kg | 50 | 2 |
| Subsequent kg | 20 | 1 |

b. SBP = 80 + (age in years × 2) mm Hg

c. Circulating blood volume = 70–80 mL/kg (90–100 mL/kg in preterms) (b/min: breaths per minute; bpm: beats per minute)

**Ans. 3** *Preoperative fasting instructions for pediatric patients:*

a. 1 hour for clear fluids

b. 4 hours for breast milk

c. 6 hours for solids

**Ans. 4** a. The hernia contains appendix called Amyand's hernia.

b. The hernia contains a Meckel's diverticulum Littre's hernia.

c. Inguinal hernias occur in 4% of infants with prematurity, low birth weight, and male sex being risk factors (M:F 6:1). Inguinal hernias are twice as common on the right side as on the left, with 10% occurring bilaterally

**Ans. 5** a. Testicular descent is usually complete by the 30th week of gestation. At birth, 4% of full-term and 30% of premature boys have an UDT.

b. Boys should be examined at birth and at 6 weeks; if a UDT is found, they should be seen at 3 months since a testis is unlikely to descend after this time. An orchidopexy is then scheduled for between 6 and 12 months.

c. A testis cannot be palpated in the canal; it can only be felt when delivered to the superficial pouch, which is also called Denis Browne's pouch (a pocket between Scarpa's fascia and EO fascia at the external ring).

d. If there is a viable intra-abdominal testis, a two-stage Fowler–Stephens orchidopexy is performed. In the first stage, testicular vessels are ligated, leaving the testis in situ, anticipating survival on the vessels accompanying the vas. 3 months later a second operation is performed; if the testis has survived, it is brought into the scrotum.

**Ans. 6** a. Right-sided intra-abdominal testis visible at the internal ring (laparoscopic view).

b. • *Single arrow:* Vas
- *Double arrow:* Testicular vessels

**Ans. 7** a. The red and blue color on one testis shows normal blood flow whereas the contralateral testis has no blood supply, consistent with a torsion. Torsion of the right testis with only modest vascular compromise in a boy with a history of intermittent pain.

b. 6–8 hours of the symptom's onset improves the chances of testicular salvage.

**Ans. 8** a. *Chlamydia trachomatis*, *Neisseria gonorrhoeae*, and *Escherichia coli*

b. Pain may subside in epididymo-orchitis on elevation of the testis (Prehn's sign).

**Ans. 9** a. IHPS

b. It is performed laparoscopically or through a supraumbilical or right upper quadrant incision.
- *Procedure:* Pyloric serosal incision given, and the "tumor" spread, leaving an intact submucosa from the duodenal fornix to gastric antrum. The incision must extend onto the stomach; short incisions cause an early recurrence.
- Procedure done for pyloric stenosis.

**Ans. 10** A. Ileum with vitellointestinal duct (a remnant becomes a Meckel's diverticulum)
B. Falciform ligament
C. Umbilical artery
D. Structure D becomes median umbilical fold.

**Ans. 11** a. Pyloromyotomy for IHPS.
b. Loss of gastric acid causes a hypochloremic, hypokalemic alkalosis
c. Correction may take 24–48 hours; 0.9% saline with 0.15% KCl in 5% glucose given at 6–7.5 mL/kg/h provides maintenance and corrects deficits in most babies. As the chloride deficit is replaced, the kidneys correct the pH.

**Ans. 12** a. Small bowel obstruction due to Ileocolic intussusception
b. Between 2 months and 2 years
c. Viral-induced hyperplasia in a Peyer's patch
d. • *Image A:* Intussusception reduction by air enema
• *Image B:* X-ray showing small bowel obstruction, a mass and a paucity of gas in the right iliac fossa. A concentric target sign is seen on an abdominal ultrasound.

**Ans. 13** a. Meckel's diverticulum
b. Technetium scan
c. A positive Meckel's scan

**Ans. 14** a. • Origin—adrenal medulla or sympathetic ganglia
• It presents with an abdominal or paravertebral mass.
• Metastasizes to—lymph nodes, bone and liver, raising urinary catecholamine levels
• Management—Small, localized tumors are excised. Advanced tumors are excised after chemotherapy.
• Survival exceeds 90% for small, localized tumors but is <50% for advanced tumors.

b. • *Origin*: Malignant renal tumor derived from embryonal cells
• *Presents:* Abdominal mass between 1 and 4 years.
• *Genetics:* A mutation in the Wilms' tumor suppressor gene (WT1) causes some cases.
• *Extension:* The tumor can extend into the renal vein and vena cava.
• *Mets:* To lymph nodes and lungs
• *Treatment:* Chemotherapy and surgery
• Survival depends on tumor spread, completeness of excision and histological appearance but exceeds 70% even with advanced tumors

# 18 Neonatal Surgery

CHAPTER

## QUESTIONS

**Q1. Answer the following:**

a. Expand VACTERL syndrome.
b. Expand CHARGE syndrome.
c. Why it is recommendable to avoid Trendelenburg position in the preterm when placing a diathermy pad.

**Q2. Which of the associated conditions to be screened in following congenital malformation?**

a. Anorectal malformation
b. Esophageal atresia
c. Congenital pulmonary airway malformation (CPAM).
d. Exomphalos

**Q3. Answer the following:**

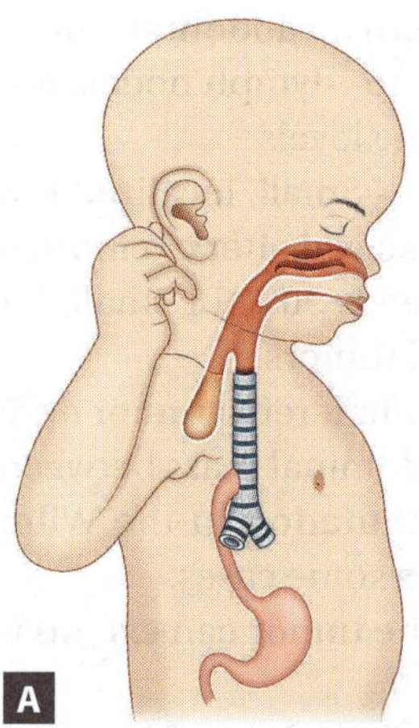


*Source:* Bailey and Love, 28th edition, page 264.

a. Explain the type of Tetralogy of Fallot (TOF) shown in image A.
b. Which type is an isolated h type TOF without atresia?
c. In which type of TOF there is no fistula.

**Q4. Answer the following:**

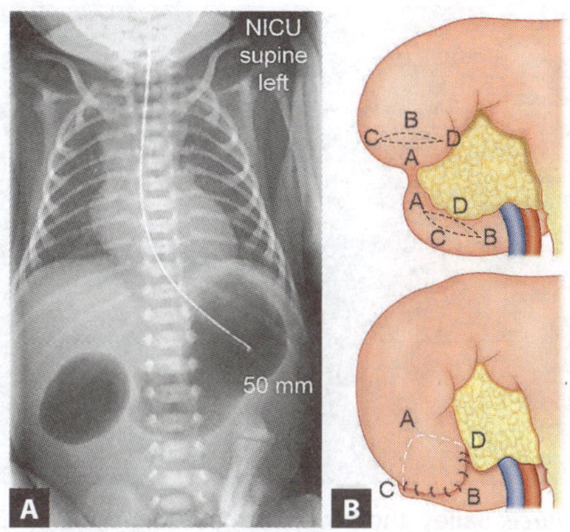


*Source:* Bailey and Love, 28th edition, page 266.

a. Explain the X-ray and his type of sign seen in
b. Above condition repair is done by which surgery
c. *TTC7A* gene associated with
d. Explain the procedure shown in image B

**Q5. Identify the images and associated condition in image A, B, C, and D.**

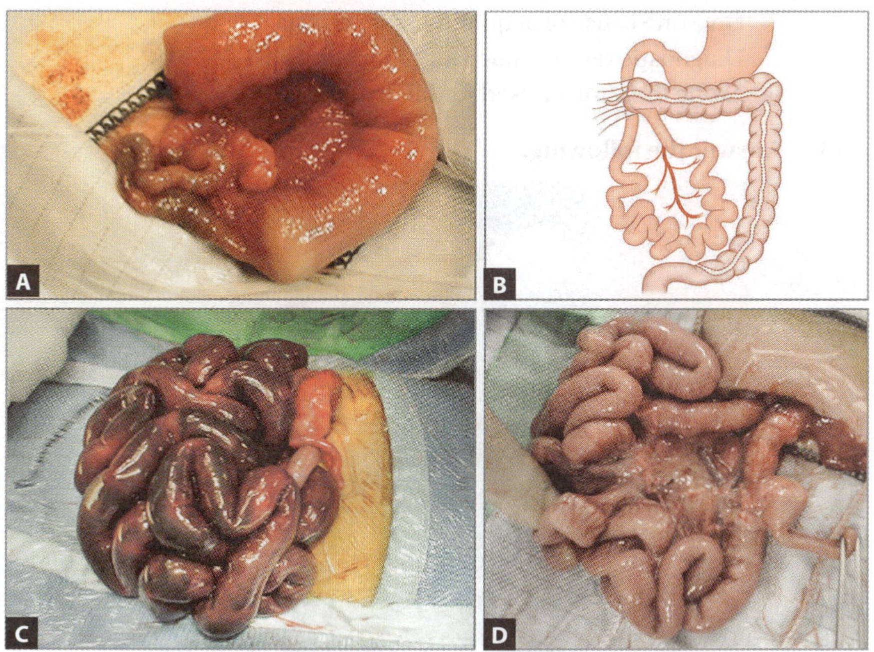


*Source:* Bailey and Love, 28th edition, page 267.

**Q6. Answer the following:**

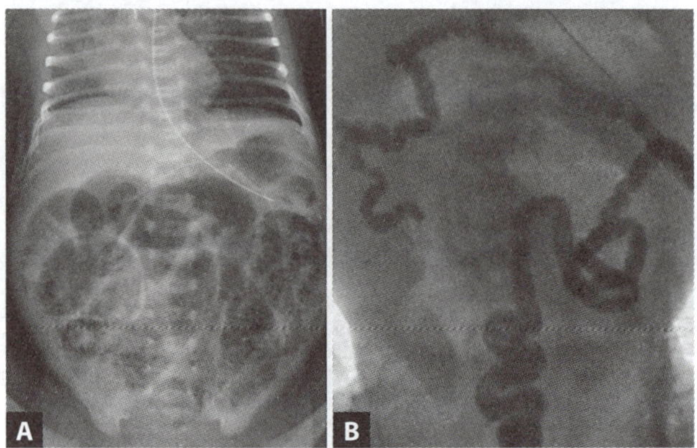


*Source:* Bailey and Love, 28th edition, page 268.

a. What is necrotizing enterocolitis (NEC)?
b. Explain the sign seen in abdominal radiograph image A and name the above condition.
c. Name the contrast used in above image B and identify the condition.

**Q7. Answer the following:**

a. Most common type of biliary atresia
b. Give one cause of acquired biliary atresia.
c. Diagnostic test of choice for biliary atresia
d. Name the surgery used for biliary atresia.

**Q8. Answer the following:**

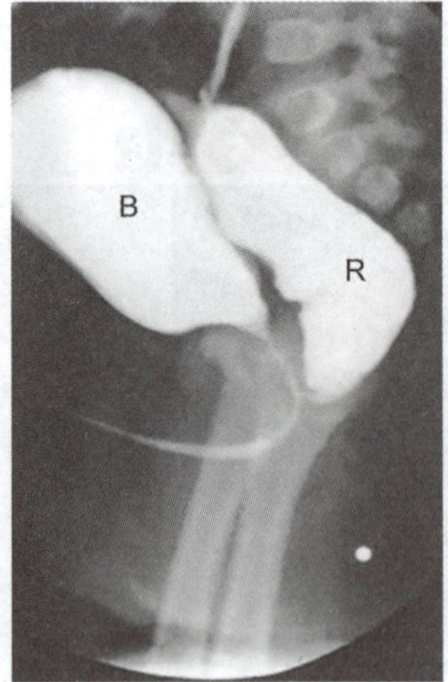


*Source:* Bailey and Love, 28th edition, page 269.

a. What is posterior sagittal anorectoplasty (PSARP) used in anorectal malformation?
b. What is depicted in above image?

**Q9. Answer the following:**

a. Name the genetic defects associated with Hirschsprung's disease.
b. How Hirschsprung's disease presents?
c. Name the surgeries for the Hirschsprung's disease.
d. Diagnostic test for Hirschsprung's disease.

**Q10. Answer the following:**

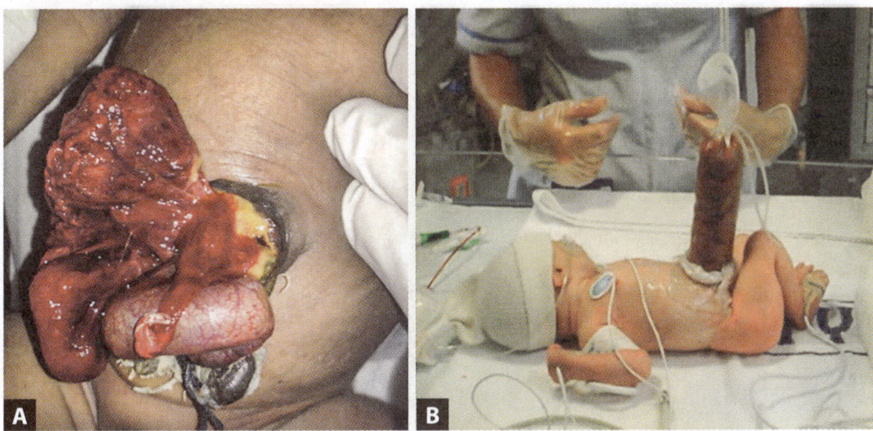


*Source:* Bailey and Love, 28th edition, pages 270 and 271.

a. Identify the condition in above images A.
b. Identify the condition in above images B.
c. What are the risk factors for above condition?

**Q11. Answer the following:**

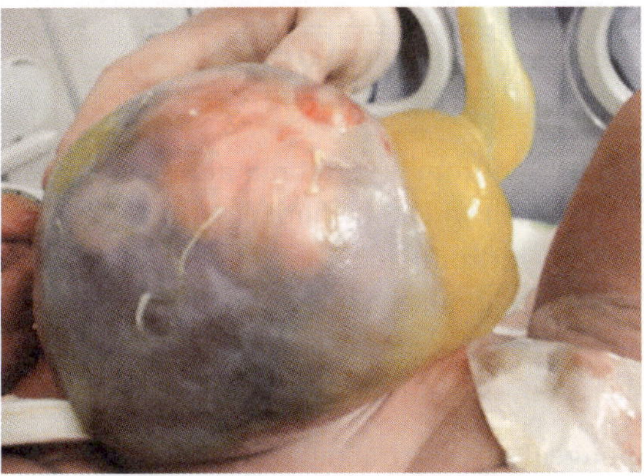

*Source:* Bailey and Love, 28th edition, page 271.

a. Identify the image and associated condition.
b. What are the three membrane layers in which prolapsed viscera covered?

**Q12. Answer the following:**

a. Name two genes associated with congenital diaphragmatic hernia.
b. Name the patch used to close larger defects.

**Q13. Answer the following:**

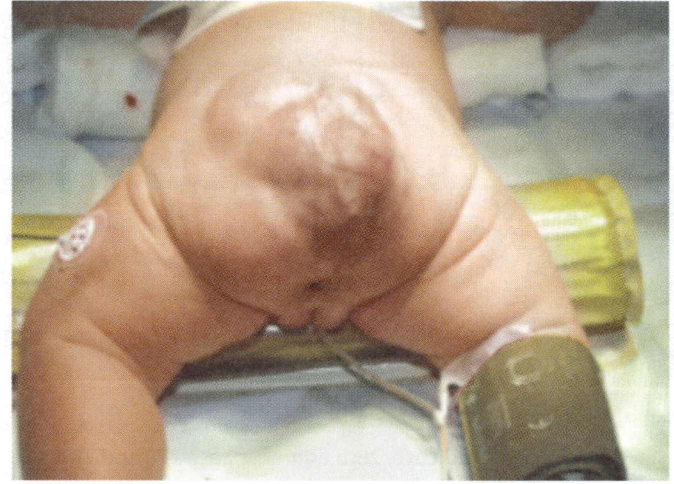

*Source:* Bailey and Love, 28th edition, page 272.

a. Identify the condition.
b. What levels are measured to detect recurrence?

## ANSWERS

**Ans. 1** a. VACTERL syndrome (vertebral, anorectal, cardiac, tracheoesophageal, renal, and limb anomalies)
b. CHARGE syndrome (coloboma, heart defects, choanal atresia, growth retardation, genital anomalies, and ear anomalies).
c. Avoid the Trendelenburg position in the preterm when placing a diathermy pad as elevation risks intraventricular hemorrhages.

**Ans. 2** a. Esophageal atresia/tracheoesophageal fistula, VACTERL, and trisomy 21

b. VACTERL, CHARGE, aneuploidy/other gene defects, duodenal atresia, anorectal malformations, tracheomalacia, and gastroesophageal reflux
c. Vertebral/chest wall deformities, intestinal duplications, cardiac anomalies, and congenital diaphragmatic hernia
d. Aneuploidy, chromosomal anomalies, cardiac defects, and Beckwith–Wiedemann syndrome

**Ans. 3** a. Type C, the upper pouch ends in the neck or upper chest but occasionally it reaches the fistula where muscle fibers are shared.
b. Type E
c. Type A

**Ans. 4** a. Double bubble in duodenal atresia (gastric and first part of the duodenum). Note the umbilical cord and clamp in the lower part of the image.
b. Repair is by open Kimura duodenoduodenostomy with or without a transanastomotic tube.
c. Multiple intestinal atresias are seen with an immune deficiency related to mutations of the *tetratricopeptide* gene (TTC7A).
d. Duodenal atresia and the incisions used to repair it: a diamond anastomosis is shown.

**Ans. 5**
- *Image A:* Small bowel atresia
- *Image B:* The narrow origin of the small bowel mesentery predisposes to midgut volvulus
- *Image C:* An acute small bowel volvulus with vascular compromise: the baby's head is to the right. Note that the terminal ileum, cecum, and appendix in the upper central abdomen are well perfused.
- *Image D:* Ladd's procedure—the duodenum is placed on the right, the colon on the left and the mesentery is broadened. The duodenum appears to lie near the colon since the wound is small. The appendix may be removed.

**Ans. 6** a. The NEC is a patchy hemorrhagic enteritis seen in about 10% of preterm babies on NICUs; all are more than a few days old and have been fed. NEC commonly involves the colon and terminal ileum, less commonly the jejunum and rarely the duodenum.
b. Abdominal radiograph showing pneumatosis. Radiological signs include pneumatosis intestinalis, gas in the portal vein and if perforated, a pneumoperitoneum.
c. Water-soluble contrast (diatrizoate) in meconium ileus showing a microcolon.

**Ans. 7**
a. Type III
b. Cytomegalovirus
c. Radionucleotide hepatobiliary iminodiacetic acid (HIDA) scan
d. The Kasai hepaticoportoenterostomy using a jejunal Roux-en-Y loop anastomosed to the portal plate.

**Ans. 8**
a. Repair of prostatic and bladder neck fistulae may be approached with a combined laparoscopic and perineal approach, whereas prostatic and bulbar urethral fistulae can both be approached in a PSARP. The stoma is closed at a third stage.
b. A rectourethral fistula, visible on a contrast study performed via a sigmoid colostomy. The bladder is filled with contrast via the fistula and the radio-opaque dot has been placed on the infant's perineum over the normal site of the anus (B: bladder; R: rectum).

**Ans. 9**
a. Genetic defects (e.g., RET, EDNRB, and EDN3) can affect the migration of neural crest-derived intestinal neurons (neurocristopathy), leading to aganglionosis and thickened nerve trunks in the distal bowel.
b. Hirschsprung's disease presents with delayed passage of meconium, abdominal distension and bilious vomiting requiring resuscitation, gastric decompression, antibiotics, and a bowel washout.
c. Swenson, Duhamel, Yancey–Soave, and transanal "pull-throughs"
d. Cot-side suction rectal biopsy

**Ans. 10**
a. Gastroschisis
b. Gastroschisis in a preformed silo
c. Risk factors include teenage pregnancy, recreational drugs, smoking, and genitourinary infection in pregnancy

**Ans. 11**
a. Exomphalos major
b. Three-layered membrane
- Peritoneum
- Wharton's jelly
- Amnion in continuity with the umbilical cord

**Ans. 12**
a. FOG2, GATA
b. GOR-TEX patch

**Ans. 13**
a. Sacrococcygeal teratoma
b. $\alpha$-Fetoprotein levels

# 19 CHAPTER

# Trauma in Children

## QUESTIONS

**Q1. Answer the following:**

a. What are the four Hs and four Ts in cardiac arrest to be considered?

b. How to estimate weight of child if weight is unknown?

**Q2. Answer the following:**

a. What is volume of packed cell volume (PCV), platelet, cryoprecipitate to be transfuse in children in terms of mL/kg?

b. In case of major hemorrhage what is dose of tranexamic acid?

## ANSWERS

**Ans. 1** a. In cardiac arrest, the four Hs and four Ts are considered: Hypoxia, hypovolemia, hypothermia/hyperthermia, hyperkalemia/hypokalemia, tension pneumothorax, cardiac tamponade, toxins, and thrombus.

b. If weight in kilograms is unknown, it can be estimated from 2 × (age in years + 4).

**Ans. 2** a.
- Packed cells 20 mL/kg
- Fresh-frozen plasma 20 mL/kg
- Platelets 10 mL/kg
- Cryoprecipitate 5 mL/kg

b. If the major hemorrhage occurred within 3 hours, a slow tranexamic acid bolus of 15 mg/kg followed by an infusion (15 mg/kg over 8 hours) should be given.

3

SECTION

# Preoperative Care

CHAPTER

# 20 Preoperative Care including the High-risk Surgical Patient

## QUESTIONS

**Q1.**

a. What does Mallampati test stands for in preoperative assessment?

b. Grade the Mallampati test.

c. Grade the Mallampati test in the given picture.

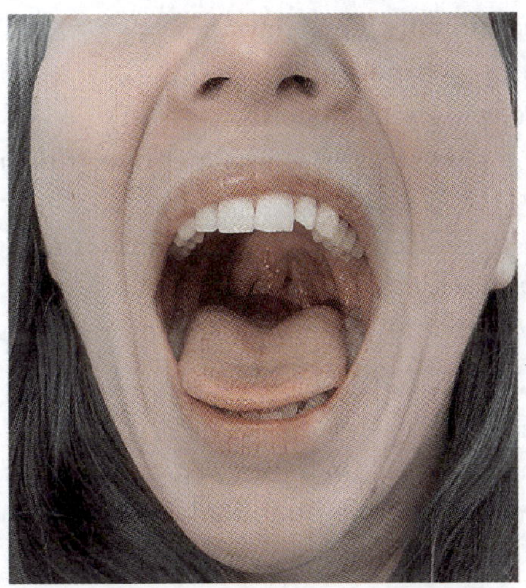

*Source:* Bailey and Love, 28th edition, page 287.

**Q2. List any four risk factors for thrombosis during preoperative assessment.**

**Q3. From a mass casualty by train accident a 56-year-old male rescued by trauma team in moribund condition and labeled with black by triage team. Answer the following.**

a. What will be the ASA grade for this patient?

b. What does ASA grade is stands for in preoperative assessment?

c. What will be the mortality rate for the ASA grade II patients in 30 days of postoperative period?

## ANSWERS

**Ans. 1** a. Airway assessment

b.

| Grade 1 | Fauces, pillars, soft palate, and uvula seen |
|---|---|
| Grade 2 | Fauces, soft palate with some part of uvula seen |
| Grade 3 | Soft palate seen |
| Grade 4 | Hard palate only seen |

c. Mallampati grade 1.

**Ans. 2**
- Age >60 years
- Obesity [body mass index (BMI) >30 kg/m$^2$]
- Trauma or surgery (especially of the abdomen, pelvis, and lower limbs)
- Total anesthesia time >90 minutes
- Reduced mobility for >3 days
- Pregnancy/puerperium
- Varicose veins with phlebitis
- Drugs, e.g., estrogen contraceptive, hormone replacement therapy (HRT), smoking
- Known active cancer or on treatment, significant medical comorbidities, and critical care admission
- Family/personal history of thrombosis, e.g., deficiencies in antithrombin III, protein S or C

**Ans. 3** a. ASA grade V

b. ASA grade—*American society of anesthesiologists system grade*
This grading system is quantitative association with the predicted percentage of postoperative mortality.

c. 0.7%

***Operative mortality by American Society of Anesthesiologists (ASA) grade.***

| ***ASA grade*** | ***Description*** | ***30-day mortality (%)*** |
|---|---|---|
| I | Healthy | 0.1 |
| II | Mild systemic disease, no functional limitation | 0.7 |
| III | Severe systemic disease, definite functional limitation | 3.5 |
| IV | Severe systemic disease, constant threat to life | 18.3 |
| V | Moribund patient unlikely to survive 24 hours with or without operation | 93.3 |
| E | Emergency operation | – |

# CHAPTER 21 Day Care Surgery

## QUESTIONS

1. **What are the criteria for day care surgery?**
2. **What are the social criteria for the day care surgery?**
3. **What are discharge criteria for day care surgery (any five)?**

## ANSWERS

**Ans. 1** Day care surgery criteria include the following:

- Low risk after immediate postoperative complications, e.g., catastrophic bleeding or airway compromise.
- Able to eat and drink or take oral nutrition postoperatively.
- Postoperative pain needs to be managed by oral painkillers.
- The patient should be able to mobilize postoperatively with or without aid.

**Ans. 2** Social criteria for day care surgery:

- Adequate housing conditions such as heating, an inside toilet, and access to a phone.
- The patient should live within a 1-hour drive of a hospital.
- A responsible adult should be able to stay with the patient for 24 hours after a regional anesthetic/general anesthetic.

**Ans. 3** Day care surgery discharge criteria:

- Steady vital signs for a minimum of 60 minutes
- Appropriate orientation in terms of place, time, and person, when applicable
- Sufficient pain management with oral analgesic supply
- Knows how to use the prescribed oral analgesic
- Ability to move and dress appropriately

- Little vomiting, nausea, or lightheadedness
- Has consumed oral fluids
- Minimal wound discharge or bleeding
- Has, if applicable, passed urine
- Has an adult in charge to drive them home
- Instructions provided verbally and in writing regarding postoperative care
- Understands when to return for a visit (if appropriate)
- Provided emergency phone number

# 22 CHAPTER

# Anesthesia and Pain Relief

## QUESTIONS

**Q1. Answer the following:**

a. Name the machine shown in this picture.
b. What is the general anesthesia tried?
c. Name any three anesthesia agents.

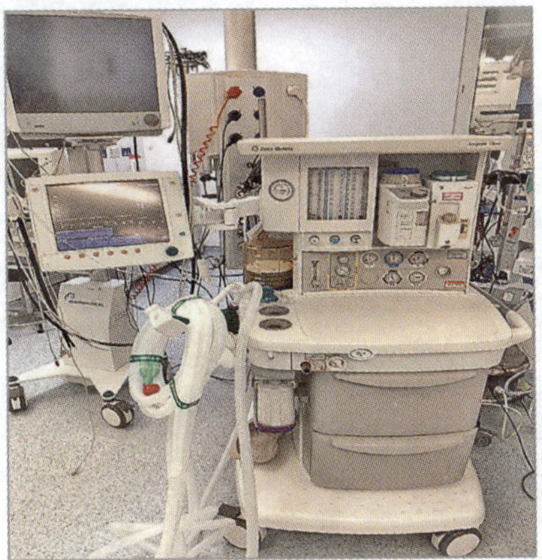

*Source:* Bailey and Love, 28th edition, page 305.

**Q2. Name the devices/instruments depicted in the given pictures.**

a.

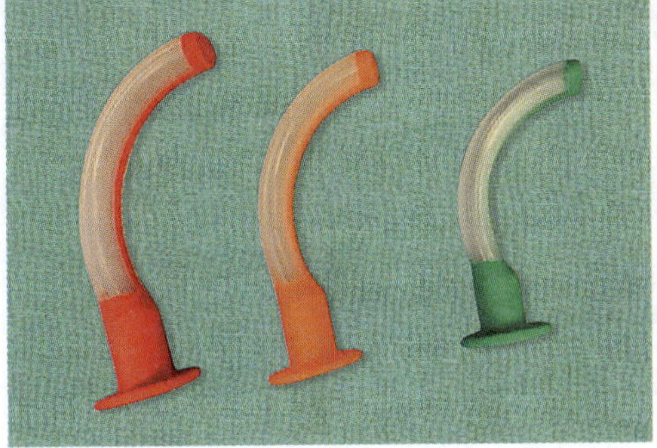

*Source:* Bailey and Love, 28th edition, page 306.

b.

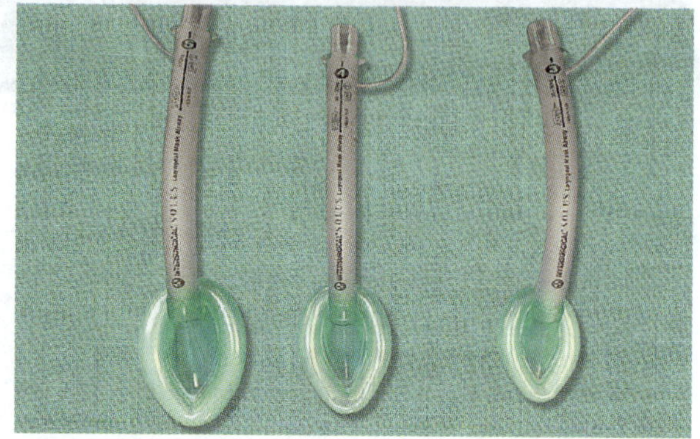

*Source:* Bailey and Love, 28th edition, page 306.

c.

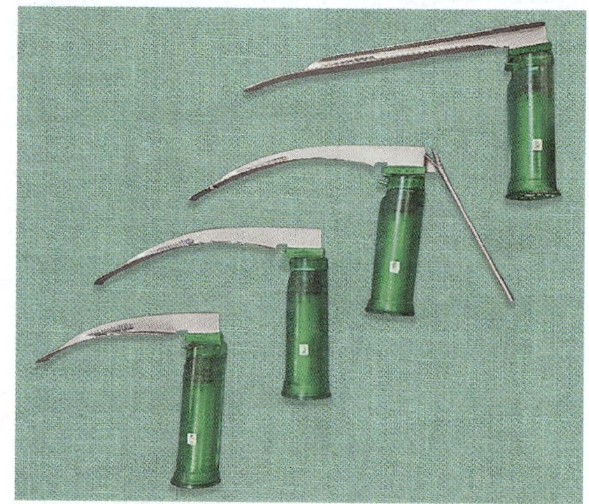

*Source:* Bailey and Love, 28th edition, page 306.

d.

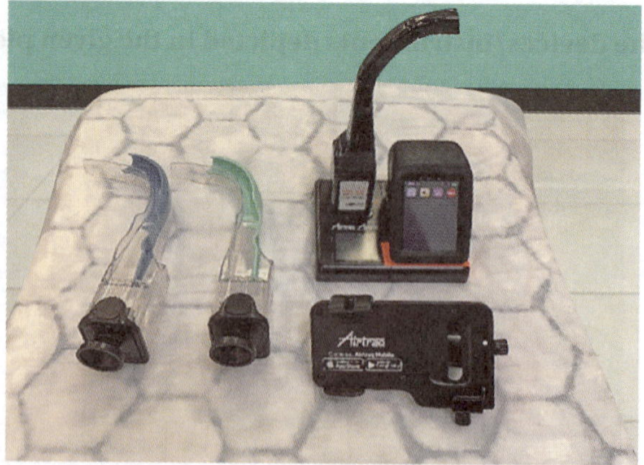


*Source:* Bailey and Love, 28th edition, page 307.

e.

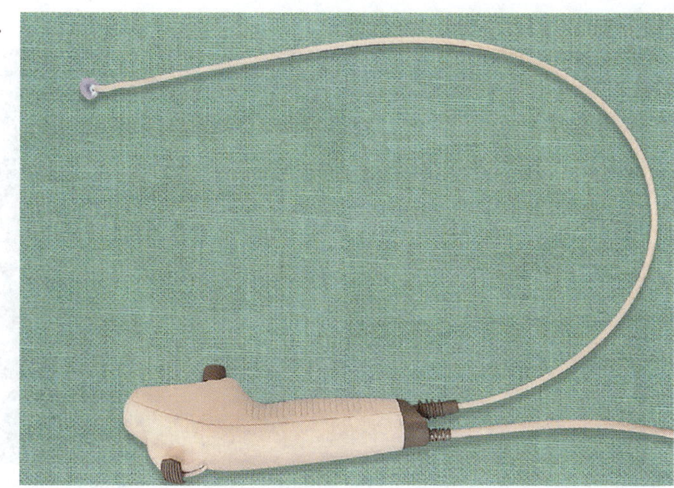

*Source:* Bailey and Love, 28th edition, page 307.

**Q3. Mention the various techniques to maintaining an airway.**

**Q4. What are the complications of intubation (any four)?**

**Q5. Name local anesthetic drugs and their maximum dose (any two).**

**Q6. A 45-year-old male has post-traumatic large infected wound over left forearm and wrist at extensor and lateral aspect. Patient is planned for debridement and dressing.**

a. Name the regional anesthesia given to this patient shown in picture (A and B).

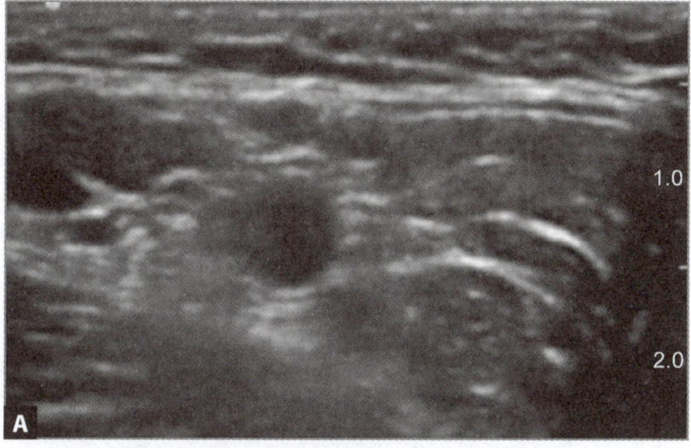


*Source:* Bailey and Love, 28th edition, page 309.

b. What is EMLA?

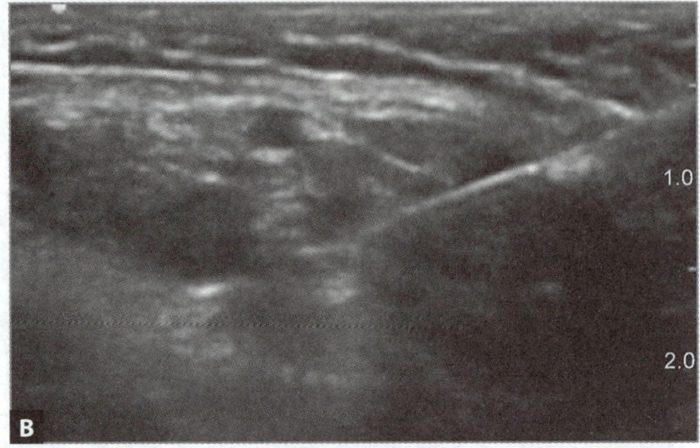


*Source:* Bailey and Love, 28th edition, page 309.

**Q7. Answer the following:**

a. Name the model depicted in this picture.

b. Where we use this model?

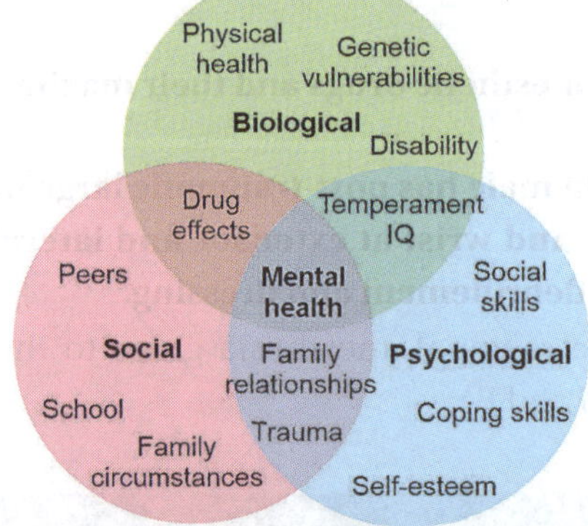


*Source:* Bailey and Love, 28th edition, page 311.

## ANSWERS

**Ans. 1** a. Anesthesia machine/Boyle's machine

b. General anesthetic triad
   1. Amnesia (loss of awareness)
   2. Analgesia (Pain relief )
   3. Muscle relaxation

c. • Propofol (di-isopropyl phenol)
   • Thiopentone (barbiturate)
   • Etomidate (steroid derivative)
   • Ketamine (phencyclidine derivative)

**Ans. 2** a. Oropharyngeal airway (first-generation)
b. i-gel—supraglottic airway
c. Single-use laryngoscope
d. Airtraq—intubating device
e. Fiberoptic intubating bronchoscope (for difficult intubation)

**Ans. 3.** Techniques using for airway maintenance:
- *Lift the chin and jaw thrust:* (For short term when aid not available)
- *Guedel airway:* (Holds tongue forward but it does not prevent the aspiration)
- *Supraglottic device:* (Easy to insert, reliable airway, and allows ventilation)
- *Endotracheal intubation:* (Secure and protect the airway)

**Ans. 4** *Complications of the intubation*
- Intubation is failed
- Accidentally bronchial intubation
- Trauma to teeth/pharynx/larynx
- Aspiration of gastric contents during intubation procedure
- Disconnection, blockage, or kinking of the tube
- Delayed—tracheal stenosis

**Ans. 5** Local anesthesia drugs

| *Name* | *Maximum dose* | *Comments* |
|---|---|---|
| Lidocaine | 3 mg/kg [7 mg/kg with adrenaline (epinephrine)] | • Early onset<br>• Short acting<br>• Good sensory block |
| Bupivacaine | 2 mg/kg | • Long lasting<br>• More cardiotoxic<br>• Never to be used intravenously |
| Prilocaine | 6 mg/kg (9 mg/kg with adrenaline) | • Least systemic toxicity<br>• Methemoglobinemia |
| Ropivacaine | 3–4 mg/kg | • Less cardiotoxic<br>• Greater sensory–motor separation |
| Levobupivacaine | 2 mg/kg | Isomer of bupivacaine, fewer cardiotoxic properties |

**Ans. 6** a. Ultrasonic guided brachial plexus block
b. Eutectic mixture of local anesthesia—2.5% lidocaine + 2.5% prilocaine

**Ans. 7** a. Biopsychosocial model of health
b. Nonpharmacological treatment for chronic pain management

CHAPTER

# 23 Postoperative Care including Perioperative Optimization

## QUESTIONS

**Q1. A 52-year-old, 80 kg, female with the American Society of Anesthesiologists (ASA) grade III underwent laparotomy for subacute intestinal obstruction. She had fever spike on postoperative day (POD) 1 followed by dyspnea. On ward round operating surgeon advised X-ray chest, as given below.**

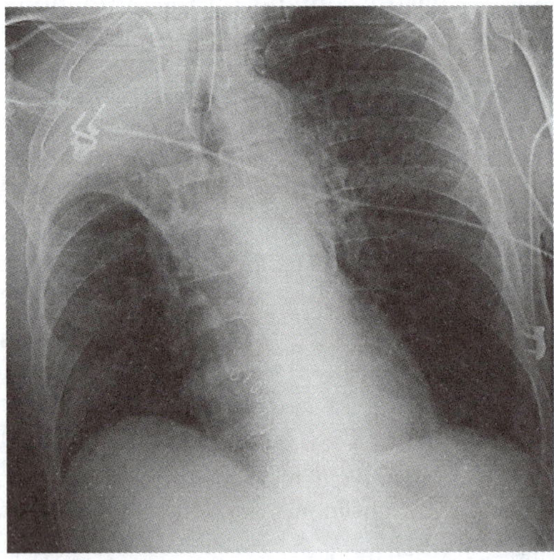

*Source:* Bailey and Love, 28th edition, page 319.

a. What is the provisional diagnosis as per the X-ray film?
b. What are the common respiratory complications in postoperative period?

**Q2. Answer the following:**

a. At postoperative day 1, what is the pathophysiology of pyrexia in elective aseptic cases?
b. Enumerate the causes of pyrexia in postoperative period (any six).

**Q3. A 62-year-old male poly trauma with head injury was is admitted in intensive care unit (ICU) from 16 days developed bed sore over presacral region as depicted in picture. Answer the following questions:**

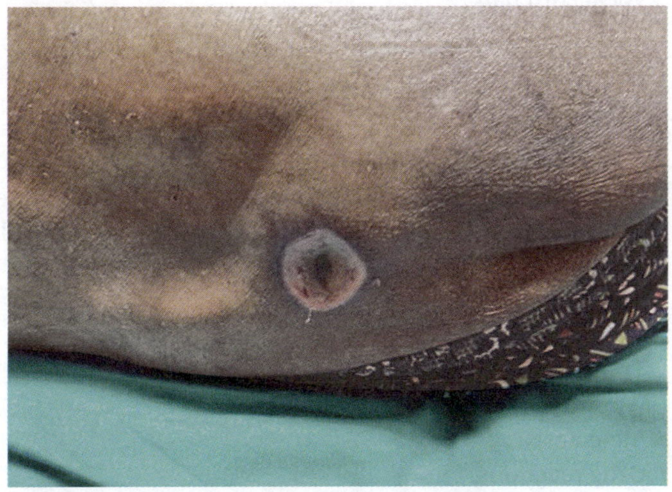

a. What is the grade of this bed sore wound?
b. What are the grades of the bed sore/pressure?
c. What is prevention and line of management of bed sore?

**Q4. Answer the following:**

a. Elaborate the term ERAS.
b. What are the key elements of ERAS?

## ANSWERS

**Ans. 1** a. Radiograph showing right upper lobe atelectasis
b. Immediate—Upper airway obstruction (most common)—due to laryngospasm, persisting relaxation of airway muscles, soft tissue edema, hematoma, vocal cord dysfunction, or a foreign body.

*Hypoventilation*

Hypoxemia—Acute pulmonary edema (fluid overload, cardiac failure, and postobstructive), bronchospasm, and pneumothorax. Aspiration and pulmonary embolism.

*Postoperative complications*

- Atelectasis
- Cough,

- Dyspnea,
- Bronchospasm,
- Hypercapnia, atelectasis, pneumonia, pleural effusion, and respiratory failure.
- Vocal cord palsy

**Ans. 2** a. Inflammatory response to surgical trauma

b. Causes of pyrexia in postoperative period

*Infective origin*

- Superficial and deep wound infection;
- Chest infection, urinary tract infection, and thrombophlebitis;
- Wound infection, anastomotic leakage, intracavitary collections, and abscesses.
- Noninfective origin
- Deep vein thrombosis (DVT);
- Transfusion reactions;
- Wound hematomas;
- Atelectasis;
- Drug reactions.

**Ans. 3** a. Category 3

b. Category 1 ulcers involve nonblanching erythema with intact skin.

- Category 2 ulcers have partial thickness skin loss and appear as a shallow open ulcer with a red-pink wound bed or an intact or ruptured serum-filled blister.
- Category 3 ulcers have full thickness skin loss, with subcutaneous fat visible in the wound, but not bone, tendon, or muscle.
- Category 4 ulcers have full thickness loss with exposed bone, tendon, or muscle.

c. *Management of pressure sores*

- Recognize patients at risk
- Wound care—debridement of dead and necrotic tissue and dressing
- Address nutritional status—High protein diet, optimize and maintain hemoglobin Hb >10 g/dL, albumin
- >3 g/dL
- Use air bed
- Keep patients mobile or regularly turned if bed-bound, frequent change position every 2 hourly
- Avoid shearing of skin while mobilizing
- Avoid direct contact of skin with plastic sheet/Mcintosh

- Treat underlying cause
  After treating underlying cause surgical management of pressure sore.
- Debridement with dressing/vacuum-assisted closure (VAC) dressing
- Wound coverage with split-thickness skin graft (STSG)/flap coverage

**Ans. 4** a. Enhanced recovery after surgery (ERAS) is an approach to the perioperative care of patients undergoing surgery for speedy recovery and reduce both the cost and the length of stay of the patient in the hospital.

b.

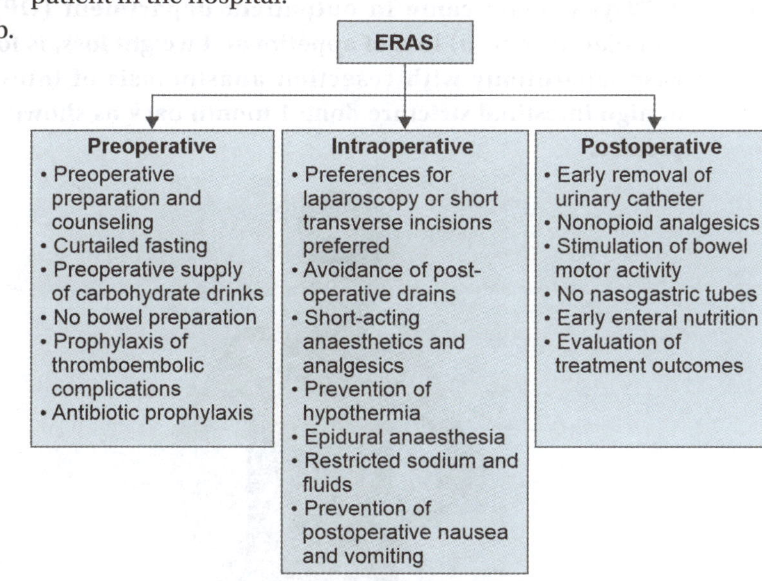

CHAPTER

# 24 Nutrition and Fluid Therapy

## QUESTIONS

**Q1.** **A 72-year-male came in outpatient department (OPD) with complaints of (c/o) loss of appetite and weight loss, is follow-up case laparotomy with resection anastomosis of intestine for benign intestinal stricture done 1 month back as shown in given picture.**

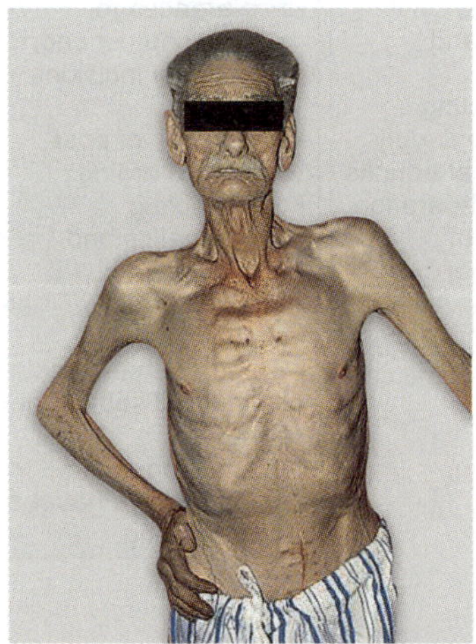

*Source:* Bailey and Love, 28th edition, page 329.

a. What are the various tools/method for nutritional assessment?
b. What is the average daily calorie requirement for a healthy person?
c. How to calculate body mass index (BMI) of person?

**Q2.** **Answer the following:**

a. Mention the normal values of sodium and potassium in plasma.
b. What is the composition of normal saline (0.9%) and Hartman's solution?

**Q3.** **Answer the following:**

a. What does Harris–Benedict equation stands for?
b. What is the daily energy requirement of a person in stress condition?

**Q4. Enumerate various modes of nutrition administration in postsurgical patient depicted in patient—A, B, C, D, E, and F.**

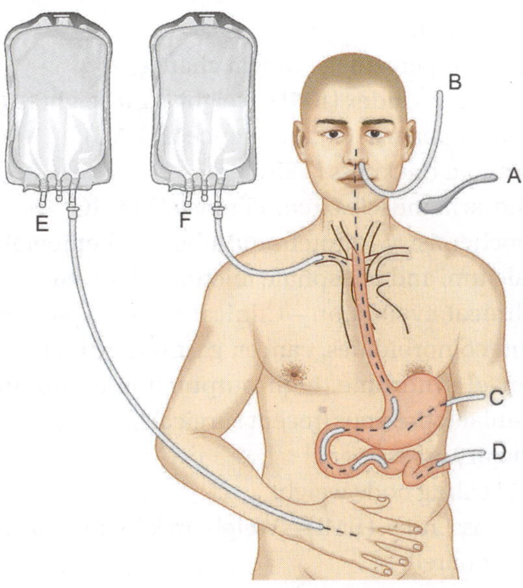


*Source:* Bailey and Love, 28th edition, page 335.

**Q5. Answer the following:**

a. What procedure is shown in the given picture?
b. What are the complications of enteral feeding?

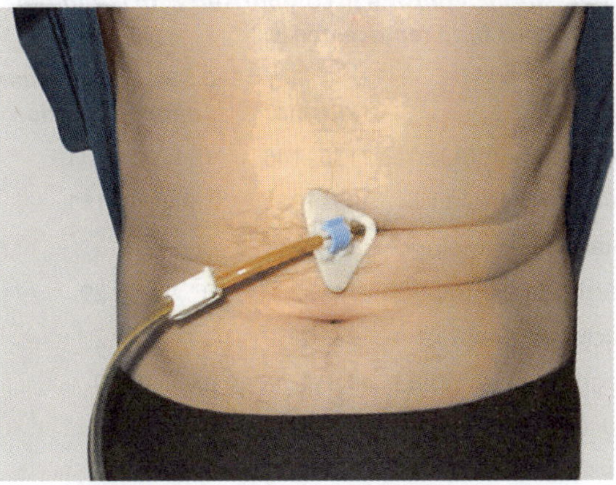

*Source:* Bailey and Love, 28th edition, page 337.

**Q6. Answer the following:**

a. What are the various access for parenteral nutrition?
b. What are the complications of parenteral nutrition?

# ANSWERS

**Ans. 1** a. Anthropometry

Weight and percentage weight change,

- Body mass index (BMI) [weight (kg)/height ($m^2$)]
- Mid-upper arm circumference (MUAC),
- Skinfold thickness (TSF)
- Mid-arm muscle circumference (MAMC)
- Biochemistry—Protein and albumin, hemoglobin, electrolytes, calcium, and phosphate micronutrient, etc.
- Clinical evaluation—Clinical history, past medical history, and comorbidities, cancer, gastrointestinal pathologies (short bowel syndrome, high-output stoma and enterocutaneous fistulae), previous/recent surgical history)
- Dietary assessment

b. 25–35 kcal/kg body weight

c. Body mass index (BMI)—Weight in kilogram divided by height in meter squared.

**Ans. 2** a. Sodium—135–145 mmol/L

Potassium—3.5–5.3 mmol/L

b. Composition of plasma in comparison with commonly used intravenous fluid replacements.

***Composition of plasma in comparison with commonly used intravenous fluid replacements.***

| | ***Plasma*** | ***0.9% Saline*** | ***Hartmann's solution*** | ***5% Dextrose*** |
|---|---|---|---|---|
| Sodium (mmol/L) | 135–145 | 154 | 131 | 0 |
| Chloride (mmol/L) | 95–105 | 154 | 111 | 0 |
| Potassium (mmol/L) | 3.5–5.3 | 0 | 5 | 0 |
| Bicarbonate (mmol/L) | 24–32 | 0 | 29 | 0 |
| Calcium (mmol/L) | 2.2–2.6 | 2 | 2 | 0 |
| Magnesium (mmol/L) | 0.8–1.2 | 0 | 0 | 0 |
| Glucose (mmol/L) | 3.5–5.5 | 0 | 0 | 227.8 (50 g) |
| Lactate | 0.5–1.0 | 0 | 29 | 0 |
| pH | 7.35–7.45 | 4.5–7.0 | 5.0–7.0 | 3.5–5.5 |
| Osmolality (mOsmol/L) | 275–295 | 308 | 273 | 278 |

**Ans. 3.** a. Harris-Benedict equation is for basal metabolic rate (BMR) calculation in normal person

*Men*

BMR = (10 × weight in kg) + (6.25 × height in cm) – (5 × age in years) + 5

*Women*

BMR = (10 × weight in kg) + (6.25 × height in cm) – (5 × age in years) – 161

b. *Daily energy intake*

Normal person—20–30 kcal for every kilogram of ideal body weight per day.

In severe stress condition—30 kcal/kg ideal body weight per day.

**Ans. 4** A. Oral

B. Nasogastric tube/duodenal/jejunal

C. Gastrostomy tube feeding (percutaneous/open surgical)

D. Jejunostomy tube feeding (laparoscopic/open surgery)

E. PPN—Partial parenteral nutrition

F. TPN—Total parenteral nutrition

**Ans. 5** a. Percutaneous endoscopic gastrostomy tube

b. *Complications of enteral feeding*

- *Tube-related*
  - Malposition
  - Displacement
  - Blockage
  - Breakage/leakage
  - Local complications (e.g., erosion of skin/mucosa)
- *Gastrointestinal*
  - Diarrhea
  - Bloating, nausea, and vomiting
  - Abdominal cramps
  - Aspiration
  - Constipation
- *Metabolic/biochemical*
  - Electrolyte disorders, including refeeding syndrome
  - Vitamin, mineral, and trace element deficiencies
  - Drug interactions

**Ans. 6** a. Central line access

- Internal jugular vein (IJV)
- Superior vena cava (SVC)
- Subclavian vein

- Femoral lines (should be avoided due to high chances of infection at this site)
- Peripherally inserted central line (PICC line)
- Basilic vein (most commonly used)
- Cephalic vein
- Brachial vein
- Median cubital vein

b. *Complications of parenteral feeding*
- *Insertion complications*
  - Pneumothorax
  - Misplacement
- *Line complications*
  - Sepsis
  - Thrombosis
- *Metabolic complications*
  - Electrolyte disorders, including refeeding syndrome
  - Blood sugar derangement
  - Liver dysfunction
  - Metabolic bone disease
  - Vitamin deficiencies

4

SECTION

# Trauma

# 25 Trauma

CHAPTER

## QUESTIONS

**Q1. Answer the following:**

a. Define trauma.

b. How much percentage of trauma represents global deaths according to WHO?

**Q2. What are the covert injuries in following trauma:**

a. Electrocution

b. Dashboard impact

c. Flexion distraction (lap belt)

**Q3. Name the five parameters that raise the suspicion of nonaccidental injury (NAI) and alert the clinician.**

**Q4. Answer the following:**

a. What is the subtle full body computed tomography (CT) effective radiation dose for all organs?

b. Enumerate stages of damage control surgery.

**Q5. Answer the following:**

a. What are the criteria for damage control surgery (DCS)?

b. What are the criteria for early total care (ETC)?

**Q6. Answer the following:**

a. What is prompt individualized safe management (PRISM) concept?

b. What is "c" in abcde?

c. What is target systolic blood pressure (SBP) in trauma resuscitation?

**Q7. Answer the following:**

a. What is role of tranexamic acid in trauma?

b. What is dose of tranexamic acid in trauma?

c. What is the role of whole body CT in trauma case?

**Q8. Answer the following:**

a. What is secondary survey?
b. What is tertiary survey?
c. What is triad of death in trauma?

**Q9. Answer the following:**

a. What is the normal value of venous lactate and role in trauma?
b. What is the value of venous lactate used for ETC and DCS?

**Q10. Answer the following:**

a. What is the relation of cerebral perfusion pressure (CPP) map and intracranial pressure (ICP) (NEET SS 2022)?
b. What is Monro-Kellie doctrine (NEET SS 2021)?
c. What is Cushing triad (NEET SS 2022)?
d. What is conning (NEET SS 2022)?

**Q11. What type of herniation is shown in the given image?**

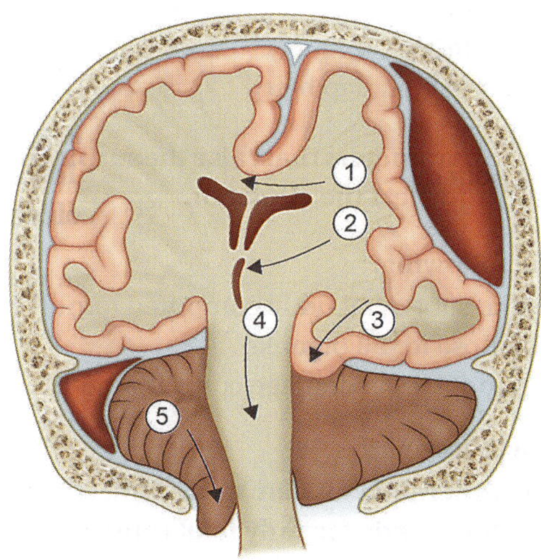


*Source:* Bailey and Love, 28th edition, page 361.

**Q12. What is the GCS in:**

a. Minor HI (head injury)
b. Moderate HI
c. Severe HI

**Q13. Answer the following:**

a. What is the discharge criteria for minor and mild head injuries?
b. According to NICE guidelines, what is the indication for CT in head injury?

**Q14. Answer the following:**

a. Concussion
b. Postconcussion syndrome

**Q15. Answer the following:**

a. Identify the sign and injury with which it is associated.
b. What results in EDH?

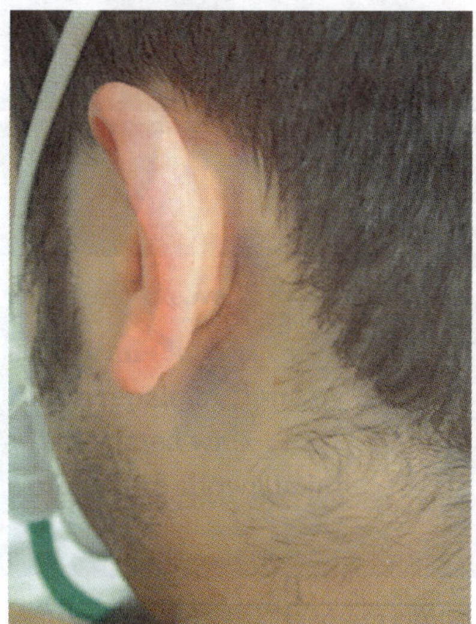

*Source:* Bailey and Love, 28th edition, page 364.

**Q16. Identify the given images:**

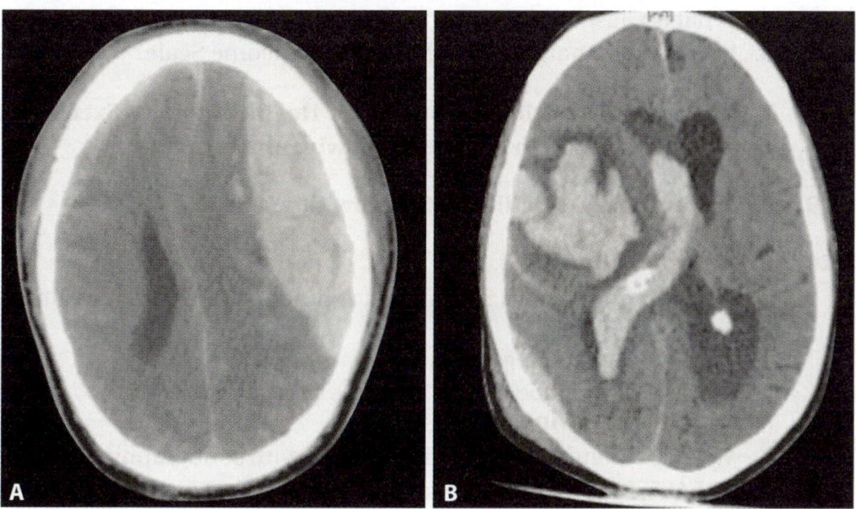


*Source:* Bailey and Love, 28th edition, page 366.

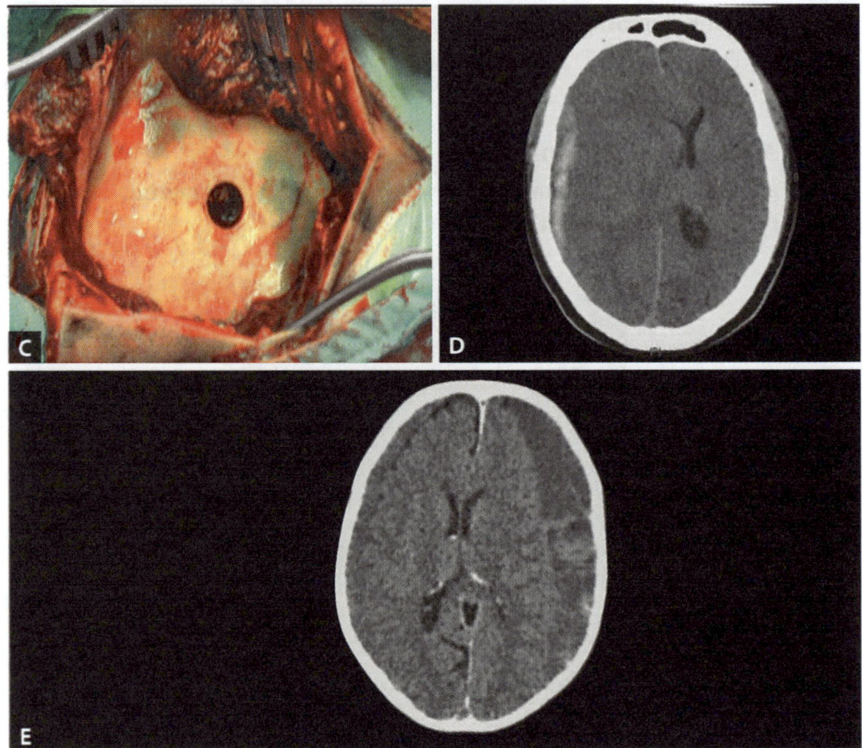


*Source:* Bailey and Love, 28th edition, page 366.

**Q17. Answer the following:**

a. What is DAI?
b. What level of exceeding ICP is suggestive of poor outcome?
c. What is Glasgow Outcome Scale?
d. What are the parameters of Glasgow Outcome Scale?

**Q18. What are the UK National Institute for Health and Care Excellence criteria for CT scan in children following the head injury?**

**Q19. Kindly enumerate pediatric Glasgow Coma Scale.**

**Q20. Answer the following:**

a. What are the clinical indicators for potential ongoing bleeding in torso trauma?
b. What is one on the floor and four more?

**Q21. Answer the following:**

a. What is extended focused assessment with sonography in trauma (e-FAST)?
b. What is utilization of e FAST?
c. What is deadly dozen threats to life from chest injury?

**Q22. Answer the following:**

a. What is open pneumothorax?
b. What are the important points in management of open pneumothorax/hemothorax?
c. What is flail chest?

**Q23. Answer the following:**

a. Identify the condition in chest X-rays (CXR) image "A" and how will you manage.
b. Identify the condition in CXR image "B" and also explain how to confirm the condition and management of the same.

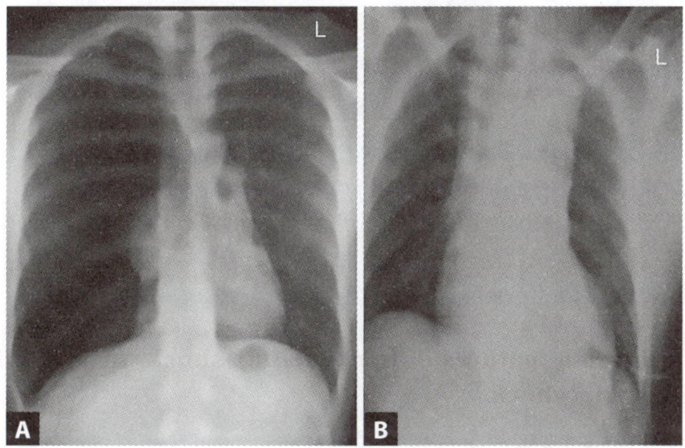


*Source:* Bailey and Love, 28th edition, pages 374 and 376.

**Q24. Answer the following:**

a. When do you consider emergency department thoracotomy (EDT) (NEET SS)?
b. What is the aim of EDT?

**Q25. Answer the following:**

a. What is diagnostic peritoneal lavage (DPL), explain the procedure?
b. What is 4p in operative management of liver injuries?

**Q26. Answer the following:**

a. What are the retroperitoneal zones depicted in diagram for the intraoperative management in blunt trauma?
b. What is tiles classification of fracture of pelvis?

**Q27. Answer the following:**

a. What are the stages of damage control surgery?
b. What are the indications of damage control surgery?

**Q28. Answer the following:**

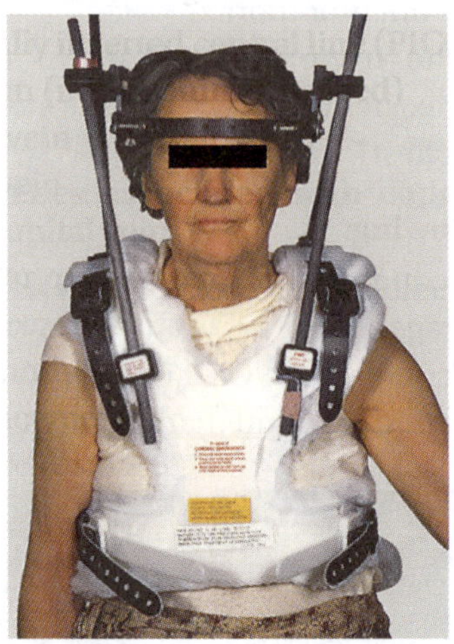

*Source:* Bailey and Love, 28th edition, page 395.

a. What is Asia impairment scale?
b. Name the external immobilizer shown in the image and its use.
c. What is Powers' ratio?
d. What is Jefferson fracture?

**Q29. Enumerate features of hypovolemic shock, neurogenic shock, and spinal shock.**

**Q30. Answer the following:**

a. Enumerate types of incomplete spinal cord injury.
b. What are the functional goal for level of injury?
   1. Level of injury C3–C4
   2. Level of injury C7
c. What is pathophysiology of spinal cord injury?

**Q31. Answer the following:**

a. What is Gustilo and Anderson open fracture classification (INISS)?
b. What is AO classification system (INISS)?
c. Explain growth plate injury classification (NEET SS).

**Q32. Answer the following:**

a. What are the advantages and disadvantages of splinting and casting?
b. What are the advantages and disadvantages of traction?
c. What are the indications of K-wire insertion?

**Q33. What are the indications for surgery in limb trauma?**

**Q34. Answer the following:**

a. What are common features of major disasters?
b. What are the factors influencing rescue and relief efforts in disaster?
c. What are the sequence of relief effort in major disaster?

**Q35. Answer the following:**

a. What is triage?
b. Enumerate triage categories.
c. Mention the principles of DCS in disaster.

**Q36. Answer the following:**

Explain briefly:

a. Tetanus
b. Necrotizing fasciitis
c. Gas gangrene

**Q37. Answer the following:**

a. Crush syndrome
b. Compartment syndrome
c. Trench foot

**Q38. Answer the following:**

a. What are the phases of DCS?
b. What are the Bureau of Indian Standards (BIS) medical support roles?

**Q39. What is a, b, c, d in the graph showing theoretical blast overpressure changes within free field?**

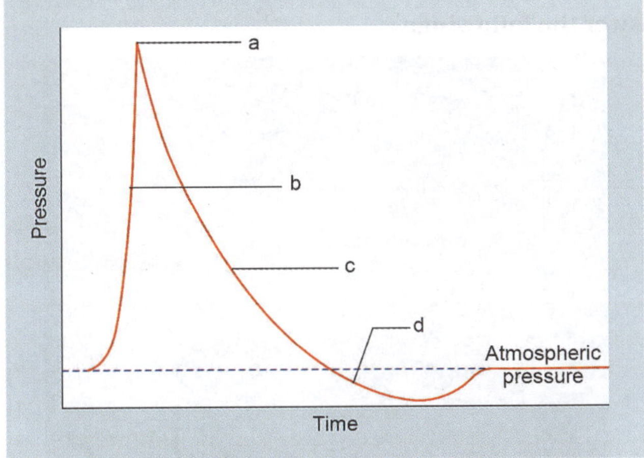


*Source:* Bailey and Love, 28th edition, page 466.

**Q40. Enumerate classification of blast injuries.**

**Q41. Answer the following:**

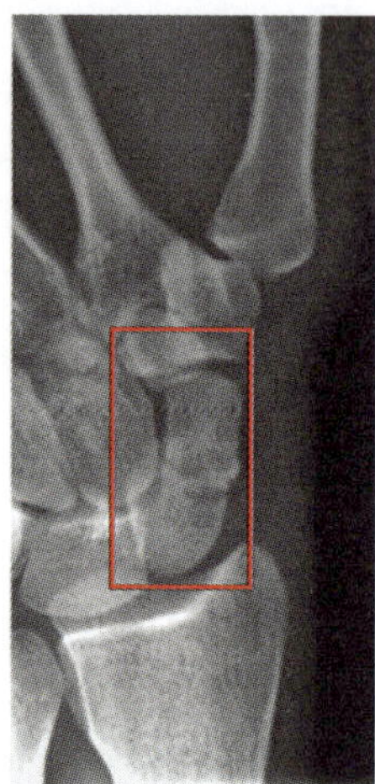

*Source:* Bailey and Love, 28th edition, page 433.

a. Identify the fracture (NEET SS 2022).
b. How will you manage this fracture?
c. What are the complications of above fracture?
d. Which scan register osteoblastic activity and may be used to demonstrate occult fracture like an undisplaced scaphoid fracture?

**Q42. Answer the following:**

a. What is the use of Seddon classification?
b. Explain the Seddon classification.

**Q43. Answer the following:**

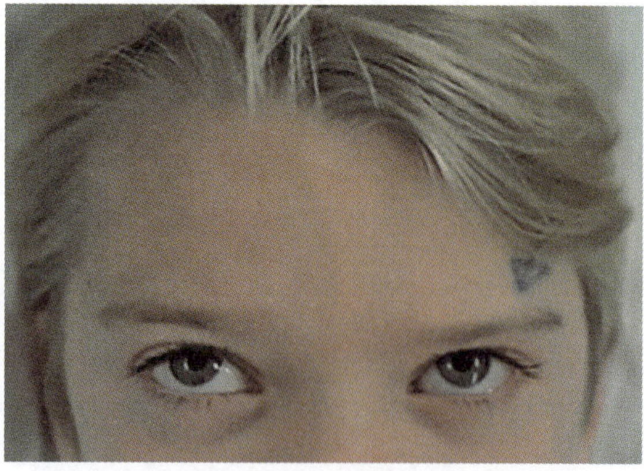

*Source:* Bailey and Love, 28th edition, page 113.

a. Explain the condition given in the image and associated issues.
b. What is the indication of surgical repair for the same?

**Q44. Answer the following:**

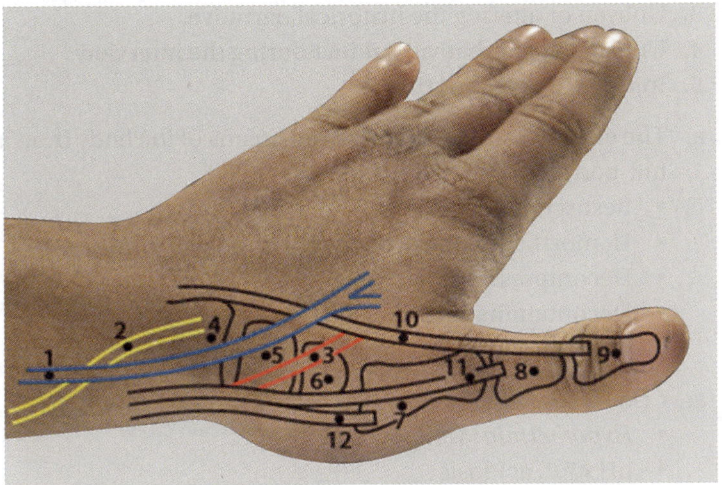


*Source:* Bailey and Love, 28th edition, page 420.

In the given surface anatomy of the anatomical snuffbox:
Kindly identify 1, 2, 3, 4, 5, 6, 7, 8, 9, 10, 11, and 12.

**Q45. Answer the following:**

a. What is LE fort fracture?
b. Enumerate type of LE fort fracture.

## ANSWERS

**Ans. 1** a. Trauma can be defined as an injury to any part of the human body as the result of energy transfer from an inflicting source. Injury including chemical, thermal, ionizing radiation, and mechanical.
b. According to the World Health Organization, there are an estimated 5 million injury fatalities worldwide, representing about 9% of global deaths.

**Ans. 2** a. Shoulder posterior dislocation
b. Posterior dislocation of hip
c. • Duodenal rupture
• Popliteal artery disruption
• Cervical spine fracture

**Ans. 3** Parameters that should alert clinician and raise suspicion of NAI:

1. External indications of damage that do not match the mechanism mentioned.
2. Long bones fracture in a child who is not yet ambulating.
3. Uneven or altering the historical narrative.
4. Unusual or combative conduct during the interview.
5. Injuries to posterior ribs.

**Ans. 4** a. The effective radiation dose to all organs of the body from a single full-body CT is 12–16 millisieverts (mSv).

b. 
- Resuscitation
- Hemorrhage control
- Decompression
- Decontamination
- Fracture splintage

**Ans. 5** a. *Criteria for DCS*

- *Hypothermia:* Temperature <34°C
- pH <7.2, acidosis
- *Serum lactate:* >5 mmol/L
- Coagulopathy
- *Blood pressure (BP):* <70 mm Hg
- Transfusion reaching 15 units
- *Injury severity score:* >36

b. *Criteria for ETC*

- Stable hemodynamics
- No need for vasoactive/inotropic stimulation
- No hypercapnia, no hypoxemia
- *Serum lactate:* <2 mmol/L
- Normal coagulation
- Normothermia
- Urinary output >1 mL/kg/h

**Ans. 6** a. The PRISM concept accepts that the decision-making process should be based on the principles of doing no "further harm to the patient", intervening promptly and utilizing the idea of individualized/personalized medicine. It is based on the understanding that every patient responds differently to the same degree of trauma, every individual has a different genetic profile and the fact that each trauma center may have different resources and staff available to deal successfully with every trauma eventuality.

b. c: Exsanguinating external hemorrhage

c. Maintaining blood flow to the brain, heart, and kidneys is the main objective of resuscitation. A target SBP of 70–90 mm Hg can be reached for a brief period of time; but, if a head injury is suspected, a higher pressure of >90 mm Hg should be the goal (NEET SS 2023).

**Ans. 7** a. Tranexamic acid—an antifibrinolytic medication lowers the chance of bleeding-related death in both blunt trauma and penetrating trauma cases.

b. 1 g intravenous (IV) over 10 minutes, followed by 1 g over 8 hours. All trauma patients with suspected significant hemorrhage, including those with an SBP of <110 mm Hg or a pulse rate >110 beats per minute, should receive tranexamic acid. The initial dose should not be given >3 hours after the accident; it should be given as soon as possible, ideally within the first hour.

c. CT from head to pelvis with IV contrast, called as whole-body CT (WBCT), is gold standard investigation in patients with signs of multiple injury or deranged physiology, but note that WBCT should not be performed on the basis of the mechanism of injury alone. Selective body system scanning has no place in the care of trauma patients with serious injuries. WBCT ought to be carried out as soon as feasible during the patient's resuscitation, whenever that is feasible.

**Ans. 8** a. In trauma, when life-threatening injuries have been identified and treated during the initial assessment, all seriously injured patients should have a comprehensive examination from head-to-toe. At this point, patients can be intubated and unresponsive, which would decrease the accuracy of the clinical evaluation.

b. "Tertiary survey"—when patient is extubated and alert to identify any "minor" injuries which are missed, such as rotator cuff tear in the shoulder or a scaphoid fracture in the wrist. These injuries can cause significant long-term disability.

c. "Triad of death"—a vicious cycle that includes acidosis, coagulopathy, and hypothermia which can lead to multiorgan failure and death.

**Ans. 9** a. <2 mmol/L

b.
- <2 mmol/L—ETC
- 2–3 mmol/L—search for a trend (rising or falling).
- >3 mmol/L—may not be receiving enough resuscitation; if necessary, either additional resuscitation or damage control operations should be performed.
- >5 mmol/L—DCS

**Ans. 10** a. CPP (75–105 mm Hg) = MAP (90–110 mm Hg) – ICP (5–15 mm Hg)

b. According to Alexander Monro (1783), the brain is housed in a "nearly incompressible" "rigid box" called the skull. Any increase in the contents—such as a hemorrhage or enlargement of the brain—may be first managed by removing fluids such as cerebrospinal fluid (CSF) and venous blood. Increased expansion is linked to an exponential increase in ICP.

c. *Cushing's triad:* Moderate head injury hypertension, bradycardia, and irregular respiration.

d. Medullary vasomotor and respiratory centers are compressed when cerebral tonsillar herniation occurs through the foramen magnum. In severe head injury (GCS 3–8) brainstem death may result without immediate intervention.

**Ans. 11**
1. Subfalcine herniation—cingulate gyrus is herniated under the falx cerebri.
2. Evident midline shift
3. Uncal herniation—the third nerve may be compressed by the temporal lobe's herniation across the tentorium cerebelli.
4. Central herniation
5. The brainstem is compromised by tonsillar herniation, which causes Cushing's triad.

**Ans. 12** a. GCS 15 with no loss of consciousness

b. GCS 9–13

c. GCS 3–8

**Ans. 13** a. Criteria for discharge for minor and moderate head injuries:

- Without any focal impairments, GCS 15/15
- If indicated as described below, a normal CT brain image
- Patient is not impaired by drugs or alcohol
- Patient with any adult who may be trusted
- *Advice about head injuries, both written and verbal*—Get medical help if:
  - Indications for CT brain
    - Persistent/worsening headache despite analgesia
    - Persistent vomiting
    - Visual disturbance
    - Drowsiness
    - Limb weakness/numbness

b. UK NICE guidelines for CT in head injury.

*Indications for CT imaging in head injury within 1 hour*

- GCS <13 (at any point )
- GCS <15 at 2 hours—Focal neurological deficit (FND)
- Suspected open, depressed, or basal skull fracture
- Post-traumatic seizure event
- >1 episode of vomiting

*Indications for CT imaging within 8 hours*

- Age >65
- History of H/o coagulopathy (e.g., use of aspirin, warfarin, or rivaroxaban)
- Dangerous mechanism of injury (RTA, fall from a height)
- Retrograde amnesia for >30 minutes

**Ans. 14** a. Concussion—alteration of consciousness as a result of closed mild HI but is generally without imaging abnormalities: loss of consciousness at the time of injury is not necessary. Main features include confusion and amnesia. Patient may be lethargic, forgetful, easily distractible, slow to interact, or may be emotionally labile. May be seen gait disturbance and incoordination.

b. Postconcussive syndrome—a loosely defined constellation of symptoms persisting for a prolonged period after injury. Patients describe physical symptoms such as headaches, lightheadedness, and visual and auditory impairments. Patient may also suffer a variety of neurocognitive and neuropsychological disturbances, including difficulty in concentration and recall, insomnia, depression, emotional lability, fatigue, and personality change.

**Ans. 15** a. *Battle's sign:* Skull base fracture may be associated with bruising over the mastoid region.

b. *Extradural hematoma:* It is a neurosurgical emergency which results from rupture of an artery, vein or venous sinus, in association with a fracture of skull. The classical injury is fracture to the thin squamous temporal bone and associated with the middle meningeal artery injury.

**Ans. 16**

- *Image A:* A large left-sided extradural hematoma (biconvex shape) exerts a mass effect; with smaller right-sided acute subdural hematoma is also evident.
- *Image B:* Frontal intracerebral hematoma on the right side extending into the lateral ventricle. With a small right posterior extradural hematoma and traumatic subarachnoid bleeding in the sulci of the hemisphere over the right side.

- *Image C:* Through a burr hole, a surgically exposed temporal bone reveals a linear skull fracture with the underlying extradural hemorrhage.
- *Image D:* Right-sided hyperdense lesion symptoms of (S/o) acute subdural hematoma (SDH) with midline shift reflects brain swelling as well as bleeding (high-energy injury).
- *Image E:* Bilateral subdural hematomas—on the left is mixed density (hypodense material—old blood, higher density—recent bleeding) probably loculated so requiring a craniotomy to evacuate. On the right is isodense which indicates intermediate age.

**Ans. 17** a. Form of primary brain injury due to the high-energy accidents that usually causes patient comatose and associated with poor outcomes. The pathological diagnosis made at postmortem, but on CT may be suggestive hemorrhagic foci in corpus callosum and dorsolateral rostral brainstem. MRI is more sensitive and helps to evaluate for diffuse axonal injury in patients who fail to improve neurologically.

b. A sustained elevated ICP >20–25 mm Hg is associated with a poor outcome, and to prevent secondary injury maintain the CPP of at least 60 mm Hg.

c. Glasgow Outcome Scale score is used to measure the degree of recovery gained after head injury. A good recovery is able to function independently and return to work rather than complete restoration to one's previous competence.

d. Glasgow Outcome Scale
   - Good recovery—5
   - Moderate disability—4
   - Severe disability—3
   - Persistent vegetative state—2
   - Dead—1

**Ans. 18** UK National Institute for Health and Care Excellence criteria for CT scan in children following head injury.

- Suspicion of nonaccidental injury (NAI)
- First seizure
- GCS <14 or <15 in under-ones
- GCS <15 at 2 hours postinjury
- Signs of fracture of the base of skull
- Focal neurological deficit
- Bruise/swelling/laceration >5 cm in under-ones

- *More than one of the following:*
  - Loss of consciousness >5 minutes
  - Abnormal drowsiness
  - Four or more episodes of vomiting
  - Dangerous mechanism
  - Amnesia >5 minutes

**Ans. 19** Pediatric Glasgow Coma Scale score.

- *Eye opening*
  - Spontaneously—4
  - To verbal stimulus—3
  - To pain—2
  - No response—1
- *Verbal response*
  - Coos/babbles—5
  - Irritable cries—4
  - Cries in response to pain—3
  - Moans in response to pain—2
  - No response—1
- *Motor response*
  - Purposeful/spontaneous movements—6
  - Withdraws to touch—5
  - Withdraws to pain—4
  - Flexes to pain—3
  - Extends to pain—2
  - No response—1

**Ans. 20** a. Clinical indicators for potential ongoing bleeding in torso trauma.

| *Physiological indicators* | *Anatomical indicators* |
|---|---|
| • ↑ Respiratory rate,<br>• Pulse rate ↑<br>• ↓ BP<br>• Rising trend of serum lactate | • Visible bleeding<br>• Injury in close proximity to major vessels<br>• Penetrating injury with a retained missile |

b. The bleeding occurs from five major sites—"one on the floor and four more"
  - External—"floor"
  - Chest
  - Abdomen (including retroperitoneum)
  - Pelvis
  - Extremities

**Ans. 21** a. Extended focused assessment with sonography for trauma (eFAST)—most common investigation.

b. This technique uses sonographic assessment. A cardiac tamponade or free blood and air in the hemithoraces should be checked in the chest. Blood in the abdominal cavity, paracolic gutters, subdiaphragmatic spaces, and pelvis should also be assessed.

c. The "deadly dozen" threats to life from chest injury.

*Immediately life threatening:*
- Airway obstruction
- Pericardial tamponade
- Tension pneumothorax
- Flail chest
- Massive hemothorax
- Open pneumothorax

*Potentially life threatening:*
- Aortic injuries
- Rupture of the diaphragm
- Myocardial contusion
- Tracheobronchial injuries
- Esophageal injuries
- Pulmonary contusion

**Ans. 22** a. Open pneumothorax—Large open defect in the chest (>3 cm), causes immediate equilibration between intrathoracic and atmospheric pressure. If the chest wall opening exceeds about two-thirds diameter of trachea, then air will therefore be pulled preferentially through the defect rather than the trachea with each inspiratory cycle. With each inspiration air accumulates in the hemithorax (rather than in lung), leading to hypoventilation on the affected side and causes hypoxia.

b. *Management of an open pneumothorax/hemothorax:*
- If lung does not reinflate, suction drain should be placed on low-pressure (5 $cmH_2O$)
- Clot occlusion of the chest drainage tube may result in "no" drainage, even in the presence of ongoing bleeding
- Second drain is sometimes necessary (but check tracheobronchial injuries)
- A chest radiograph or e-FAST—help to identify the presence of blood

- Active mobilization and physiotherapy should begin as early as possible.

c. Flail chest is a condition associated with blunt trauma with multiple rib fractures defined as 3 or >3 rib fractures in 2 or more places.
Clinically diagnosed with paradoxical motion of the chest wall (on inspiration—loose segment of the chest wall displaced inwards and on expiration—loose segment moves outwards)
High risk of development of hemothorax or pneumothorax
*Diagnosis:* CT scan is gold standard
*Management*
- $O_2$ administration
- Analgesia
- Physiotherapy
- Chest tube in selective patients (hemothorax, pneumothorax, etc.)
- Surgery in selective patients to stabilize the flail segment using internal fixation

**Ans. 23** a. (A) Radiological appearance of a tension pneumothorax.
*Tension pneumothorax*
*Management*
- Clinical diagnosis as soon as possible (Do not delayed by waiting for radiological confirmation)
- Decompression in the safe triangle—defined by posteriorly latissimus dorsi muscle, anteriorly lateral border of pectoralis major, and inferiorly line perpendicular to the nipple going to the back, just anterior to mid-axillary line—or, in extremis, a finger thoracostomy at the same location.

b. (B) Chest radiograph showing a widened mediastinum.
Erect CXR can suggest thoracic aortic disruption. M/C radiological finding is widened mediastinum.
Diagnosis is confirmed by a CT scan of mediastinum.
In the hypotensive patient, widening of the mediastinum and aortic injury is not the cause of the hypotension. Invariably, these patients have other injuries causing hypotension as patients with complete aortic disruption rarely, if ever, survive to reach hospital.

In the presence of thoracic aortic injury, initial management consists of control of the systolic arterial blood pressure (to <120 mm Hg). Thereafter, an endovascular intra-aortic stent can be placed, or the tear can be operatively repaired by direct repair or by excision and grafting using a Dacron graft.

**Ans. 24** a. Emergency department thoracotomy (EDT)—for those patients with penetrating injury with signs of life are still present. In the prehospital phase patients who have received cardiopulmonary resuscitation (CPR) of their care are unlikely to survive, and electrical activity should present.

The EDT is considered futile in some situations:

- Presence of penetrating thoracic trauma CPR for >15 minutes (despite endotracheal intubation)
- In the presence of blunt thoracic trauma CPR for >10 minutes (despite endotracheal intubation)
- In blunt trauma when no signs of life at the scene.

b. Aim of EDT is to perform the following:

- Internal cardiac massage in the cardiovascularly "full" patient.
- Bleeding control from injury to the lung or heart.
- Intrathoracic bleeding control from other sources.
- Massive air leak control
- Thoracic aorta clamping to preserve the blood supply to the heart and brain, and cutting of the arterial blood supply distally in major distal penetrating injury of moribund patients.

**Ans. 25** a. This test is used to assess the presence of blood or any contaminants in the abdominal cavity.

- After insertion of the nasogastric (NG) tube and urinary catheter, a cannula is inserted below the umbilicus, directed posteriorly and caudally. Blood is aspirated through the cannula (>10 mL is positive), and following this, from the 1 L bag approximate 500 mL of warmed Ringer's lactate solution is allowed to run into the abdomen with remaining 500 mL is placed on the floor and the intra-abdominal fluid is allowed to drain under the influence of gravity.

In the nasogastric tube or urinary catheter presence of frank blood or similar contents denotes a positive DPL. In laboratory diagnosis, the presence of >100,000 red cells/μL or >500 white cells/μL is positive (this is equivalent to 20 mL of free blood in the abdominal cavity), as is raised amylase level. If laboratory facilities are not available, the urine dipstick may be useful. A diaphragm injury is indicated by the lavage fluid draining through a chest drain. e-FAST has now largely taken the place of DPL.

b. *Four Ps in the operative management of liver injuries:*

- *P*ressure
- *P*ringle
- *P*lug
- *P*ack

**Ans. 26**

a.

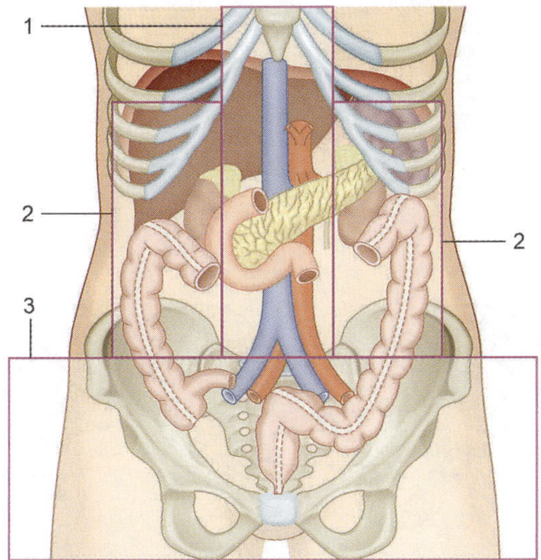


The retroperitoneum zones include:

- Zone 1—central
- Zone 2—lateral
- Zone 3—pelvic

b. *Tile classification*—the pelvic ring fractures can be classified into three types, use based on the severity of the fracture (and reflecting the energy required to cause it).

*Type A*

Type A are the most common fractures and are completely stable. They result from lateral compression, which causes compression fractures of the pubic rami or compression fracture of the sacrum posteriorly.

*Type B*

These fractures are partially stable, and there is disruption of the anterior pelvis and partial disruption of the posterior pelvis. The pelvis can open and close "like a book", but because the sacroiliac ligaments remain intact there is no vertical displacement. Internal or external stabilization is required. Blood loss can be significant.

*Type C*

This fracture is completely unstable. Both the anterior pelvis and the entire posterior pelvic complexes are disrupted and the disrupted pelvic bones are free to displace horizontally and vertically. In both type B and type C pelvic injuries, there is a high risk of associated abdominal injuries (bowel perforation or mesenteric laceration) and rupture of the diaphragm.

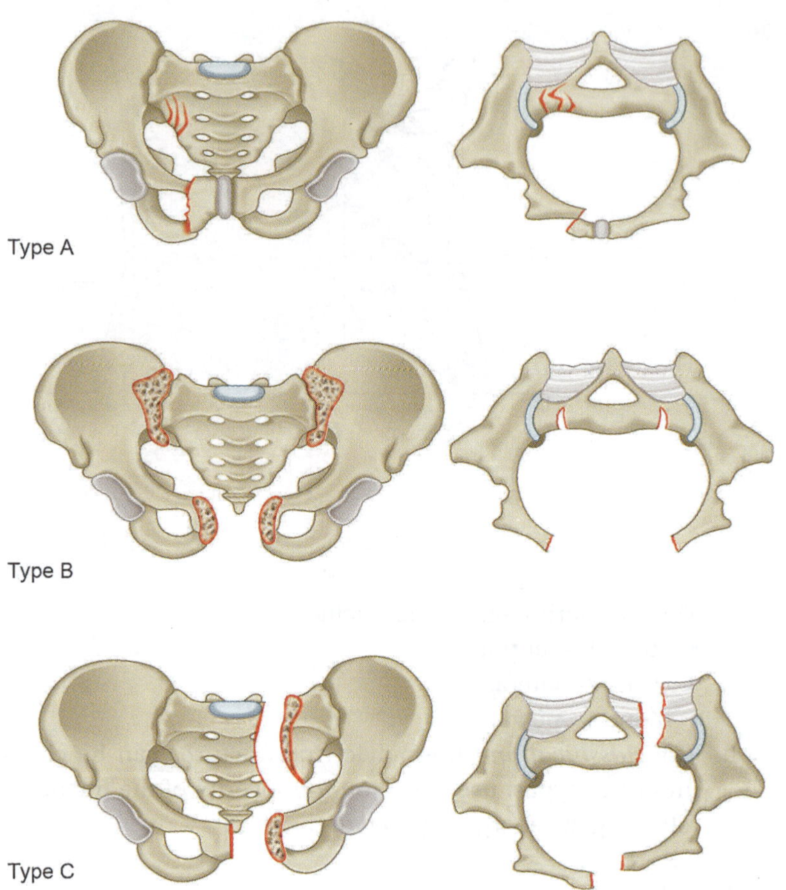


**Ans. 27**

a. Damage control surgery stages.

| *Stage* | *Intervention* |
|---|---|
| I | Patient selection |
| II | Control of hemorrhage and control of contamination |
| III | Resuscitation continued in intensive care unit (ICU) |
| IV | Definitive surgery |
| V | Abdominal closure |

b. *Indications for the damage control surgery (DCS):*

| Anatomical | Physiological (decline of physiological reserve) |
|---|---|
| • Inability to achieve hemostasis<br>• Complex abdominal injuries, e.g., liver, pancreas, etc.<br>• Combined vascular, solid, and hollow organ injuries, e.g., aortic injury or caval injury<br>• Inaccessible major venous injury, e.g., retrohepatic vena cava<br>• Demand for nonoperative control of other injuries, e.g., fractured pelvis<br>• Anticipated need for a time-consuming procedure | • Temperature <34°C<br>• pH <7.2<br>• Serum lactate >5 mmol/L (normal: <2.5 mmol/L)<br>• Prothrombin time >16 seconds<br>• Partial thromboplastin time >60 seconds<br>• >10 units blood transfused<br>• Systolic blood pressure (SBP) <90 mm Hg for >60 minutes |

**Ans. 28** a. Extent of spinal cord injury is defined by the American Spinal Injury Association (ASIA) Impairment scale (modified from the Frankel classification):
- Complete spinal cord injury
- Sensations present, motor absent
- Sensations present, motor present but not useful (MRC grade <3/5)
- Sensations present, motor useful (MRC grade ≥3/5)
- Normal functions

b. External immobilization using a halo jacket. Halo Brace can be used to perform a closed realignment and immobilization of the cervical fractures.

c. Powers' ratio is used to assess skull translation.

d. Jefferson fracture—(Atlas fracture)
Fracture of atlas (C1) vertebrae ring may association with transverse ligament rupture

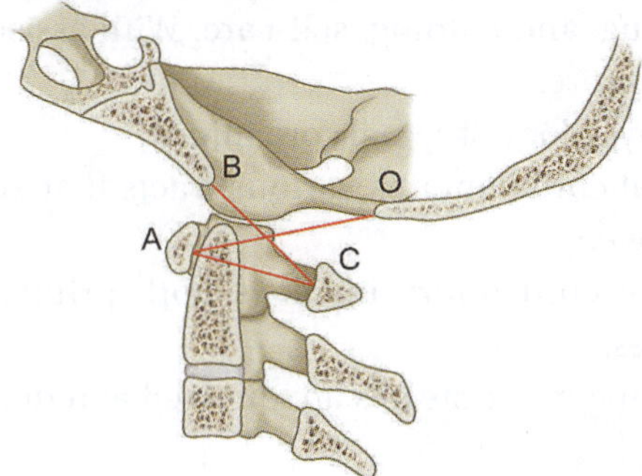


Powers' ratio. BC/OA ≥1 indicates anterior translation; ≤0.75 indicates posterior translation.

**Ans. 29**

| Hypovolemic shock | Neurogenic shock | Spinal shock |
|---|---|---|
| • Hypotension, tachycardia with cold clammy peripheries and most often due to hemorrhage<br>• Adequate resuscitation care should be administered | • This shows up as warm peripheries, bradycardia or a normal heart rate, and hypotension<br>• This is because cervical spinal cord injuries at or above the sympathetic outflow (T5) threshold cause unopposed vagal tone<br>• Inotropic support should be used in its treatment, and fluid overload should be avoided | • Spinal shock is a temporary physiological disorganized functioning of the spinal cord that starts within minutes following the injury. The length of effect is variable, but it can last 6 weeks or longer<br>• Characterized by hyporeflexia, reduced tone, and paralysis. The bulbocavernosus reflex returns after it has been resolved |

**Ans. 30** a. *Types of incomplete spinal cord injuries:*

- Central cord syndrome
- Brown–Séquard syndrome (hemisection)
- Anterior spinal syndrome
- Posterior cord syndrome
- Cauda equina syndrome

b. 1. Power wheelchair with mouth or chin control. Verbalize care, communicate through adaptive equipment. May be ventilator dependent.

2. Manual wheelchair, independent transfer, dressing (with aids), feeding, and bathing, self-care. With assistance bladder and bowel care.

c. Pathophysiology of spinal cord injury

- Spinal cord contains various tracts that are topographically arranged.
- Spinal cord injury involves both primary and secondary phases.
- Therapeutic strategies are directed at reducing the secondary injury.

**Ans. 31** a. Gustilo and Anderson open fracture classification.

| Type | |
|---|---|
| I | A low-energy open fracture with a wound <1 cm long and clean |
| II | An open fracture with a laceration >1 cm long without extensive soft-tissue damage, faps, or avulsion |
| III | High-energy injury irrespective of the size of the wound. Extensive damage to soft tissues, including muscles, skin, and neurovascular structures, and a high degree of contamination. Multifragmentary and unstable fractures |
| *Subgroups of type III* | a. Adequate soft-tissue cover of a fractured bone after stabilization<br>b. Inadequate soft-tissue cover of a fractured bone after stabilization (i.e., fap coverage required)<br>c. Open fracture associated with an arterial injury requiring repair |

b. The AO (Arbeitsgemeinschaft für Osteosynthesefragen) system provides a comprehensive classification of all fractures. The first number defines the bone injured and the second number the segment of bone injured: Proximal metaphysis, diaphysis, and distal metaphysis. The letter and number that follows further defines the nature of the injury.

*The AO classification system: The first two numbers specify the fracture site.*

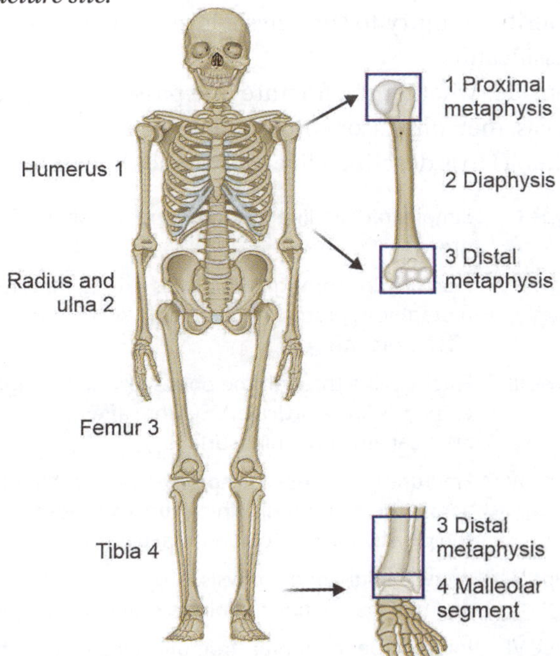


*The AO classification system: The letter defines the nature of the fracture.*

**Diaphyseal types** | **Metaphyseal types**

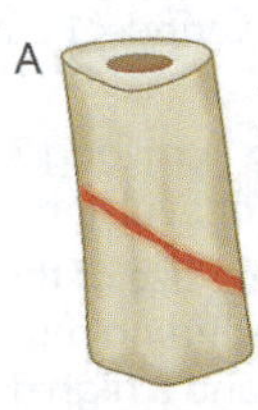


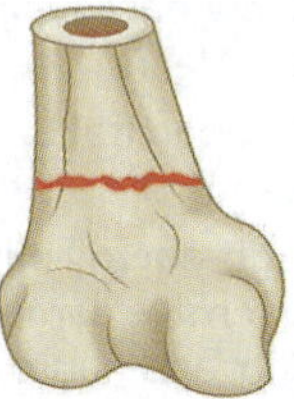


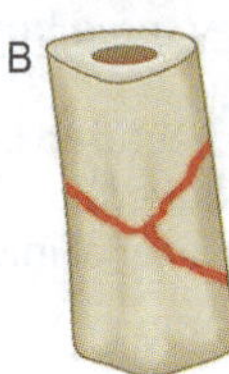


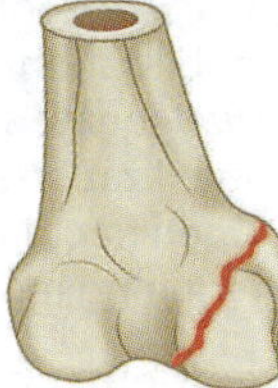


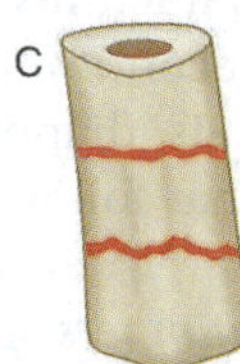


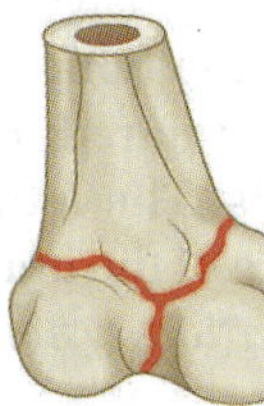


c. Severity of injury to the physis is classified in the Salter–Harris classification.
Consider whether the fracture line passes through the epiphysis, physis, metaphysis, or combinations of all the above.
Salter–Harris described five and Mercer Rang added the sixth.

| | |
|---|---|
| Type I | Simple fracture line just involving the physis. Seldom affects growth |
| Type II | Fracture line through the physis exiting through the metaphysis, producing a metaphyseal fragment. Seldom affects growth |
| Type III | Fracture line through the physis exiting through the epiphysis (intra-articular). Seldom affects growth, but intra-articular affecting joint surface |
| Type IV | Fracture-line across the epiphysis, across the physis, and across the metaphysis. This injury can cause focal fusion of the physis, leading to abnormal growth |
| Type V | A crush injury of the physis. Growth disturbance is common and may be the first radiological sign of an injury |
| Type VI | Injury to perichondral structures by direct trauma. Rare injury, high chance of abnormal growth |

*The Salter–Harris classification of growth plate injuries.*

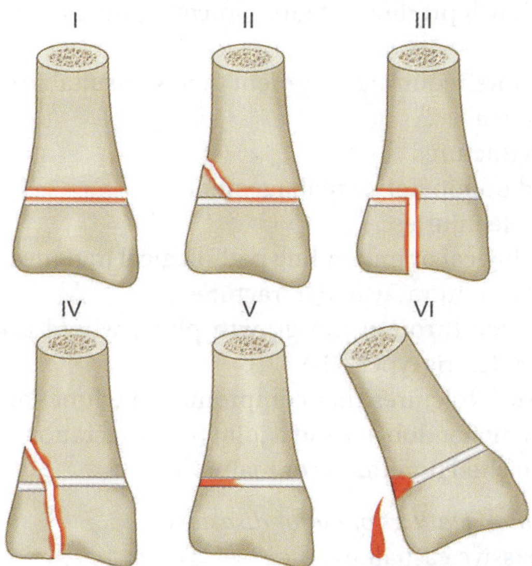


**Ans. 32** a. Advantages and disadvantages of splinting and casting.

| *Advantages* | *Disadvantages* |
|---|---|
| • Cheap<br>• Adjustable<br>• No need to remove implants<br>• No wound<br>• No interference with the fracture site | • Restricted ability to reach the soft tissue<br>• Cumbersome (particularly in the elderly)<br>• Prevents functionality<br>• Inadequate mechanical stability<br>• "Plaster disease"—joint stiffness and muscle wasting |

b. Advantages and disadvantages of traction.

| *Advantages* | *Disadvantages* |
|---|---|
| • No wound in zone of injury<br>• No interference with fracture site<br>• Materials cheap<br>• Adjustable | • Restricts mobility of patient<br>• Expensive in hospital time<br>• Skin pressure complications<br>• Pin-site infection<br>• Thromboembolic complication |

c. *Indications for K-wire insertion:*

- Temporary immobilization of a small joint
- Temporary fixation
- Definitive fixation—with small fracture fragments (e.g., wrist and hand injuries)
- Tension band wiring (fractures of patella and olecranon)

**Ans. 33** Indications for surgery in limb trauma. The main indication is that operation will produce a better outcome; the principles are given in the text.

- A fracture requiring treatment that is unsuitable for nonoperative measures
- Open fractures
- Failed nonoperative management
- Multiple injuries
- Pathological or impending pathological fractures
- Displaced intra-articular fractures
- Fractures through the growth plate, where arrest is possible (Salter–Harris types III–V)
- Avulsion fractures that compromise the functional integrity of a ligament/tendon around a joint (e.g., olecranon fracture)
- Established nonunions or malunions

**Ans. 34** a. *Common features of major disasters:*
- Massive casualties
- Infrastructure damage
- Shelter for large number of people required
- Panic and uncertainty among the population
- Limited access to the disaster area
- Communication breakdown

b. *Factors influencing rescue and relief efforts:*
- Status of communications
- Location, whether rural or urban
- Accessibility of the location
- Time frame in which disaster occurs
- Economic state of development of the area

c. *Sequence:*
- Establish chain of command
- Setup the lines of communication
- Carry out damage assessment
- Mobilize the resources
- Initiate the rescue operation
- Triage casualties
- Start emergency treatment
- Arrange evacuation
- Start definitive management

**Ans. 35** a. Triage (French verb trier) means "to sort" and is the cornerstone of the management of mass casualties. Aim is to identify those patients who will benefit the most by getting treatment the earliest, ensuring "the greatest good for the greatest number".

b. Triage categories.

c. *Principles of DCS in disaster:*
- Do the bare minimum required to all safe transfer to a definitive care center
- Take step to prevent further deterioration during transfer
- Secure airway
- Control bleeding (may require compression, laparotomy, craniotomy, thoracostomy, major vessels repair of the limb)
- Prevent the pressure build up (may require chest drain, fasciotomy, laparotomy, burr holes)
- Prevent infection and contamination of tissue (debridement of dead tissue)

| Priority | Color | Medical need | Clinical status | Examples |
|---|---|---|---|---|
| First (I) | Red | Immediate | Critical, but likely to survive if treatment given early | Severe facial trauma, tension pneumothorax, profuse external bleeding, hemothorax, flail chest, major intra-abdominal bleed, and extradural hematomas |
| Second (II) | Yellow | Urgent | Critical, likely to survive if treatment given within hours | Compound fractures, degloving injuries, ruptured abdominal viscus, pelvic fractures, and spinal injuries |
| Third (III) | Green | Nonurgent | Stable, likely to survive even if treatment is delayed for hours to days | Simple fractures, sprains, and minor lacerations |
| Last (0) | Black | Unsalvageable | Not breathing, pulseless, so severely Severe brain damage, very extensive burns, major injured that no medical care is likely to help | Severe brain damage, major disruption/loss of chest or abdominal wall structures, and very extensive burns |

**Ans. 36** a. Tetanus
- Causative agent *Clostridium* tetani
- Spores—soil
- Thrives in dead or contaminated tissue
- Produces tetanospasmin (exotoxin)
- Causes muscles spasm

- Make sure patients are immunized
- For heavily contaminated wounds give antithymocyte globulin (ATG)

b. Necrotizing fasciitis
- β-hemolytic *Streptococcus* or is polymicrobial
- Also known as Fournier's or Meleney's gangrene
- Progress is rapid and renal failure is an early complication
- Treat with radical surgical excision repeated every 24 hours
- Give oxygen and penicillin

c. Gas gangrene
- Causative agent—*Clostridium perfringens*
- Spores—present in soil
- Thrives in anaerobic conditions and produces many exotoxins
- Treatment—radical and regular surgical excision
- Give oxygen and penicillin
- Early amputation (may be life-saving)

**Ans. 37** a. Crush syndrome
- Result of reperfusion
- Acute kidney injury (AKI) and renal failure from myoglobinuria is a complication.
- Late fasciotomy may make things worse not better.

b. When a trauma causes a rise in the pressure inside a muscle compartment. This happens in muscles that are fascia-enclosed, such as the intrinsic muscles of the hand and foot, the calf, and the forearm. Pressure within the compartment increases until it surpasses venous drainage pressure due to a tight bandage or plaster, bleeding from a fracture, or severe violent trauma. If the pressure rises further, it will cut off perfusion of the muscle.

*Important points:*
- Most prevalent in soft-tissue crush injuries or closed fractures.
- Pain during passive muscular extension is indicative of a diagnosis.
- Intracompartmental pressure studies are not reliable.
- It is imperative to do a fasciotomy as soon as there is any indication.

c. Frostbite and immersion injuries (trench foot) occur when a part of body freezes. The cells are disrupted and the tissue dies. It is essentially a "cold" burn and is classified similarly to a conventional burn based on the depth it impacts.

Frostbite (trench foot)

*Important points:*
- Can be superficial or deep (like a burn)
- Gentle rewarming

- Allow natural demarcation of margins
- Protect against further infection and trauma

**Ans. 38** a. *DCS: To restore physiology over anatomy, divided into several phases:*

| | |
|---|---|
| Phase 1 | An understanding of the extent of the injury and the requirement for both surgical and resuscitative damage control techniques<br>Rapid-sequence intubation and anesthetic induction, early rewarming, and timely transfer to the operation theater (OT) are characteristics of phase 1 |
| Phase 2 | Immediate laparotomy, abdominal packing, interim wound closure, and quick bleeding, and contamination control |
| Phase 3 | ICU for ongoing resuscitation with physiological and biochemical parameter normalization |
| Phase 4 | Re-exploration in the OT to perform definitive repair of all injuries. There may be a need for numerous procedures at different times. If physiology deteriorates even at this point, nonessential operations may be shortened or postponed |

b. Medical support roles

| | |
|---|---|
| R1 | Unit-level medical care including first aid and primary health care |
| R2 | Intermediary device for stabilization, damage control, and resuscitation |
| R3 | Multispecialty hospital treatment that has been deployed |
| R4 | Definitive hospital care within the home or allied nation |

**Ans. 39** a. Blast overpressure
b. Quasi-instantaneous pressure rise
c. Positive pressure phase
d. Negative pressure phase

**Ans. 40**

| *Classification* | *Injury type* | *Examples* |
|---|---|---|
| Primary blast | Overpressure | Blast lung, intestine blast injury, and tympanic membrane injury |
| Secondary blast | Penetrating/ fragmentation | All penetrating injuries |
| Tertiary blast | Blunt | Amputations caused by trauma, blunt and crush injuries |
| Quaternary blast | Miscellaneous | Burns, inhalation injury |
| Quinary blast | Effect of device additions | Radiation sickness, infection |

**Ans. 41** a. Scaphoid oblique.

b. Immobilize the wrist for 10–14 days later.

- Check if tenderness remains, repeat the scaphoid views.
- Early diagnosis may be made with a bone scan, magnetic resonance imaging (MRI), or CT.
- Undisplaced fracture can be treated nonoperatively with below-elbow cast.

c. Complications of scaphoid fractures include: Nonunion, avascular necrosis, malunion, and carpal instability.

d. Technetium-99

**Ans. 42** a. Peripheral nerve injury

b. Classification of nerve injuries into the following:

| | |
|---|---|
| Neurapraxia | No loss of nerve sheath continuity or peripheral Wallerian degeneration. (Pressure is removed from the nerve, recovery potential is good but may take months) |
| Axonotmesis | Nerve sheath remains intact, with internal nerve fiber damage and associated Wallerian degeneration. The neural tube (endoneurium) can guide the regenerating nerve fibers to their target. Good potential for recovery; nerve fiber regrowth is @ 1 mm per day |
| Neurotmesis | Complete division of the nerve, nerve sheath, and nerve fiber. Functionally, poor outcome without surgical intervention to restore continuity of the nerve sheath |

**Ans. 43** a. Oculocardiac reflex secondary to a "white eye" blow-out left orbital floor.

b. Indications—enophthalmos or persistent diplopia resulting from restricted eye motility as a result of EOM entrapment within the line.

**Ans. 44**
1. Cephalic vein (blue)
2. Radial nerve (yellow)
3. Radial artery (red)
4. Lower end of radius
5. Scaphoid
6. Trapezium
7. First metacarpal
8. Proximal phalanx
9. Distal phalanx
10. Extensor pollicis longus
11. Extensor pollicis brevis
12. Abductor pollicis longus.

**Ans. 45** a. Maxillary fractures are classified according to their anatomical level, as originally described by René Le Fort.

b. *Le Fort I* line extending from the pterygoid plates through the lateral wall of the maxillary sinus and piriform aperture of the nose.

*Le Fort II* involves the whole of the dentition bearing portion of the maxilla and the nasal bones. The fracture line extends from the pterygoid plates to the inferior orbital rim and across the bridge of the nose.

*Le Fort III* essentially is where the whole of the midface is separated from the skull base. Line runs from the pterygoid plates to the base of the zygomatic arch, the lateral walls of the orbit through the FZ suture and the nasal bridge.

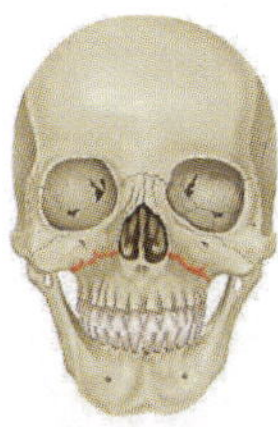

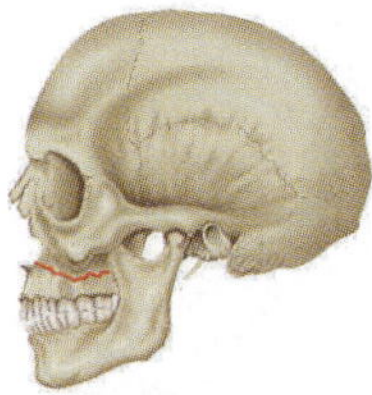

**Le Fort I**
Fracture line extending from the pterygoid plates through the lateral wall of the maxillary sinus and piriform aperture of the nose

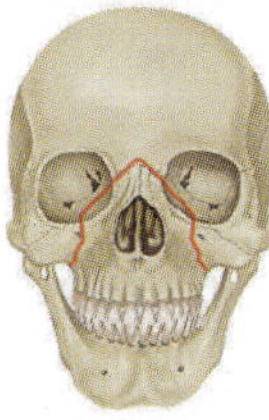

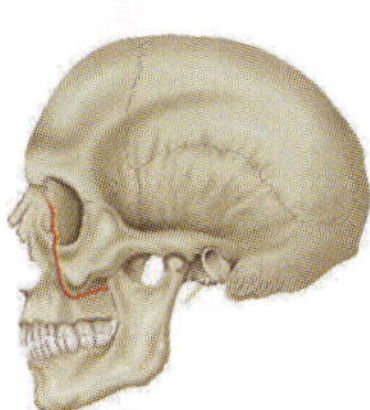

**Le Fort II**
Fracture line extends from the pterygoid plates to the inferior orbital rim and across the bridge of the nose

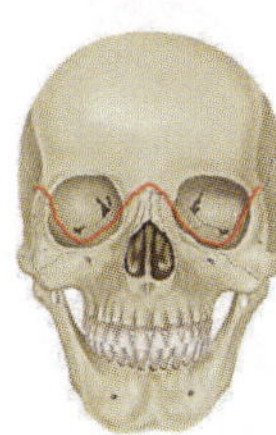

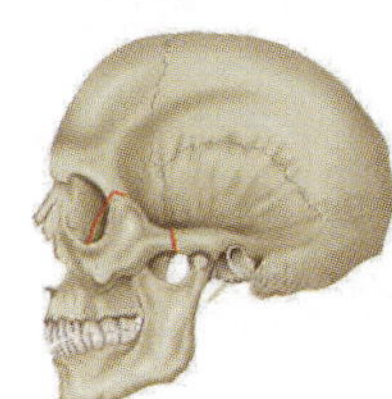

**Le Fort III**
Fracture line runs from the pterygoid plates to the base of the zygomatic arch, the lateral walls of the orbit through the FZ suture and the nasal bridge

5

SECTION

# Elective Orthopedics

# 26 CHAPTER Elective Orthopedics

## QUESTIONS

**Q1. Where is the presentation of limp in the following?**

a. Osteoarthritis (OA)
b. Cerebral palsy

**Q2. What is the pathology behind following limp?**

a. Trendelenburg limp
b. High stepping gait
c. Spastic

**Q3. Explain the terminology used to describe the direction of movement.**

a. Circumduction
b. Pronation and supination
c. Retraction
d. Inversion and eversion

**Q4. What is sensory and motor supply of the following root levels?**

a. C5
b. C6
c. C7
d. C8
e. T1

**Q5. What is sensory and motor supply of the following root levels?**

a. L1
b. L2
c. L3
d. L4
e. L5
f. S1

**Q6. What is Beighton score and how it is calculated?**

**Q7. Name the test shown in the figure and this test is used for:**

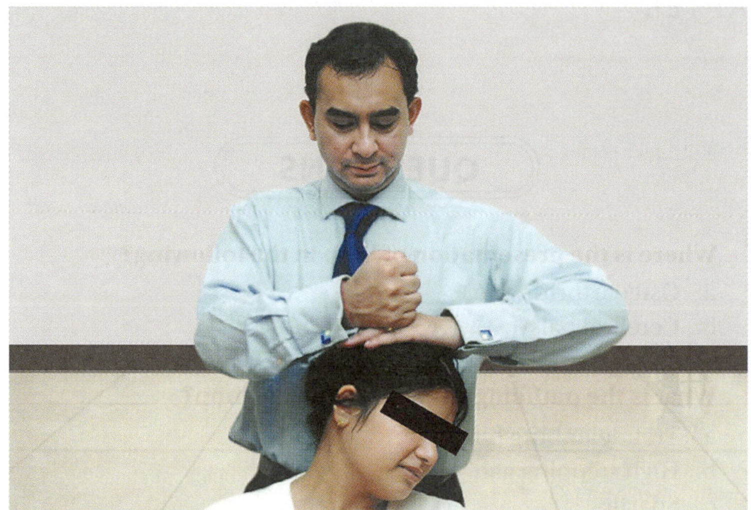

*Source:* Bailey and Love, 28th edition, page 477.

**Q8. As per the Medical Research Council, what is the muscle power grading system?**

**Q9. Explain the test used in the following figures:**

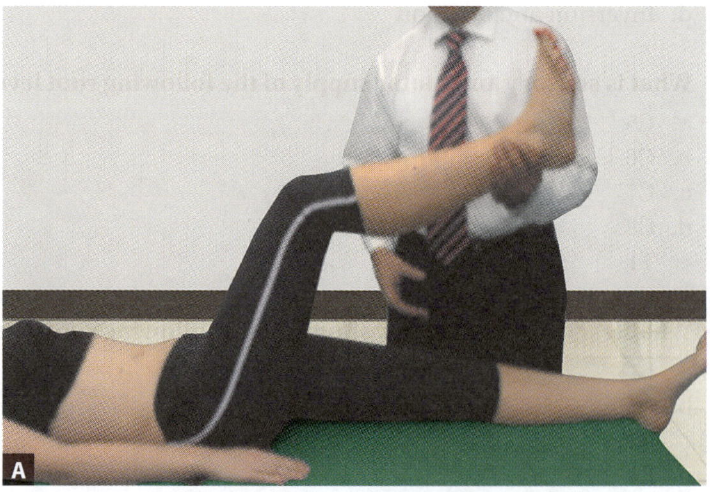


*Source:* Bailey and Love, 28th edition, page 479.

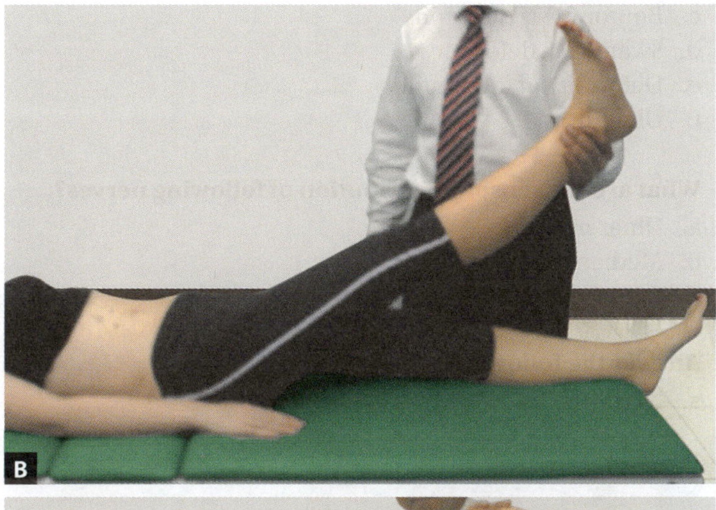


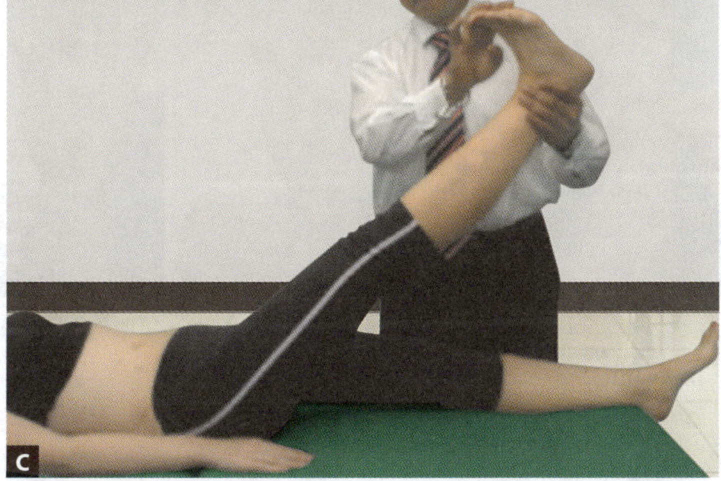


*Source:* Bailey and Love, 28th edition, page 479.

**Q10. Which patterns of muscle wasting are present in the following conditions?**

a. Median nerve palsy (C8)
b. Ulnar nerve palsy (T1)

**Q11. Name the bony anatomical site and association with the following:**

a. Heberden's node
b. Bouchard's node

c. Boutonnière deformity
d. Swan neck deformity
e. Deformity of the thumb
f. Ulnar drift

**Q12. What are the sensory distribution of following nerves?**

a. Ulnar nerve
b. Median nerve
c. Radial nerve

**Q13. Answer the following:**

a. Name the test shown in images.

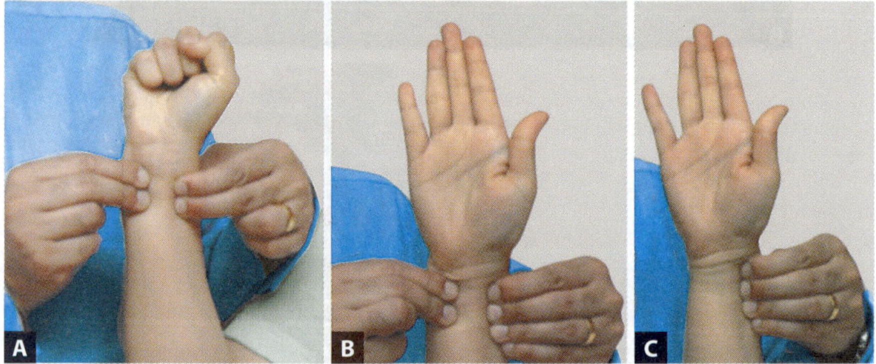


*Source:* Bailey and Love, 28th edition, page 481.

b. Name the test shown in image.

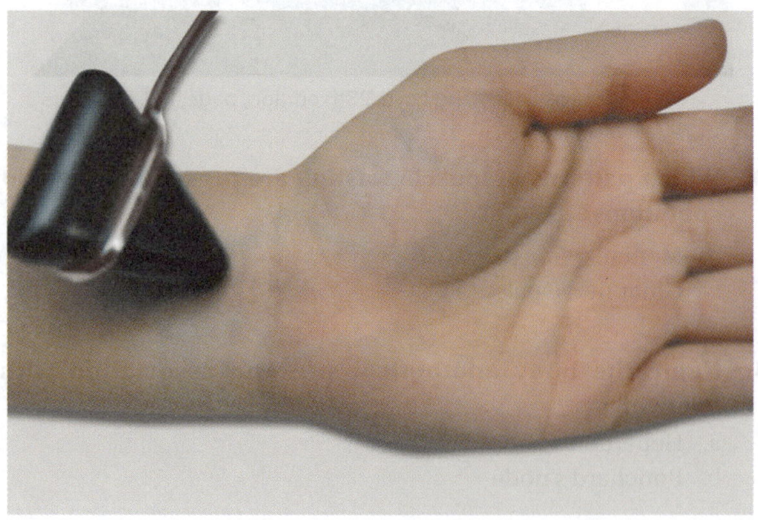

*Source:* Bailey and Love, 28th edition, page 482

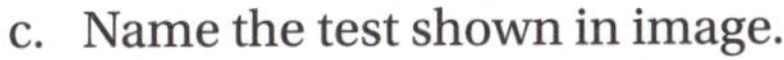

c. Name the test shown in image.

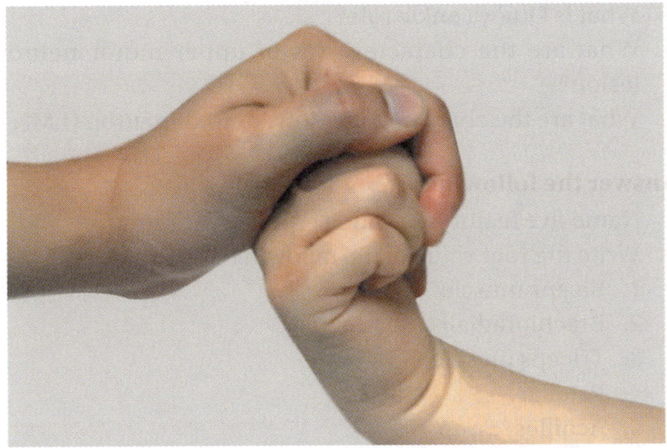

*Source:* Bailey and Love, 28th edition, page 482.

d. Name the test shown in image.

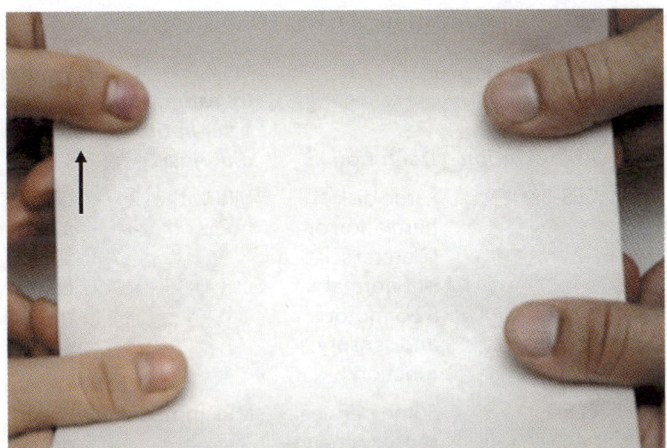

*Source:* Bailey and Love, 28th edition, page 483.

**Q14. Explain the given special hand test technique and their significance.**

a. Allen's test
b. Tinel's test
c. Phalen's test
d. Froment's sign

**Q15. Answer the following:**

a. Name the tests to distinguish flexible from fixed flat foot.
b. What is Morton's neuroma?

**Q16. Answer the following:**

a. What is Ottawa ankle rule?
b. What are the characteristics of upper motor neuron (UMN) lesion?
c. What are the characteristics lower motor neuron (LMN) lesion?

**Q17. Answer the following:**

a. Name five features of cauda equina syndrome.
b. Write the root value of the following:
   1. Biceps muscle
   2. Brachioradialis muscle
   3. Triceps muscle
   4. Patellar
   5. Achilles

**Q18. Answer the following:**

a. What is cauda equina classification (CES)?
b. Write the classification of CES.

| ***Name*** | ***Abbreviation*** | ***Definition*** | ***Investigation after initial diagnosis*** | ***Treatment if MRI positive for compression of CES*** |
|---|---|---|---|---|
| CES suspected | CES-S | Large disk herniation or bilateral sciatica but normal S2-5 motor and sensory function | MRI within 24 hours | Discuss risks and benefits of surgery versus conservative treatment |
| CES early | CES-E | Some perineal sensory change but normal bladder and bowel function | MRI immediate | Urgent decompression |
| CES incomplete | CES-I | Impaired bladder function or sensation but executive/ voluntary control of bladder maintained | MRI immediate | Urgent decompression |

*Contd...*

*Contd...*

| Name | Abbreviation | Definition | Investigation after initial diagnosis | Treatment if MRI positive for compression of CES |
|---|---|---|---|---|
| CES retention | CES-R | Bladder retention and overflow incontinence | MRI immediate | Urgent decompression on next daytime list if patient presents overnight |
| CES complete | CES-C | Complete loss of cauda equina function | MRI in working hours | Decompression, if improvement considered possible |

**Q19. Name the procedure shown in the figures and name of implant.**

a.

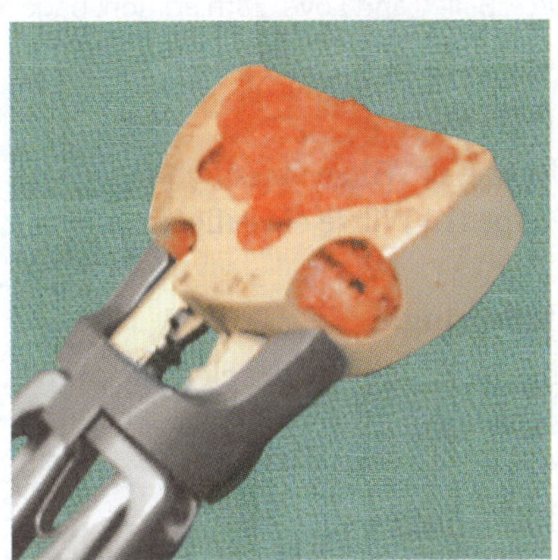

*Source:* Bailey and Love, 28th edition, page 515.

b.

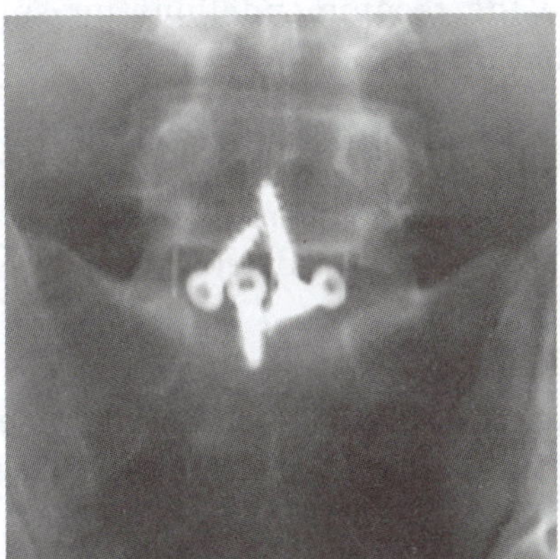

*Source:* Bailey and Love, 28th edition, page 515.

c.

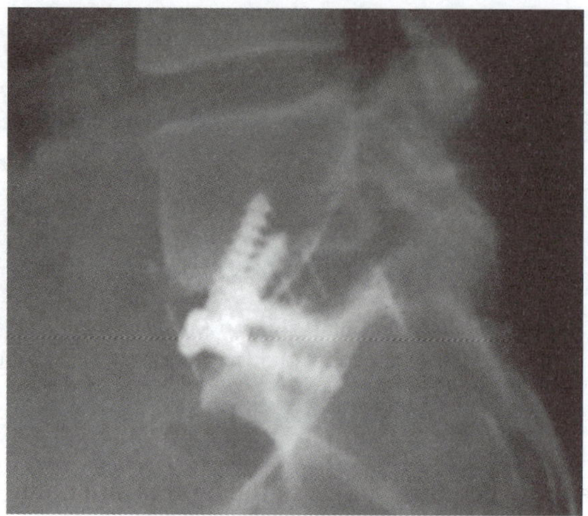

*Source:* Bailey and Love, 28th edition, page 515.

**Q20. Answer the following:**

a. What is the use of Wiltse classification?
b. Write the types of Wiltse classification.

**Q21. Answer the following:**

a. What is the use of Meyerding classification?
b. Write the grades of Meyerding classification.

**Q22. Answer the following:**

a. Which is the most common malignancy that metastasize to spine?
b. What are the recommendations for spinal surgery in the rheumatoid arthritis?

**Q23. Answer the following:**

a. What is Sprengel's shoulder?
b. What are the radiological differences between RA and OA?

**Q24. Answer the following:**

a. Name three tests for carpal tunnel syndrome.
b. Identify the clinical images and make probable diagnosis.

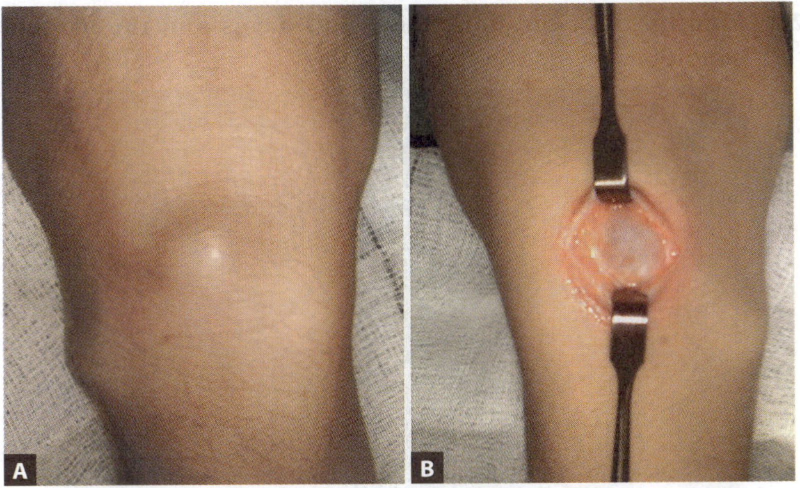


*Source:* Bailey and Love, 28th edition, page 548.

**Q25. Answer the following:**

a. What is the use of Steinberg's classification?
b. Write the stages of Steinberg's classification.

**Q26. Answer the following:**

a. How many major bones in foot?
b. How many layers of the muscles in the sole of foot?
c. Blood supply of foot

**Q27. Answer the following:**

a. What is characteristic of pes cavus?
b. Identify the image and probable associated condition.

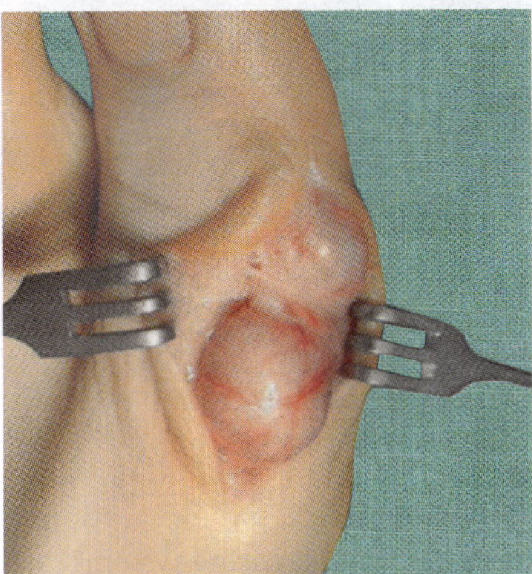

*Source:* Bailey and Love, 28th edition, page 576.

**Q28. Identify the condition shown in images and the associated condition.**

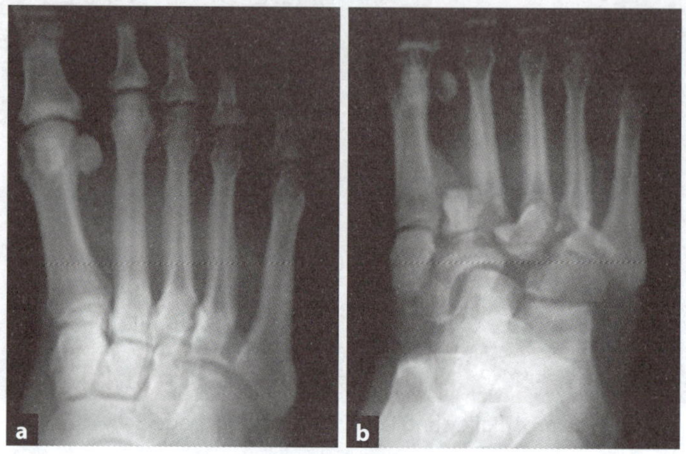

*Source:* Bailey and Love, 28th edition, page 577.

**Q29. Why is a patient with diabetes prone to infection?**

**Q30. Identify the image in the given figures.**

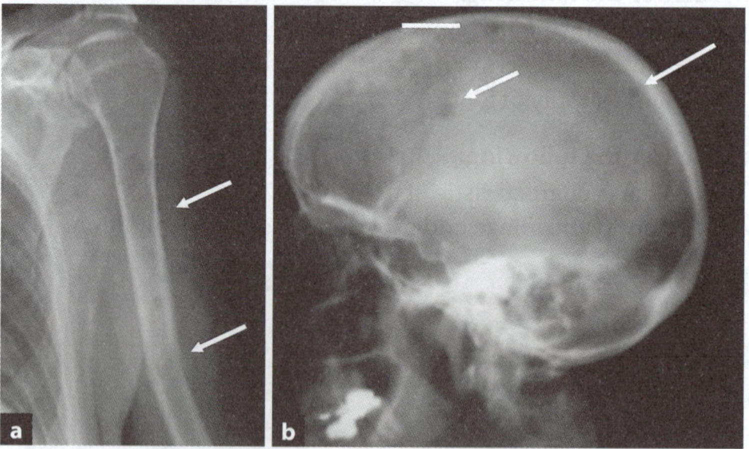

*Source:* Bailey and Love, 28th edition, page 580.

**Q31. Answer the following:**

a. Enneking staging system used for
b. Write the grades of it.

**Q32. Answer the following:**

a. What is the use of Mirels scoring system?
b. Write the scoring system.

**Q33. Answer the following:**

a. What is the use of BACH classification system?

b. Write the classification system.

**Q34. Answer the following:**

a. What are the laws governing the remodeling of bone?

b. What are the common causes of rickets?

**Q35. Answer the following:**

a. What is the treatment of club foot?

b. Identify the given clinical image and associated imaging and give probable diagnosis.

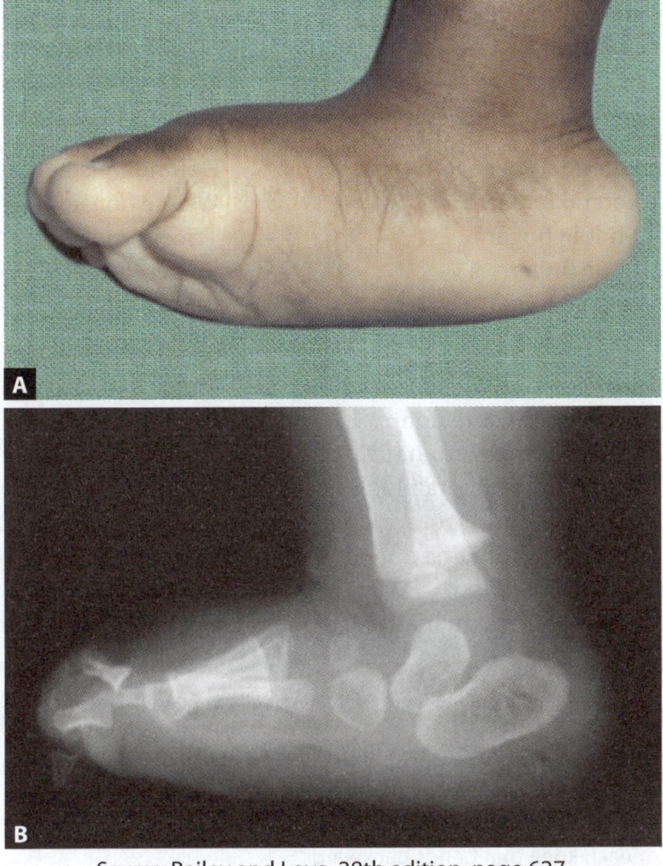


*Source:* Bailey and Love, 28th edition, page 627.

**Q36. What are the clinical predictors according to Kocher et al. (2004) for the diagnosis of septic arthritis?**

## ANSWERS

**Ans. 1**
a. Head dips. Cadence dash/dash
b. Head movement lacks coordination. No regular cadence.

**Ans. 2**
a. Hip abductors weakness
b. Foot drop due to common peroneal nerve (CPN) palsy.
c. Cerebral palsy

**Ans. 3**
a. Circumduction—using flexion, abduction, extension, and adduction in combination with the limbs without rotation
b. Supination—forearm movement in which the palm faces front and when the forearm pronates, the palm faces posteriorly.
c. Retraction—the head, jaw, or shoulders moving backward.
d. Inversion—the foot directs the sole of the foot laterally during an eversion movement and medially during an inversion movement.

**Ans. 4**

| | *Sensory* | *Motor* |
|---|---|---|
| a. | Lateral upper arm | Deltoid muscle |
| b. | Lateral forearm | Wrist extension |
| c. | Middle finger | Triceps muscle |
| d. | Little finger | Finger flexors |
| e. | Medial forearm | Interossei |

**Ans. 5**

| | *Sensory* | *Motor* |
|---|---|---|
| a. | Anterior thigh region | Psoas muscle |
| b. | Anterior thigh/groin region | Quadriceps muscles |
| c. | Anterior and lateral thigh region | Quadriceps muscles |
| d. | Medial leg and foot region | Tibialis anterior muscle |
| e. | Lateral leg and first dorsal web space of foot | Extensor hallucis longus muscle |
| f. | Lateral and plantar aspect of foot | Gastrocnemius/perineals |

**Ans. 6** *Beighton score:*

| | ***Points*** |
|---|---|
| While standing forward bending, the patient can place their palms on the ground with legs straight | 1 point |
| For each elbow that bends backward | 1 point |
| For each knee that bends backward | 1 point |
| For each thumb that touches the forearm when bent backward | 1 point |
| For each little finger that bends backward beyond 90° | 1 point |
| Total score out of 9 | |

Beighton score (a screening technique for hypermobility).

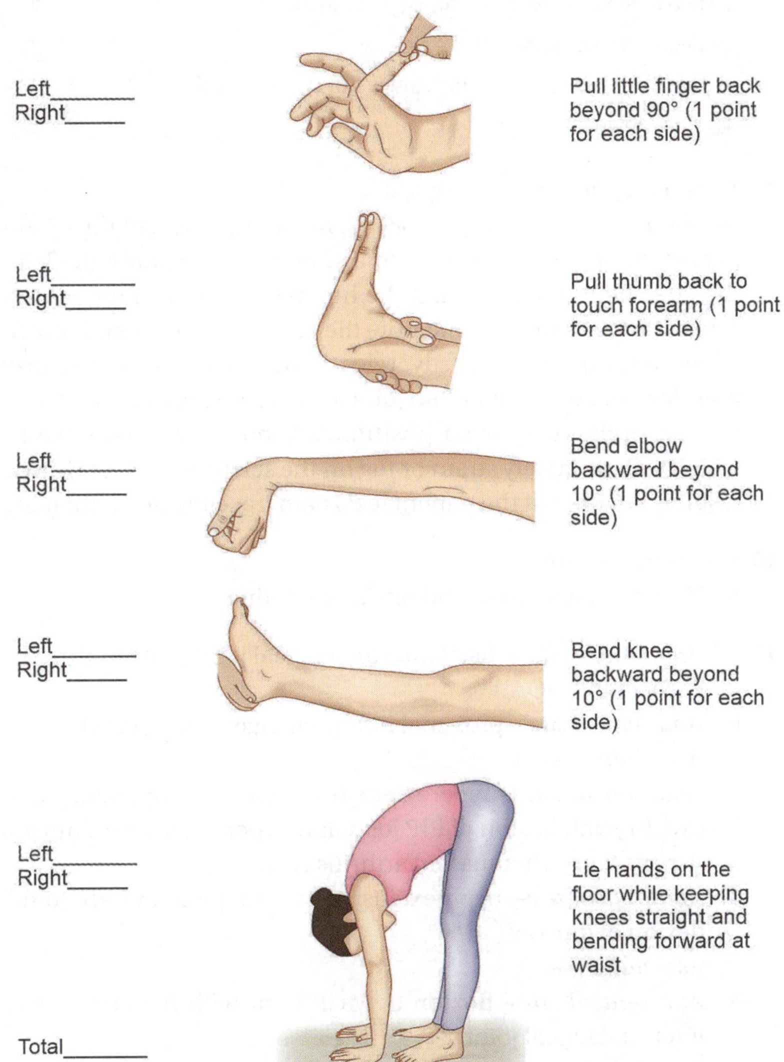


*Source:* Bailey and Love, 28th edition, page 475.

**Ans. 7** Spurling's test

- *Use*—cervical spine nerve root entrapment.
- *Method*—the examiner extends and presses downward on the top of the patient's head while they turn their head to the side that is afflicted.

**Ans. 8**

| | *Grade* |
|---|---|
| No movement | 0 |
| Flicker of movement | 1 |
| Active movement with the gravity elimination | 2 |
| Active movement against the gravity | 3 |
| Active movement against resistance but power less than full | 4 |
| Normal power | 5 |

**Ans. 9** Test—Lasègue's straight leg test.

Method—tension along the sciatic nerve (the roots of the L5 and S1 nerves) increases in this test. In a supine posture, raise the leg with the knee bent to ensure that the hip may move without pain. Next, extend your leg straight and note the angle at which your hamstrings allow your hip to flex. Lastly, release the tension in your hamstring muscles by allowing your hip joint to stretch. This will put your ankle in a securely dorsiflexed position without using excessive force, which will ultimately strain or tug on the sciatic nerve. A positive test result is obtained if the patient feels pain traveling down their leg.

**Ans. 10** a. Thenar wasting

b. Hypothenar wasting and intrinsic wasting

**Ans. 11** a. *Anatomical site*—distal interphalangeal joint (DIPJ)
Association—OA

b. *Anatomical site*—proximal interphalangeal joint (PIPJ)
*Association*—OA

c. *Anatomical site*—hyperextension at metacarpophalangeal joint (MCP) joint, flexion of PIP joint and hyperextension of dip joint.
*Association*—rheumatoid arthritis (RA)

d. *Anatomical site*—hyperextension at MCP joint and PIP joint and flexion of dip joint
*Association*—RA

e. *Anatomical site*—flexion at MCP joint with hyperextension of interphalangeal joint
*Association*—RA

f. *Anatomical site*—subluxation of the MCPJ
*Association*—RA

**Ans. 12** a. Little finger and ring finger's ulnar portion.

b. The thumb, index finger, middle finger, and ring finger's radial half.

c. Thumb base on the dorsal side of the hand.

**Ans. 13** a. Allen's test
b. Tinel's test
c. Phalen's test
d. Froment's sign

**Ans. 14** a. Allen's test technique—raise your hand and obstruct the ulnar and radial arteries simultaneously with digital pressure. Next, instruct the patient to repeatedly clench their fist. The tips of your fingers should turn pale. Now, release each artery separately and observe the return of color.
Significance—to assess the arcade's patency and the hand's sufficient blood flow from the radial and ulnar arteries.
b. Tinel's test technique—tapping over the nerve, tingling may be an indication of nerve compression.
*Significance*—to determine whether a peripheral nerve is compressed.
c. *Phalen's test technique*—to stretch the elbows and position the wrist at its maximum flexion.
*Significance*—medial nerve compression, which results in paresthesia.
d. *Froment's test technique*—ask the patient hold a piece of paper between their thumb and index finger on both hands. Hold the same paper in a comparable manner. Ask patient to resist the pulling as you attempt to pull the paper away.
*Significance*—a positive test results in flexion of the thumb interphalangeal (IP) joint, which implies ulnar nerve-supplied adductor pollicis muscle weakening. Moreover, the thumb posture is explained by the median nerve, which innervates the flexor pollicis brevis.

**Ans. 15** a. Windlass and Jack's tests
b. Morton's neuroma—when the digital nerve crosses the ligament that connects the metatarsals in the front foot, the tissue surrounding it thickens and leads to the toes. Most frequently occurs between the third and fourth toes. The first sign of a neuroma is burning sensation in the base of the foot that extends to the afflicted toes.

**Ans. 16** a. The Ottawa ankle rules:
- Bone tenderness along 6 cm distal to the posterior margin or at the tip of medial malleolus.
- Bone tenderness along 6 cm distal to the posterior margin or at the tip of lateral malleolus.

- Unable to support weight when the event occurred or while being examined.

b. UMN lesions characteristics:
- Increased tone—spastic
- Muscle spasms
- Hyperreflexia
- Motor weakness
- Positive Hoffmann's sign
- Disuse atrophy
- Upgoing plantar response
- Ankle and patellar clonus

c. *LMN lesions characteristics:*
- Decreased tone—flaccid
- Denervation fasciculations
- Hyporeflexia
- Motor weakness
- Severe atrophy
- Loss of sensation
- Extensor plantar response

**Ans. 17** a. Cauda equina syndrome
- Low backache
- Saddle anesthesia
- Unilateral or bilateral sciatica
- Lower extremities motor weakness
- Variable rectal and urinary symptoms

b. 1. C5/C6
2. C5/C6
3. C7/8
4. L3/4
5. S1/2

**Ans. 18** a. CES is a very serious and urgent condition, arising from compression of the cauda equina nerve roots, which supply the perineum and genital regions and bladder, bowel, and sexual function. Massive central lumbar disk protrusion at the L4/5 or L5/S1 level is the most common cause. Postoperative epidural hematoma, spinal tumors, lumbar fractures, and spinal stenosis are further causes.

b. Classification of cauda equina syndrome (CES).

| Name | Abbreviation | Definition | Investigation after initial diagnosis | Treatment if MRI positive for compression of CES |
|---|---|---|---|---|
| CES suspected | CES-S | Large disk herniation or bilateral sciatica but normal S2-5 motor and sensory function | MRI within 24 hours | Discuss risks and benefits of surgery versus conservative treatment |
| CES early | CES-E | Some perineal sensory change but normal bladder and bowel function | MRI immediate | Urgent decompression |
| CES incomplete | CES-I | Impaired bladder function or sensation but executive/ voluntary control of bladder maintained | MRI immediate | Urgent decompression |
| CES retention | CES-R | Bladder retention and overflow incontinence | MRI immediate | Urgent decompression on next daytime list if patient presents overnight |
| CES complete | CES-C | Complete loss of cauda equina function | MRI in working hours | Decompression, if improvement considered possible |

**Ans. 19** The anterior lumbar interbody fusion.

a. Before implantation, the PEEK cage is filled with bone transplant (poly-ethyl-ethyl-ketone)
b. The anteroposterior postoperative radiograph.
c. Lateral postoperative imaging.

**Ans. 20** a. Spondylolisthesis

b.

| Type 1 | Dysplastic | Congenital deficiency of the L5/S1 articulation |
|---|---|---|
| Type 2 | Isthmic | • Lesion of the pars interarticularis<br>Three subtypes:<br>• 2A—lytic defect of the pars<br>• 2B—elongated or attenuated pars<br>• 2C—acute pars fracture |

*Contd...*

*Contd...*

| | | |
|---|---|---|
| Type 3 | Degenerative spondylolisthesis | Facet arthrosis or disk degeneration-related segmental instability |
| Type 4 | Traumatic | Acute fracture other than pars interarticularis in the posterior components |
| Type 5 | Pathological | Generalized bone disease that causes the pars to attenuate (e.g., neoplastic, metabolic) |
| Type 6 | Postsurgical | When the lumbar spine has decompressed |

**Ans. 21** a. Degree of slip of spondylolisthesis.

b. Meyerding classification

| | |
|---|---|
| Grade I | 1–25% |
| Grade II | 26–50% |
| Grade III | 51–75% |
| Grade IV | 76–100% |

**Ans. 22** a. Breast 21%

b. Recommendations for spinal surgery in RA

- When the posterior atlantodental interval (PADI) is 14 mm or smaller, atlantoaxial subluxation (AAS) occurs.
- AAS with a minimum 5 mm basilar invagination.
- Subaxial subluxation with a sagittal canal diameter of at least 14 mm.

**Ans. 23** a. Because of aberrant scapular descent from the embryonic midcervical location, this congenital anomaly is the most prevalent. A small, high, rotated scapula that is still attached to the cervical spine by an omovertebral body, a fibrous band, or a bony bar is the typical appearance.

b. Radiographic differences between rheumatoid arthritis and osteoarthritis.

| *RA* | *OA* |
|---|---|
| • Ankylosis<br>• Joint deformity or malalignment<br>• Marginal erosion<br>• Periarticular soft-tissue swelling<br>• Narrowing of joint space<br>• Periarticular osteoporosis/ subchondral erosions | • Less common ankylosis<br>• Less pronounced deformities<br>• Marginal osteophytes<br>• Less pronounced swelling<br>• Narrowing of joint space<br>• Subchondral sclerosis and cysts |

**Ans. 24** a. 1. Tinel's test, percussion over the carpal tunnel
2. Phalen's test, distal paresthesia with full prolonged wrist flexion
3. Duken's test, occurrence of symptoms due to digital pressure over carpal tunnel

b. Ganglion cyst over dorsal aspect of the wrist and intraoperative appearance.

**Ans. 25** a. Steinberg's classification—for avascular necrosis of the femoral head according to the type of radiological alteration shown on MRI and radiography.

b. *Stage description*
0—MRI, bone scan, or normal or nondiagnostic radiograph
I—anomalous MRI, normal radiograph, or bone scan
II—cysts and sclerosis
III—crescent sign and subchondral collapse
IV—femur head flattening and a normal acetabulum
V—acetabular involvement VI obliteration of the joint space

**Ans. 26** a. 26 bones
b. In sole—4 layers
c. Anterior and posterior tibial arteries plus the peroneal artery.

**Ans. 27** a. Patients may exhibit hand symptoms, cavovarus foot, aches and pains, thin calf musculature, and gradual minor muscle wasting.
- Pes cavus require further neurological investigation.
- Approximately, 80% of pes cavus occurrences are linked to neurological conditions.
- Charcot-Marie-Tooth disease is the most frequent cause.
- *Unilateral pes cavus:* Consider tumors or diastematomyelia.

b. Angioleiomyoma of hallux.

**Ans. 28** Charcot foot.
a. At the time of a minor injury and
b. 6 weeks later.

Diabetes patients frequently experience foot issues as a result of neuropathy and microvascular alterations. Patients are at increased risk of infection, ulceration, and trauma can lead to collapse of the foot, also known as Charcot neuroarthropathy.

**Ans. 29** Patients with diabetes are prone to infection due to:
- Peripheral vascular disease (PVD)
- Peripheral neuropathy
- Impaired resistance to infection

**Ans. 30** a. Pathological fracture in the left humerus due to multiple myeloma.
b. Multiple myeloma with numerous deposits in the skull.

**Ans. 31** a. Bone tumors.

b. The Enneking staging system for bone tumors.

| | | |
|---|---|---|
| Low grade | • Intracompartmental<br>• Extracompartmental | • 1A<br>• 1B |
| High grade | • Intracompartmental<br>• Extracompartmental | • 2A<br>• 2B |
| Any grade | • Metastases | • 3 |

*Source:* Bailey and Love, 28th edition, page 589.

**Ans. 32** a. For risk of pathological fracture.

b. Refer Bailey and Love, 28th edition, page 593.

| | **Score** | | |
|---|---|---|---|
| | ***1*** | ***2*** | ***3*** |
| *Site* | Upper limb | Lower limb | Peritrochanteric |
| *Pain* | Mild | Moderate | Functional |
| *Size* | <One-third | One-third—two-thirds | >Two-thirds |
| *Lesion* | Blastic | Mixed | Lytic |

Score >8 high-risk of fracture—urgent prophylactic fixation should be considered.

<8 Low-risk fracture

**Ans. 33** a. Osteomyelitis

b. The BACH classifcation

| | ***Bone involvement*** | | ***Antimicrobial options*** | ***Coverage of soft tissue*** | ***Host status*** |
|---|---|---|---|---|---|
| Uncom-plicated | B1<br>Cavitary involvement (including medullary, cortical, and nonsegmen-tal cortico-medullary) | | Ax<br>Unknown/ culture negative<br>A1<br><4 resistant tests<br>≥80% susceptibility tests sensitive | C1<br>Direct closure possible, plastic surgery expertise not required | H1<br>Patient fit well or has well controlled disease |
| Complex | B2<br>Segmental involvement, any infection with joint involvement | | A2<br>>4 resistant tests<br><80% susceptibility tests sensitive | C1<br>Direct closure not possible Plastic surgery expertise required | H2<br>Patient with either poorly controlled disease, se-vere disease, or recurrent osteomyelitis |

Contd...

*Contd...*

| | Bone involvement | | Antimicrobial options | Coverage of soft tissue | Host status |
|---|---|---|---|---|---|
| Limited options | B3<br>Whole bone involvement | | A3<br>Sensitivity to either 0 or 1 susceptibility test | | H3<br>Unfit for anesthetic<br>Patient declines surgery<br>Surgery not indicated |

*Source:* Bailey and Love, 28th edition, page 605.

**Ans. 34** a. Hueter-Volkmann principle

- Compressive forces inhibit growth.
- Tensile stresses to encourage the growth of Wolff's law

*Wolff's law*

- Stresses exerted determine the deposition and resorption of bone.

b. *Nutritional*—intake of calcium and vitamin D

*Environmental*—insufficient exposure to the sun

*Gastrointestinal disease*—Crohn's disease and gluten-sensitive enteropathy

*Genetic*—X-linked hypophosphatemia (excess FGF23 production)

*Renal disease*—there may be secondary hyperparathyroidism, renal tubular abnormalities, and end-stage renal disease.

**Ans. 35** a. *Treatment of club foot:*

- Ponseti method—if serial casting is considered as avoiding formal surgical correction, it is successful in 95% of feet.
  The typical order in which they are performed is:
  C—correction of the forefoot cavus by elevation of the first ray.
  A—gradual forefoot abduction to 60°, and simultaneous
  V—correction of the varus hindfoot
  E—correction of hindfoot equinus usually follows a percutaneous Achilles tenotomy, which is an integral part of treatment.
- TATT—for older children to correct dynamic supination (If Ponseti method fails)
- Surgical release addresses posterior, medial, plantar, and lateral structures, that causes a stiffer foot than one treated conservatively.

b. *Congenital vertical talus:*

A. "Rocker-bottom foot" (lateral view)

B. X-ray showing hindfoot equinus deformity and indicating a dorsal subluxation of the forefoot and nonossified navicular bone with regard to the talus head.

**Ans. 36** The clinical predictors of Kocher et al. (2004) for the diagnosis of septic arthritis:

- History of (H/o) fever >38.5°C
- Nonweight bearing
- Erythrocyte sedimentation rate (ESR) >40 mm/h
- White blood cell (WBC) >12 × $10^9$/L

6

SECTION

# Skin, Plastic and Reconstructive

# 27 CHAPTER Skin and Subcutaneous Tissue

## QUESTIONS

**Q1. Answer the following:**

a. Enumerate the layers of epidermis in sequence.
b. What is the embryological origin of melanocytes and in which layer of epidermis it is present?
c. Name the only smooth muscle present in epidermis and function of the muscle.

**Q2. A 55-year-old lady came with c/o generalized skin lesion as shown, gradually increasing in size as well as in numbers; her mother and 2 siblings also have the same lesions. Answer the following.**

a. What is the likely diagnosis?
b. Describe the etiopathogenesis.
c. Enumerate the associated lesions in this patient.

**Q3. An obese [body mass index (BMI) 30.1 kg/m$^2$] 18-year-old girl came in clinic with axillary lesion as shown in picture. Answer the following.**

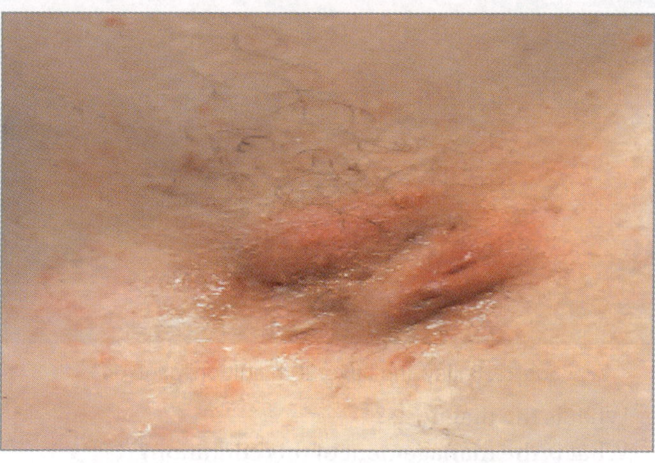

*Source:* Bailey and Love, 28th edition, page 642.

a. What is the likely diagnosis?
b. M/C causative agent and etiopathogenesis?
c. What is the management?

**Q4. A 52-year-old female came with purple undermined edges cutaneous ulcerative lesion over leg and breasts as shown in photograph a and b. She is known case of inflammatory bowel disease.**

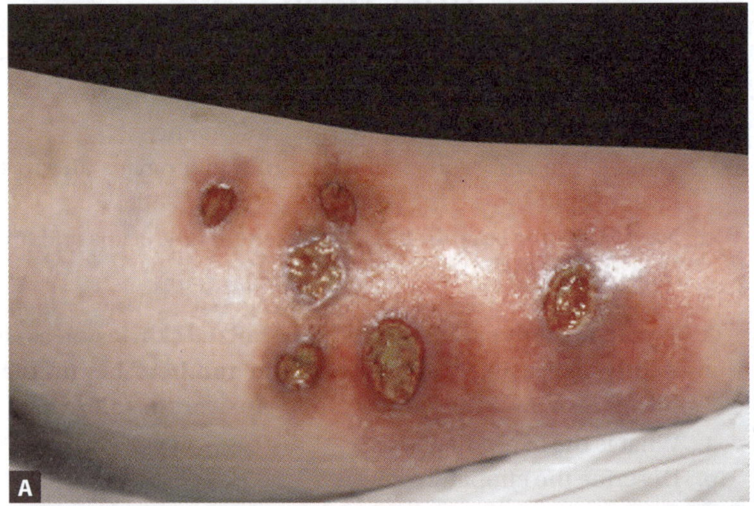


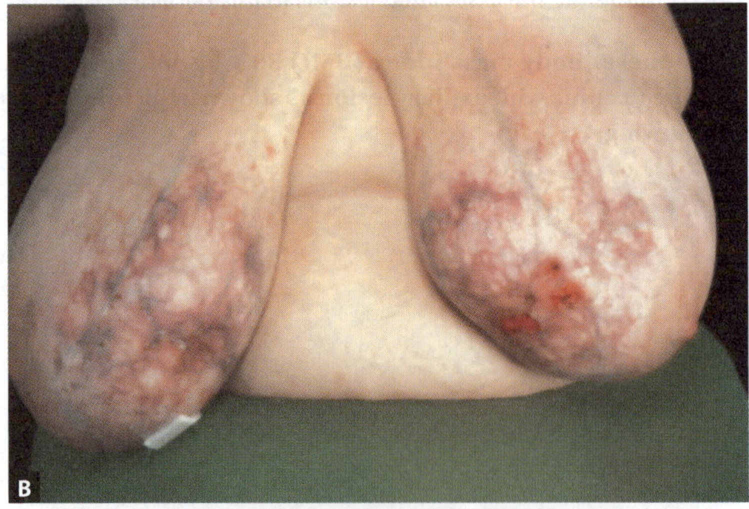


*Source:* Bailey and Love, 28th edition, page 643.

a. What is the diagnosis?
b. What is the management of this condition?

**Q5. Identify the diagnosis in images A, B, and C.**

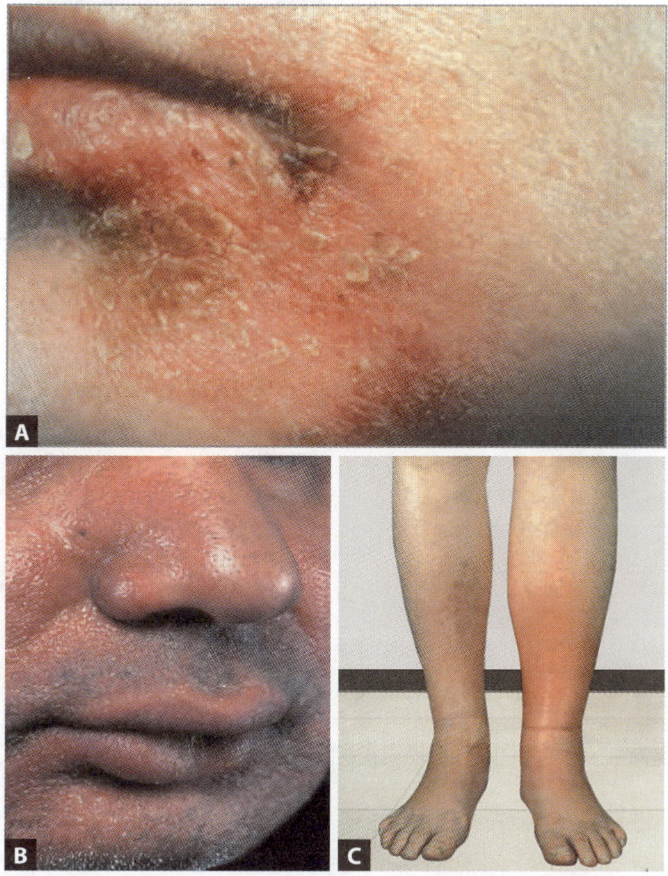

*Source:* Bailey and Love, 28th edition, pages 643 and 644.

**Q6. Identify the skin lesions depicted in given pictures.**

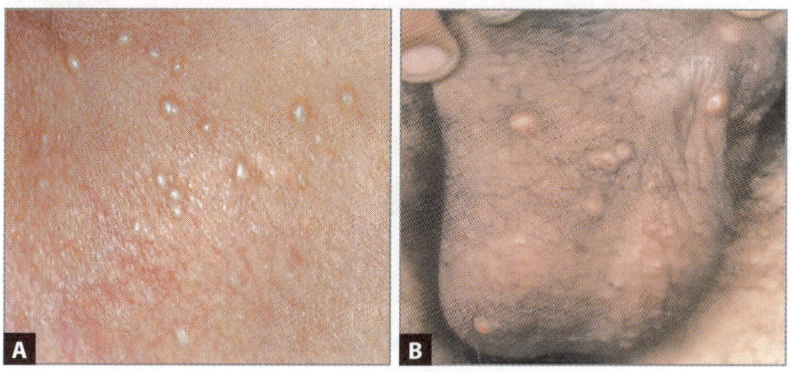

*Source:* Bailey and Love, 28th edition, pages 645 and 646.

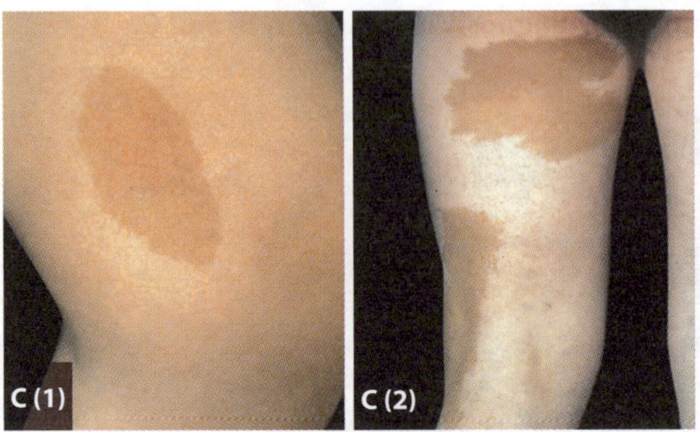


*Source:* Bailey and Love, 28th edition, page 648.

## Q7. Identify the skin lesions depicted in given pictures.

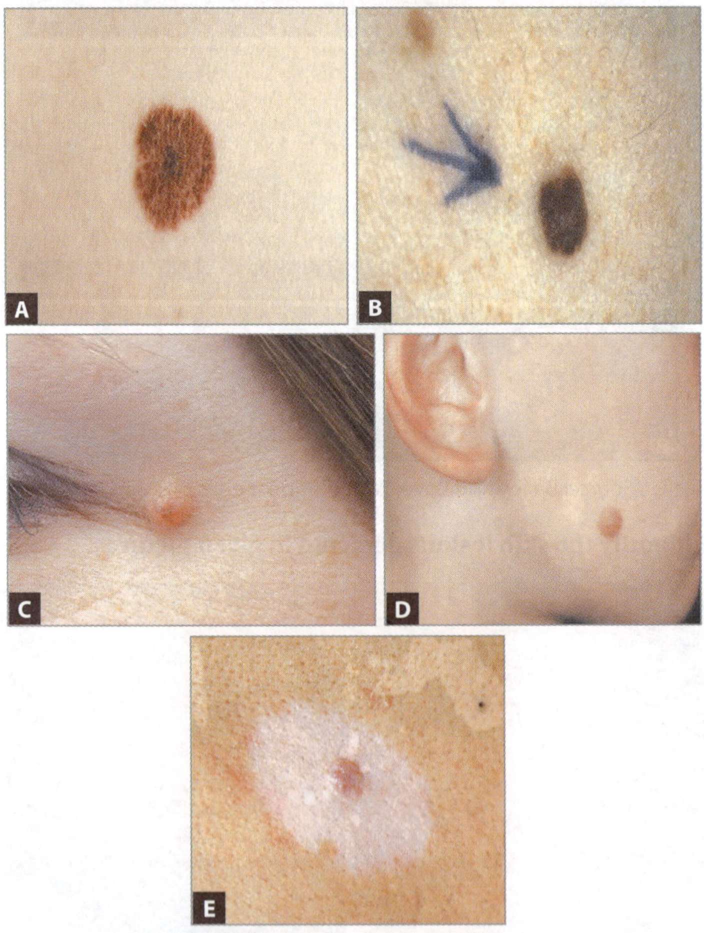


*Source:* Bailey and Love, 28th edition, pages 646 and 647.

**Q8. Identify the skin lesions in the given pictures.**

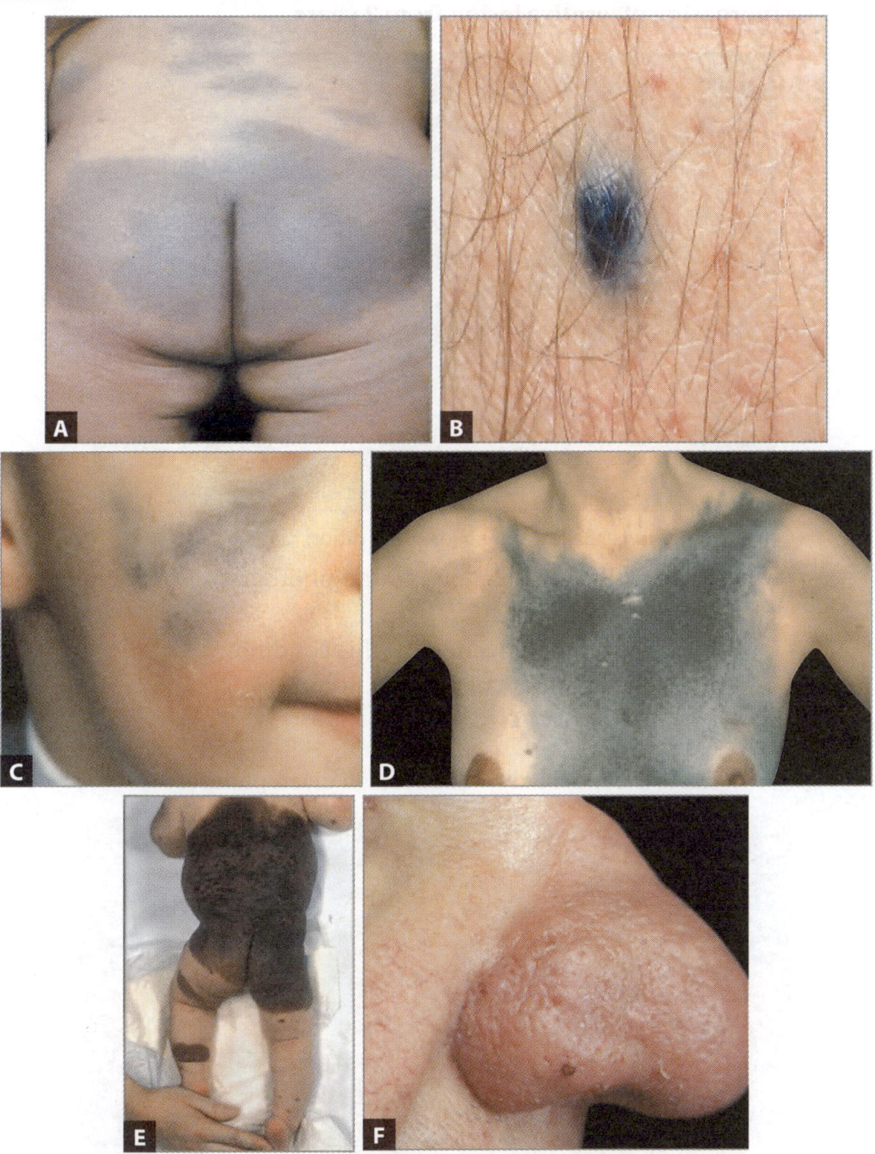


*Source:* Bailey and Love, 28th edition, pages 648 to 651.

**Q9. A 57-year-old female, labor by occupation came with c/o gradually increasing ulcerative lesion from 2 years.**

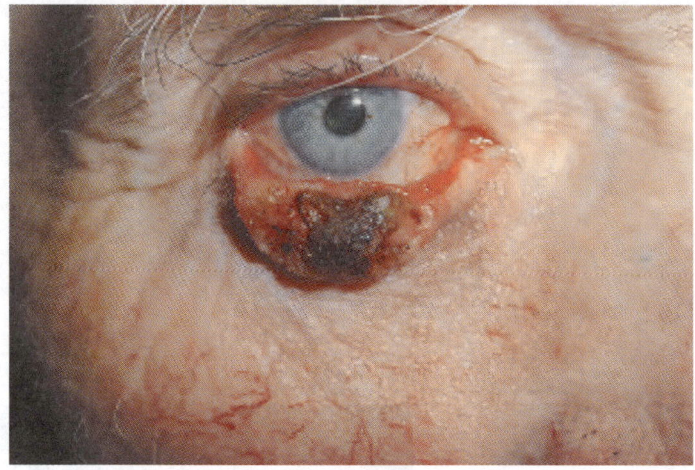

*Source:* Bailey and Love, 28th edition, page 652.

a. What is the likely diagnosis in the photograph shown here and mention the variants?
b. What is the etiopathogenesis of this condition?
c. What is the treatment of this condition?

**Q10.**

a. What is the most likely diagnosis in given pictures?

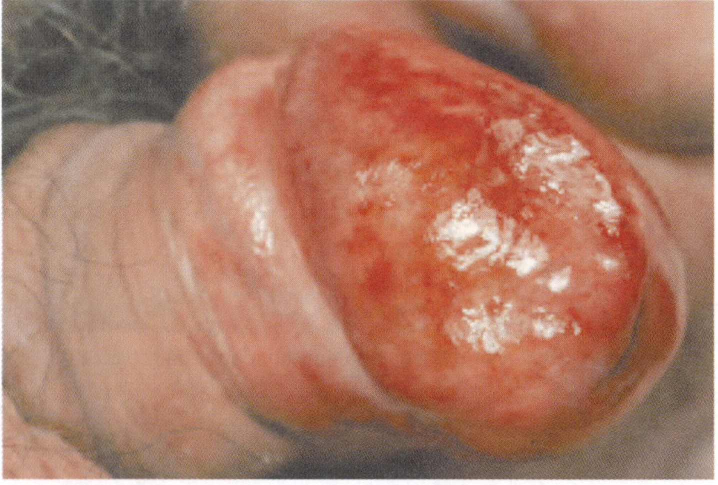

*Source:* Bailey and Love, 28th edition, page 654.

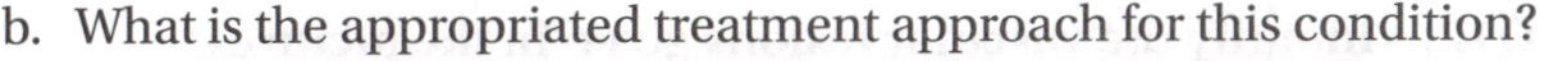

b. What is the appropriated treatment approach for this condition?

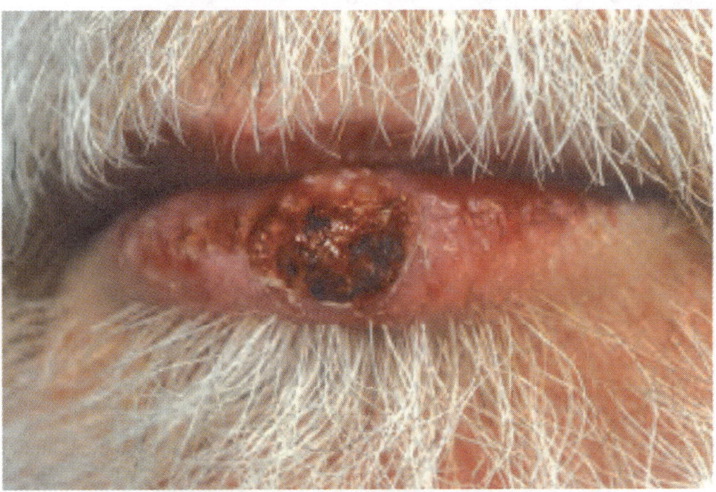

*Source:* Bailey and Love, 28th edition, page 655.

**Q11. A 32-year-old fair colored female came with skin lesion as shown in photograph, which is rapidly increasing in size. She is clinically diagnosed with malignant melanoma.**

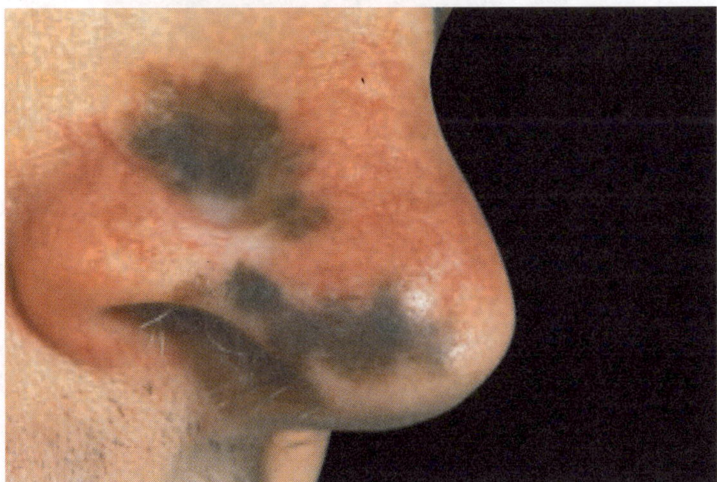

*Source:* Bailey and Love, 28th edition, page 656.

a. What are the macroscopic features in nevi suggestive of malignant melanoma?
b. Enumerate the variants of melanoma.
c. What is the appropriate management for this condition?

**Q12. Identify the vascular lesions given in the pictures.**

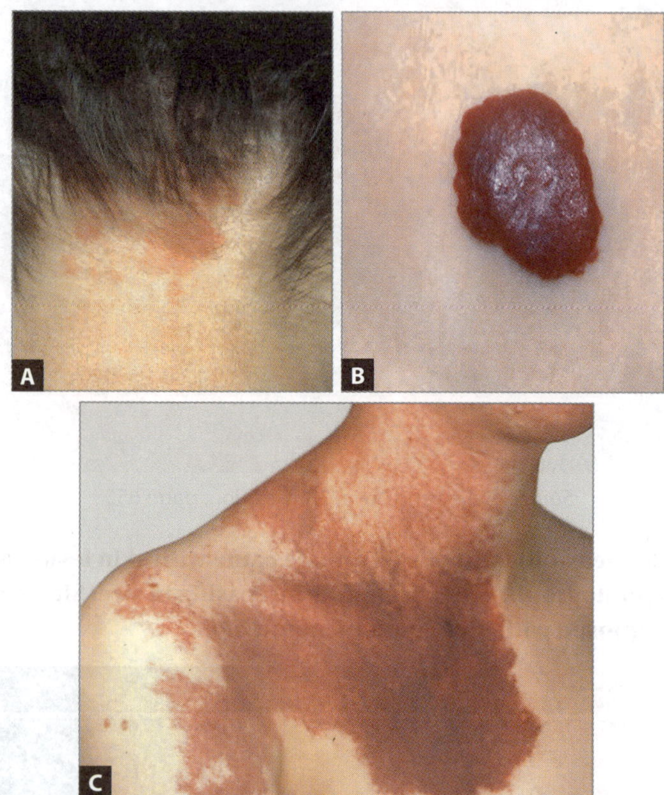


*Source:* Bailey and Love, 28th edition, pages 660 and 661.

**Q13.**

a. Define ulcer.

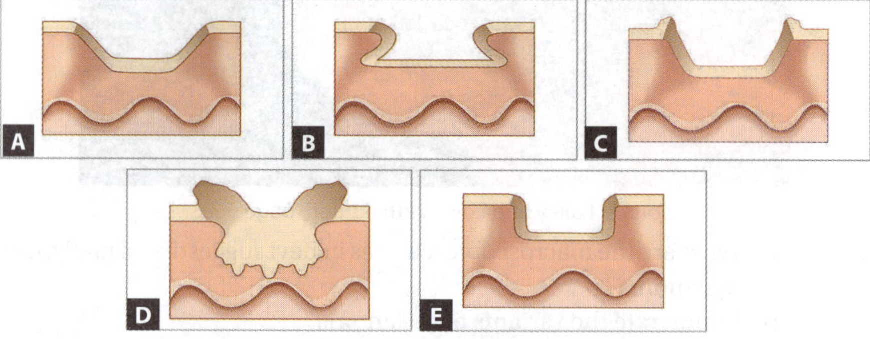


*Source:* Bailey and Love, 28th edition, page 663.

b. Identify type of ulcers by clinical edges of the ulcer and give one example of each as shown in diagram.

# ANSWERS

**Ans. 1** a. 
- Stratum basalis (deep)
- Stratum spinosum
- Stratum granulosum
- Stratum lucidum
- Stratum corneum (superficial)

b. Melanocytes are dendritic cells which originate from neural crest. Located in the basal epidermis.

c. Arrector pili muscle—Hair elevation at the time of stress and cold.

**Ans. 2** a. Neurofibromatosis

b. This condition is autosomal dominant, develops from genetic mutation with variants.

Neurofibromatosis type I (NF1)/Von Recklinghausen's disease—Chromosome-17
Neurofibromatosis type II (NF2)—Chromosome-22
Schwannomatosis—Chromosome-22

c. More than five café-au-lait spots
Armpit or groin freckling
Lisch nodules

**Ans. 3** a. Hidradenitis suppurativa (HS)

b. Etiopathogenesis—Caused by follicular occlusion followed by folliculitis, with secondary infection by skin flora (most commonly *Staphylococcus aureus* and Propionibacterium acnes)

c. 
- Lifestyle modification—stop smoking and lose excess weight.
- Conservative management—antiseptic soaps, tea tree oil, and wearing noncompressive and aerated undergarments.
- Medical treatments include topical and oral antibiotics and anti-androgen drugs.
- Surgical management (in selected cases)—Radical excision of lesion with reconstruction.

**Ans. 4** a. Pyoderma gangrenosum (PG)

b. Management—Local wound care with topical antibiotic application Steroid therapy—Surgical debridement is rarely indicated (may exacerbate the condition—mostly patients are immune-compromised).

**Ans. 5**
- *Image A:* Impetigo (honey-colored crust)
- *Image B:* Erysipelas (sharply demarcated erythema and edema on face)
- *Image C:* Cellulitis affecting left leg

**Ans. 6**
- *Image A:* Milia (small, hard, and keratin retention cysts mostly over the face)
- *Image B:* Multiple scrotal epidermal cysts (cystic lesion fixed to the skin with central punctum)
- *Image C:* Cafe-au-lait spots (coffee-colored macules of variable size, two topographical variants:
  1. Smooth border –"coast of California"
  2. Irregular border "coast of Maine"

**Ans. 7**
- *Image A:* Junctional nevus (deeply pigmented macules or papules)
- *Image B:* Compound nevus (maculopapular, pigmented lesion, and becomes most prominent at adolescence)
- *Image C:* Intradermal nevus (intradermal nevi are faintly pigmented)
- *Image D:* Spitz nevus (reddish brown nodules, occasionally deeply pigmented)
- *Image E:* Halo nevus (halo of depigmentation around any benign nevus)

**Ans. 8**
- *Image A:* Mongolian spot (congenital blue gray macule found on the sacral region, pigmentation initially deepens and regresses completely by age 7 years)
- *Image B:* Blue nevus (benign skin lesion, four times more common in children and affecting the extremities and face)
- *Image C:* Nevus of Ota (dermal, melanocytic hamartoma, blue or gray macule in the trigeminal V1 and V2 dermatomes)
- *Image D:* Nevus of Ito (dermal melanocytosis in the shoulder region)
- *Image E:* Giant congenital pigmented nevus (GCPN) or giant hairy nevus (hamartoma of nevo-melanocytes, tendency to dermatomal distribution)
- *Image F:* Rhinophyma (end-stage sequela of nasal acne rosacea, nasal sebaceous gland hypertrophy, and hyperplasia more affect elderly men).

**Ans. 9**
a. Ulcerating basal cell carcinoma on the lower eyelid.
   - Variants—localized nodular
     - Nodulocystic
     - Cystic
     - Pigmented
     - Nevoid
   - *Generalized—superficial:* Multifocal and superficial spreading; *Infiltrative:* Morpheic, ice pick, and cicatrizing.

b. Etiopathogenesis—slow-growing and locally-invasive, malignant tumor of pluripotential epithelial cells arises from basal epidermis due to-excessive sun exposure/ultraviolet ray. Arsenical compounds, coal tar, aromatic hydrocarbons, ionizing radiation, and genetic skin cancer syndromes.

c. Surgical management—Wide local excision + reconstruction
Mohs' micrographic surgery
Nonsurgical—topical treatments (5-fluorouracil, imquimod) in biopsy-proven, elderly, or infirm patients.

**Ans. 10** a. i. Erythroplasia of Queyrat—squamous cell carcinoma on the glans penis (Paget's disease of the penis)
ii. Lower lip squamous cell carcinoma

b. Treatment approach
- Detailed history with clinical examination
- Investigations—routine hematological and biochemical blood investigations

Tissue diagnosis—Biopsy
Radiological imaging—X-ray chest
Definitive management
- Surgical excision using surgical loupe magnification.
- 4 mm clearance—squamous cell carcinoma (SCC) measures <2 cm across,
- 1 cm clearance margin if >2 cm.
- Follow-up up to 5 years

**Ans. 11** a.
- Change in size, shape, and color
- Thickness (elevation/nodularity, or ulceration)
- Satellite lesions (pigment spreading into surrounding area)
- Tingling/itching/serosanguinous discharge (usually late signs)

b.
- Superficial spreading melanoma (SSM)
- Nodular melanoma (NM)
- Lentigo maligna melanoma
- Acral lentiginous melanoma (ALM)
- Others—Amelanotic melanoma, desmoplastic melanoma

c. History and clinical examination
- Excision biopsy with 2–3 mm margin of skin and a cuff of subdermal fat (for tissue diagnosis and Breslow thickness)
- Surgery—Wide local excision with regional lymph node dissection (if sentinel lymph node present)
  - In situ melanoma—wide excision of 5 mm margin
  - Melanoma <1 mm deep—1 cm margin
  - Deeper lesions—2 cm only margin is recommended
  - Targeted combination therapy in stage IV melanoma using dabrafenib or vemurafenib/trametinib, ipilimumab, or nivolumab.

**Ans. 12**
- *Image A:* Salmon patch (a pinkish macule, usually at the nape of neck and disappears at 1 year)
- *Image B:* Capillary hemangioma (strawberry nevus) (most common "birth mark", most commonly on head and neck, 10% resolve each subsequent year, with 70% resolved by 7 years old.)
- *Image C:* Capillary vascular malformations "port-wine" stains (appear at birth as flat, smooth, intensely purple-stained, frequently on head and neck, often within the maxillary and mandibular dermatomes of the trigeminal nerve.)

**Ans.13** a. An ulcer is a discontinuity of the covering epithelium—skin or mucous either due to molecular death or traumatic removal.

b. A. Sloping edges—Healing ulcer/Venous ulcer
   B. Undermined edge—Tuberculous ulcer
   C. Rolled out (everted) edge—Basal cell carcinoma (rodent ulcer)
   D. Everted edge and irregular thickened—Epithelioma
   E. Punched-out edge and thin base—Syphilis, gummatous ulcer, and deep trophic ulcers.

# 28 CHAPTER Burns

## QUESTIONS

**Q1. A 36-year-old factory worker came in emergency with 1 hour ago burn injury over face, neck, chest, and both shoulder region. Patient has complaints of (c/o) severe burning pain, with hoarseness of voice, on examination conscious, blood pressure (BP) 110/80 mm Hg, pulse 95/min, and $SpO_2$—94% on room air.**

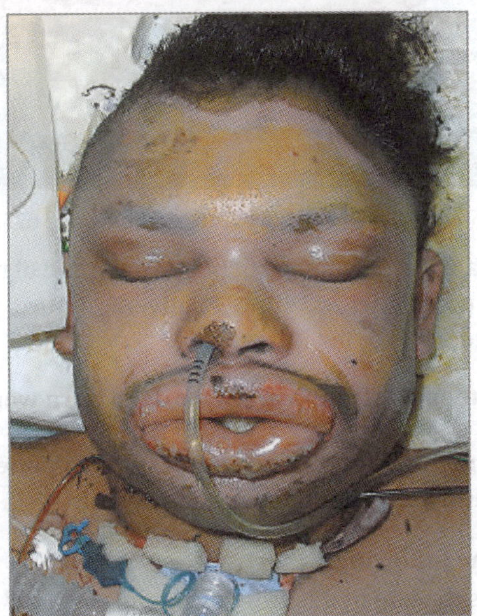

*Source:* Bailey and Love, 27th edition, page 618.

a. In any burn patient what are the warning signs of burns to the respiratory system?
b. What are the major determinants of the outcome of a burn (any five)?
c. What is the line of management for this patient?
d. What is the Parkland formula for fluid resuscitation?

**Q2.** **Brief the various approaches to assess the burn surface area.**

**Q3.** **Classify the burn according to the depth with identifying clinical features.**

**Q4.** **A 32-year-old gentleman came in emergency with full thickness burn over both upper limbs, both lower limbs, chest, abdomen, and genitals. Patient is conscious, oriented, BP—100/70, pulse 96/min, $SpO_2$ 96% on room air with left radial pulse not palpable.**

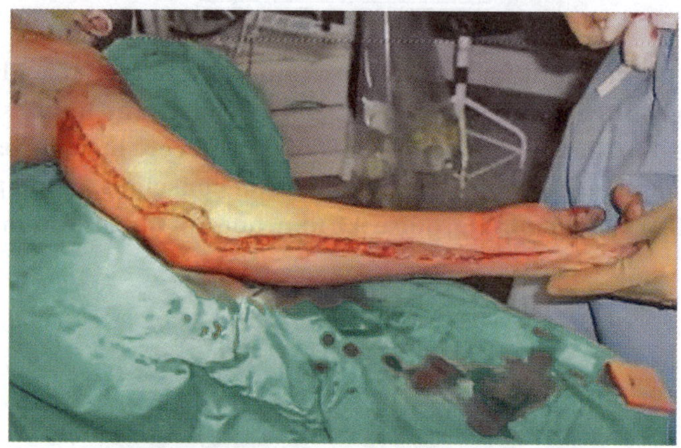

*Source:* Bailey and Love, 27th edition, page 625.

a. Calculate the percentage of burn as per rule of nine.
b. What procedure is done in given picture and appropriate management for left upper limb?

**Q5.** **Enumerate topical application for deep burn wounds.**

**Q6.** **What is the nutrition management in burn patients, give Curreri formula and Sutherland formula for feeding?**

**Q7.** **Answer the following:**

a. What is the aim of the dressing in burn wound?
b. What is "Biobrane"?
c. What are the preferred dressing materials for burn wounds?

**Q8.** **Describe the electric burn injury and management.**

**Q9.** **Classify the superficial burn as per etiology.**

**Q10.** **Write the differences between superficial acid burn and alkali burn.**

## ANSWERS

**Ans. 1** a. *Warning signs of burns to the respiratory system:*
- Burns around the face and neck
- A history of being trapped in a burning room
- Change in voice
- Stridor

b. *Major determinants of the outcome of a burn (any five):*
- Etiology of burn (chemical/electric/thermal)
- Percentage surface area involved
- Depth of burns
- Presence of an inhalational injury
- Age of the patient
- Nutritional status of patient
- Other comorbidities and immune status of patient

c. *Line of management:*

A: Airway control—early elective intubation is safest (preferably fiber optic laryngoscopy) in late cases cricothyroidotomy/ tracheostomy.

B: Breathing and ventilation—nebulizers and warm humidified oxygen.

C: Circulation—two wide bore intravenous peripheral cannula and starts crystalloids.

D: Disability—neurological status

E: Exposure with environmental control

F: Fluid resuscitation

d. Parkland formula = Total percentage body surface area × weight (kg) × 4 = volume (mL) (half of this volume is given in the first 8 hours and the second half is given in the subsequent 16 hours.)

**Ans. 2**
- "Rule of nines" (can be used as a rough guide to total body surface area (TBSA)]
  Each upper limb—9% TBSA,
  Each lower limb—18%,
  The torso 18% each side,
  The head and neck 9%
- Lund and Browder chart—useful in larger burns and pediatric age group.
- Patient's whole hand is 1% TBSA, and is a useful in small burns.

**Ans. 3**
- Superficial partial-thickness burns
  - Blistering and/or loss of the epidermis
  - Underlying dermis is pink and moist

  - Blanching present
  - Pinprick sensation normal
- Deep partial-thickness burn
  - Epidermis lost
  - No blanching
  - Sensation reduced
- Full-thickness burns
  - Hard, leathery feel
  - Appearance may vary from normal skin to charred black
  - No capillary return
  - Completely anesthetized

**Ans. 4** a. 73%

b. After resuscitation emergency, surgery:
  - Left upper limb mid axial escharotomy
  - Extend the wound beyond the deep burn, avoiding major nerves
  - Apply hemostatic dressing elevate the limb, postoperatively
  - Followed by burn wound care with antibacterial dressing
  - Pain management
  - Fluid resuscitation/blood transfusion if require
  - Antibiotic coverage
  - Elevate the limb postoperatively
  - Nutritional assessment and replenish as per requirement

**Ans. 5** Topical treatment of deep burns
- 1% silver sulfadiazine cream
- 0.5% silver nitrate solution
- Mafenide acetate cream
- Serum nitrate, silver sulfadiazine, and cerium nitrate

**Ans. 6** Burns patients need extra feeding
- Adult with a burn >15% (10% in children) of TBSA has an increased nutritional requirement
- All 20% or greater of TBSA should receive a nasogastric tube
- Start feeding within 6 hours of the injury
- Prefer enteral feeding over parenteral feeding

*Curreri formula*

*Age 16–59 years:* (25) W + (40) TBSA

*Age 60+ years:* (20) W + (65) TBSA

*Sutherland formula*

*Children:* 60 kcal/kg + 35 kcal%TBSA

*Adults:* 20 kcal/kg + 70 kcal%TBSA

**Ans. 7** a. Aims of dressing in burn wound

- Decrease pain
- Protect wound
- Isolate wound

b. Biobrane is a bilaminar dressing made up of

- Inner layer—knitted nylon threads coated with porcine collagen.
- Outer layer—rubberized silicone impervious to gases (but not fluids and bacteria).
- Ideal wounds for Biobrane—burn wounds should be fresh (<24 hours), sensate, show capillary blanching and refill.

c. Nonadherent dressing such as Vaseline gauze or Mepitel

- Biobrane is a bilaminar dressing
- Duoderm or hydrocolloid dressings

**Ans. 8** Low-voltage injuries—small, localized, and deep burns

- Can cause cardiac arrest through pacing interruption
- High-voltage injuries damage by flash (external burn) and conduction (internal burn)
- *Sources of damage:* (1) Flash; (2) Flame; (3) Current
- Can cause—*Myocardium* damage
- Due to damage of underlying muscles compartment
- Syndrome/myoglobinuria followed by acute kidney injury

*Management:*

A: Airway control

B: Breathing and ventilation

C: Circulation

D: Disability

E: Exposure with environmental control

F: Fluid resuscitation

- Maintain a high urine output of up to 2 mL/kg body weight per hour
- Acidosis correction by bicarbonate
- Pain management
- Wound management
- For compartment syndrome fasciotomies or amputation

**Ans. 9** Burn etiology

- Thermal burn—Cold/heat burn
- Electric burn
- Chemical burn—Acidic/alkali burn
- Ionizing radiation burn

**Ans. 10** Difference between acid burn and alkali burn

| | *Acid burn* | *Alkali burn* |
|---|---|---|
| Etiology | Strong acids—$H_2SO_4$, HCl, etc. | Strong base—KOH, NaOH |
| Pathology | Coagulation necrosis | Saponification followed by liquefaction necrosis |
| Burn | 2nd degree | Deep |
| Edema | Mild | Marked |
| Eschar | Hard | Soft |
| Management | Copious lavage with water<br>• Calcium gluconate gel topically<br>• Early excision and later split skin graft (SSG) | Copious lavage with water<br>• Wound management |

7

SECTION

# Head and Neck

# CHAPTER 29 Cranial Neurosurgery

## QUESTIONS

**Q1. Identify the clinical condition and probable associated condition and reason behind it.**

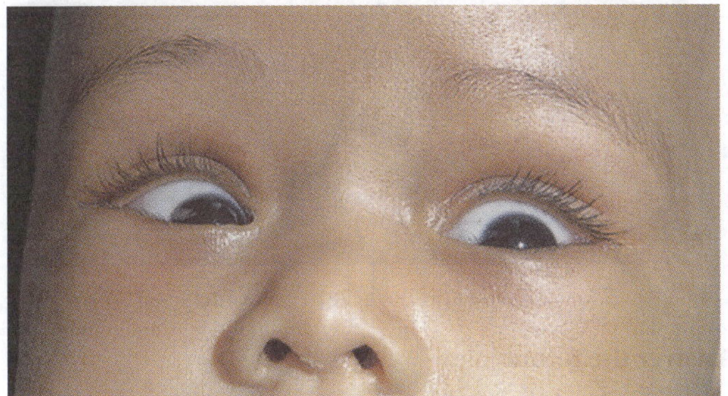

*Source:* Bailey and Love, 28th edition, page 702.

**Q2. Identify the graph and P1, P2, and P3.**

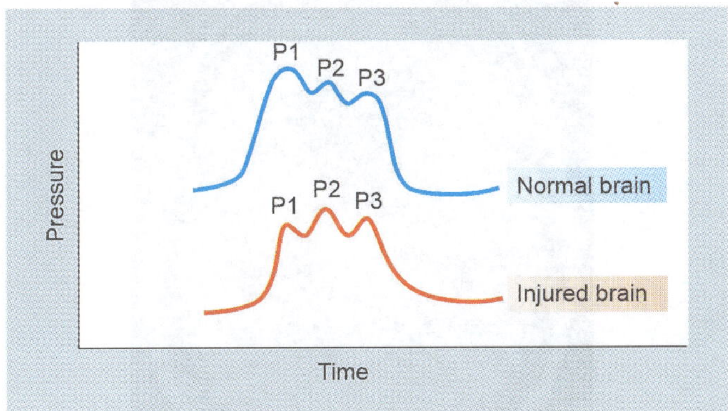


*Source:* Bailey and Love, 28th edition, page 703.

**Q3. Answer the following:**

a. What are the etiologies of hydrocephalus?
b. Identify the specimen and probable associated condition.

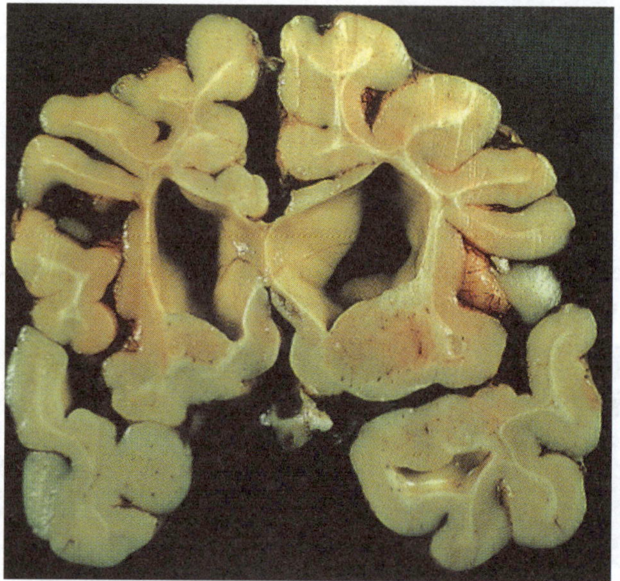

*Source:* Bailey and Love, 28th edition, page 704.

**Q4. Answer the following:**

a. What is normal pressure hydrocephalus?
b. Identify the image and probable associated condition.

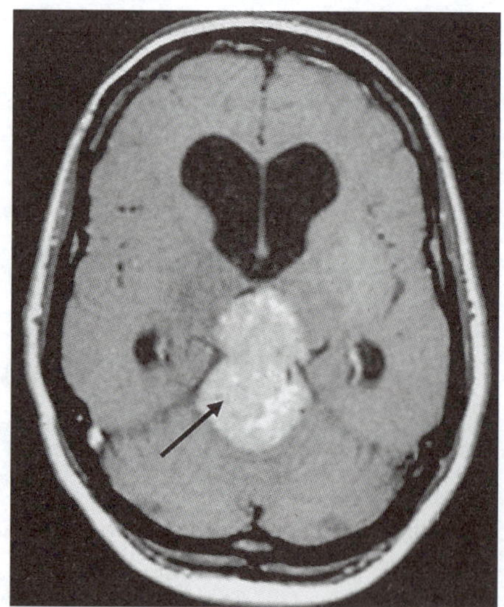

*Source:* Bailey and Love, 28th edition, page 704.

**Q5. Identify the image and associated complication.**

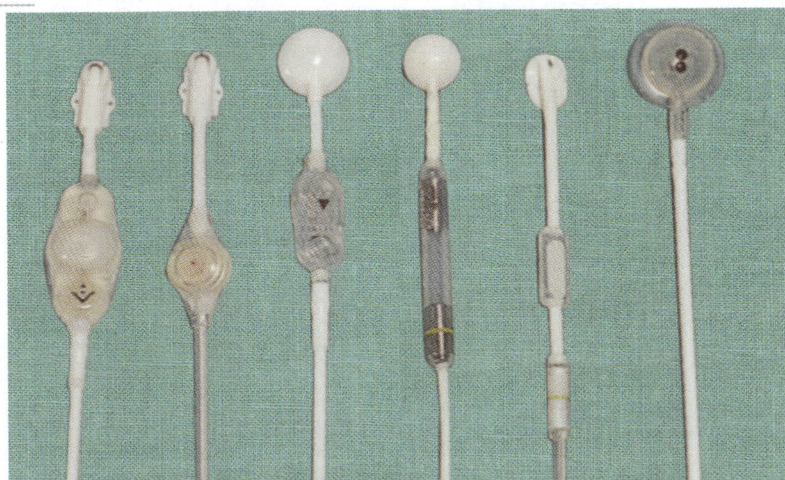

*Source:* Bailey and Love, 28th edition, page 705.

**Q6. Answer the following:**

a. Identify the image and associated condition.

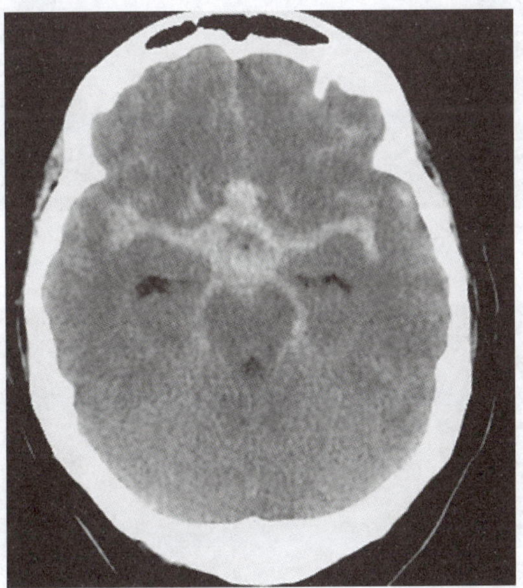

*Source:* Bailey and Love, 28th edition, page 709.

b. What is grading protocol of above condition according to World Federation of Neurosurgical Societies (WFNS)?

c. What is Terson syndrome?

## Q7. Identify the image and associated condition and procedure

a.

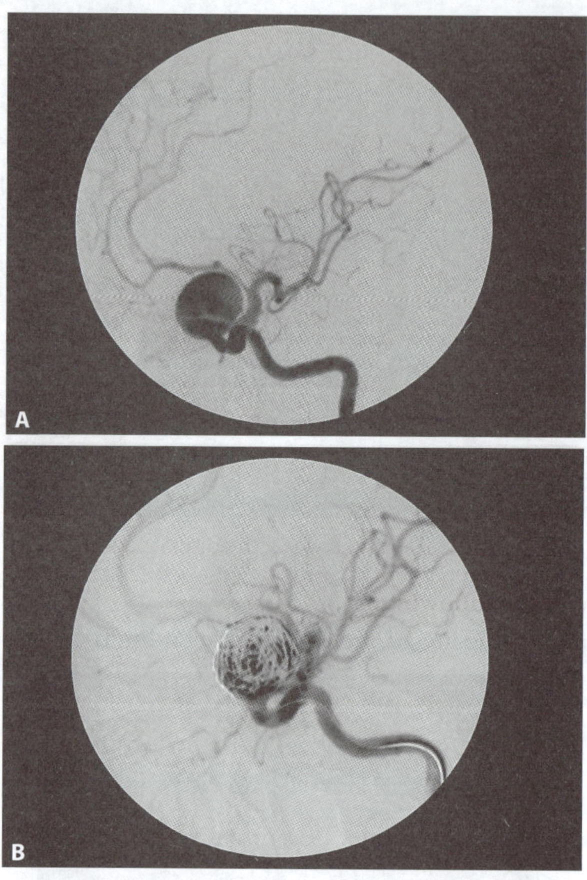


*Source:* Bailey and Love, 28th edition, page 710.

b.

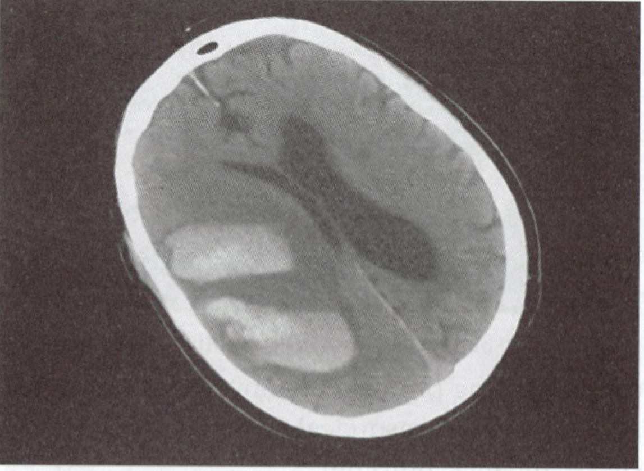

*Source:* Bailey and Love, 28th edition, page 711.

**Q8. Answer the following:**

a. Identify the image and associated condition.

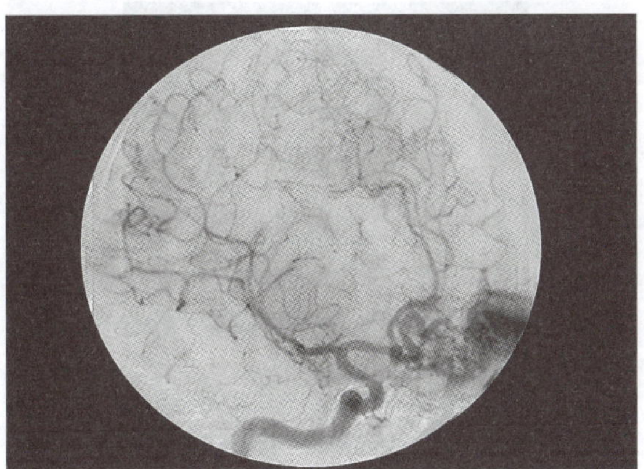

*Source:* Bailey and Love, 28th edition, page 712.

b. Identify the image and associated condition.

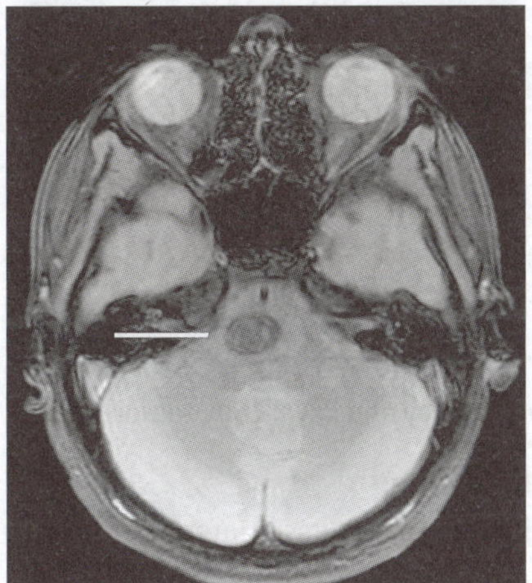

*Source:* Bailey and Love, 28th edition, page 712.

**Q9. Complete the table associated with chromosomal abnormalities associated with brain tumors. By identifying A, B, C, D, E, F, G, H, and I.**

| *Syndrome* | *Gene defect* | *Tumor* |
|---|---|---|
| Neurofibromatosis type 1 | A | B |
| Neurofibromatosis type 2 | C | D |
| Cowden's disease | E | F |
| Hereditary nonpolyposis colorectal cancer | G | H |
| Li–Fraumeni syndrome | I | J |

**Q10. Answer the following:**

a. Identify the image and associated condition.

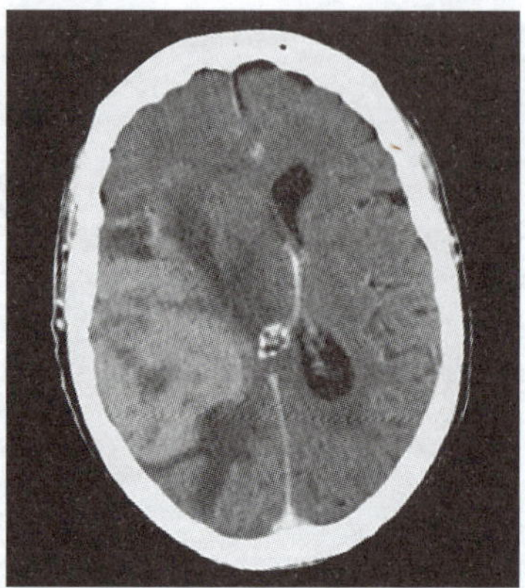

*Source:* Bailey and Love, 28th edition, page 715.

b. Identify the specimen and associated condition.

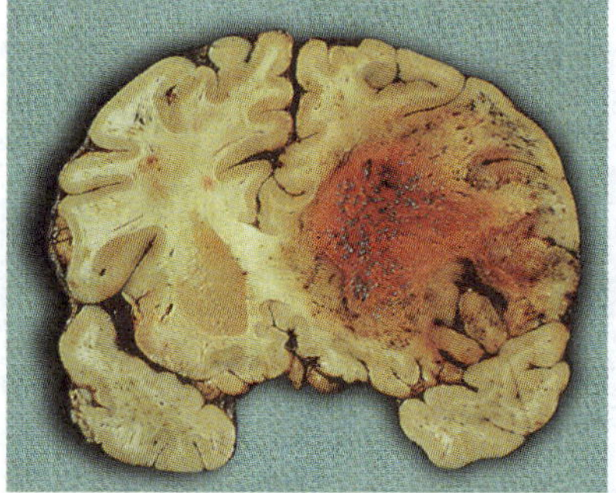

*Source:* Bailey and Love, 28th edition, page 715.

**Q11. Answer the following:**

a. Identify the image and associated condition.

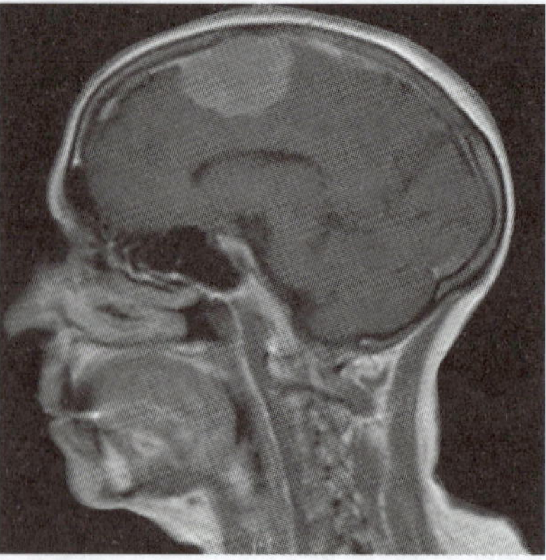

*Source:* Bailey and Love, 28th edition, page 717.

b. Identify the image and associated condition.

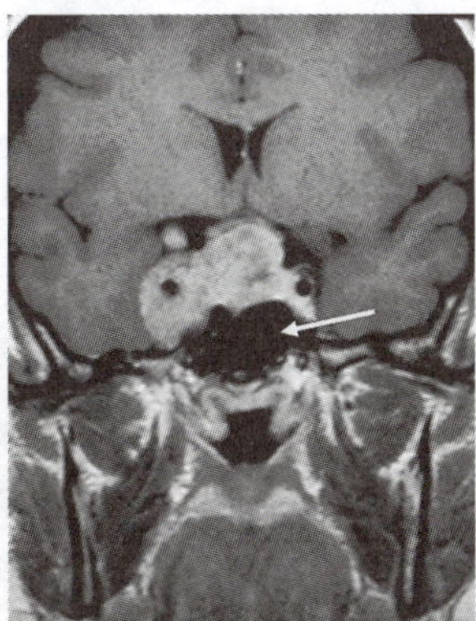

*Source:* Bailey and Love, 28th edition, page 717.

**Q12. Answer the following:**

a. Identify the type of neural tube defect shown in image.

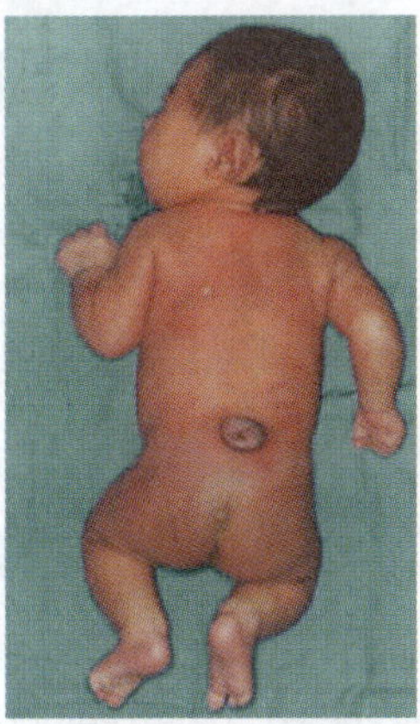

b. What is neural tube defect?

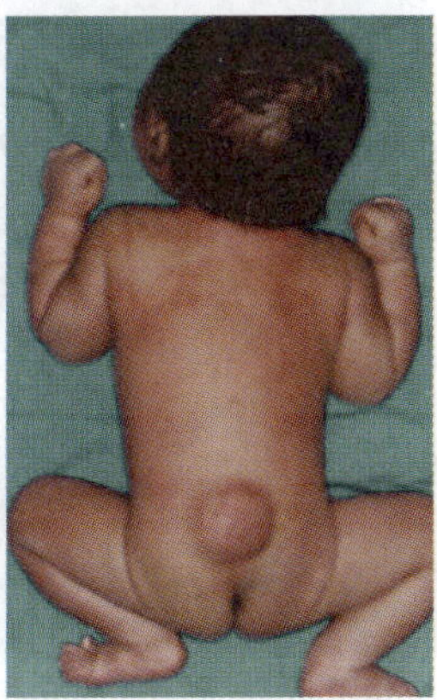

**Q13. Enumerate two posterior fossa malformation.**

**Q14. Answer the following:**

a. What is craniosynostosis?
b. What is I, II, III, IV, and V?
c. Identify the clinical image and associated type of craniosynostosis.

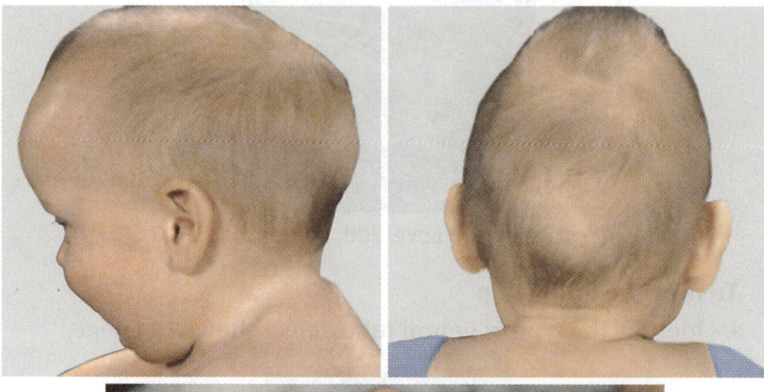

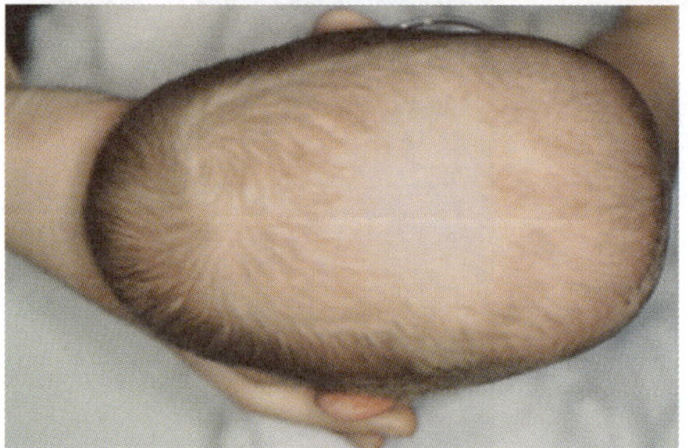

*Source:* Bailey and Love, 28th edition, page 720.

d. Identify the imaging modality and associated condition.

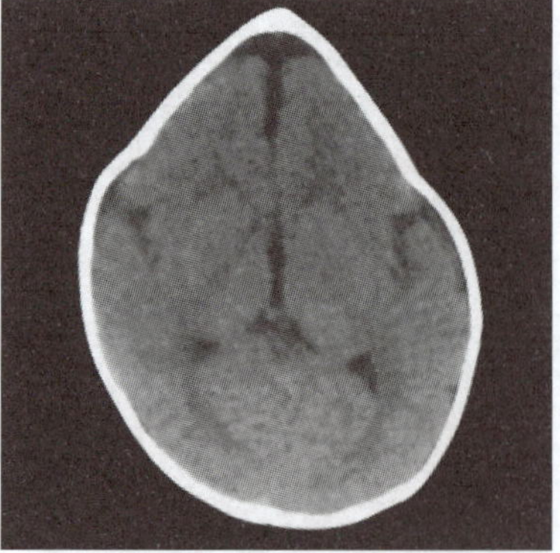

*Source:* Bailey and Love, 28th edition, page 720.

**Q15. Answer the following:**

a. Wada test
b. What is functional neurosurgery?
c. What is Creutzfeldt-Jakob disease (CJD)?

**Q16. What is brain stem death?**

## ANSWERS

**Ans. 1** Parinaud's syndrome with sunsetting—before the skull sutures close, infants with increased intracranial pressure (ICP) may present differently, with noticeable scalp veins, a greater circumference of the skull, and tense, bulging fontanelles. Features of Parinaud's syndrome in infants and older children suggestive of, loss of up gaze known as sunsetting due to raised cerebral spinal fluid (CSF) pressure results in dorsal midbrain compression.

**Ans. 2** Intracranial pressure waveform

| | | |
|---|---|---|
| P1 | Percussion wave | Equates to the pulse of the arteries |
| P2 | Tidal wave | A prominent P2 wave is linked to reduced cerebral compliance in the setting of traumatic brain injury, among other conditions |
| P3 | Dicrotic wave | Represents venous pulsation |

**Ans. 3** a. Etiology of HCP (hydrocephalus)

| *Obstructive HCP* | *Communicating hydrocephalus* |
|---|---|
| • Ventricular lesion<br>• Ventricular wall lesion<br>• Distant ventricular lesion but with a mass effect | • Posthemorrhagic<br>• CSF infection<br>• Raised CSF protein<br>Excessive CSF production (rare)—choroid plexus papilloma/carcinoma |

b. Pathological specimen of hydrocephalic brain

**Ans. 4** a. • *NPH:* Important cause of dementia (easily reversible)
- *Causes:*
  - Idiopathic
  - Previous brain insults [due to subarachnoid hemorrhage (SAH), head injury, meningitis, and tumor]

The trio of incontinence, cognitive deterioration, and gait disturbance is observed in patients. Imaging shows ventriculomegaly, although other dementia diseases may potentially cause cortical atrophy to account for this.

The diagnosis is based on drainage and/or lumbar infusion tests that show improved clinical outcomes and/or changed compliance related to CSF drainage.

Treatment—insertion of a VP shunt

b. Pineal region tumor (arrow) causing obstructive hydrocephalus.

**Ans. 5** *Examples of ventriculoperitoneal shunt valves:* Shunts complications—disconnection, infection, blockage, and overdrainage.

- About 75% of shunt infections manifest within a month, reflecting introduction at the time of shunt placement. Shunt infections have been known to cause fever, headaches, and meningitis.
  - A lumbar puncture or a CSF tap from the shunt reservoir can confirm the diagnosis.
  - Management—shunt removal, external ventricular drainage, or a series of lumbar punctures along with antibiotic treatment. The shunt can be inserted at a different location once CSF analysis confirms the infection has resolved and the protein concentration is normal.
- Individuals who had blocked shunts displayed hydrocephalus symptoms. A CT scan can confirm the diagnosis. Slow refilling or challenging compression may be encountered with shunt reservoirs. Most blockages are caused by cellular and proteinaceous debris, particularly after infection; blood clots, adhesions of the choroid plexus, and valve mechanism failure are other potential reasons.
- Low-pressure headaches, which are usually worse when standing, can be caused by overdrainage. Subdural hygroma or subdural hemorrhage can develop from fluid or blood collection in the subdural space brought on by ventricular collapse. The underdevelopment of the ventricles and subarachnoid spaces in children receiving shunt treatment leads to poor brain compliance, a condition known as the slit ventricle syndrome. Coughing and straining may result in symptoms of elevated ICP in these patients because typical ICP fluctuations are exacerbated.

**Ans. 6** a. Diffuse SAH due to ruptured ACA (anterior communicating artery) aneurysm extending to the prepontine region, ambient cisterns around the brainstem and into both Sylvian fissures.

b. Subarachnoid hemorrhage grading protocol as per the WFNS

| Grade | Glasgow Coma Scale | Focal deficits |
|---|---|---|
| I | 15 | – |
| II | 13–14 | – |
| III | 13–14 | + |
| IV | 7–12 | ± |
| V | 3–9 | ± |

c. Terson syndrome—combination of SAH and vitreous hemorrhage, occurs in 15-20% of patients.

**Ans. 7** a. *Image A:* Internal carotid artery (ICA) giant aneurysm
*Image B:* Giant aneurysm—angiographic embolization (coiling). The single misplaced coil that enters the middle cerebral artery (MCA) and then the distal ICA.

b. Large acute intracerebral hemorrhage (ICH) in the right frontal and parietal lobes region, with surrounding edema and the midline shift.

*Intracerebral hemorrhage:*

- In 10-15% of strokes
- The patient has focal deficits, elevated ICP, and a headache.
- Because high blood pressure can be persistent, it should only be treated and managed.
- Anticoagulants ought to be stopped.
- Clot evacuation is a possibility for treating elevated ICP in fit patients, but it cannot correct deficits.
- To rule out an underlying vascular or neoplastic lesion, imaging may be necessary.

**Ans. 8** a. This angiography shows the arteriovenous malformation (AVM) supplied by the middle cerebral, anterior cerebral, and middle meningeal arteries at 4 o'clock (AVMs are responsible for small proportion of SAH and ICH. Vessels and calcification may be apparent on CT scan or MRI and the lesions are confirmed on angiography).

b. Brainstem cavernoma [cavernoma—discrete venous anomalies within brain tissue, visible on MRI scan but not on angiography that can bleed repeatedly and causing progressive deficit. They can be managed by surgical removal if required.)

**Ans. 9** A. Neurofibromin (chromosome 17)
B. Astrocytomas; neurofibromas
C. Schwannomin (chromosome 22)
D. Acoustic neuromas (bilateral), meningiomas

E. PTEN (chromosome 10) (PTEN—phosphatase and tensin homolog)
F. Astrocytomas
G. Multiple
H. Astrocytomas
I. p53 (chromosome 17)
J. Astrocytomas

**Ans. 10** a. A heterogeneous right frontoparietal lesion with mass effect and midline shift is shown on a contrast-enhanced CT scan; this lesion is most likely glioblastoma multiforme. MRI scan with and without contrast will aid evaluation.

b. Pathological specimen of glioblastoma multiforme

The most typical glial tumors are anaplastic astrocytoma (WHO grade III) and glioblastoma (WHO grade IV) are examples of high-grade gliomas.

*INISS Pointer:* Integrated molecular diagnostic categories have been added to the WHO 2016 classification of gliomas. Gliomas with low-grade histology frequently exhibit characteristic alterations, such as 1p/19q chromosomal codeletion, which is unique to oligodendrogliomas, and point mutations in the isocitrate dehydrogenase (IDH) enzymes. Grade IV tumors, or IDH wild-type "primary" glioblastomas, and occasionally IDH mutant "secondary" glioblastomas, are classified as glioblastomas by the WHO. These may be the consequence of tumors that have already been detected transforming into low-grade gliomas that remain clinically silent. IDH wild-type status is a strong predictor of aggressive malignant propensity even in the absence of high-grade histological features.

**Ans. 11** a. On T1-weighted MRI an extra-axial, A lesion with a durally based origin is developing in the falx area. A meningioma is this condition.

b. The optic chiasm is compressed superiorly by a non-functioning pituitary macroadenoma (arrow), which also reaches into the right cavernous sinus and covers the right carotid artery.

**Ans. 12** a.
- Myelomeningocele (open spina bifida)
- Meningocele (closed spina bifida)

b. *Neural tube defect:* Neural tube closure failure is linked to folate deficiency, family history, and some anticonvulsant medications. Amniocentesis, a diagnostic procedure, and serum $\alpha$-fetoprotein levels, or USG, can be used for prenatal screening.

The following conditions are among the range linked to the posterior neuropore's inability to close:

- *Spina bifida occulta:*
  - Spinous process absent at birth, with no meninges or brain tissue exposed. The base of the spine has a distinctive shallow depression covered in hair.
  - Associated with tethered cord syndrome, which involves thickening of filum terminale, resulting in traction on the spinal cord.
  - Presented with progressive deficits, bladder dysfunction, spasticity, or scoliosis
  - Treatment—spinal cord detethering and surgical exploration
- *Meningocele:*
  - A meningeal sac that is skin-covered and solely made up of CSF herniates via an anterior or posterior bone defect.
  - *Myelomeningocele:* A meningeal sac that herniates and exposes either the spinal cord, the nerves, or both. There is always a Chiari II deformity associated with this syndrome. Open myelomeningocele needs to be surgically repaired as soon as possible because it poses a high risk of infection.
- *Lipomyelomeningocele:* Through the bone defect, adipose tissue linked to the spinal cord herniates into the sacrolumbar soft tissue. This could be linked to bladder problems and necessitate surgical correction of the resulting cord tethering. Failure to close the anterior neuropore results in anencephaly, which is always fatal and replicates the range of spinal dysraphisms in the skull. Failure of fusion, usually in the occipital area, results in craniofacial bifidum. This may associate with herniation of meninges and CSF (meningocele) and brain substance (encephalocele).

**Ans. 13**

- *Chiari malformations:* Cerebellar herniation through foramen magnum
  - *Normal:* Through the foramen magnum, up to 5 mm of the cerebellar tonsillar descent.
  - *Chiari I:* Tonsillar descend of >5 mm. Typically presents in young adults with cough, headaches, and neurological disturbance which reflects brainstem/cerebellar compression and/or formation of a fluid-filled syrinx in the spinal cord as result of disordered CSF flow. The preferred treatments are foramen magnum decompression and shunting.
  - *Chiari II:* Hydrocephalus and myelomeningocele are linked to the tonsils and vermis falling. Clinically presented in infancy.

- *Dandy–Walker malformations:* Infants with hydrocephalus, developmental delay, and macrocephaly exhibit this. The majority of individuals has problems in other organ systems and the central nervous system. Imaging can show a hypoplastic cerebellar vermis, with a massive thin-walled cyst occupying the posterior fossa. Treatment involves shunt placement.

**Ans. 14** a. Types of craniosynostosis.

| *Type* | *Suture involved* | *Clinical features* |
|---|---|---|
| Scaphocephaly | I | Narrow boat-shaped head |
| Brachycephaly | II | Shortened/broad forehead |
| Microcephaly | III | Small head |
| Plagiocephaly | IV | Asymmetric skull |
| Trigonocephaly | V | Pointed narrow forehead |

b. I. Sagittal suture
 II. Coronal suture
 III. All sutures involved
 IV. Unilateral coronal/lambdoid suture
 V. Metopic suture

c. Sagittal suture synostosis-characteristic look with scaphocephaly

d. An axial CT scan reveals significant trigonocephaly as a result of the metopic suture's early fusion.

**Ans. 15** a. *Wada test:* The goal of the neuropsychological evaluation is to determine the risk of language and memory deficits following temporal lobe epilepsy surgery, as well as to appraise the patient's preoperative function and search for concordant focused impairments.

- Sodium amytal is injected into each ICA, with testing speech and memory simultaneously to pinpoint the function.
- The purpose is to confirm language laterality, meaning that resection on the side of the lesion won't have a major impact on verbal memory functions.

b. *Functional neurosurgery:* Uses nerve and brain tissue stimulation or ablation to treat pain, mobility problems, and epilepsy.

- Surgical methods for treating intractable epilepsy include removing one or more seizure foci or implanting a vagal nerve stimulator.
- DBS (deep brain stimulation) using implanted electrodes has replaced lesioning of these structures for management of the drug refractory Parkinson's disease.

- Microvascular decompression, or MVD, is a treatment option for TGN (trigeminal neuralgia). Nerve tract injuries can also trigger reactions in other neuropathic pain syndromes.

c. Creutzfeldt-Jakob disease—uncommon transmissible spongiform encephalopathy, which is always fatal and causes dementia to proceed quickly. A prion, which is a misfolded protein, is the causal agent and cannot be eliminated by standard sterilization methods.

**Ans. 16** *Brain stem death:* Defined as irreversible loss of brainstem and cerebral function. The brainstem death is legally equivalent to death. This is a precondition for harvesting the organs for transplant from the heart-beating donors.

*Diagnosis criteria:*

- Finding the reason behind the irreversible coma
- Elimination of the reversible coma causes
- *Clinical demonstration:* Brainstem function is absent.

This calls for two tests to be conducted by two clinicians in order to prove that the following are absent:

- Response to the pain
- Respiratory drive (apnea despite a $PCO_2$ >6.7 kPa)
- Gag reflex
- Pupillary light reflex
- Vestibulo-ocular reflex
- Corneal reflex
- Oculocephalic reflex

CHAPTER

# 30 The Eye and Orbit

## QUESTIONS

**Q1. Identify the image and associated condition.**

a.

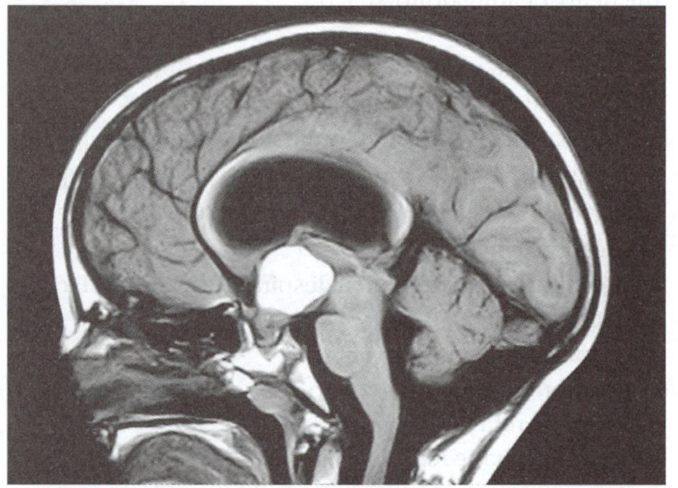

*Source:* Bailey and Love, 28th edition, page 735.

b.

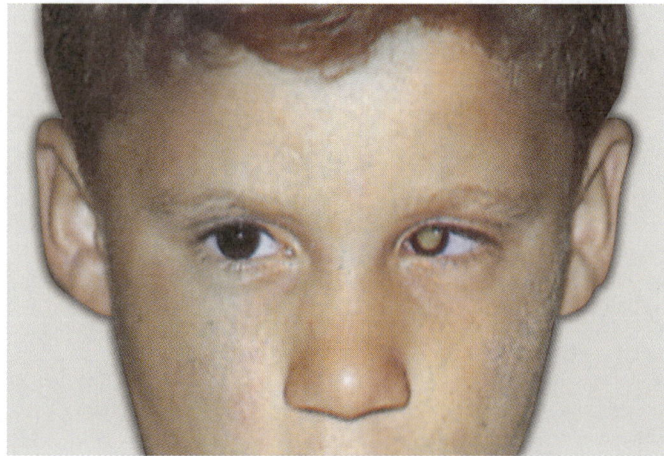

*Source:* Bailey and Love, 28th edition, page 728.

## ANSWERS

**Ans. 1** a. Magnetic resonance imaging scan with sagittal view—craniopharyngioma. A mass in the suprasellar cistern with high-signal intensity because of the proteinaceous fluid that the cyst.

b. Retinoblastoma giving rise to white pupillary reflex.

CHAPTER

# 31 Developmental Abnormalities of the Face, Mouth, and Jaws: Cleft Lip and Palate

## QUESTIONS

**Q1. Classify the craniofacial abnormalities.**

**Q2. A 38-year-old primigravida female came in OPD with her husband has history of cleft lip repair at his age of 6 month.**
**What are the prenatal management of the craniofacial abnormalities?**

**Q3. What congenital condition depicted in pictures?**

a. 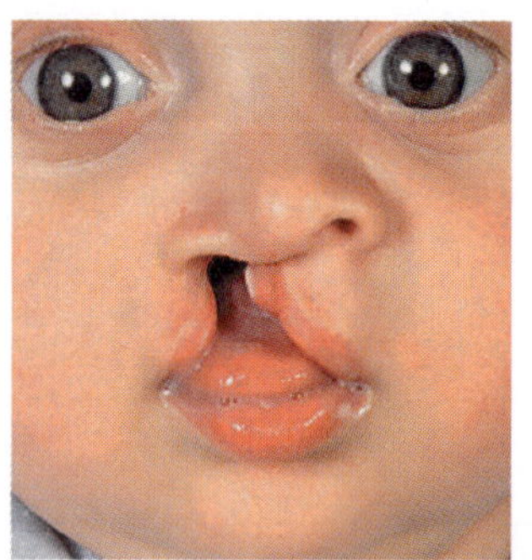

b. 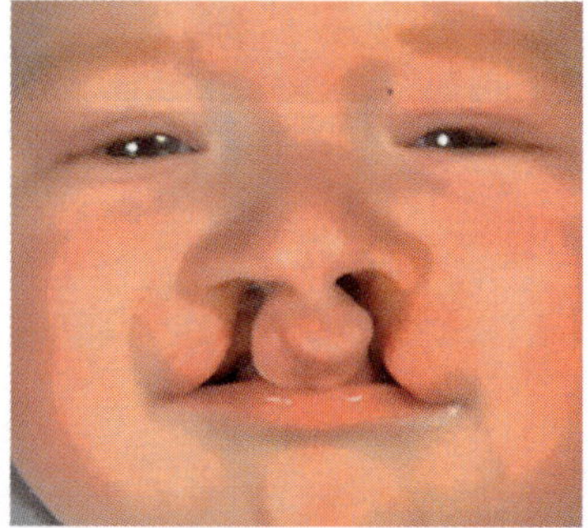

c. 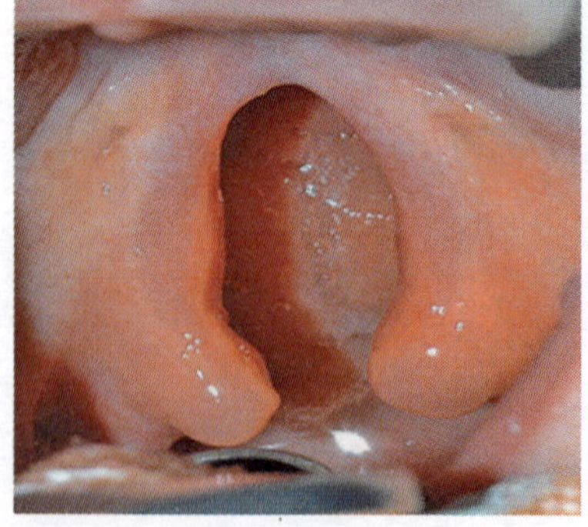

*Source:* Bailey and Love, 28th edition, page 741.

**Q4. Elaborate this classification depicted in picture.**

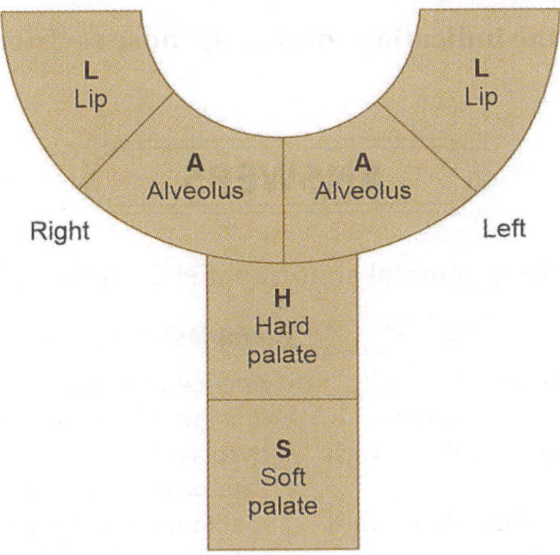


*Source:* Bailey and Love, 28th edition, page 741.

**Q5. A 2-month-old baby in OPD presented with complete right unilateral complete cleft lip, alveolus, hard palate, and soft palate as shown in picture.**

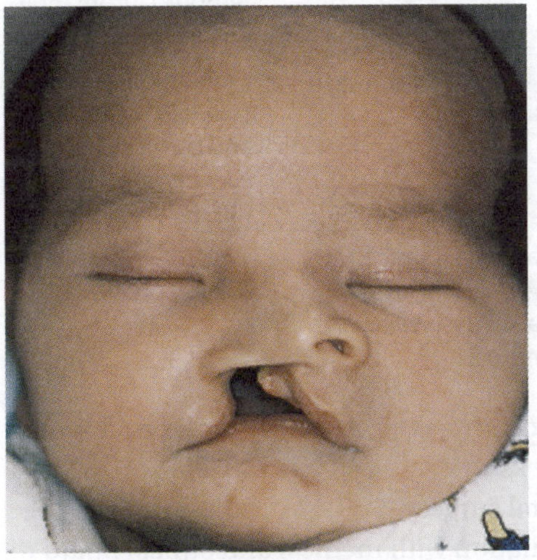

*Source:* Bailey and Love, 28th edition, page 743.

How will you code this patient as per LAHSAL classification in your prescription?

**Q6. What is Veau classification system?**

**Q7. Brief the immediate/neonatal care for a patient with a cleft and/or palate.**

**Q8. What is the preferred age for cleft lip and palate repair?**

**Q9. What are the indications of cleft lip/nose revision surgery?**

## ANSWERS

**Ans. 1** Types of developmental abnormalities of the face, mouth, and jaws.

| *Types* | *Examples* |
|---|---|
| • Cerebrocranial dysplasias<br>• Cerebrofacial dysplasias<br>• Craniofacial dysplasias with clefting<br>• Craniofacial dysplasias with dysostosis | • Anencephaly, microcephaly<br>• Rhinencephalic and oculo-orbital dysplasias<br>• Lateronasomaxillary, medionasomaxillary, intermaxillary, and maxillomandibular clefting<br>• Sphenoidal, sphenoidal frontal, frontal, frontofrontal, frontonasoethmoidal, internasal, nasal, premaxillomaxillary, nasomaxillary, maxillozygomatic, zygomatic, zygoauromandibular, temporoauromandibular, mandibular, and intermandibular |
| • Craniofacial dysplasias with synostosis | • *Craniosynostosis:* Lambdoid and sagittal<br>• *Craniofaciosynostosis:* Metopic, coronal, and bicoronal<br>• *Faciosynostosis:* Vomeropremaxillary (Binder syndrome) |
| • Craniofacial dysplasias with dysostosis and synostosis<br>• Craniofacial dysplasias with dyschondrosis | • Crouzon, Apert, and Pfeiffer syndromes<br>• Anencephaly |

**Ans. 2**
- *Prenatal screening:* Anomaly markers, anomaly scan at the age of 20 weeks
- Prenatal surgery
- Termination with medical and ethical board decision
- Best supportive care in preparation for the birth with additional demands and needs
- Counseling and meeting of parents who have experienced the same condition is often very valuable.

**Ans. 3** a. Unilateral (right) cleft lip

b. Bilateral cleft lip

c. Isolated cleft palate

**Ans. 4** *LAHSAL classification:*

- L—right lip
- A—right alveolus
- H—hard palate
- S—soft palate
- A—left alveolus
- L—left lip

Capital letter for complete cleft (LAHSAL)
Small letter for incomplete cleft (lahsal)
Dot (.) for no cleft

**Ans. 5** Complete right unilateral cleft lip [LAHS..]

**Ans. 6** Veau classification system for cleft lip and palate

| Class | Description |
|---|---|
| I | Soft palate only |
| II | Hard and soft palate to the incisive foramen |
| III | Complete unilateral of soft, hard, lip, and alveolar ridge |
| IV | Complete bilateral of soft, hard and/or lip, and alveolar ridge |

**Ans. 7** Babies born with a cleft may have issues with feeding and airway with nonsurgical management in the initial phase:

- Maintain airway
- Appropriate feeding with proper position/expressed milk with specialized feeders
- Rule out other congenital syndromes
- A cleft multidisciplinary team is required to meet all the needs of a child.

**Ans. 8**

- Cleft lip repair—3–6 months of the age
- Cleft palate repair—6–12 months of the age

**Ans. 9** Indications of cleft lip/nose revision surgery are dependent on the site and severity of the residual deformity.

Relative indications for lip revision include:

- Misaligned vermilion
- Lip asymmetry

Relative indications for residual nasal deformity include:

- Incorrect alar base position
- Poor nasal tip projection
- Deviation of cartilaginous nasal septum into the noncleft nostril

# CHAPTER 32 The Pharynx, Larynx, and Neck

## QUESTIONS

**Q1. As given in schematic diagram.**

a. Collection of lymphatic tissues in pharynx known as

b. Name the structures A, B, and C given in picture.

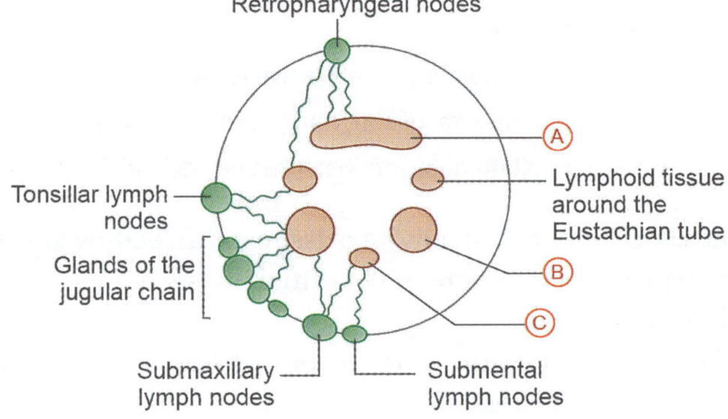


*Source:* Bailey and Love, 28th edition, page 775.

**Q2. Name the structures A, B, C, and D given in upper aerodigestive tract diagram.**

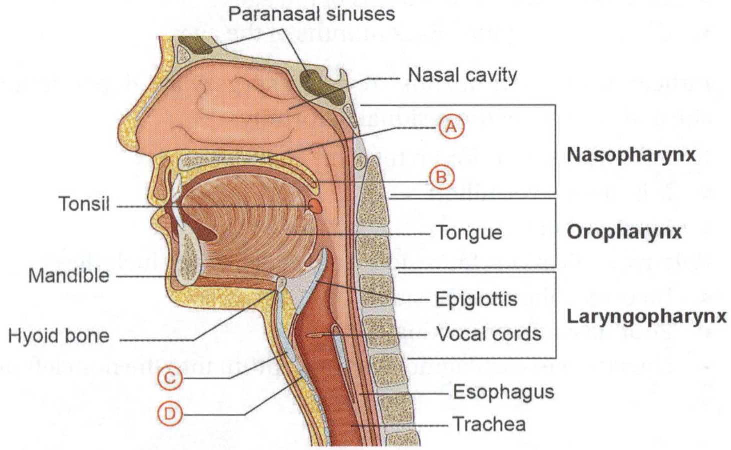


*Source:* Bailey and Love, 28th edition, page 776.

**Q3. Answer the following:**

a. Name the structures A, B, and C given in diagram.
b. What are the major functions of larynx (any 3)?

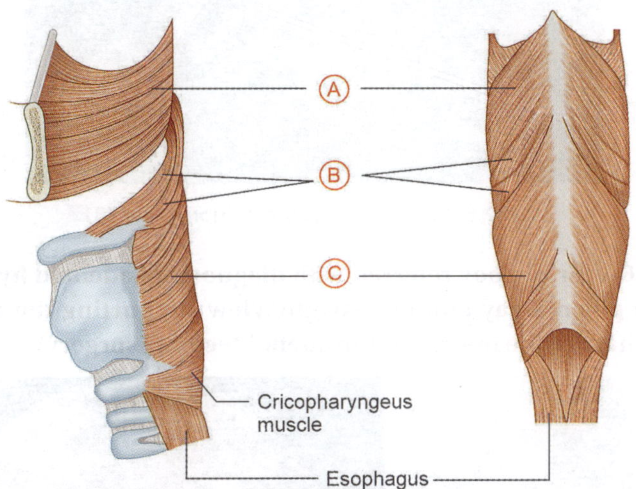


*Source:* Bailey and Love, 28th edition, page 775.

**Q4. Mention the level of lymph nodes A, B, C, D, E, F, and G given in diagram.**

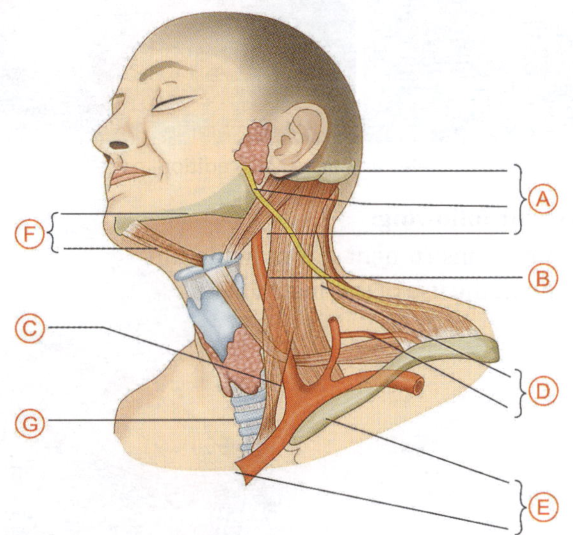


*Source:* Bailey and Love, 28th edition, page 778.

**Q5. Answer the following:**

a. Name the instrument shown in picture.
b. Mention the larynx and pharynx examination techniques along with their advantages and disadvantages (1-1 each).

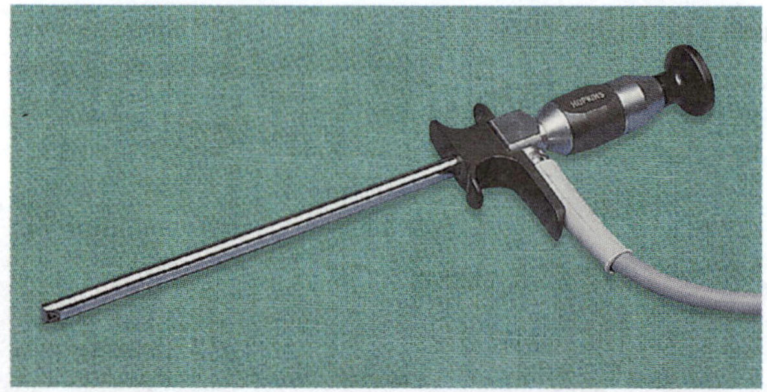

*Source:* Bailey and Love, 28th edition, page 781.

**Q6. A 6-year-old boy referred with diagnosis of adenoid hyperplasia. In given X-ray and endoscopic view supporting the diagnosis. What are the indications of adenoidectomy surgery?**

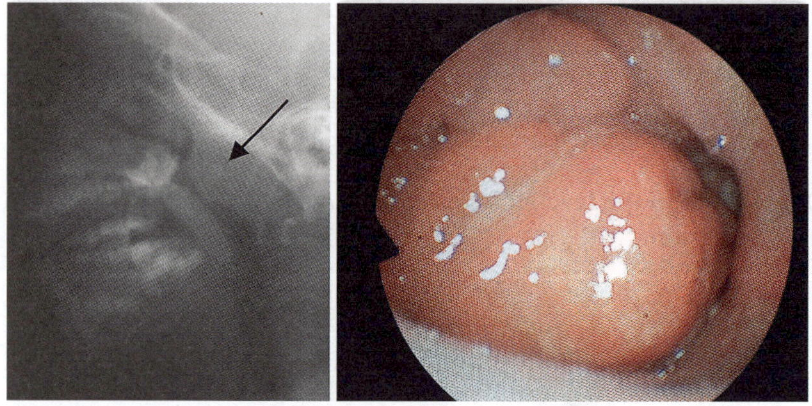

*Source:* Bailey and Love, 28th edition, page 782.

**Q7. Answer the following:**

a. Name the instrument shown in picture.
b. Mention the use of this instrument.

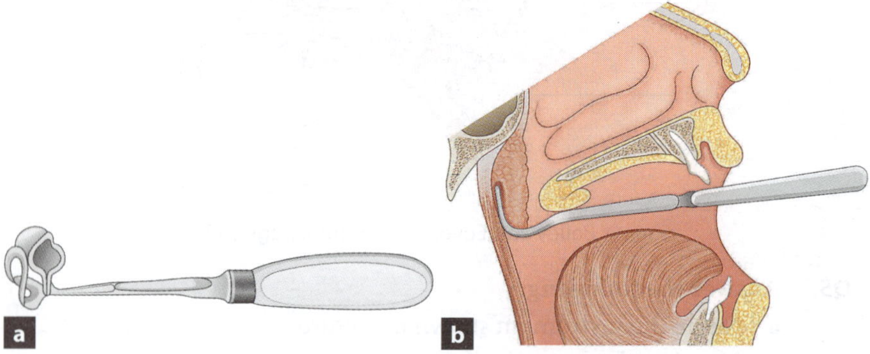


*Source:* Bailey and Love, 28th edition, page 782.

**Q8. A 10-year-old boy presented with a stuffy nose with postnasal drip. The clinical picture and CT report pictures as shown.**

a. Most likely diagnosis
b. Surgical approaches for this condition

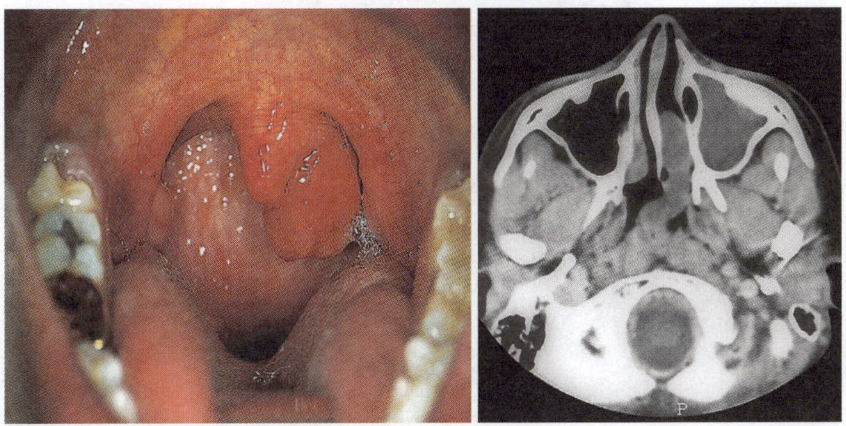

*Source:* Bailey and Love, 28th edition, page 784.

**Q9. What are the probable diagnoses as shown in pictures?**

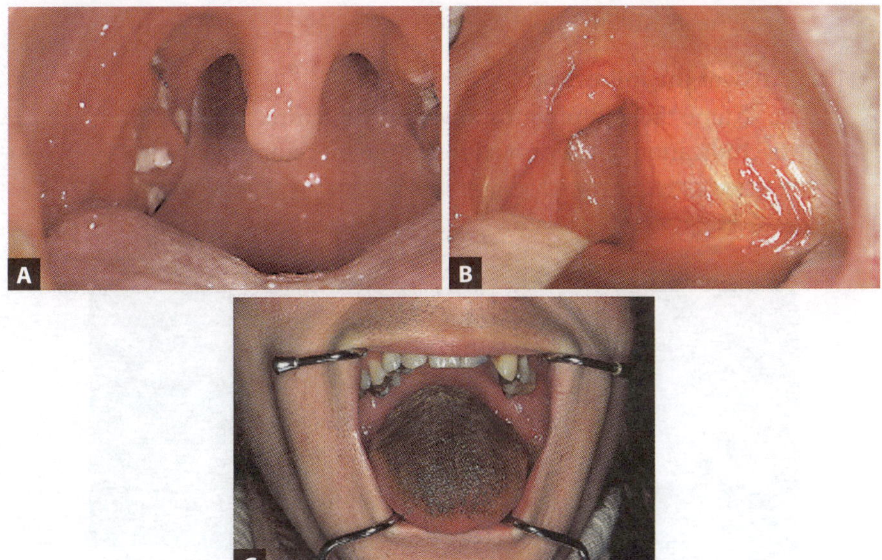


*Source:* Bailey and Love, 28th edition, pages 785, 788.

**Q10. Answer the following:**

a. Mention the indications of tonsillectomy.
b. Complications of tonsillectomy

**Q11. A 60-year-old women presented with regurgitation of undigested food 1 hour after a meal occasionally associated with bending down.**

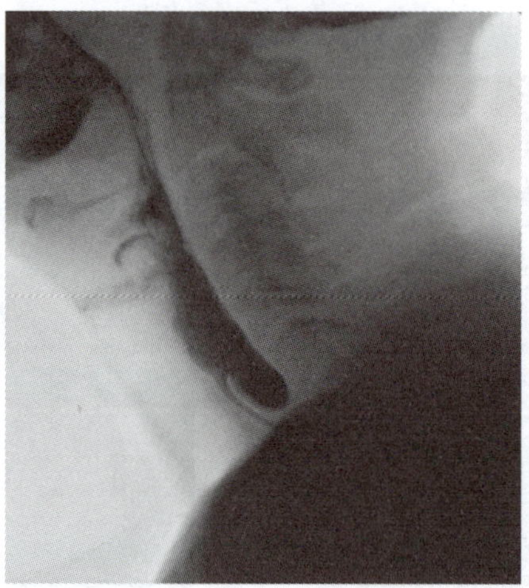

*Source:* Bailey and Love, 28th edition, page 789.

a. Name the condition and which investigation performed as depicted in picture.
b. What is Killian's dehiscence?

**Q12. Answer the following:**

a. Name the equipment shown in the picture.
b. Indication of the procedure where this equipment use

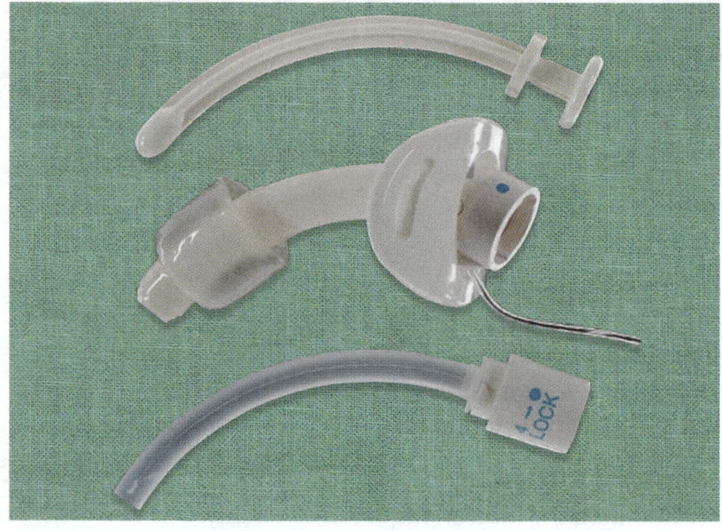


*Source:* Bailey and Love, 28th edition, page 798.

**Q13. Answer the following:**

a. Name the position of the as depicted in diagram "A" and name the surgeries where intraoperative this position often use.
b. Name the flap of trachea in tracheostomy procedure as shown in diagram "B".

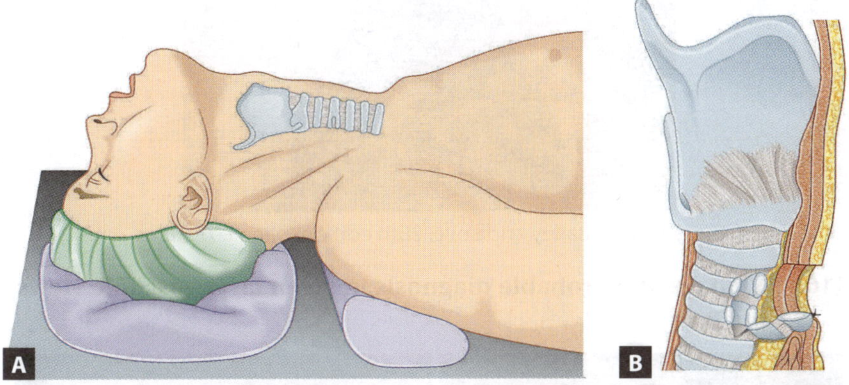


*Source:* Bailey and Love, 28th edition, pages 796, 797.

**Q14. Answer the following:**

a. Name the procedure shown in pictures.
b. Mention the advantages and disadvantages of the tracheostomy over the endotracheal intubation (each any 3).

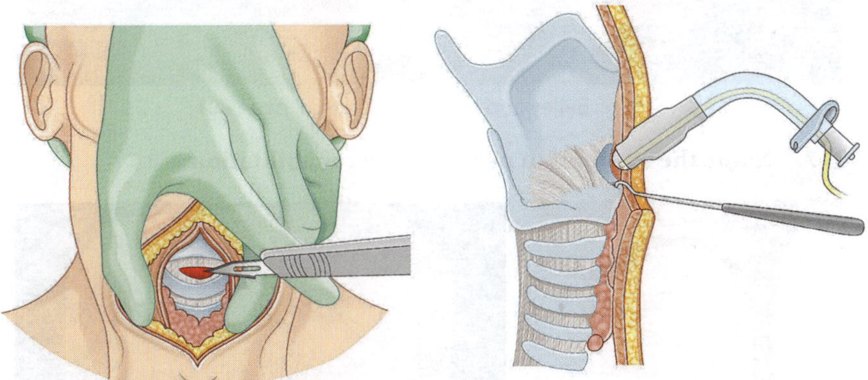

*Source:* Bailey and Love, 28th edition, page 800.

**Q15. A 38-year-old gentleman, teacher by occupation presented with hoarseness of voice. Laryngoscopic findings are shown in picture.**

a. What is the probable diagnosis?
b. Line of management for this patient

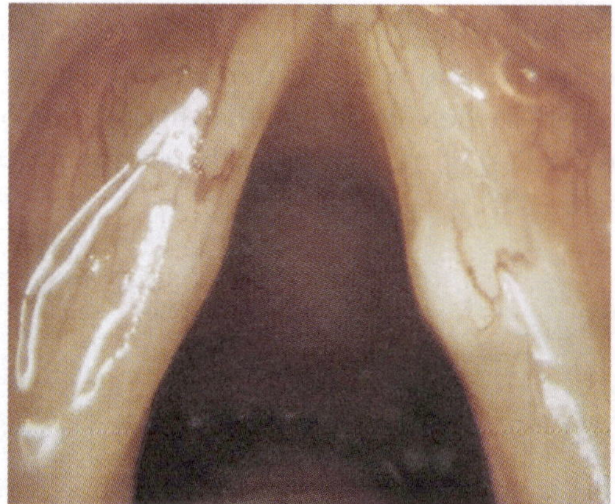

*Source:* Bailey and Love, 28th edition, page 801.

**Q16. What are the probable diagnosis in given laryngoscopic views A and B.**

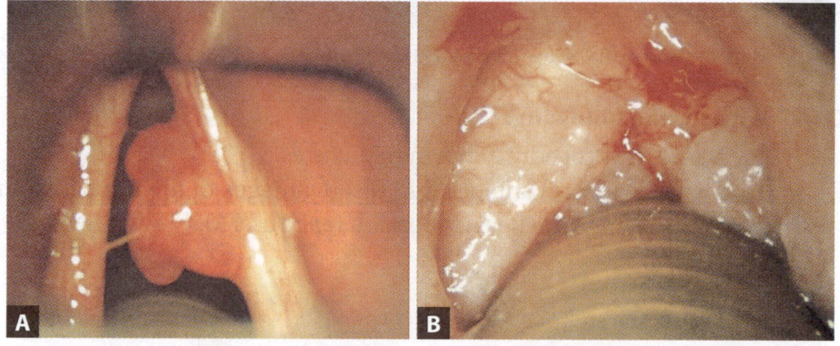


*Source:* Bailey and Love, 28th edition, page 801.

**Q17. Name the equipment uses in voice rehabilitation.**

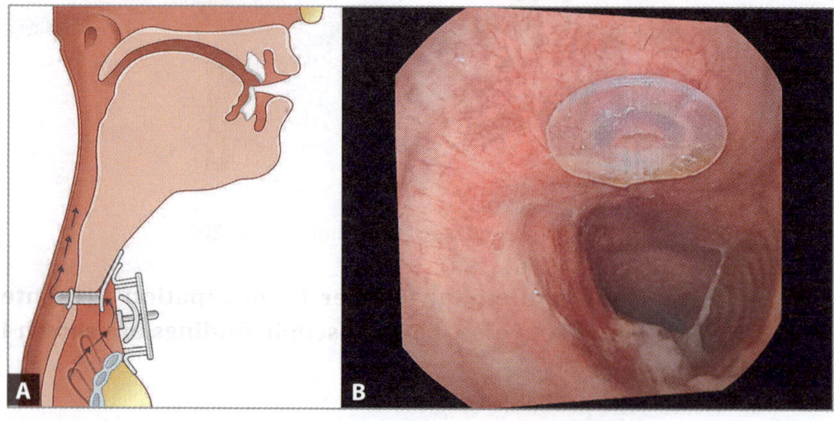


*Source:* Bailey and Love, 28th edition, page 804.

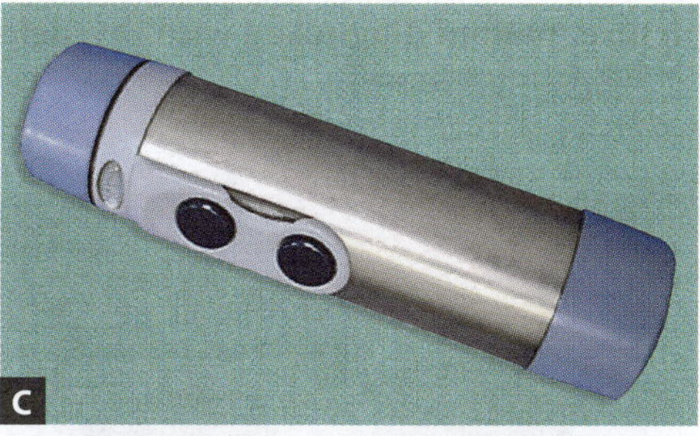

*Source:* Bailey and Love, 28th edition, page 804.

**Q18. A 14-year-old boy presented with discharging sinus at lower third part of lateral side of neck.**

Identify the pictures A, B, and C.

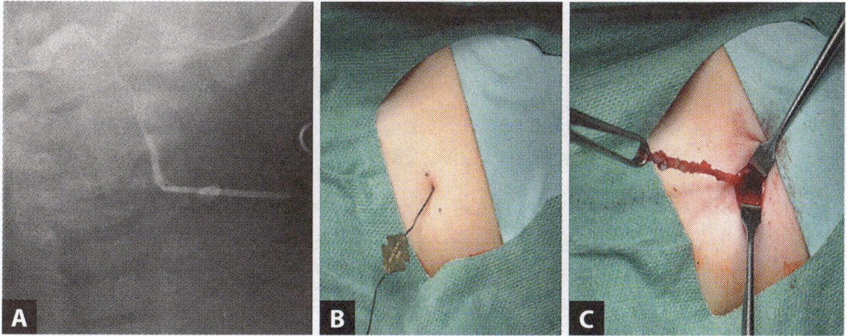

*Source:* Bailey and Love, 28th edition, page 806.

**Q19. A 1-year-old boy presented with swelling over neck, gradually increasing in size. On examination, swelling transilluminating cystic swelling over right side of the neck as shown in picture.**

a. What is the diagnosis?
b. Definitive management for this patient.

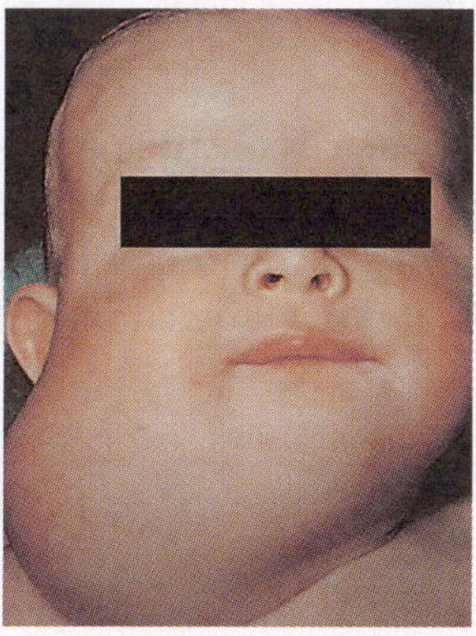

*Source:* Bailey and Love, 28th edition, page 806.

**Q20. In given picture, patient diagnosed with thyroglossal fistula.**

a. Cause of thyroglossal fistula
b. Management for this

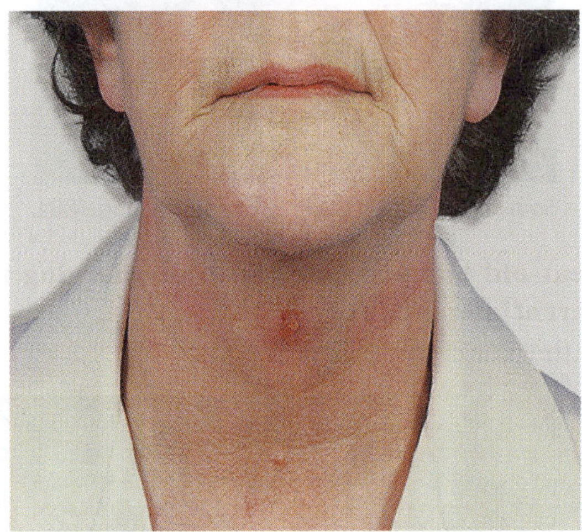

*Source:* Bailey and Love, 28th edition, page 807.

## ANSWERS

**Ans. 1** a. Waldeyer's ring
b. A. Adenoids
B. Faucial tonsils
C. Lingual tonsils

**Ans. 2** A. Hard palate
B. Soft palate
C. Thyroid cartilage
D. Cricoid cartilage

**Ans. 3** a. A. Superior pharyngeal constrictor muscle
B. Middle pharyngeal constrictor muscle
C. Inferior pharyngeal constrictor muscle

b. *Functions of the larynx:* Protection of the lower respiratory tract by:
- Laryngeal inlet closure
- False cords closure
- Glottis closure
- Cough reflex
- Cessation of respiration

- *Phonation:* Sound is produced by the quasiperiodic vibration of vocal folds.
- *Respiration:* Regulation of pressure
- Fixation of chest

**Ans. 4** A. Level II
B. Level III
C. Level IV
D. Level V
E. Level VII
F. Level I
G. Level VI

**Ans. 5** a. Rigid Hopkins' rod or endoscope
b. *Methods for examining the larynx and throat:*

- *Flexible nasolaryngoscopy:*

| *Advantages* | *Disadvantages* |
|---|---|
| Well-tolerated examination procedure | Requires fiberoptic light source |
| Able to examine nasal passages and postnasal space | |

- *Rigid endoscopy:*

| *Advantages* | *Disadvantages* |
|---|---|
| Suitable for use with a stroboscope to assess the voice | Requires fiberoptic light source |
| High-definition view during examination | Bulky and difficult (if prominent gag reflex present) |

- *Laryngeal mirror:*

| *Advantages* | *Disadvantages* |
|---|---|
| No need for fiberoptic light source | Can not record the examination |
| | Low-resolution image |
| | Difficult (if prominent gag reflex present) |

**Ans. 6** *Indications of adenoidectomy surgery:*
*Absolute indications:*

- OSA associated with the postnasal obstruction
- Prolonged serous or recurrent acute otitis media (typically if duration exceeds 3 months)

*Relative indications: Recurrent* rhinosinusitis/postnasal discharge

**Ans. 7** a. St Clair Thomson adenoid curette
b. Curettage of the adenoids

**Ans. 8** a. Antrochoanal polyp
b. Surgery—complete removal—endoscopic approach through the middle meatus of:
- Maxillary sinus
- Open approach—Caldwell-Luc procedure

**Ans. 9**
- *Image A:* Acute follicular tonsillitis
- *Image B:* Quinsy/peritonsillar abscess
- *Image C:* Hairy tongue in HIV (human immunodeficiency virus)-positive patient

**Ans. 10** a. *Indications for tonsillectomy:*

| | |
|---|---|
| Absolute | • Chronic respiratory tract obstruction, sleep apnea, and cor pulmonale<br>• Tonsillar malignancy (suspected) |
| Relative | • Recurrent acute tonsillitis<br>• Chronic tonsillitis<br>• Peritonsillar abscess (quinsy)<br>• Asymmetrical tonsils<br>• Diphtheria carriers<br>• Tonsillitis causing febrile convulsions<br>• Systemic disease caused by β-hemolytic *Streptococcus* (nephritis and rheumatic fever) |

b. *Complications of tonsillectomy:*
- Hemorrhage (immediate/late)
- *Pain/otalgia:*
  - Infection
  - Velopharyngeal insufficiency
- Postoperative airway obstruction
- Injury to oral cavity or oropharyngeal structures

**Ans. 11** a. Pharyngeal pouch on barium swallow
b. Killian's dehiscence is a weak area of posterior pharyngeal wall between the oblique fibers of the thyropharyngeus muscle and the transverse fibers of cricopharyngeus muscle at the lower end of the inferior constrictor muscle.

**Ans. 12** a. Cuffed tracheostomy tube and inner cannula
b. *Indications for tracheostomy:*
- Acute upper airway obstruction
- Potential upper airway obstruction

- Protection of the lower airway
- Patients requiring prolonged artificial respiration

**Ans. 13** a. *Rose position:*
- Hyper-extension of neck and head
- *Surgeries in rose position:*
  - Tracheostomy
  - Thyroid surgery
  - Tonsillectomy
  - Adenoidectomy
  - Uvulopalatopharyngoplasty/cleft palate surgery, etc.

b. Björk flap

**Ans. 14** a. Cricothyroidotomy

b. 
- *Advantages:*
  - Anatomical dead space reduced by approximately 50%
  - Work of breathing reduce
  - Alveolar ventilation increase
  - Level of sedation needed for patient decrease
  - Patients may able to talk and eat with the tube in place.
- *Disadvantages:*
  - Loss of moisture and heat exchange in upper respiratory tract
  - The tracheal epithelium desiccation
  - Production of mucus due to presence of foreign body sensation in the trachea
  - Block the tube due to more viscid mucus and thick crust
  - Chances of aspiration

**Ans. 15** a. Vocal nodules/Singer's nodule

b. *Speech therapy:*
- Symptomatic management for pain
- Surgical removal—microlaryngoscopic dissection or laser techniques
- Postoperative speech therapy

**Ans. 16** a. Vocal fold polyp

b. Laryngeal papillomas

**Ans. 17**
- *Image A:* Blom-Singer valve—an external stoma valve and tracheoeso-phageal fistula created surgically
- *Image B:* Provox voice valve prosthesis (in rear wall of trachea)
- *Image C:* Electrolarynx

**Ans. 18**
- *Image A:* Radiopaque dye on a plain radiograph taken in the fistula tract
- *Image B:* Probing of the fistula tract
- *Image C:* Excision of the fistula tract

**Ans. 19** a. Cystic hygroma

b. *Definitive treatment for cystic hygroma:*
- Complete excision of cyst at early stage
- Injection sclerotherapy agent (alternative option) may reduce the size of the cyst

**Ans. 20** a. Cysts in the thyroglossal duct are a continuation of the track and can be located anywhere along the midline, from the root of the tongue to the thyroid isthmus.

b. *Sistrunk's operation:* The entire thyroglossal tract is removed, including a core of tissue on both sides, the hyoid bone's body, and the suprahyoid tract, which travels from the base of the tongue to the vallecula near the location of the primitive foramen cecum.

33

CHAPTER

# Oral Cavity Cancer

## QUESTIONS

**Q1. Mention the risk factors for oral cavity malignancy (any 5).**

**Q2. Name the neck triangles A, B, and C as shown in diagram.**

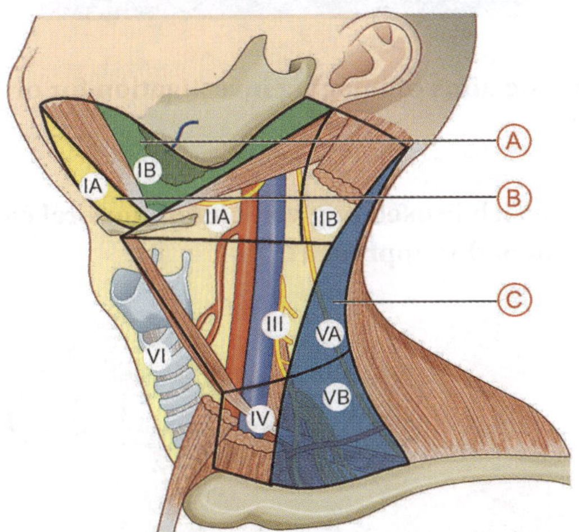


*Source:* Bailey and Love, 28th edition, page 816.

**Q3. What are the boundaries and contents of submandibular triangle?**

**Q4. What are the histological parameters in routine oral cavity squamous cell carcinomas (OCSCC) report?**

**Q5. A 38-year-old gentleman presented with lesion at angle of mouth, lower lip, and oral cavity from 3 months and gradually increasing to the present size as shown in picture.**

Patient has history of tobacco chewing. Answer the following.

a. What are the signs of oral cavity neoplasm?

b. Outline of management for this patient.

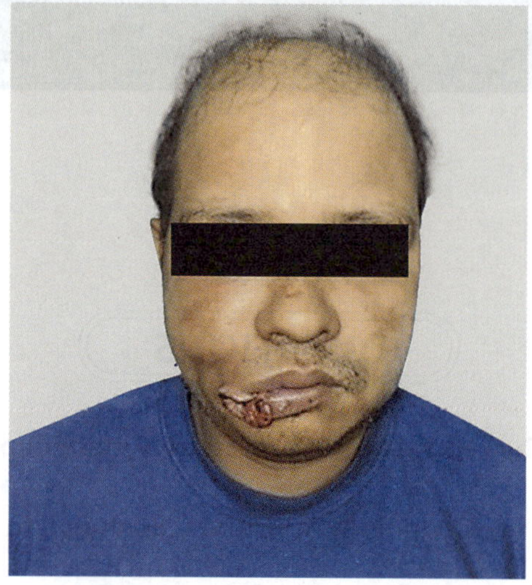

**Q6. What are the aims of imaging investigation for oral cavity cancer lesions?**

**Q7. What approach is used in given picture for oral cavity carcinoma and benefit of this approach?**

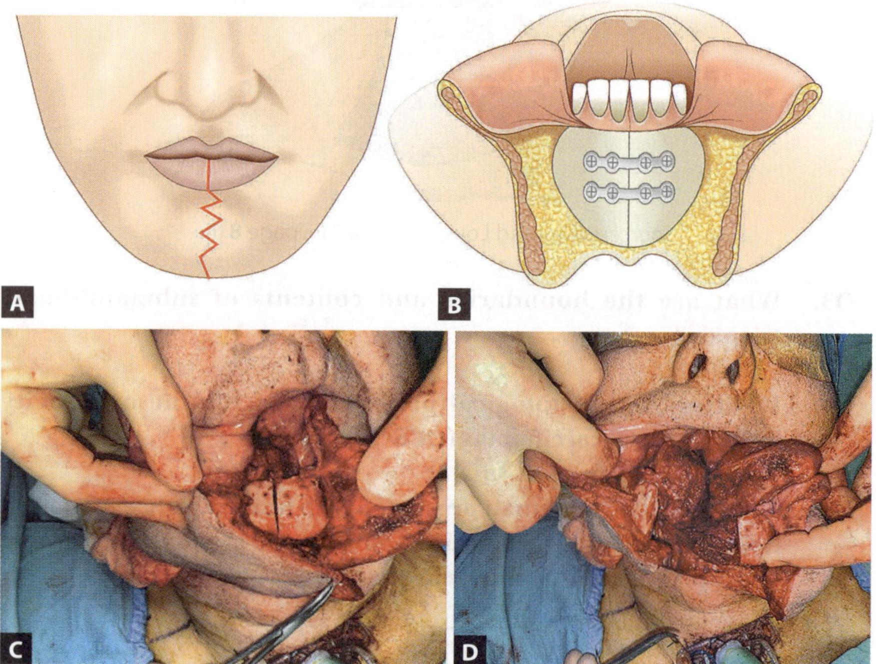


*Source:* Bailey and Love, 28th edition, page 822

**Q8. Name the approach as depicted in picture.**

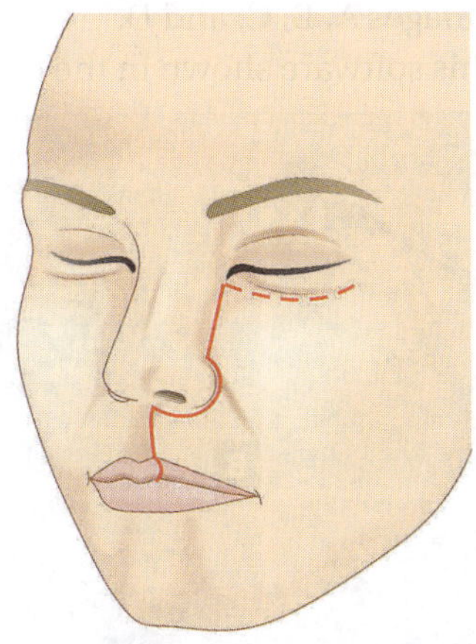

*Source:* Bailey and Love, 28th edition, page 822.

**Q9. What is the reconstruction ladder for oral cavity lesions primary defect?**

**Q10. A 66-year-old man presented with nonhealing ulcerated lesion over left lateral border of the tongue from 3 months.**

What is the probable clinical diagnosis and what procedure has performed on given clinical pictures?

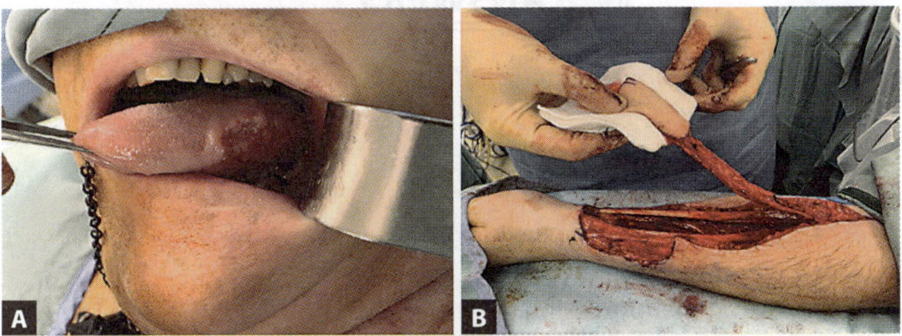


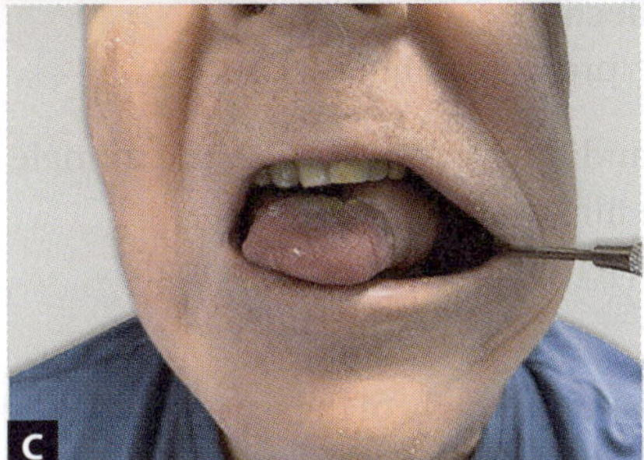


*Source:* Bailey and Love, 28th edition, page 824.

**Q11. Answer the following:**

a. Identify the images A, B, C, and D.

b. Brief about this software shown in the picture.

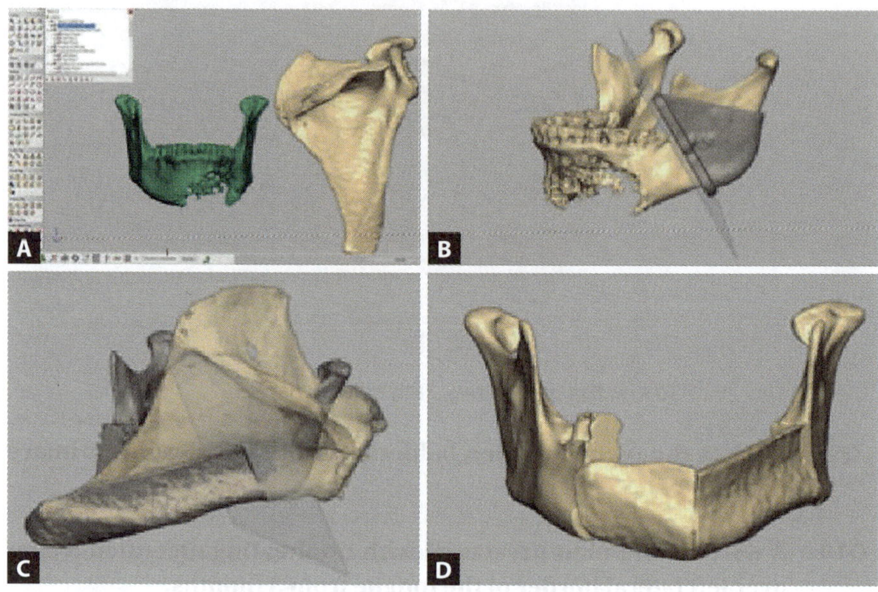


*Source:* Bailey and Love, 28th edition, page 828.

## ANSWERS

**Ans. 1** *Risk factors for oral cavity malignancy:*

- Smoking
- Alcohol
- Betel quid
- Human papillomavirus (HPV)
- Hereditary conditions
- Immunosuppression
- Chronic infection
- Potentially/premalignant lesions

**Ans. 2** A. Left submandibular triangle/digastric triangle

B. Left submental triangle

C. Left occipital triangle/posterior triangle

**Ans. 3** *Submandibular triangle boundaries:*

- Anterior—anterior belly of digastric muscle
- Posterior—posterior belly of digastric muscle
- Superior—Inferior border of the mandible

- *Contents:*
  - Viscera—submandibular gland, lymph nodes, and caudal part of parotid gland
  - Vessels—facial vessels, lingual vessels, and submental vessels
  - Nerves—hypoglossal nerve (CN XII) and mylohyoid nerve

**Ans. 4** Histological parameters routinely described in OCSCC include:

- Histology category
- Tumor classification or distinction
- The invasion pattern
- Depth of invasion (DOI) and thickness of tumor
- Intraneural [perineural invasion (PNI)] invasion
- Invasion of lymph nodes [lymphovascular invasion (LVI)]
- Engagement of the bones
- Metastases to nodes

**Ans. 5** a. *Signs and symptoms of the oral cavity neoplasm:*

| *Signs* | *Symptoms* |
|---|---|
| • Ulcer that does not heal (>2 weeks)<br>• Long-lasting lymphadenopathy or neck mass<br>• Pigmentation lesion that gradually enlarges<br>• Injunction accompanied by induration<br>• Long-lasting red or white sore<br>• Nonhealing "inflammatory" wound<br>• Soft-tissue lesion accompanied by radiological abnormalities<br>• Inexplicable tooth movement | • Motor neuron deficit<br>• Persistent pain<br>• Unknown cause of trismus<br>• Dysphagia |

b. *Line of management for oral cavity lesion:*

- Detailed history
- *Examination:* Oral cavity, neck, and head to toe
- Biopsy; for tissue diagnosis
- Research on radiographic and clinical staging
- Functional status and comorbidity
- Treatment plan preparation and discussion with the tumor board and multidisciplinary team (MDT)
- Demographical staging
- Adjunctive therapies, when applicable
- *Surgical management:* For this patient, wide local excision + MRND + locoregional/free flap coverage

**Ans. 6** *Aims of imaging are as follows:*

- For the main tumor's anatomical extent (T stage)
- The tumor's "resectability" according to how it affects important structures.
- Identification of metastases within a region
- Metastasis illness detection preventing recovery
- Finding simultaneous primary lung and upper aerodigestive tract tumors
- Tracking the progression of the illness after non-surgical treatment
- Identification of illness relapse

**Ans. 7** *Lip-split mandibulotomy:* This method, which is the most often utilized access procedure, offers superior access to lesions in the oropharynx, posterior oral cavity, and tongue base.

**Ans. 8** Weber–Fergusson approach which offers superior access to the periorbital region and the maxilla, should the lesion extend infraorbitally.

**Ans. 9** *Reconstruction ladder for oral cavity lesions primary defect:*

- Recovery by secondary healing
- Principal closure
- Skin transplantation
- Local flap coverage
- Regional flap coverage
- Microvascular free flaps reconstruction

**Ans. 10**

- Probably tongue carcinoma over left lateral border of the tongue.
- Radial forearm free flap (RFFF) used to reconstruct left lateral tongue defect after the partial glossectomy

**Ans. 11** a. *Virtual surgical planning (VSP) software:*

- *Image A:* A virtual mandible with an obvious bony defect
- *Images B and C:* Resection cutting plane with the scapula overlaid
- *Image D:* Final reconstruction plan with a two-part (osteotomized) scapula osseous component.

b. Potential advantages of VSP include shorter operating times, more precision, and better cosmetic and functional results. Based on CT images, this software provides simulated cutting and reconstruction guidelines for the donor sites as well as the tumor before surgery.

# 34 Disorders of Salivary Glands

CHAPTER

## QUESTIONS

**Q1. What are the degenerative disorders of the salivary glands?**

**Q2. What is Milan system for reporting salivary gland cytopathology?**

**Q3. Answer the following:**

a. What are the important anatomical relations to the submandibular gland?
b. What is the management of established Frey's syndrome?

**Q4. Answer the following:**

a. The patient had a solid to nodular, variable-consistency mass that has been progressively growing and painless for 10 years.

The most likely diagnosis is:

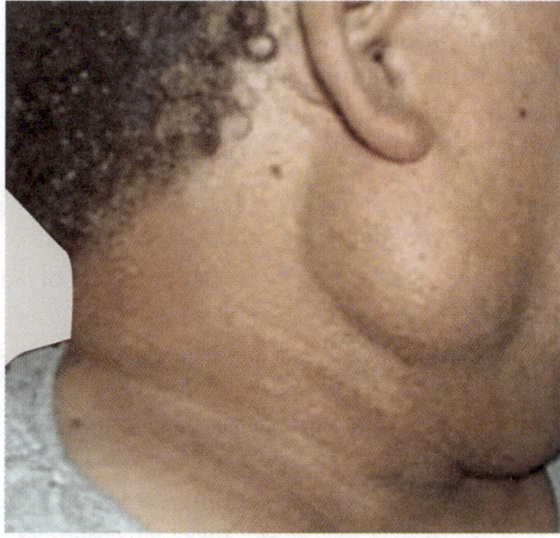

b. What are the clinical features and treatment of pleomorphic adenoma?
c. What is the probable diagnosis based on the given image?

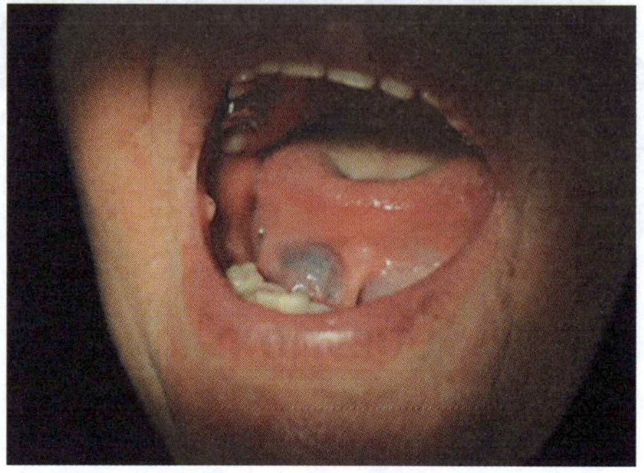

## ANSWERS

**Ans. 1** *Primary Sjögren's syndrome:*

- Severe xerostomia
- No connective tissue disorder
- Commonly dysfunction of exocrine gland

*Secondary Sjögren's syndrome:*

- In middle age
- Underlying connective tissue condition
- Male to female ratio: 1:10

*Benign lymphoepithelial lesion:*

- Diffuse parotid swelling (20% bilateral)
- 5% develops lymphoma

**Ans. 2**

| *Diagnostic criteria* | *Risk of the malignancy* | *Management* |
|---|---|---|
| Non-diagnostic | 25% | Correlation/repeat of radiological and clinical findings |
| Non-neoplastic | 10% | Radiological correlation and clinical follow-up |
| AUS | 20% | Repeat FNAC/Surgery |
| *Neoplasm:*<br>• IVA Benign<br>• SUMP | <br><5%<br>35% | <br>• Conservative surgery/clinical follow-up<br>• Conservative surgery* |
| Suspicious for malignancy | 60% | Surgery* |

*Contd...*

*Contd...*

| *Diagnostic criteria* | *Risk of the malignancy* | *Management* |
|---|---|---|
| Malignant | More than 90% | Surgery (extent is determined by the kind and grade of cancer) |

*Determining the extent of operation may be aided by an intraoperative frozen section

(AUS: atypia of undetermined significance; FNAC: fine-needle aspiration cytology; SUMP: salivary gland neoplasm of uncertain malignant potential)

**Ans. 3** a. *Important anatomical relations to the submandibular gland:*
- Anterior facial vein and facial artery
- Lingual nerve
- Hypoglossal nerve
- Marginal mandibular nerve (branch of facial nerve)

b. *Management of Frey's syndrome:*
- Antiperspirants that contain aluminum chlorohydrate
- Tympanic neurectomy-induced denervation
- Botulinum toxin injection into the afflicted area of skin

**Ans. 4** a. *Pleomorphic adenoma:*
- Less common in submandibular and sublingual glands (rare in small salivary glands)
- Most common benign salivary gland tumor and MC tumor of main salivary glands
- MC location is parotid tail (superficial lobe)
- Recurrences are multicentric but typically unicentric.
- Usually, does not affect the nerve in the face.

b. • *Clinical features:*
  - Painless swelling without noticeable alterations in size
  - Presented at typical sites below, in front and behind the ear lobule
  - Lobular tumor, slow growing affecting women around 40 years of the age
  - Involves the deep lobe and has components in the neck and oral cavity. It may also push the tonsils and pillars of fauces toward the midline (known as dumbbell tumor).

- *Diagnosis:*
  - Fine-needle aspiration cytology (FNAC) is the diagnostic tool
  - Superficial parotidectomy—Patey's operation
  - Excision of complete gland in pleomorphic adenoma of submandibular gland
  - Lazy "S" and modified Blairs or Sistrunk incisions are used for parotidectomy incisions.

c. Ranula

8

SECTION

# Endocrine and Breast

CHAPTER

# 35 Thyroid

## QUESTIONS

**Q1. Answer the following:**

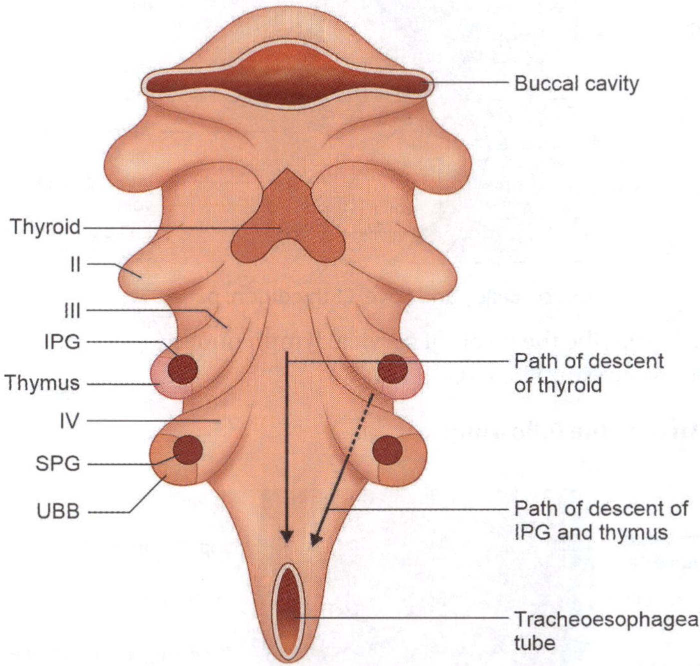


*Source:* Bailey and Love, 28th edition, page 850.

a. Describe the depicted image.
b. Describe surgical anatomy of thyroid gland (TG).

**Q2. Answer the following:**

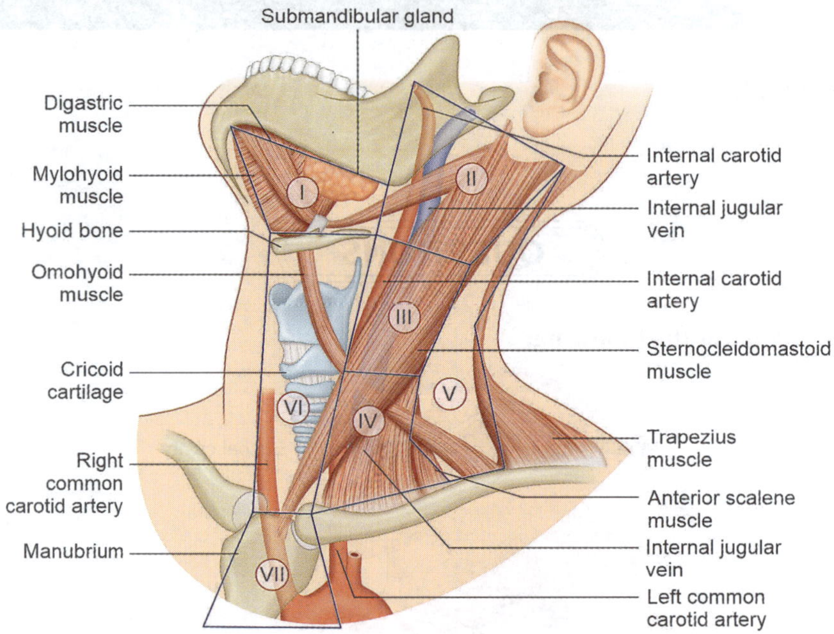


*Source:* Bailey and Love, 28th edition, page 851.

a. Describe the levels of cervical lymph nodes.
b. Nerve supply of TG.

**Q3. Answer the following:**

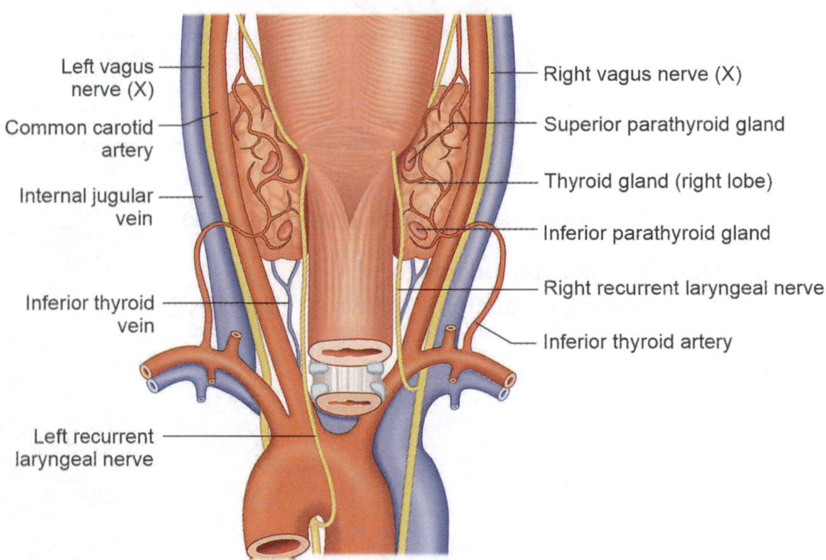


*Source:* Bailey and Love, 28th edition, page 851.

a. What is the course of this nerve?
b. Describe the nerve injuries which supply TG.
c. Describe CERNEA classification.
d. Describe MC site of injury of this nerve.

**Q4. After total thyroidectomy operation, just after extubation patient developed stridor.**

a. What is the cause?
b. Management of this situation.

**Q5. Answer the following:**

a. Describe the synthesis of thyroid hormone (TH).
b. Describe diseases related to physiology of TH.
c. Describe in brief about thyroid function tests (TFTs).
d. Describe in brief about hypothyroidism and hyperthyroidism.
e. Describe in brief about Refetoff syndrome.

**Q6. Describe in tabular form about the TFTs in normal and pathological states.**

**Q7. Answer the following:**

a. Describe in brief about thyroid investigations.
b. What is the role of ultrasonography (USG) neck in thyroid disease?
c. What is the role of fine needle aspiration cytology (FNAC)/fine needle non-aspiration cytology (FNNAC) in thyroid disease?

**Q8. Answer the following:**

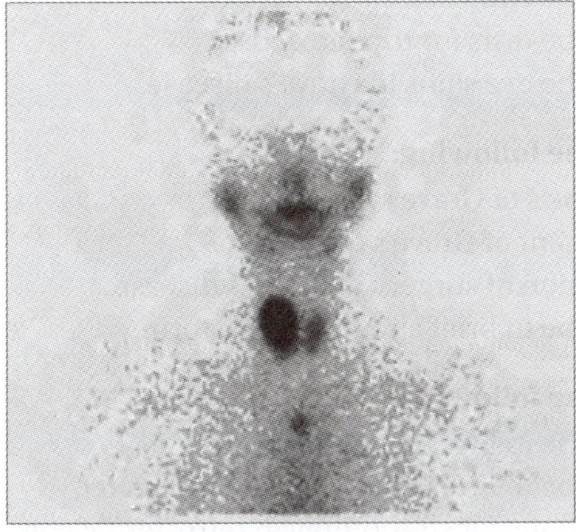

*Source:* Bailey and Love, 28th edition, page 854.

a. What is depicted in the image?
b. Describe radioactive iodine uptake (RAIU) study in thyroid disease.

c. What are the uses of RAIU in thyroid disease?
d. What are the side effects of RAI?
e. What are the contraindications for RAI?

**Q9. Answer the following:**

a. Classification of thyroid swellings
b. Clinical features of thyroid swellings
c. Indications for operation in thyroid swellings

**Q10. Answer the following:**

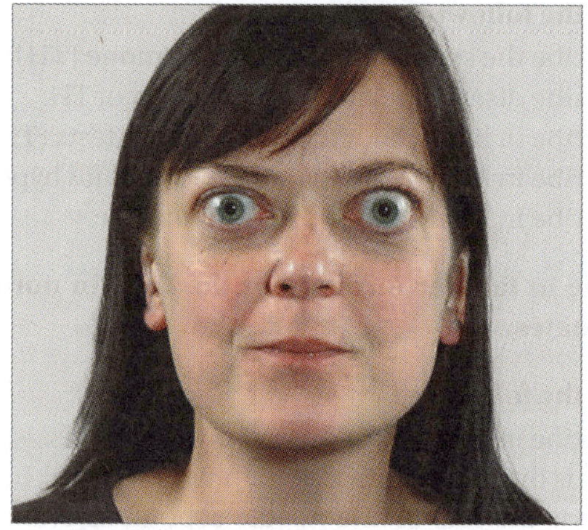

*Source:* Bailey and Love, 28th edition, page 861.

a. Describe Grave's disease.
b. Describe clinical tests in thyroid.
c. Describe tests for thyrotoxicosis.
d. Describe eye signs in Grave's disease.

**Q11. Answer the following:**

a. Diagnosis of Grave's disease
b. Treatment of Grave's disease
c. Indication of surgery in Grave's disease
d. Describe in brief about thyroid storm.

**Q12. Answer the following:**

a. Describe in brief about thyroiditis.
b. Describe in brief about retrosternal goiter.
c. Indications for sternotomy in retrosternal goiter

**Q13. Answer the following:**

a. Describe in brief about thyroglossal cyst (congenital).
b. Sistrunk incision is used for

**Q14. Thyroid carcinoma:**

a. Describe Dunhill's classification.
b. Predisposing factors for thyroid carcinoma
c. Syndromes associated with thyroid cancers

**Q15. Answer the following:**

a. Staging of thyroid CA
b. Difference between papillary carcinoma and follicular carcinoma
c. Scoring system for prognosis of thyroid CA

**Q16. Answer the following:**

a. Describe in brief about Hurthle cell carcinoma.
b. Describe in brief about medullary Ca of thyroid.
c. Describe in brief about anaplastic carcinoma.
d. Describe in brief about postoperative management of Dunhill's differentiated Ca.

**Q17. Thyroid surgery:**

a. What are the types of thyroidectomy?
b. Describe in brief about steps in thyroid surgery.
c. What are the postoperative complications of thyroid surgery?

**Q18. During thyroid surgery, surgeon finds a yellow tissue with the dissected thyroid. What to do?**

**Q19. Name various approaches for minimally invasive surgery or by robotic surgery for thyroid.**

**Q20. Describe in brief about monitoring of recurrent laryngeal nerve (RLN) injury.**

## ANSWERS

**Ans. 1** a. Embryology of thyroid and parathyroid—diagram of an anterior view of the pharynx in a 4-week embryo showing the relationship of the third and fourth pharyngeal pouches to final position of the thyroid and parathyroid glands (IPG: inferior parathyroid; SPG: superior parathyroid; UBB: ultimobranchial body)

b. • *Butterfly-shaped organ:*
   - Derived from thyroglossal tract (originating from foramen cecum) which comes down and divides into thyroid bud.
   - Ultimobranchial body gives rise to parafollicular cells

- *Arterial supply:*
  - Superior thyroid artery (STA) arises from external carotid. Enters the gland and then divides into branches.
  - Inferior thyroid artery (ITA) arises from thyrocervical trunk of subclavian artery and divides into multiple branches before entering the gland.
  - Inferior thyroid artery—supplies all four parathyroid glands.
  - Rarely, one more artery-from arch of aorta-arteria thyroidea ima is seen.
- *Ligation of STA and ITA:*
  - *Old concept:* Ligate STA close to gland to prevent injury to external laryngeal nerve (ELN), ITA ligated away from gland to prevent injury to RLN.
  - *New Concept:* To prevent hypocalcemia due to parathyroid loss of blood supply. Now we ligate the ITA very close to the gland as individual vessels (remember both STA and ITA are ligated close to gland).

    *Most common site of ectopic thyroid:* Lingual thyroid (failure to descend from foramen cecum of tongue)

*Venous drainage:*

- Superior thyroid vein (STV)—drains to internal jugular vein (IJV)
- Inferior thyroid vein (ITV) drains to brachiocephalic vein.
- Middle thyroid vein (MTV) drains into IJV.
- Fourth vein—Kocher's vein drains into IJV or brachiocephalic vein

**Ans. 2** a. Seven levels of neck nodes:

| | |
|---|---|
| 1. Submental and submandibular nodes | |
| 2. Upper jugular | Extend from base of skull to hyoid bone |
| 3. Middle jugular | Extend from hyoid bone to cricoid cartilage |
| 4. Lower jugular | Extend from cricoid cartilage to suprasternal notch |
| 5. Supraclavicular or posterior group | |
| 6. Prelaryngeal/pretracheal (prelaryngeal as Delphian nodes) | Extend from hyoid bone to sternal notch |
| 7. Upper mediastinal nodes | |

b. *Vagus nerve:* Two types:
   1. Recurrent laryngeal nerve
   2. Superior laryngeal nerve

**Ans. 3** a. *Thyroid gland nerve innovation course:*
*Recurrent laryngeal nerve course:*
- RLN arises from vagus nerve as it descends down, it gives the branches—right and left RLN.
- RLN hooks and comes back.
- Right RLN hooks around right subclavian artery.
- Left RLN hooks around ligamentum arteriosum.
- RLN is nonrecurrent in 5% cases.
- RLN is both motor and sensory.

Motor—all muscles of vocal cord including posterior crico-arytenoid:
- Helps in abduction of vocal cord (opening)
- Also called safety muscle of larynx

Sensory—below the mucosa of vocal cord.

b. *Injuries to nerves:*
- *Internal laryngeal nerve (ILN):* Paroxysmal nocturnal cough/aspiration (due to loss of sensation above vocal cords)
- *External laryngeal nerve (ELN):* Huskiness of voice at the rate of loss of timber of voice or loss of pitch
- *U/L RLN:* Hoarseness of voice
- *B/L RLN:* Stridor

*External laryngeal nerve injury:*
- Most common nerve injured: ELN

c. Classification of ELN course in relation to superior pole of thyroid—CERNEA classification
- >1 cm from the superior pole
- <1 cm from the superior pole
  - Above the gland
  - On the gland, hence has a high chance of damage.

d. *Recurrent laryngeal nerve:*
- Most common site of injury Beahrs' triangle. Boundaries of Beahrs' triangle
  - Laterally—common carotid artery
  - Medically by tracheoesophageal groove
  - Superiorly ITA
- *Extraedge:*
  - Tubercle of Zuckerkandl, most posterior lateral portion part of thyroid, also known as pointing tip toward RLN.

- Close to Berry's ligament, which is a condensation of pretracheal fascia:
  - Connecting thyroid to trachea
  - Reason for movement of thyroid with deglutition

**Ans. 4** a. Its due to B/L RLN injury (leads to stridor postoperative) (first sign due to B/L nerve going for cadaveric position)

b. *Stridor management:*

- Step 1—immediate reintubation
- Wait for 24–48 hours (many neuropraxias will recover with steroids).
- Extubate with entire team ready for tracheotomy.
- If there is stridor again and both nerves not functioning, tracheostomy done.
- After few months, if it is permanent damage we must go for some special procedures:
  - Advice arytenoidectomy/lateralization of cord (types of thyroplasty)

**Ans. 5** a. RDA for I2—0.1–0.15 mg/day

*Steps in synthesis (Mnemonic—TOBC):*

- Trapping
- Oxidation (iodine to iodide via thyroid peroxidase)
- Binding iodide with thyroglobulin [to form monoiodothyroglobulin (MIG) or di-iodothyroglobulin (DIG)]
- *Coupling:*
  - MIG + DIG = T3, half-life = 24 hours
  - DIG + DIG = T4, half-life = 7 days.
  - T3 is the active form.
  - Peripherally T4 is converted to T3.

b. *Diseases related to physiology:*

- *Deficiency of iodine:* Most common cause of hypothyroidism in the world
- Congenital thyroid peroxidase deficiency—Pendred syndrome
  - Sensory neural hearing loss
  - Congenital hypothyroidism
- *Hashimoto thyroiditis: Inhibitory antibody against:*
  - Thyroid peroxidase (TPO)-most common cause (MCC)
  - Thyroglobulin
  - Thyroid-stimulating hormone receptor (TSHR)
  - MCC of hypothyroidism in western countries
- *Grave's disease:* Stimulatory antibody to TPO, TG, and TSHR which results in increased T3 and T4 production

c. *Thyroid profile:*
   - Free T3—3-9 µmol/L
   - Free T4—8-24 nmol/L
   - TSH—<3 mU/L
   - TPO value—>25 U/mL
   - Anti-TG >1:100

d. *Hypothyroidism:*
   - Free T3—N/decreased
   - Free T4—N/decreased
   - TSH—increased

   *Hyperthyroidism*:
   - TSH—decreased
   - FT3—N/increased
   - FT4—N/increased

   *Extraedge*:
   - Most sensitive investigation of choice for hypothyroidism/ hypothyroidism—TSH value
   - Subclinical cases—free T3

e. Refetoff syndrome—increased T4 along with normal or increased TSH. Due to peripheral T4 resistance syndrome

**Ans. 6** Results of TFTs in normal and pathological states.

| *Thyroid functional state* | *TSH (0.3–3.3 mU/L)* | *Free T4 (10–30 nmol/L)* | *Free T3 (3.5–7.5 µmol/L)* |
|---|---|---|---|
| Euthyroid | Normal | Normal | Normal |
| Thyrotoxic | Undetectable | High | High |
| Myxedema | High | Low | Low |
| Suppressive T4 therapy | Undetectable | High | High (often normal) |
| T3 toxicity | Low/undetectable | Normal | High |

**Ans. 7** a.
   - TFT
   - USG neck
   - FNAC/FNNAC
   - Radioactive iodine uptake study

b. *USG—neck:*
   - Helps to identify if it is thyroid/not.
   - Consistency (solid/cystic)
   - Lymph node

   *TIRADS (Thyroid Imaging Reporting and Data System) grading system:*
   - Composition of gland and tumor
   - Echogenicity

- Size
- Echogenic foci
- Margin

c. *FNAC/FNNAC:*
- FNNAC—tissue is collected in needle hub (no negative pressure created)
- After that take gas in syringe and push it on glass slide
- Bethesda classification—based on FNNAC/FNAC
- Thy1—nondiagnostic
- Thy 1c—cystic lesion: Cd completely disappear.
- Nonrecurrent/less than three times recurrence
- Recurrent less than three times—surgery
- Incompletely disappear—surgery is treatment of choice.
  - Thy 2—benign
  - Thy 3—follicular neoplasm
  - Thy 4—suspicious of malignancy
  - Thy 5—definite malignancy

**Ans. 8** a. Technetium thyroid scan showing appearance of a 1-cm "toxic" adenoma in the right thyroid lobe with suppression of uptake in the left lobe. The intense uptake gives a false impression of the size of the swelling.

b. Radioactive iodine uptake study:
- Mixed with milk and taken orally:
  - I131: t½—8 days
  - I123: t½—12–14 hours
  - I132: t½—2.5 hours
  - Tc-99m: t½—6 hours
- Gland traps RAI and emits beta-radiation—used for diagnostic and therapeutic purposes.
- Caught on gamma cameras—to see for uptake—called as thyroid scan.

c. *Uses of RAIU in thyroid disease:*

| ***Diagnostic uses (Most common used is low-dose I123)*** | ***Therapeutic uses (Most common used is I131)*** |
|---|---|
| • <16% uptake—hypothyroidism; >48% uptake—hyperthyroidism; 1–48% uptake—Normal<br>• Warm nodule—increased activity than the surrounding tissue 5% are malignant. Cold nodule—decreased activity than the surrounding. Tissue 20% are malignant | Treatment of choice for:<br>• Grave's disease<br>• To destroy thyroid cancer mets |

*Contd...*

*Contd...*

| ***Diagnostic uses (Most common used is low-dose I123)*** | ***Therapeutic uses (Most common used is I131)*** |
|---|---|
| • To locate ectopic thyroid<br>• *Thyroglossal cyst:*<br>– *IOC in adults:* USG neck<br>– *IOC in children:* RAIU study—to rule out if this is the only functioning thyroid tissue.<br>• After total thyroidectomy for malignancy—look for metastasis<br>– Not done before thyroidectomy as uptake will be only in thyroid tissue | *Extraedge:* Post-RAI—what happens to physiology?<br>• *After RAI ablation:* Most Grave's disease patient becomes euthyroid in 2 months.<br>• *After 6 months:* 50% remains euthyroid<br>• Remaining 50% becomes hypo-/hyperthyroid |

d. *Side effects of RAI*:

| ***Immediate (usually recover)*** | ***Long-term tumors*** | ***Long-term damage*** |
|---|---|---|
| Neck pain | Leukemia | Infertility |
| Thyroiditis | Papillary Ca of thyroid | Abortion |
| Sialadenitis | Anaplastic Ca of thyroid | Pulmonary fibrosis |
| Cerebral edema | Breast Ca | Bone marrow suppression |
| Vocal cord paralysis | Gastric Ca | Ovarian/testicular failure |
| Bone marrow suppression | Lung Ca | Hypoparathyroidism |
| | Salivary tumors | |
| | Bladder Ca | |

e. *Contraindications for RAI:*
- Severe ophthalmopathy
- Pregnancy and lactation
- Children
- Nodules +
- Smoking females

*Extraedge: After RAI I131:*
- Isolate patient for 8 days
- Do not spit/urinate/kiss in public

RAIU is also used to know the cause for hyperthyroidism.

| *Excessive T3 and T4 production: Increased RAIU* | *Normal production but increased release: N/decreased RAIU* |
|---|---|
| • Grave's disease<br>• Secondary toxicosis<br>• Jod–Basedow effect<br>• Struma ovarii<br>• Hydatidiform mole<br>• TSH secreting pituitary adenoma<br>• Drugs—amiodarone | • Thyroiditis (in acute inflammatory phase—increased release of hormone)<br>• Thyrotoxicosis factitia (excessive thyroxine tablet taken)<br>• Hamburger toxicosis (south Americans eat thyroid of cow in burger) |

**Ans. 9** a. *Classification of thyroid swellings:*

| *Diffuse* | *Nodular* | *Inflammatory* | *Neoplastic* |
|---|---|---|---|
| • Physiological<br>• Grave's disease<br>• Colloid goiter | • Colloid goiter<br>• Solitary nodular<br>• Multinodular | • Hashimoto's<br>• Reidel's<br>• De Quervain's | • Papillary Ca<br>• Follicular Ca<br>• Medullary Ca<br>• Anaplastic Ca |

b. *Clinical features:*

| *Hypothyroidism* | *Hyperthyroidism* |
|---|---|
| Obese | Slim |
| Less intake | Increased intake |
| Cold intolerance | Heat intolerance |
| Constipation | Diarrhea (increased bowel movement) |
| Menorrhagia—amenorrhea (anemia) | Oligomenorrhea |
| • Tendon reflex—decreased<br>• Pseudomyotonic reflex/hung up ankle reflex—delayed ankle jerk | • Tendon reflex—increased<br>• Fine tremors |
| • Loss of eyebrow<br>• Macroglossia<br>• Mask-like faces<br>• Depression | Eye signs—exophthalmos (early):<br>• Pretibial myxedema—deposition of mucopolysaccharides in front of tibia<br>• Acropachy—subperiosteal bone resorption of fingers—look-like clubbing<br>Both are late features |
| *Cause:*<br>• Cretinism (pediatrics)<br>• Myxedema (adults) | *Cause:*<br>• Grave's disease (1′ toxicosis)<br>• Plummer's disease (2′ toxicosis) due to multinodular goiter (MNG) >SNT (for examinations) |

*Contd...*

*Contd…*

| ***Hypothyroidism*** | ***Hyperthyroidism*** | |
|---|---|---|
| Treatment: 50–100 µg tablet thyroxine (supplement dose) | Grave's | Plummer's |
| | 1′ | 2′ |
| | Diffuse enlargement with simultaneous toxic features | Long-standing solitary nodular thyroid |
| | | Suddenly go for toxic features |
| | *Affect:* CNS+ eye sings+ | *Affect:*<br>Old guys<br>CVS+:<br>• Sinus atrial Tachycardia (mc)<br>• Atrial extrasystole<br>• Atrial fibrillations<br>• Congestive cardiac failure<br>• Thyroid storm<br>• Lerman scratch sound (systolic scratch sound in left second ICS on expiration)—rub between pleura and pericardium |

c. *Indications for operation in thyroid swellings:*

| Neoplasia | FNAC positive Thy3–5 | |
|---|---|---|
| | Clinical suspicion | Age |
| | | Male sex |
| | | Hard texture |
| | | Fixity |
| | | Recurrent laryngeal nerve palsy |
| | | Lymphadenopathy |
| | | Recurrent cyst |
| | | |
| Toxic adenoma | | |
| Pressure symptoms | | |
| Cosmesis | | |
| Patient's wishes | | |

**Ans. 10** a. *Grave's disease*:
- MCC of hyperthyroidism
- *Autoimmune disease:* HLAB8, HLADR3, and HLADQ1
- Diffuse enlargement, soft consistency, highly vascular
  - *Palpation:* Thrill in superior pole
  - *Auscultation:*
    - Arterial bruit
    - Venous hum+ (due to increased sympathetic activity causing hyperdynamic circulation)

b. *Clinical tests in thyroid (all clinical examination videos will be showed in clinical examination section):*
- Examined from behind
- Short neck—Pizzillo's method (hand behind neck and hyper-extension of neck)
- Retrosternal goiter—Pemberton's sign (to look for superior vena cava compression—lift both arm with arm touching ears—look for facial congestion)
- *Lahey's test:* Four-finger examination (push on one side and palpate with four fingers)
- Crile's test—for doubtful nodule (using only thumb—ask patient to swallow; feel for nodule)
- Trail's sing—prominent sternocleidomastoid muscle (SCM) muscle (thyroid swelling pushes trachea)
- Berry's sign—nonpalpable carotid artery against vertebrae (due to engulfment of the tumor)

c. *Tests for toxicosis:*

| ***CNS*** | ***CVS*** | ***Eye signs*** |
|---|---|---|
| • Increased reflexes<br>• Tremors—fine<br>• Fasciculation in tongue (with tongue inside mouth) | Sleeping pulse rate<br>Crile's grading method<br>• Phenobarbitone night dose and measure | Exophthalmos |

d. *Eye signs:*
- *Mild exophthalmos due to only sympathetic activity:*
  - von Grafe's lid lag sign—ask patient to follow vertical movement—lid lags behind
  - Dalrymple's sign/lid retraction sign—visible upper sclera
  - Stellwag's sign—starring look

- *Moderate due to retro-orbital accumulation:*
  - *Joffroy's sign:*
    - Absence of forehead wrinkle on looking up
    - Ask patient to look at the ceiling (patient eye is already out)
- *Severe due to intraocular accumulation and paralysis of muscle:*
  - Mobius sign—Inability to converge (paralysis of intraocular muscle)
- Malignant—though treatment given—exophthalmos increases
  - Epiphora
  - Congestion
  - Redness
- *Other signs:*
  - Jellwek's sign—pigmentation in upper eyelid
  - Naffziger sign—see through supraorbital ridge—normally eyes not seen.
    - If seen, it is exophthalmos or proptosis.
  - *Gifford test (eversion of upper eyelid to differentiate exophthalmos and proptosis):*
    - Exophthalmos—Müller muscle spasm+ —inability to evert upper eyelid
    - Proptosis—pathology behind eyeball—able to evert upper eyelid

**Ans. 11** a. *Diagnosis:*
- T3, T4 increased, and TSH decreased
- RAIU increased
- Autoimmune antibodies increased: Anti-TG, Anti-TPO—75% cases
- Long-acting thyroid stimulator (LATS) is elevated in 90% cases. Also known as thyroid-stimulating antibody or TSH-R stimulating Ab.
- *FNAC is not beneficial:*
  - Hemorrhagic aspirate
  - Therefore, not advised in Grave's disease.

b. *Management of Grave's disease:* First—preparation of the thyrotoxic patient to euthyroid state, then give:
- Radioactive iodine ablation therapy—gold standard
- Surgery

Preparation of the thyrotoxic patient to euthyroid state—If not done properly, thyroid storm (MC cause is inadequate preparation for surgery)

| ***Antithyroid drugs*** | ***Quick preparation*** | ***Lugol's iodine*** |
|---|---|---|
| *Inhibit:*<br>• Trapping of iodine<br>• Oxidation of iodine<br>• Peripheral conversion T4 to T3 | • Decrease sympathetic overactivity of the gland<br>• Early preparation is possible | *Mechanism:*<br>• Decrease vascularity of the gland<br>• Makes the gland firm |
| • Carbimazole leads to reversible agranulocytosis<br>• Ask history of sore throat<br>• First sign of decreased WBC count | *Beta-blockers:*<br>• Propranolol (short acting)—40 mg TDS<br>• Nadolol (long-acting) 160 mg OD | 5% iodine<br>+<br>10% potassium iodide (KI) 10 drops TDS |
| Methimazole—10–30 mg TDS | | |
| Propylthiouracil—used in pregnancy—do not cross placental barrier | | |
| Take for 3 months to become euthyroid | | Last 10 days before surgery |
| Block and replacement therapy: Antithyroid drugs—high-dose carbimazole + thyroxine | | |
| Last dose of carbimazole given night before surgery | *Note:* Continue beta-blocker 7 days postoperative including intraoperative period | |

c. *Total thyroidectomy—advised in Grave's disease:*
*Indications:*
- RAI is contraindicated.
- Suspicious of cancer
- Goiter >80 g
- Compressive symptoms
- Patient not responding to radioactive iodine
- Rapid control is needed.

d. *Thyroid storm:* MCC—inadequate preparation of thyroid patient other causes:
- Illness
- Stress
- Amiodarone

*Characterized by:*
- CNS problems—agitation/depression
- CVS problems—dysfunction—congestive cardiac failure (CCF)
- 10% mortality

*Clinical features*:
- Tachycardia
- Hyperpyrexia
- Dehydration
- CCF (symptoms+)
- Hyperexcitability
- Atrial fibrillation

*Treatment of thyroid storm:*

| ***Basic life support*** | ***Antithyroid drugs*** | ***Special drugs*** |
|---|---|---|
| $O_2$ | IV propranolol | Steroids—hydrocortisone 200 mg (adrenal is exhausted) |
| Tepid sponging | Lugol's iodine | Diazepam (they are hyperexcitable) |
| IV fluids | PTU | Diuretics (they have CCF) |
| Glucose | Carbimazole | Digoxin (if in AF) |
| | Potassium iodide (KI)—in IV | |

**Ans. 12** a. *Thyroiditis:*
- Most common in females 30–40 years
- Inflammation of TG

| ***Hashimoto*** | ***Reidel (fibrosis)*** | ***De Quervain*** | ***Acute*** |
|---|---|---|---|
| Most common type | | | Most common in children |
| As known as chronic lymphocytic/ autoimmune thyroiditis | Associated with:<br>• Invasive fibrosing thyroiditis<br>• Dupuytren's contracture<br>• Retroperitoneal fibrosis | • As known as postviral or subacute (after few weeks of viral infection)<br>• Associated with HLAB35 | • Bacterial infection<br>• Most common *Streptococcus*<br>• No HLA association |
| *Abs (inhibitory):*<br>• TPO-MC<br>• TG<br>• TSH-R | | | Persistent pyriform sinus fistula important cause of recurrent acute bacterial thyroiditis |

*Contd...*

*Contd…*

| ***Hashimoto*** | ***Reidel (fibrosis)*** | ***De Quervain*** | ***Acute*** |
|---|---|---|---|
| *FNAC:*<br>• Hurthle cells/ Ashkenazy cells (abundant cytoplasm with varying size of nucleus)<br>• Lymphocytes+ | FNAC cannot be Dunwoody hard mimics cancer. Do tru-cut biopsy (done in anaplastic and Riedel) | | |
| *C/F:*<br>• Pain +<br>• Thyrotoxicosis (due to increased release not production)<br>• Burn out leading to hypothyroidism<br>• When patient presents—painless enlarged thyroid with hypothyroidism | Always hypothyroid—produce compressive symptoms | • Predominantly hyperthyroid with pain for long period<br>• Later become hypothyroid<br>*DD:*<br>Grave's—increased RAIU<br>*De Quervain:*<br>• Decreased RAIU<br>• Increased erythrocyte sedimentation rate (ESR) | • Severe neck pain + odynophagia<br>• Increased ESR<br>• Increased WBC |
| *Complications:*<br>• Hypothyroidism<br>• Compressive symptoms<br>• Premalignant-lymphoma and papillary carcinoma | | | • Laryngitis<br>• Perichondritis<br>• Sepsis<br>• Tracheal rupture<br>• Esophageal rupture<br>• IJV thrombosis |
| *Treatment:*<br>• Tablet thyroxine<br>• Painkiller for pain (surgery is not advised except in compressive symptoms) | • Tablet thyroxine<br>• Steroids<br>• Antiestrogen tamoxifen<br>• Mycophenolate mofetil | • Analgesics<br>• Steroids | • Antibiotics<br>• Remove pyriform sinus fistula |

b. *Retrosternal goiter:*

Why goiter extends downward?

- Pretracheal fascia attaches from hyoid to aortic arch (superior mediastinum)
- SCM prevents upward movement.

*Types:*

| ***Primary mediastinal*** | ***Secondary mediastinal (retrosternal goiter)*** |
|---|---|
| • Arising from ectopic thyroid gland present inside chest<br>• Blood supply from thoracic vessels<br>• Sternotomy is required. | • Typical retrosternal extension—99% patients<br>• Blood supply from superior and inferior thyroid artery<br>• Approach through neck incision—put finger and hook it = TOBOGANN maneuver<br>• Pemberton sign+ (hands on ear—flushing of face) |

*Management:*
- *Investigation of choice (compulsory):* CECT thorax/neck
- *Elderly:* Asymptomatic—wait and watch

c. *Indications for sternotomy:*
- Previous neck surgery
- Recurrent retrosternal goiter
- Posterior mediastinal extension
- 1′ mediastinal goiter (blood supply from mediastinal blood vessels)
- Adhesions in mediastinum

**Ans. 13** a. *Thyroglossal cyst (congenital):*
- Persistence of tract
- *Clinical features:*
  - 5–25 years (though congenital)
  - Females
  - Moves with protrusion of tongue
  - Most common site—subhyoid
- *Complications:*
  - Infection—most common
  - Rupture/I and D leads to TG fistula = acquired
  - Malignancy—papillary Ca
- *IOC:* USG neck
- *Pediatric case:* RAIU study
  - If this is the only thyroid—wait till child becomes adult.
  - If normal TG is present—Sistrunk operation
- Remove whole tract + central hyoid bone

b. *Sistrunk operation:* Lymphedema of limbs, thyroglossal cyst (congenital)

c. *Sistrunk incision:* Parotid surgery

**Ans. 14** Thyroid carcinoma

a. *Dunhill classification:*

| *Differentiated* | *Medullary* | *Undifferentiated* |
|---|---|---|
| Papillary Ca—80% | 2.5% | Anaplastic—5% |
| Follicular Ca—10% | | Lymphoma (NHL)—2.5% |
| Hurthle cell Ca | | |

*Sequence-based question:* Papillary > follicular > anaplastic > medullary = lymphoma

b. *Predisposing factors*:
- *Long-standing multinodular goiter:* Follicular Ca
- *Irradiation:* Papillary Ca
- *Hashimoto's:* NHL and papillary Ca
- *Thyroglossal cyst:* Papillary Ca
- *Genetic mutation and syndromes:*
    - *RET oncogene:* Medullary Ca
    - *RAS oncogene:* Follicular > papillary
    - *PTEN:* Follicular Ca
    - *P53:* Anaplastic Ca

c. *Syndromes:*
- Cowden syndrome
- Familial adenomatous polyposis
- MEN 2A and MEN 2B
- Carney's triad
- McCune Albright syndrome

| *MEN 2A (Sipple syndrome)* | *MEN 2B* |
|---|---|
| Medullary Ca thyroid | Medullary Ca thyroid |
| Pheochromocytoma | Pheochromocytoma |
| Hyperparathyroidism | Marfanoid habitus |
| Hirschsprung disease | Neuromas (mucosal) |
| *Prophylactic thyroidectomy done for both patients* | |
| <5 years | <1 year |

**Ans. 15** a. *Staging of thyroid CA:*
- *T-staging:*
    - *T1a:* <1 cm
    - *T1b:* 1–2 cm
    - *T2:* 2–4 cm
    - *T3:* >4 cm, muscle/soft tissue+

- *T4a:* Removable structures—RLN/trachea/larynx/esophagus
- *T4b:* Nonremovable structures—carotid vessels/mediastinum/prevertebral fascia

- *Nodes*:
  - *N1a:* Level VI (delphic nodes)
  - *N1b:* More than level VI

b.

| ***Papillary carcinoma*** | ***Follicular carcinoma*** |
|---|---|
| Most common thyroid cancer | Most common in iodine deficiency areas |
| *Pathology:*<br>• Multifocal—one lobe many foci<br>• Multicentric—B/L<br>• May or may not have capsule | • Single<br>• Well-defined capsule |
| *Spread:*<br>• Lymph node mets "lateral aberrant thyroid"<br>• Metastatic node from an occult papillary CA<br>• *Distant mets:* Lungs<br>*FNAC (3p):*<br>• Psammoma bodies (concentric calcification)<br>• Pale empty orphan Annie eye nucleus<br>• Papillary projections | Hematogenous<br>*Most common site:* skull—pulsatile osteolytic secondaries<br>*Distant mets:* Skull<br>• Inconclusive (cannot define benign/malignant)<br>• Capsular invasion cannot be detected with FNAC |
| *Predisposing factors:*<br>• Irradiation<br>• Hashimoto's<br>• Thyroglossal cyst | Long-standing multinodular goiter |
| *Prognosis: Excellent:* 95% 10-year survival | Good prognosis |
| *Treatment:* Total thyroidectomy+ modified radical neck dissection (if nodes +ve) | *Management:*<br>• If >4 cm—do total thyroidectomy directly<br>• If Thy 3 (<4 cm), then do hemithyroidectomy—cut and send for HPE (not frozen—miss malignancy)—result in 2–3 days<br>*Based on result:*<br>• If benign: Discharge patient<br>• If malignant: On Day 3, do completion total thyroidectomy |

d. *Scoring system for prognosis:* AGES, AMES, and MACIS

| | **Low risk** | **High risk** |
|---|---|---|
| Age | <40 years | >40 years |
| sex | Female | Male |
| Mets | Absent | Present |
| Grade | Well differentiated | Poorly differentiated |
| Size | <2 cm | >4 cm |
| extent | Confined | Out of capsule + |
| Completion of surgery | Completed | Not completed R1—microscopic residual tissue |

**Ans. 16** a. *Hurthle cell carcinoma:*

- *Rare variant of follicular carcinoma:*
  - Malignancy indicated by capsular invasion
  - FNAC not useful
- *Differentiating features:*
  - From oxyphil cells of thyroid
  - Do not take up RAIU.
  - Multifocal and multicentric
  - Lymph node mets +
  - Bad prognosis—20% mortality in 10 years
- *Treatment:* Total thyroidectomy + modified radical neck dissection (mRND) + central neck node dissection
- *Central neck node dissection:* Removal of level six nodes—advised in medullary Ca of thyroid
- Central neck nodes are seen between:
  - Hyoid bone superiorly
  - Clavicle inferiorly
  - SCM laterally

b. *Medullary Ca of thyroid:*

- Incidence 2.5%
- Parafollicular C-cells (ultimobranchial body)
- *RET oncogene mutation:* MEN2A and MEN2B

| **Sporadic** | **Familial** |
|---|---|
| 80% M/C type | 20% |
| Unilateral | Bilateral—multicentric and multifocal |
| | MEN2A, MEN2B, familial medullary carcinoma thyroid syndrome |

*Properties:*

- *Neuroendocrine tumor (secretory):*
    - Calcitonin—tumor marker for follow up (>0.08 ng/mL is significant)
    - CEA—for prognosis
    - ACTH—Cushing syndrome
    - Serotonin—diarrhea
    - PGE2 and PGF2-alpha
    - Histaminidase
- Rule out pheochromocytoma—24-hour urinary VMA increased. If present—operate.
- Pheochromocytoma first
- FNAC shows amyloid stroma.
- Extraedge—recent advances
- *Epidermal growth factor receptor (EGFR) antibodies:* Vandetanib
- *Anticarcinoembryonic antigen (CEA) antibodies:* Labetuzumab
- *Treatment:* Total thyroidectomy + central neck node dissection (irrespective of node –/+) +
- mRND (If node +)
- MC site of distant metastasis—liver (like other neuroendocrine)
- *Prophylactic thyroidectomy:*
    - *MEN2A:* <5 years
    - *MEN2B:* <1 year

c. *Anaplastic carcinoma—p53 mutation:*
- Old women
- Aggressive
- Bad prognosis
- In 6 months, they die
- FNAC—cannot be done—stony hard
- Tru-cut biopsy has to be done.
- MCC of death—respiratory obstruction
    - If a know case of anaplastic Ca coming with stridor—let him die peacefully.
    - Not a know case of anaplastic Ca with stridor—isthmectomy/tracheostomy is done.

d. *Postoperative management of Dunhill's differentiated Ca:*
- Total thyroidectomy followed by RAIU study to look for mets. If mets are present RAI ablation therapy given:
    - *RAI dose:* 30–100 mci
    - *Indication for RAI ablation therapy:*
        - Distant mets+
        - Extrathyroid spread+

        - Size >4 cm tumor
        - Lymph node mets are+
        - Papillary Ca—variants
    - Tall cell variant
    - Insular variant
    - Columnar variant
- External beam radiotherapy (EBRT) for follicular Ca
- *Chemotherapy:*
    - Doxorubicin
    - Paclitaxel
- *Hormone therapy:* Papillary Ca (TSH suppression with thyroxine tablets—0.3 mg)

**Ans. 17** a. *Types of thyroidectomy:*
- Lobectomy/hemithyroidectomy—remove isthmus + one lobe.
- Subtotal thyroidectomy—leave behind 8 g in each tracheoesophageal groove.
- Near total thyroidectomy/Hartley-Dunhill procedure—2–4 g is left behind on one side.
- Total thyroidectomy—nothing is left behind.

b. *Steps in thyroid surgery:*
- Reverse Trendelenburg position (head up)—decrease bleeding from neck
- Neck extended position/dog barking position
- Skin crease incision
- Subplatysmal flap—raise above and below
- Open deep fascia of neck
- Strap muscle is cut/retracted
- First ligated vessel—middle thyroid vein
- Then ligate artery near the gland:
    - Superior thyroid artery—prevent ELN injury
    - Inferior thyroid artery—preserve parathyroid gland blood supply
- Place drain for 24 hours—look for bleed

c. *Postoperative complications:*
- Stridor—B/L RLN injury/neuropraxia—reintubate—wait for 48–72 hours by giving steroids and anti-inflammatory drugs
    - If stridor disappear—extubate
    - If persistent stridor—extubate and do tracheostomy
    - Permanent B/L RLN injury—do lateralization of cord/arytenoidectomy
- *Life-threatening complication in postoperative:*
    - Hematoma—due to slippage of ligature of STA
    - Management—remove suture In bed side—then prepare OT

- Nowadays we do not get it as we have drain.
- If bleed is seen in drain—shift patient to OT and capture the bleed.

- *Nerve injuries:*
  - U/L RLN—hoarseness of voice
  - B/L RLN—stridor
  - ELN (MC)—huskiness of voice (timber is lost)
  - ILN—paroxysmal nocturnal cough/aspiration
- Laryngomalacia—after the removal of thyroid, the larynx collapses
- Thyroid storm
- *Respiratory dyspnea:*
  - Hematoma
  - B/L RLN injury
  - Vocal cord edema
  - Laryngomalacia (tracheomalacia)
  - Laryngismus stridulus (hypocalcemia)
- Hypocalcemia

**Ans. 18** Surgeon finds a yellow tissue with the dissected thyroid. What to do?

- Saline float test—place tissue in normal saline.
  - If sinks, it is parathyroid gland
  - If floats, it is fat/lymph node
  - Intraoperative—place parathyroid gland in SCM muscle pocket
  - Postoperative—place parathyroid gland in nondominant brachioradialis as implant.

**Ans. 19** Minimally invasive surgery or by robotic surgery by various approaches:

- Axillary approach
- Submammary approach
- Supraclavicular approach
- Breast approach

**Ans. 20** *Monitoring of RLN injury:*

| *Continuous* | *Intermittent* |
|---|---|
| Electrode on vagus nerve | Electrode on vocal cords at ET tube |
| When we give traction on RLN, it is detected and we get signal | Indicates after vocal cords lie in cadaveric position |
| Prevents injury | Injury is detected (after palsy) |

# 36 CHAPTER Parathyroid Gland

## QUESTIONS

**Q1. Answer the following:**

a. Parathyroid gland were first described by
b. The first parathyroidectomy was performed by
c. Parathyroid gland develop from which pharyngeal pouches
d. Blood supply of superior and inferior parathyroid gland arises from
e. Why inferior parathyroid gland, and thymus there is more variation in there anatomical position.
f. Most common position of superior parathyroid gland.
g. Half-life of parathyroid hormone (PTH)

**Q2. Answer the following:**

a. Band keratopathy is pathognomonic of which disease.
b. Most common clinical manifestation of symptomatic primary hyperparathyroidism (PHPT)

**Q3. Answer the following:**

a. Define hypercalcemic crisis. First-line treatment in advanced malignancy and serum calcium level 3 mmol/L and also explain mechanism of action of that drug.
b. Name two genes regulating the cell cycle, have been recognized as playing important role in parathyroid adenomas of PHPT.
c. Name the scientist who developed technique of selective venous sampling for parathyroid localization.

**Q4. Answer the following:**

a. What are the three different protocols for sestamibi scan?
b. What is MIBI in sestamibi?
c. Mechanism of sestamibi scan.

**Q5. Name the scan and finding of the scan.**

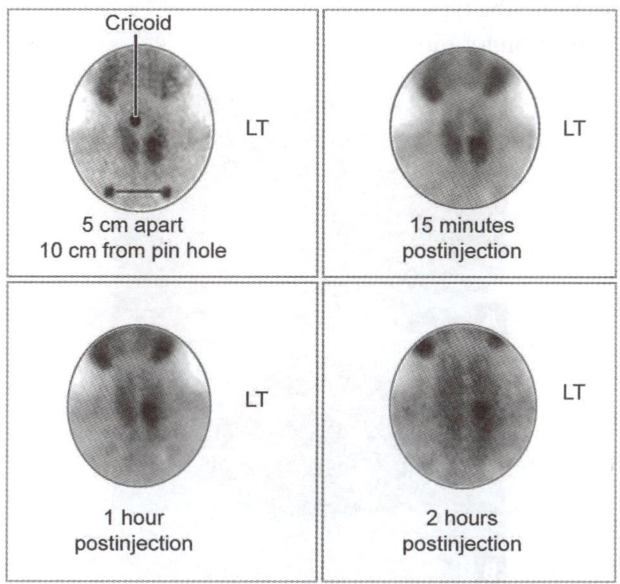


*Source:* Bailey and Love, 28th edition, page 877.

**Q6. Type of scan and kindly opine marked structure.**

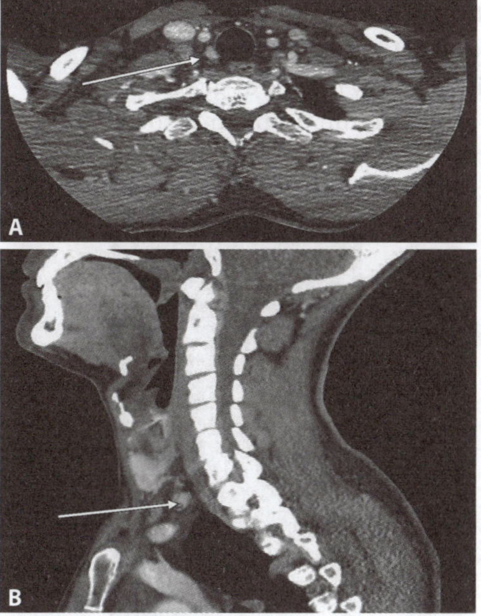


*Source:* Bailey and Love, 28th edition, page 878.

**Q7. Considering the following images A and B.**

a. Mention the type of surgery
b. Indication for the surgery

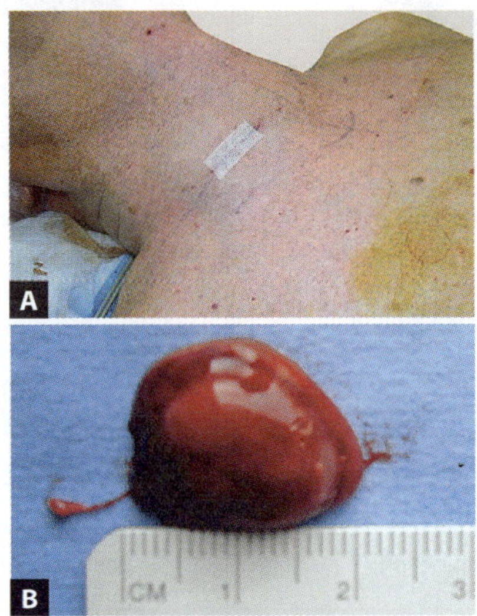


*Source:* Bailey and Love, 28th edition, page 879.

**Q8. A 57yr Old lady is k/c/o chronic kidney disease presented with pain over right foot and generalized body ache. Routine lab parameters s/o - high serum phosphate, elevated PTH, low calcium and vitamin D.**

a. Identify the x-ray finding as given below
b. What could be the problem associated condition in this CKD patient?

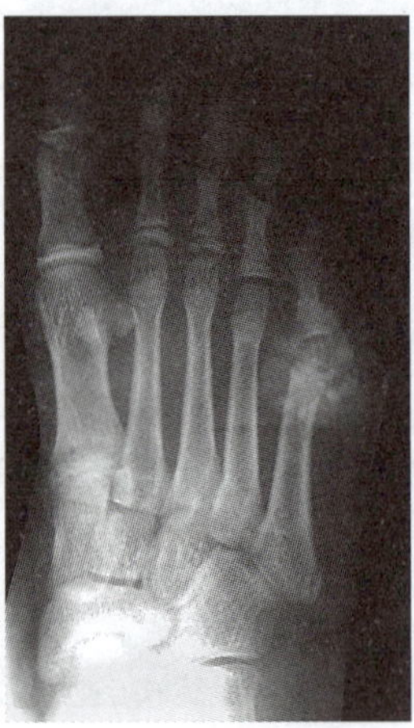

*Source:* Bailey and Love, 28th edition, page 884.

**Q9. Answer the following:**

a. What are the key points to be consider to explain patient and their relatives while taking patient for parathyroidectomy.

b. Define Miami criteria

**Q10. Answer the following:**

a. Name the surgeon got Nobel prize in physiology or medicine in 1909 for his research on the thyroid (INISS 2022).

b. What is Chvostek's and trousseau's sign?

**Q11. Answer the following:**

a. Mechanism of action of bisphosphonates

b. Mechanism of action of denosumab

**Q12. Answer the following:**

a. What are calcimimetics and their mechanism of action.

b. Genes associated with multiple endocrine neoplasia 1 (MEN 1), MEN 2A, and MEN 4

c. Hyperparathyroidism–jaw tumor syndrome associated with gene

**Q13. Criteria for genetic testing according to current NHS England National Genomic Test Directory testing criteria from March 2019 for familial hyperparathyroidism.**

**Q14. Answer the following:**

a. Define secondary hyperparathyroidism.

b. Explain pathogenesis of secondary hyperparathyroidism.

c. Explain Casanova test.

**Q15. Answer the following:**

a. Define calciphylaxis.

b. Pathogenesis of calciphylaxis

c. Definitive treatment of secondary hyperparathyroidism

**Q16. Answer the following:**

a. Indication for surgical intervention in secondary hyperparathyroidism

b. Indications of surgery in tertiary hyperparathyroidism

**Q17. Identify the procedure and structure marked with arrows.**

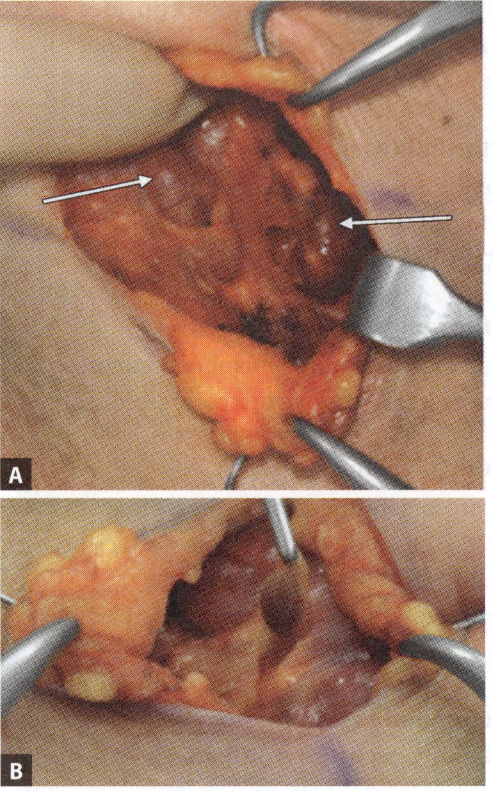


*Source:* Bailey and Love, 28th edition, page 880.

## ANSWERS

**Ans. 1** a. In 1850, Sir Richard Owen provided a description of the dissection of an Indian rhinoceros' neck at the Zoological Gardens in London.

b. Albert Gahne, a tram conductor, presented with severe primary hyperparathyroidism and osteitis fibrosa cystica. Mandi conducted the first parathyroidectomy in Vienna.

c. Between the fifth and the twelfth weeks of pregnancy, the third and fourth pharyngeal pouches give rise to the four parathyroid glands. The third pharyngeal pouch is the source of the thymus and inferior parathyroid gland. The dorsal part of the fourth pharyngeal pouch is where the superior parathyroid glands originate.

d. The inferior thyroidal artery supplies blood to the superior and inferior parathyroid glands.
e. The third pharyngeal pouch is the origin of the thymus and inferior parathyroid gland. As inferior parathyroid gland has longer normal embryological descent. So the variation is more in their anatomical position. That is the reason, in >50% of cases the inferior parathyroid gland are located at the inferior pole of the thyroid gland, on the anterior, lateral, or posterior surface.
f. The superior parathyroid glands are found in the posterior side of the thyroid lobe in >80% of patients. They have a diameter of 2 cm and are centered 1 cm around the point where the recurrent laryngeal nerve and inferior thyroid artery meet, closely surrounding the cricothyroid junction.
g. 3–5 minutes

**Ans. 2** a. Band keratopathy—causative factor for primary hyperparathyroidism, as a result of calcium phosphate crystals being deposited in the cornea
b. The most prevalent clinical sign of symptomatic primary hyperparathyroidism is the presence of kidney stones (PHPT).

**Ans. 3** a. Up to 5% of hospitalized patients and 0.5% of the general population have been reported to have hypercalcemia. With a slight to moderate rise of serum calcium (<3 mmol/L and 3–3.5 mmol/L, respectively), the majority are asymptomatic and respond well to treatment of the underlying etiology with related dietary modifications. A tiny percentage of patients will show symptoms when their total calcium level is >3.5 mmol/L. This is called a hypercalcemic crisis and needs to be treated aggressively with medicine.

Agents that limit the release of calcium from skeletal reserves may be necessary for individuals with advanced cancer and blood calcium levels >3 mmol/L. Bisphosphonates are used as part of first-line treatment. These are pyrophosphate analogs that inhibit osteoclast activity in areas of high bone turnover. Because of their low absorption in the gastrointestinal tract, they are administered intravenously in the acute context. Calcium excretion from the kidneys can be increased and osteoclastic activity can be decreased by calcitonin. Because of its brief duration of action, it is typically employed as a stopgap measure to lower calcium levels until the long-term effects of bisphosphonates become apparent. Because of its brief duration of action, it is typically employed as a stopgap measure to lower calcium levels until the long-term effects of bisphosphonates become apparent. They might therefore also be involved in illnesses linked to an overabundance of vitamin D.

b. MEN1 and CCND1

c. A radiologist at the National Institutes of Health in the United States, John L Doppman (1928–2000) invented the method of selective venous sampling for parathyroid localization.

**Ans. 4** a. There are three different protocols for sestamibi scanning—(1) single-isotope dual-phase scan, (2) dual-isotope subtraction imaging, and (3) single-photon emission computed tomography (SPECT).

b. 2-methoxy-2-methylpropylisonitrile

c. Because sestamibi builds up in mitochondria, it excretes at varying rates based on the quantity of mitochondria present in a given tissue. Oxyphilic cells with a high mitochondrial content are frequently found in significant concentrations in parathyroid adenomas. Compared to the thyroid gland, they retain tracer, which is why adenomas are linked to a delayed washout.

**Ans. 5** Sestamibi scan demonstrating right inferior adenoma.

**Ans. 6** Four-dimensional computed tomography scanning demonstrating a right inferior parathyroid adenoma (arrows).

**Ans. 7** a. Lateral approach minimally invasive parathyroidectomy

b. The parathyroid adenoma removed

The idea that >80% of people with PHPT have a solitary adenoma is the foundation of minimally invasive procedures. The process, which has no precise definition, is generally understood to involve making an incision little larger than 3 cm in order to remove a localized aberrant parathyroid gland.

**Ans. 8**
- Soft-tissue calcium deposits.
- Secondary hyperparathyroidism. Radiograph showing ectopic calcification.

**Ans. 9** a. The risks associated with having a parathyroidectomy must be disclosed to the patient, including the potential for recurrent laryngeal nerve injury (risk <1%), irreversible hypoparathyroidism (risk 0.5%), and persistent (5%) or recurring hyperparathyroidism (risk 0.5%).

b. To ascertain the degree of resection, the Miami criteria were created. Single-gland disease appears to be reliably predicted by a PTH decline into the normal range and to less than half the highest preoperative PTH at 10 minutes.

**Ans. 10** a. Emil Theodor Kocher, 1841–1917, surgeon, Berne, Switzerland, awarded the Nobel Prize in Physiology or Medicine in 1909 for his research on the thyroid.

b. In hypoparathyroidism:
- Chvostek's sign refers to contraction of the ipsilateral facial muscles on percussion of the facial nerve below the zygoma.
- Trousseau's sign refers to the development of carpopedal spasm secondary to occlusion of the arm (usually with a blood pressure cuff).

**Ans. 11** a. Analogs of pyrophosphate, known as bisphosphonates, are found in regions with elevated bone turnover. By suppressing apoptosis and osteoclast activity, they promote bone mineralization and decrease bone turnover.

b. Denosumab is a monoclonal antibody that works as a receptor activator of nuclear factor-κB (RANK) ligand inhibitor. Data from the DENOCINA trial suggest that it may be a valid treatment option for patients in whom surgery is undesirable.

**Ans. 12** a. PTH secretion is negatively regulated by the extracellular calcium-sensing receptor on the surface of parathyroid cells. When the receptor is activated, PTH secretion is reduced, which lowers bone turnover. Calcium-sensing receptor sensitivity to extracellular calcium is increased by calcimimetics, including cinacalcet, which modifies the set point and reduces PTH synthesis.

b.
- MEN 1 mutations occur in the *MEN1* gene, which encodes the protein Menin. Menin acts as a tumor suppressor.
- MEN 2A connected to changes in the RET proto-oncogene's codon 634
- *MEN 4:* It results from a pathogenic mutation in the cyclin-dependent kinase inhibitor *CDKN1B* gene that inactivates.

c. Hyperparathyroidism-jaw tumor (HPT-JT) is a rare cause of PHPT. It develops as a result of inactivating mutations in the parafibromin-encoding *HRPT2/CDC73* gene on chromosome 1q21–q31.

**Ans. 13** The current NHS England National Genomic Test Directory testing criteria from March 2019 for familial hyperparathyroidism state that testing should be considered for patients with PHPT and a creatinine clearance ratio > 0.02 who meet one of the following criteria:
- Presenting before the age of 35 years
- Presenting before the age of 45 years with one of:
  - Proven multigland involvement

- Hyperplasia on histology
- Ossifying fibroma(s) of the maxilla or mandible
- At least one first-degree relative with unexplained hyperparathyroidism

The testing criterion for familial hypocalciuric hypercalcemia (FHH) is a creatinine clearance ratio <0.02.

**Ans. 14** a. A disruption in calcium homeostasis that results in an increase in PTH secretion as a compensatory mechanism is defined as secondary hyperparathyroidism. It is sometimes called renal hyperparathyroidism since it mainly results from chronic kidney disease. Additional underlying causes include chronic lithium use, vitamin D deficiency, gastrointestinal malabsorption, and liver illness.

b. Renal failure is linked to the pathophysiology of secondary hyperparathyroidism. Hyperphosphatemia is caused by abnormalities in the renal tubular absorption of phosphate. PTH secretion is stimulated and parathyroid cells are directly affected by this. Recent translational research has identified fibroblast growth factor 23, or FGF23, as a new phosphaturia hormone. In order to offset chronic phosphate retention, this is gradually produced by osteocytes. This decreases 1,25-dihydroxyvitamin D levels, which in turn causes a decrease in intestinal calcium absorption and an increase in PTH secretion.

c. Selective venous sample for PTH in the neck and the brachial vein on the side of the graft can be helpful in situations of recurrent disease when there is no indication of active disease in the neck and a prior allograft has been transplanted to the forearm. This is called the Casanova test, and a ratio larger than 20:1 indicates that the transplanted arm is where the recurring disease (graft hyperplasia) is situated.

**Ans. 15** a. Skin necrosis and vascular calcification are two outcomes of the disseminated calcification condition known as calciphylaxis (calcific uremic arteriolopathy). About 4% of patients receiving surgical surgery for secondary hyperparathyroidism had this condition. Expanding, painful cutaneous purpuric lesions, mostly on the extremities but often on the lower belly, are the initial signs of this condition. Ischemic necrosis and the development of gangrene are caused by the underlying tissue calcification within the arteriolar and tiny arterial walls. This ultimately results in overwhelming sepsis and death.

b. The development of the condition in uremic individuals may be related to irregularities in smooth muscle cell biology and a decrease in the serum levels of α2-Heremans-Schmid glycoprotein, a calcification inhibitory protein. It has been demonstrated that an immediate parathyroidectomy can lessen pain, enhance wound healing, and lower the patient's chance of amputation. Additionally, it has been linked to a rise in median survival.

c. The only proven treatment for secondary hyperparathyroidism is still renal transplantation.

**Ans. 16** a.

| ***Indications for surgical intervention in secondary hyperparathyroidism*** | |
|---|---|
| ***Essential components*** | ***Clinical findings*** |
| • Persistently high serum level of intact PTH >500 pg/mL<br>• Hypercalcemia (serum Ca >2.5 mmol/L or 10 mg/dL) or hyperphosphatemia (serum $PO_4$ >6 mg/dL) that is resistant to medical treatment<br>– Estimated volume of the largest gland >300–500 $mm^3$ or long axis >1 cm | It is advised that individuals get a parathyroidectomy if they exhibit any of the following symptoms:<br>• Severe osteitis fibrosa with associated high bone turnover<br>• Subjective symptoms (arthralgia, irritability, muscle weakness, and discomfort in the bones and joints)<br>• Progressive ectopic calcification<br>• Calciphylaxis<br>• Progressive reduction in bone mineral content<br>• Anemia resistant to ESA<br>• Dilated cardiomyopathy/cardiac failure |

(ESA: erythropoietin-stimulating agent; PTH: parathyroid hormone)

b. Indications for surgical intervention in tertiary hyperparathyroidism:

- Subacute severe hypercalcemia (>3 mmol/L)
- Impaired graft function
- Hyperplasia of parathyroid gland nodules(s)
- Progressive symptoms (>2 years after transplant)
- Worsening bone disease (pain, fracture, and bone loss)
- Renal stones/nephrocalcinosis
- Soft-tissue or vascular calcifications

**Ans. 17** Surgical removal of the parathyroid glands, exposing the left superior and inferior glands in situ (shown by white arrows) (A) and on its vascular pedicle, the left superior gland became mobilized (B).

# 37

# The Adrenal Glands and Other Abdominal Endocrine Disorders

CHAPTER

## QUESTIONS

**Q1. Answer the following:**

a. Weight of normal adrenal gland
b. Blood supply of adrenal gland (INI SS 2023)
c. Adrenal gland located in retropertoneum near the upper pole of kidney, within the Gerota's facia. The Gerota's fascia name given by whom?

**Q2. Answer the following:**

a. What is extra adrenal paraganglia?
b. Paraganglioma (PGL)
c. Chemodectomas

**Q3. Answer the following:**

a. Cortex and medulla derived from which layer
b. Functionally active incidentaloma determined by

**Q4. Answer the following:**

a. What are the radiological features suspicious of adrenal malignancy?
b. Laparoscopic adrenalectomy recommended for

**Q5. Answer the following:**

a. Most common mutation associated with aldosterone producing adenoma
b. Genes associated with familial hypercholesterolemia (FH) type I
c. Genes associated with FH type II–IV

**Q6. Identify the mode of imaging and associated condition.**

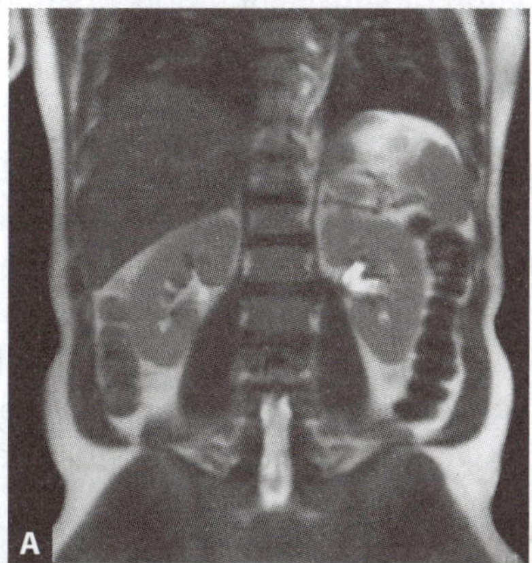


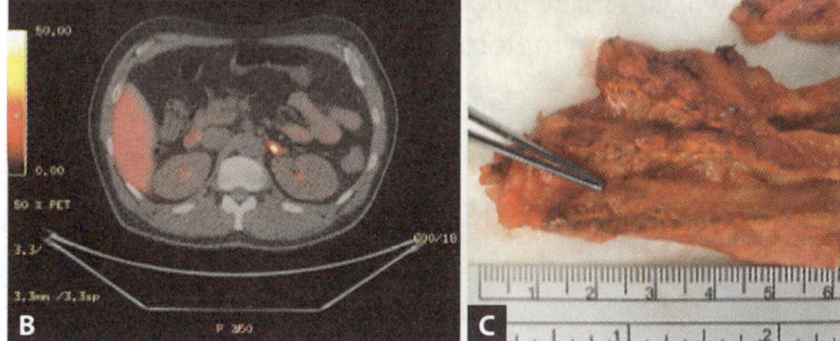


*Source:* Bailey and Love, 28th edition, page 892.

**Q7. Answer the following:**

a. Most common clinical feature in Cushing syndrome
b. Biochemical method to diagnose Cushing syndrome
c. Medical treatment of Cushing syndrome

**Q8. Answer the following:**

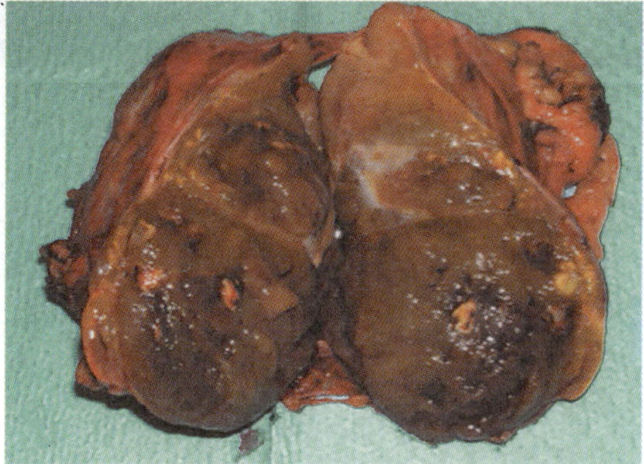

*Source:* Bailey and Love, 28th edition, page 895.

a. Identify the specimen and its associated condition.
b. At presentation of above condition what are the three common scenarios?
c. Modified Weiss criteria (INISS 2022)

**Q9. Answer the following:**

a. Most common defect in congenital adrenal hyperplasia (CAH) (INISS NOV 2023)
b. What are the inherited endocrine tumor syndrome associated with pheochromocytomas and paragangliomas (PPGLs)?
c. What are the characteristics of Von Hippel-Lindau (VHL) disease?
d. What are the characteristics of neurofibromatosis 1 (NF1)

**Q10. Answer the following:**

a. How will you make biochemical diagnosis of PPGL?
b. Most common symptom of PPGL

**Q11. Answer the following:**

a. Identify the imaging modality and associated condition.

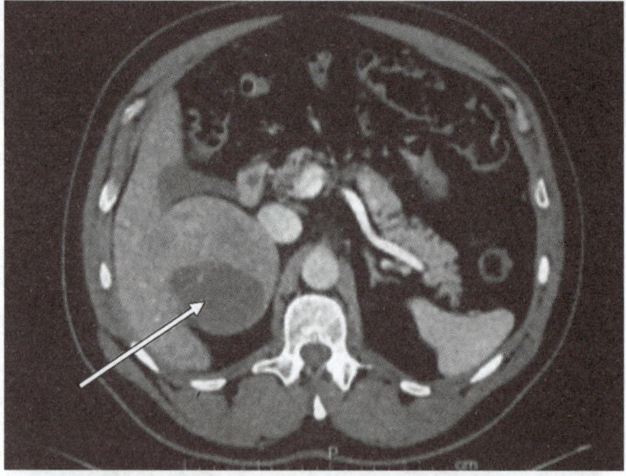

*Source:* Bailey and Love, 28th edition, page 901.

b. Identify the imaging modality, intraoperative finding, and associated condition.

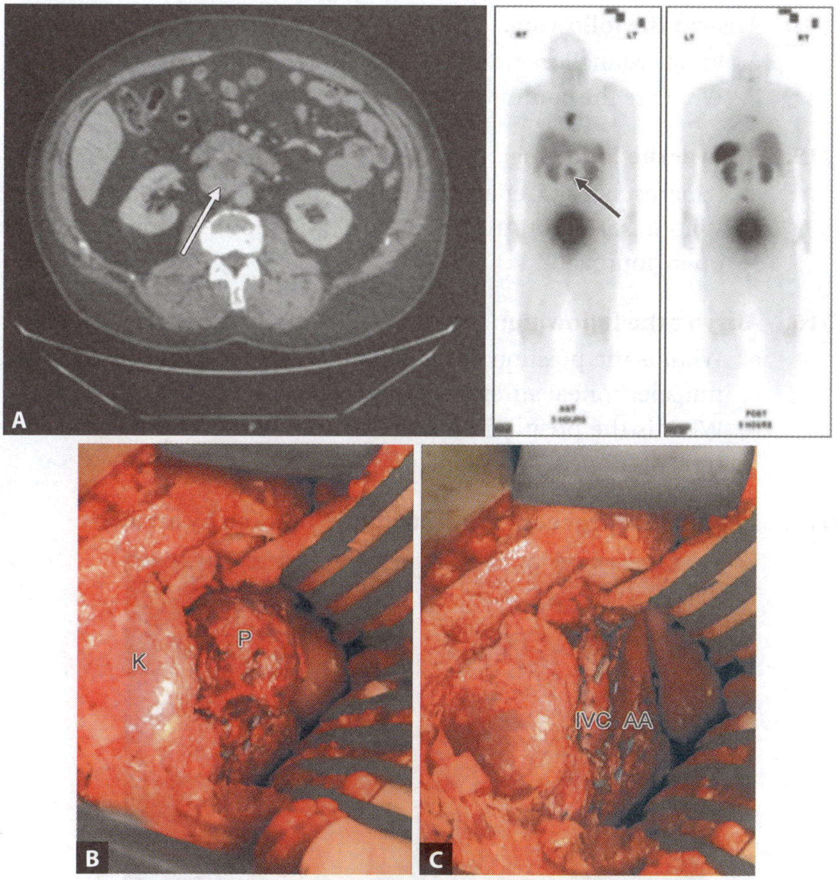

*Source:* Bailey and Love, 28th edition, page 901.

**Q12. How will you manage pheochromocytoma in pregnancy?**

**Q13. Identify the imaging modality and its associated condition.**

How will you diagnose and treat this condition?

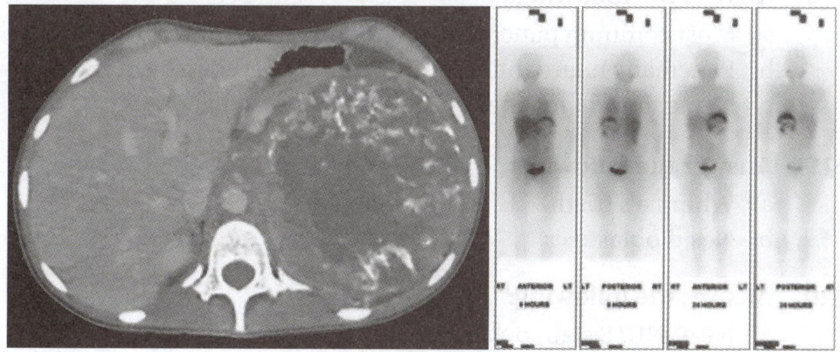

*Source:* Bailey and Love, 28th edition, page 903.

**Q14. Answer the following:**

a. What is ganglioneuroma (GN)?
b. What are the common locations of GN?

**Q15. Answer the following:**

a. Laparoscopic adrenalectomy first done by [INISS 2022]
b. Who described retroperitoneoscopic modification of posterior open approach?

**Q16. Answer the following:**

a. What is the position of patient and number of port used in right transperitoneal adrenalectomy?
b. What is the position of patient and number of port used in left transperitoneal adrenalectomy?

**Q17. Identify the procedure and structure marked by arrow.**

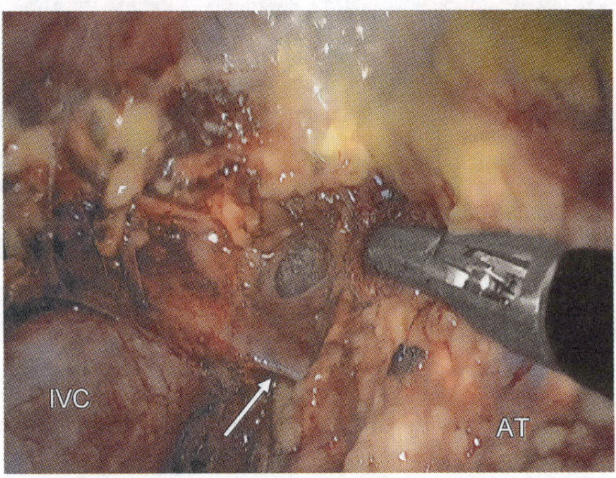


*Source:* Bailey and Love, 28th edition, page 904.

**Q18. Answer the following:**

a. Most common pancreatic neuroendocrine tumors (P-NETS) is
b. Pancreatic neuroendocrine cells are believed to be derived from
c. Name four main types of cells in islets of Langerhans.

**Q19. Answer the following:**

a. Whipple's triad
b. Nesidioblastosis

**Q20. Answer the following:**

a. NF-P-NETS stain positive for
b. NF P NETS distribution ratio for pancreas head to body to tail

**Q21. Answer the following:**

a. What is carcinoid syndrome?
b. Cardinal feature of carcinoid
c. Most common location of neuroendocrine tumor

**Q22. Identify the image and associated condition.**

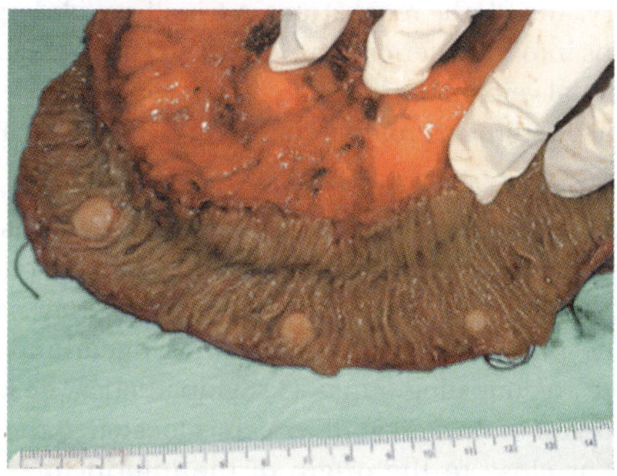

*Source:* Bailey and Love, 28th edition, page 910.

**Q23. Answer the following:**

a. Clinical manifestation of multiple endocrine neoplasia type 1 (MEN 1)
b. What are the genotype-phenotype associations for disorders arising from ret gene mutation?

**Q24. Identify the condition and associated condition.**

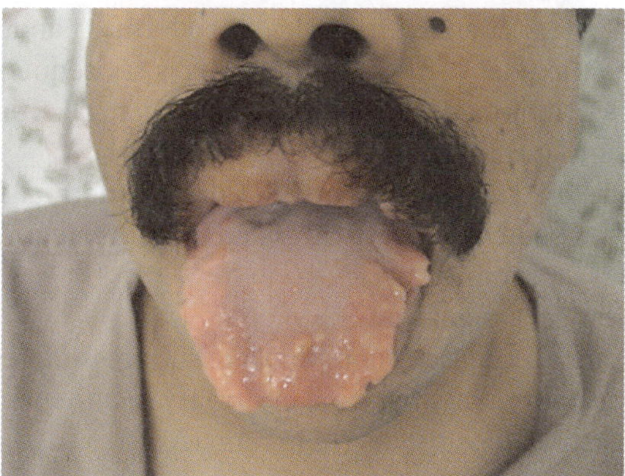

*Source:* Bailey and Love, 28th edition, page 913.

**Q25. What is the age of prophylactic surgery owning to strong genotype—phenotype relationship (NEET SS 2023)**

## ANSWERS

**Ans. 1** a. The weight of a normal adrenal gland is approximately 4 g.

b. Each adrenal gland is supplied by multiple small arterial branches from three main vessels—(1) the aorta, (2) the inferior phrenic artery, and (3) the renal artery. A usually single large adrenal vein drains into the inferior vena cava (IVC) on the right side and into the renal vein on the left side.

c. Dumitru Gerota (Professor of surgery, Bucharest, Romania)

**Ans. 2** a. Paraganglia are neuroendocrine cells associated with the autonomic nervous system. They can be adrenal (medulla) or extra-adrenal. Extra-adrenal paraganglia occurs throughout the sympathetic nervous system and along some branches of the parasympathetic glossopharyngeal and vagus nerves. There are four subgroups—(1) Sympathetic: The largest cluster is the organ of Zuckerkandl, which is located at the aortic bifurcation or close to the origin of the inferior mesenteric artery; (2) chemoreceptor: Including aortic and carotid bodies that assist in the regulation of respiration; (3) visceral-autonomic: In the urinary bladder and peripheral blood vessels; and (4) intravagal: Situated within or adjacent to the vagal trunk.

b. Neoplasms of extra-adrenal paraganglia are called PGLs.

c. Tumors of chemoreceptors are usually referred to as chemodectomas and those from parasympathetic ganglia are termed glomus tumors.

**Ans. 3** a. The cortex is derived from the mesoderm. At about the fifth week of life the fetal cortex develops; this is subsequently surrounded by a second wave of mesothelial cells that will eventually form the definitive cortex.

The adrenal medulla is derived from ectodermal chromaffin cells that are believed to have migrated from the neural crest.

b. This is determined by:

- Clinical assessment
- 1 mg overnight dexamethasone suppression test (DST)
- Measurement of plasma or urinary metanephrines
- Plasma aldosterone-renin ratio (ARR)
- Sex hormones and steroid precursors

**Ans. 4** a. *Radiological features suspicious of adrenal malignancy:*

- Diameter >40 mm and >10 HU density
- Contrast enhanced washout computed tomography (CT)

- Relative <40%
- Absolute <60%
- *MRI chemical shift:* No change in signal intensity on out-of-phase imaging
- *Fludeoxyglucose (FDG)-positron emission tomography (PET):* Positive uptake

b. Laparoscopic adrenalectomy is recommended for unilateral adrenal masses with radiological findings suspicious of malignancy and a diameter <60 mm, but without evidence of local invasion.

**Ans. 5** a. The most common mutations are those of the potassium channel encoded by the *KCNJ5* gene; these are present in approximately 40% of patients with aldosterone-producing adenoma (APA).

b. FH type I or glucocorticoid-remediable aldosteronism (GRA) arises as a result of a *CYP11B1/CYP11B2* chimeric gene and presents with (typically normokalemic) hypertension when the patient is in their early twenties.

c. FH types II–IV (caused by germline CLCN2 pathogenic variants, KCNJ5 pathogenic variants and CACNA1H pathogenic variants, respectively) all result in early-onset PA within affected kindreds.

**Ans. 6** A patient with confirmed Conn's syndrome. Magnetic resonance imaging (A) failed to demonstrate a lesion but a 30-SUVmax lesion was demonstrated on a 11C-metomidate PET–CT scan (B). (C) Surgical specimen sliced to reveal a 6-mm APA in the medial limb. The patient's hypertension resolved with laparoscopic left adrenalectomy.

**Ans. 7** a. Obesity 90% (hypertension 85%, facial plethora 70%, and hirsutism 75%)

b. Endocrine Society 2008 guidance states that two of the following tests should be abnormal for diagnosis:

- *Late-night salivary cortisol (two measurements):* Raised levels signify a loss of diurnal rhythm
- *24-hour urinary free cortisol (UFC) excretion (two measurements):* More than three times the upper limit signifies overspill into the urine
- *Overnight 1-mg DST:* Nonsuppressed morning cortisol >50 nmol/L
- Raised serum adrenocorticotropic hormone (ACTH) signifies pituitary-dependent disease; if it is adrenal in origin, the ACTH is suppressed (<5 pg/mL).

c. Metyrapone or ketoconazole therapy reduces steroid synthesis and secretion by CYP11B1 inhibition and can be used to prepare patients with severe hypercortisolism preoperatively or as primary therapy if surgery is not possible. In patients who are critically ill with Cushing's syndrome, intravenous etomidate infusion (even at non-hypnotic doses) can reduce serum cortisol levels to normal within 24 hours, providing a suitable window for surgery. This requires monitoring in an intensive care unit setting.

**Ans. 8** a. Adrenocortical carcinoma tumors are often large (>10 cm) with a cut surface that ranges from orange to brown. Necrosis is usually present.

b. 23

c. Modified Weiss histopathology system:
- This system may be used to guide the management
- It comprises five criteria:
  1. >6 mitoses/50 high-power fields
  2. ≤25% clear tumor cells in cytoplasm
  3. abnormal mitoses
  4. Necrosis
  5. Capsular invasion

If a criterion is absent, it is scored 0; if present, it scores 2 for the first two criteria and 1 each for the last three. A total score ≥3 is suggestive of malignant behavior.

**Ans. 9** a. The most frequent defect (95%) is the 21-hydroxylase deficiency, which has an incidence of 1 in 5,000 live births.

b. Tumors that arise from the neuroectodermal tissue of the adrenal medulla are termed phaeochromocytomas (PCCs) and those arising from the extra-adrenal parasympathetic and sympathetic ganglia are termed PGLs. PCCs and PGLs are collectively abbreviated to PPGL.

Overall, about 70% of PPGLs are sporadic and the rest occur as part of inherited endocrine tumor syndromes, which include:
- Hereditary PPGL syndromes
- MEN 2
- VHL
- NF1

c. An autosomal dominant disease characterized by central nervous system and retinal hemangiomas (60–80%), renal cysts (50–70%), clear cell renal cell carcinoma (30%), P-NETS (8–17%), PPGL (20%), endolymphatic sac tumors (6–15%), and epididymal/broad ligament cyst adenoma (50%).

- VHL is defined by its genotype as type I (deletions) without PPGL and type II (missense mutations), which is associated with PPGL. Patients develop PCC much more frequently than PGL. VHL tumors overproduce only noradrenaline.

d. This is a syndrome characterized by the development of café-au-lait spots (100%), axillary freckling (90%), neurofibromas (84%), Lisch nodules of the iris (70%), typical osseous lesions (14%), and optic glioma (4%). PPGL (PCC 96%) are found in 7% of affected patients. NF-1 is a tumor-suppressor gene and loss-of-function mutations lead to cell proliferation and cancer development.

**Ans. 10** a. The diagnosis of PPGL is confirmed by elevated catecholamine metabolites (metanephrines) in plasma and/or raised 24-hour urinary excretion of fractionated metanephrines. Metanephrines are produced as a result of intratumor conversion of catecholamines by the enzyme catecholamine O-methyltransferase. Measurement of plasma and urinary metanephrines is more sensitive (99% and 97%, respectively) than plasma and urinary catecholamine measurement (86% and 84%, respectively). Measurements of one or more of these substances that are four times greater than the upper limit of the reference range are 100% diagnostic. Plasma dopamine can be regarded as a marker of tumor burden in malignant PPGL.

b. Hypertension 80–90%

**Ans. 11** a. A cross-section CT scan of a large pheochromocytoma (PCC) showing characteristic central necrosis (arrow).

b. (A) A cross-section CT scan showing a paraganglioma (PGL) anterior to the abdominal aorta (white arrow) and an in-octretide scan demonstrating uptake by the tumor (black arrow). Operative photographs before (B) and after (C) extraction of the tumor (AA: abdominal aorta; IVC: inferior vena cava; K: right kidney; P: paraganglioma).

**Ans. 12** PCC in pregnancy may be silent and presents as a hypertensive emergency or it may mimic an amnion infection syndrome or preeclampsia. Without adequate α-blockade, mother and unborn child are threatened by a hypertensive crisis during delivery. In the first and second trimesters, the mother should be scheduled for laparoscopic adrenalectomy after adequate α-blockade; the risk of a miscarriage during surgery is high. In the third trimester, elective cesarean with delayed consecutive adrenalectomy 6 weeks later should be performed. The maternal mortality rate is 50% when a PCC remains undiagnosed.

**Ans. 13** Huge left-sided neuroblastoma (NB) with central necrosis on CT scan and MIBG (metaiodobenzylguanidine) scan.

Neuroblastoma (NB) is the most common and deadliest solid extracranial malignancy in children. It is derived from the primitive nerve cells (neuroblasts) of the sympathetic nervous system, derived from the neural crest. It is often termed the "clinical enigma" as the prognosis ranges from spontaneous regression to treatment resistance, metastasis, and death.

*Diagnosis*: NBs may secrete catecholamines, leading to elevated 24-hour urinary metanephrines. Serum lactate dehydrogenase is a useful tumor marker. An unequivocal diagnosis is from histology of either the tumor or bone marrow aspirate. Imaging is undertaken to stage the disease using CT or MRI and MIBG. In children with regional or metastatic disease, biopsy is necessary for diagnosis and prognostication.

*Treatment*: Patients are classified as low, intermediate, or high risk. Low-risk patients are treated by surgery alone whereas intermediate-risk patients are treated by surgery with adjuvant multiagent chemotherapy. For those patients with localized disease, surgical resection is curative. Postchemotherapy surgery may be performed for complete resection. Patients assigned to the low-risk, intermediate-risk, and high-risk groups have overall 3-year survival rates of 90%, 70–90%, and 30%, respectively.

**Ans. 14** a. GNs are benign differentiated tumors of neural crest-derived cells in the autonomic nerves.

b. GNs are benign and are most often located in the mediastinum (20%), retroperitoneum (10%), and adrenal gland (30%). However, GNs can arise anywhere sympathetic nervous tissue is found, such as tongue, bladder, uterus, bone, and skin. They are composed of an admixture of ganglion cells and Schwannian stroma/cells.

**Ans. 15** a. Gagner

b. Walz

**Ans. 16** a. The patient is positioned right side up, with table break. Four ports are used. The liver is retracted cranially and the peritoneal fold between the liver and the tumor is divided from the lateral border of the IVC to the right triangular ligament with the preferred energy device.

b. The patient is positioned left side up, with table break. Three ports are used.

**Ans. 17** View of the right adrenal vein draining (arrow) into the IVC during posterior retroperitoneoscopic adrenalectomy (AT: adrenal tumor).

**Ans. 18** a. Insulinoma 70–80%

b. Derived from pluripotent stem cells that differentiate into endocrine cells.

c. There are four main types of cell in the islets of Langerhans, which can be classified according to their secretions: all P-NETS.

1. β cells producing insulin (65–80% of the islet cells)
2. α cells producing glucagon (15–20%)
3. δ cells producing somatostatin (3–10%)
4. Pancreatic polypeptide (PP) cells containing polypeptide (1%)

**Ans. 19** a. Insulinoma cornerstone of diagnosis remains Whipple's triad:

- Symptoms induced by fasting
- Hypoglycemia at the time of symptoms
- Symptoms relieved by administration of glucose

b. Nesidioblastosis is a rare disorder, mainly encountered in children that is characterized by replacement of normal pancreatic islets by diffuse hyperplasia of islet cells.

**Ans. 20** a. Stain positively for chromogranin A and synaptophysin

b. Pancreas with a head to body to tail ratio of 7:1:1.5

**Ans. 21** a. In the presence of liver metastases, NET metastases secrete 5-HT into the IVC, avoiding hepatic first-pass metabolism and leading to symptoms of 5-HT excess, known as carcinoid syndrome.

b. The cardinal features are sweating, flushing, bronchospasm, and restrictive cardiomyopathy secondary to fibrotic right heart valvular disease (Hedinger syndrome).

c. Appendix 40%

**Ans. 22**
- Multiple neuroendocrine tumors in the small bowel
- They arise from the enterochromaffin cells and secrete serotonin and substance P. They are either solitary or multiple (30%) and the primary tumor can be small (5–20 mm).

**Ans. 23** a. *Tumor site:*

- PHPT (four-gland disease)—95 frequency (%)
- *Pancreatic islet cell tumors:*
  - Gastrinoma
  - NF-P-NET
  - Insulinoma
  - Glucagonoma
  - VIPoma
  - Somatostatinoma

- *Pituitary tumors:*
    - Prolactin (60%)
    - Growth hormone (25%)
    - ACTH (5%)
    - Nonfunctioning
- Adrenocortical tumors mainly nonfunctioning
- NET lung, thymus, and stomach
- Lipomas
- MEN 1 is also associated with meningiomas and facial angiofibromas

b. Genotype–phenotype associations for disorders arising from *RET* gene mutations.

| *Syndrome* | *Frequently affected RET gene codons* | *MTC (%)* | *PHPT (%)* | *PCC (%)* |
|---|---|---|---|---|
| MEN 2A | 609, 634, 790, 804 | 90–100 | 20–30 | 10–70 |
| FMTC | 533, 630, 768, 844 | 90–100 | — | — |
| MEN 2B | 883, 918 | 100 | — | 10–60 |

(FMTC: familial medullary thyroid carcinoma; MEN: multiple endocrine neoplasia; MTC: medullary thyroid carcinoma; PCC: pheochromocytoma; PHPT: primary hyperparathyroidism)

**Ans. 24** Ganglioneuromatosis of the oral mucosa in MEN2B

**Ans. 25**

| *Risk level, codon* | *Age of RET testing* | *Age of required first calcitonin* | *Age of prophylactic surgery* |
|---|---|---|---|
| D, 918, 804 | As soon as possible, within first year of life | 6 months if not already done | As soon as possible, within first year of life |
| C, 634 | <3–5 years | >3–5 years | Before 5 years |
| B, 609, 611, 618, 620 | <3–5 years | >3–5 years | Consider before 5 years, may delay |
| A, 833, 819, 891, 912 | <3–5 years | >3–5 years | Between 10 and 15 years |

# 38 CHAPTER The Breast

## QUESTIONS

**Q1. Answer the following:**

a. Define terminal ductal lobular unit (TDLU).
b. Most of the ductolobular tissue located in which quadrant?

**Q2. Identify a, b, c, d, e, and f.**

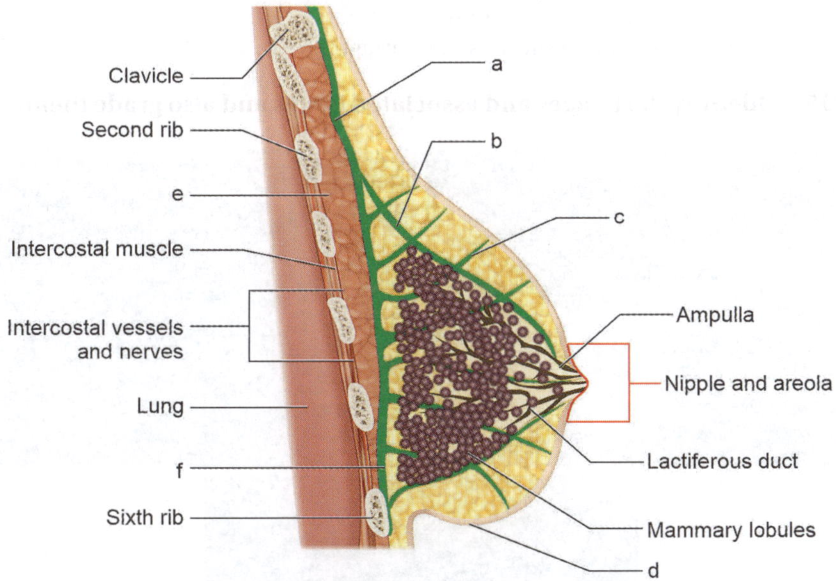


*Source:* Bailey and Love, 28th edition, page 915.

**Q3. Answer the following:**

a. Explain lymphatics of breast.
b. What are the surgical classifications of axillary lymph nodes?

**Q4. Identify the imaging modality and associated condition.**

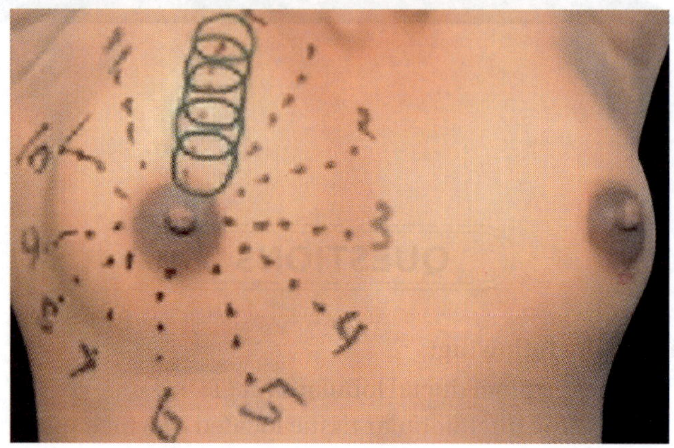

*Source:* Bailey and Love, 28th edition, page 916.

a. What is triple assessment?
b. Identify the method used in image.

**Q5. Identify the images and associated issues and also grade them.**

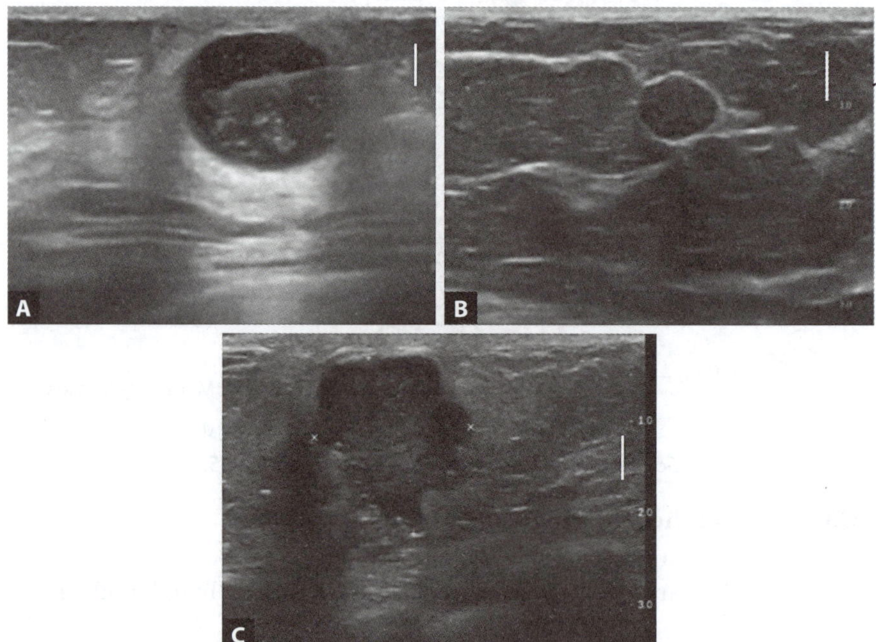

*Source:* Bailey and Love, 28th edition, page 916.

**Q6. Expand abbreviation BI-RADs and explain categories.**

**Q7. Answer the following:**

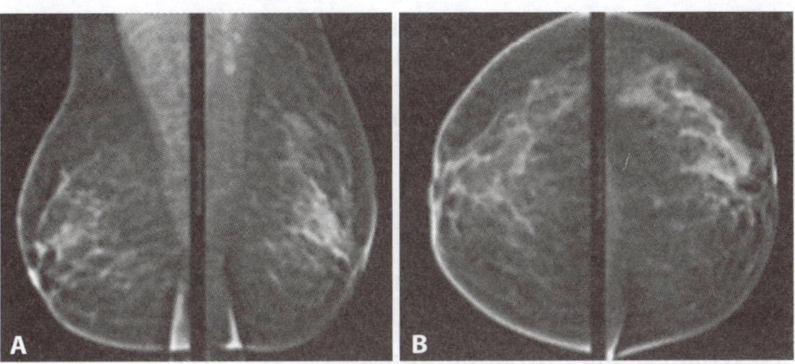


*Source:* Bailey and Love, 28th edition, page 917.

a. What are the two planes in mammography?
b. What is the approximate dose of radiation in mammography?
c. Identify the type of modality and feature in given image.

**Q8. Identify the images A, B, and C and associated condition.**

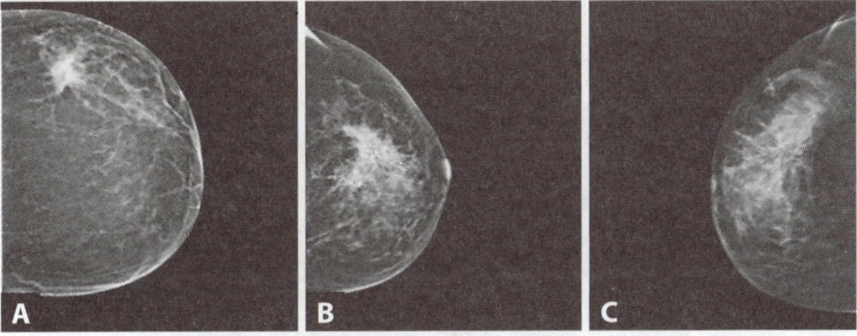


*Source:* Bailey and Love, 28th edition, page 917.

**Q9. Identify the images A, B, and C and associated condition.**

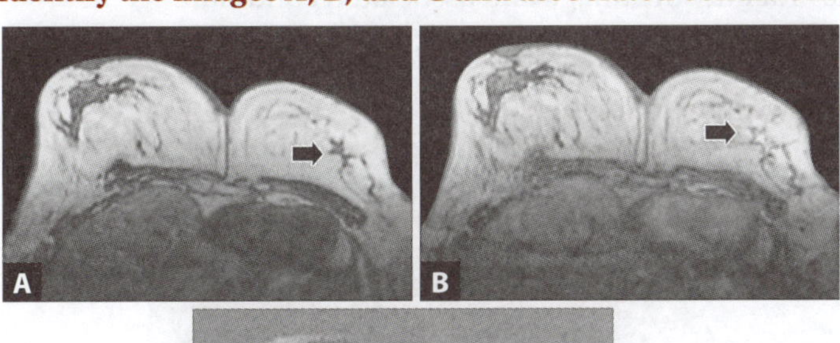


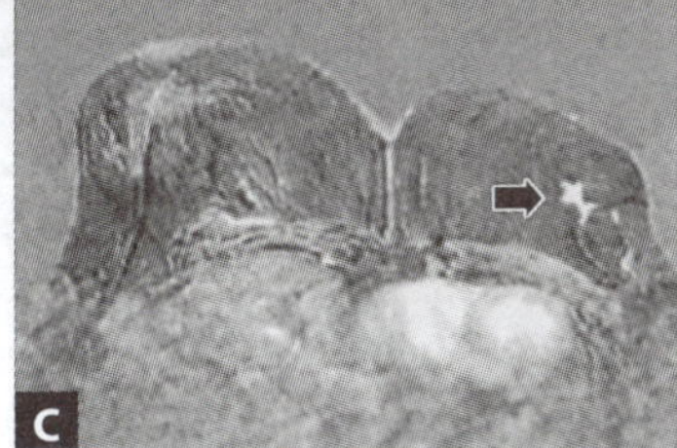

**Q10. Answer the following:**

a. What is juvenile papillomatosis?
b. What is Tietze's syndrome?

**Q11. Explain treatment of breast pain.**

**Q12. Answer the following:**

a. Cardiff-Lucknow nodularity scale used for
b. What are the noninflammatory causes of discrete breast lump?

**Q13. Answer the following:**

a. What is giant fibroadenoma?
b. What is RR for Ca breast in complex fibroadenoma with family history?
c. Indication of surgery in fibroadenoma

**Q14. Answer the following:**

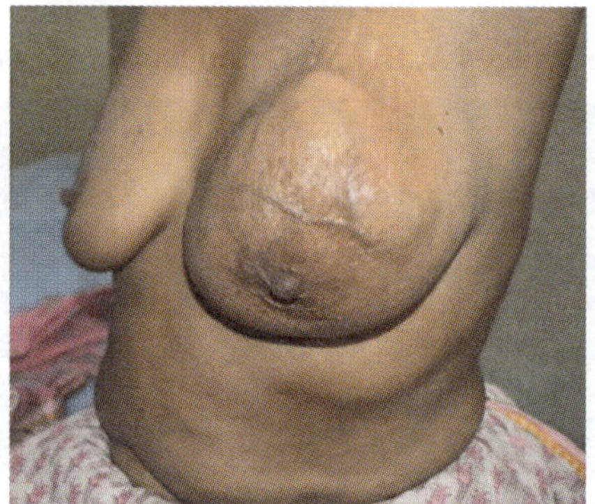

*Source:* Bailey and Love, 28th edition, page 922.

a. Identify the image and associated condition.
b. How will you manage this condition?

**Q15. Answer the following:**

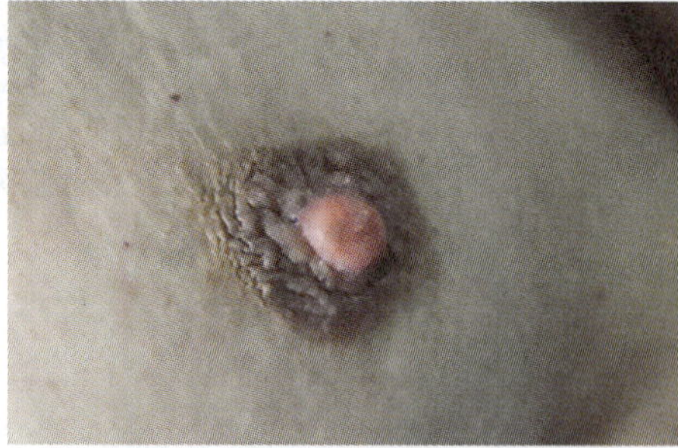

*Source:* Bailey and Love, 28th edition, page 924.

a. Identify the above condition and associated condition.
b. How will you treat associated condition?

**Q16. Answer the following:**

a. Identify the associated syndrome in image.

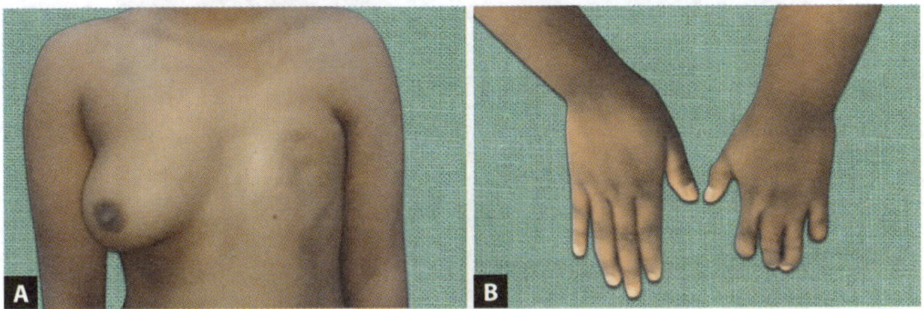


*Source:* Bailey and Love, 28th edition, page 926.

b. Identify the associated condition in image and pathology behind it.

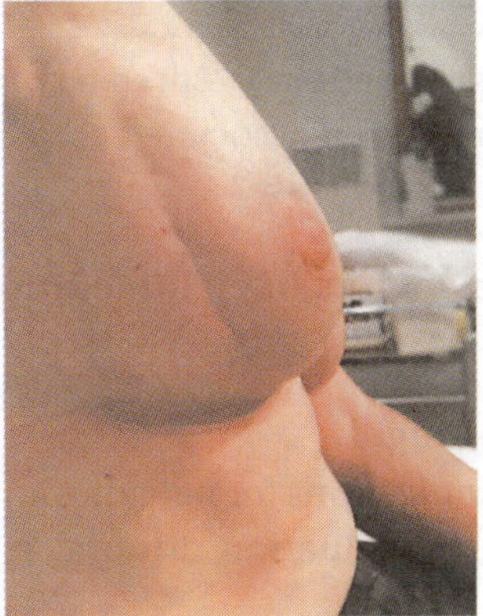

*Source:* Bailey and Love, 28th edition, page 930.

**Q17. Answer the following:**

a. Enumerate modifiable risk factor for breast cancer.

b. Enumerate nonmodifiable risk factor for breast cancer.

**Q18. Write molecular classification of breast cancer.**

**Q19. Identify the image a and b and associated condition.**

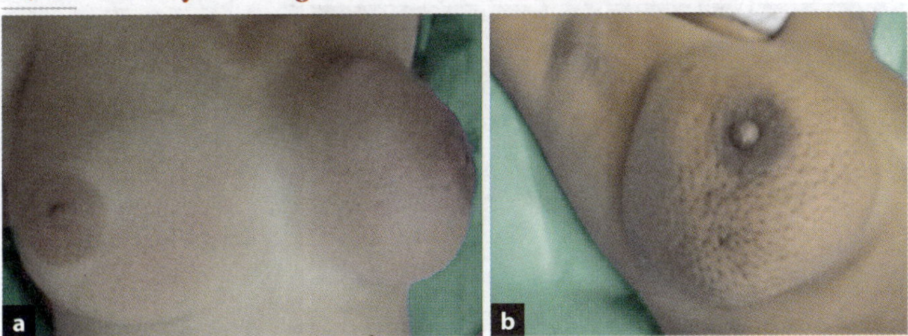


*Source:* Bailey and Love, 28th edition, page 932.

**Q20.**

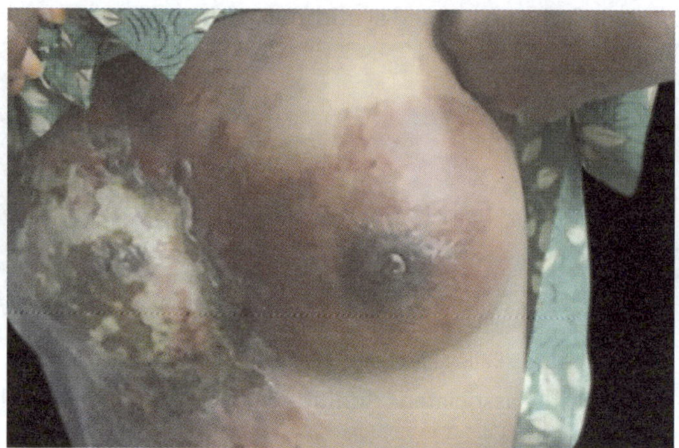

*Source:* Bailey and Love, 28th edition, page 933.

a. Identify the image and associated condition.
b. What is cancer en cuirasse?

**Q21. What are the key points of eighth edition of AJCC TNM staging system?**

**Q22. Answer the following:**

a. What are the indications for neoadjuvant chemotherapy (NACT)?
b. What response evaluation criteria in solid tumors (RECIST) categories?

**Q23. Explain the surgical technique used to treat breast cancer.**

a. Modified radical mastectomy
b. Level I oncoplasty
c. Level II oncoplasty
d. Wide local excision (WLE)

**Q24. Identify the procedure and dye used in below image.**

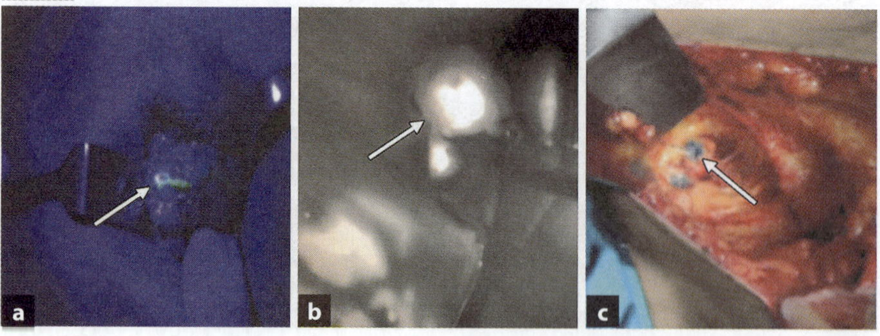


*Source:* Bailey and Love, 28th edition, page 937.

**Q25. Identify structure a, b, c, d, e, f, and g.**

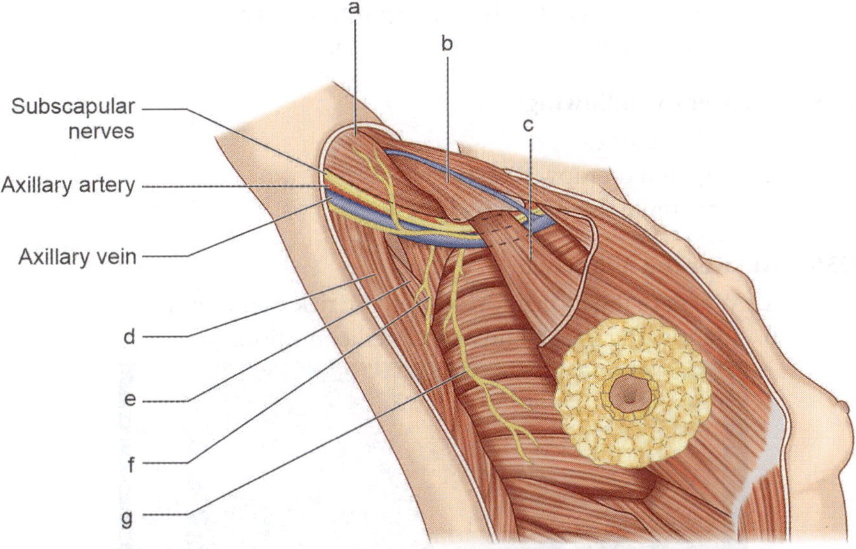


*Source:* Bailey and Love, 28th edition, page 938.

**Q26. Identify the reconstructive flap used in image a and b.**

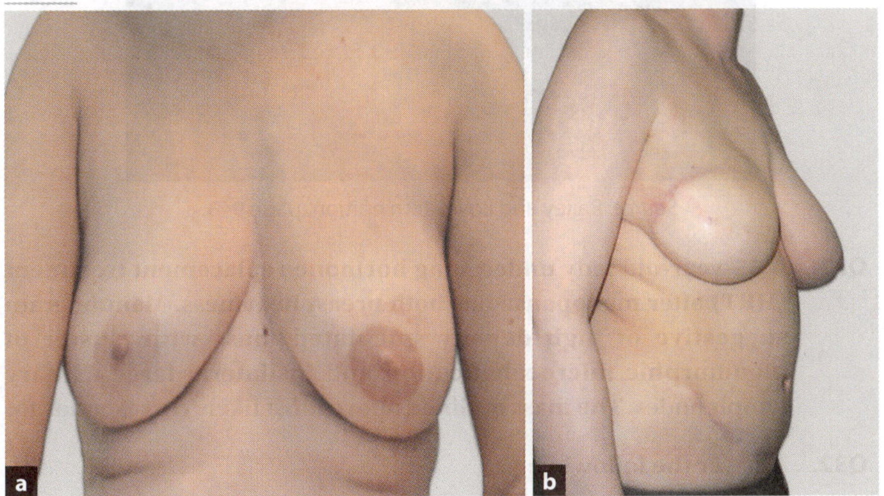


*Source:* Bailey and Love, 28th edition, page 939.

**Q27. Answer the following:**

a. What is indications of radiotherapy?
b. What is the dose of radiotherapy after breast cancer surgery (BCS) given to breast?
c. What is accelerated partial breast irradiation (ABPI) and its indication?

**Q28. Answer the following:**

a. What are the chemotherapy regimens for Ca breast?
b. Adjuvant chemotherapy indicated for

**Q29. Answer the following:**

a. ROR Includes
b. Targeted therapy in Ca breast
c. Hormonal therapy in Ca breast

**Q30. Answer the following:**

a. What are the indications of genetic risk evaluation?
b. Identify the image and associated condition.

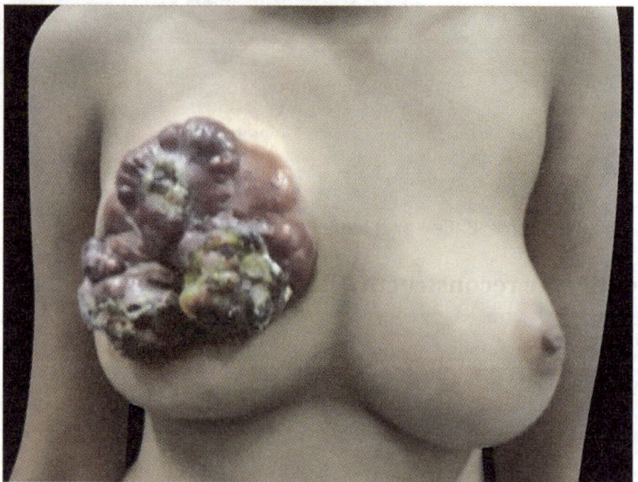

*Source:* Bailey and Love, 28th edition, page 943.

**Q31. A 55-year-old lady undergoing hormone replacement treatment (HRT) after menopause has both breast heaviness. Mammogram suggestive of high density spiculated mass with cluster of pleomorphic microcalcification and ipsilateral large axillary lymph nodes. The mass outlined above most likely corresponds to:**

**Q32. Answer the following:**

a. Ipsilateral supraclavicular lymph nodes are positive in a patient of CA breast. Stage is
b. CA breast stage T4b involve
c. Breast mass of 6 × 3 cm size with hard mobile ipsilateral axillary lymph node and ipsilateral supraclavicular lymph node
d. A 43-year-old woman arrives with a 3 cm node in the supraclavicular fossa and a 5 cm lump in her right breast. Write TNM stage she belongs to as per the latest AJCC staging system.

**Q33. Answer the following:**

a. According to the AJCC, the patient with a 1.2 cm breast mass and three axillary lymph nodes without metastases is at which stage?
b. TNM staging of breast carcinoma with positive bilateral supraclavicular lymph nodes is?
c. A 45-year-female patient with a family history of breast carcinoma, showed diffuse microcalcification on mammography. Intraductal carcinoma in situ (DCIS) was seen on biopsy. Most appropriate management is

**Q34. Answer the following:**

a. A 36-year-old patient underwent breast conservation therapy and chemotherapy for a 1.5 × 1.2 cm ER positive breast cancer with one positive axillary lymph node. She is now on tamoxifen. How will you follow up the patient?
b. A 45-year-old female presented with a history of painless breast lump of size 6 × 5 cm in left upper quadrant with no axillary lymph nodes. A tru-cut biopsy was suggestive of ductal carcinoma in situ. She undergoes surgery with resection of all tumor tissue with adequate margins and postoperative HPE showing DCIS with high-grade necrosis with 4 mm clearance on margins. What needed next?
c. A patient underwent breast conservation surgery (BCS) for a 3 cm lesion along with sentinel lymph node biopsy, which showed one-third of sentinel lymph nodes are positive for macrometastasis. Next step of management is:

**Q35. Answer the following:**

a. A woman discovered a lump and red discharge coming from her left breast. Histopathology revealed duct ectasia. Treatment for this:
b. Using a small fine probe, single lactiferous duct is excised. What is the name of the procedure?

**Q36. A 50-year-old lady presented with the given tumor in the OPD. Tumor was found to be malignant on biopsy. What is the best treatment option?**

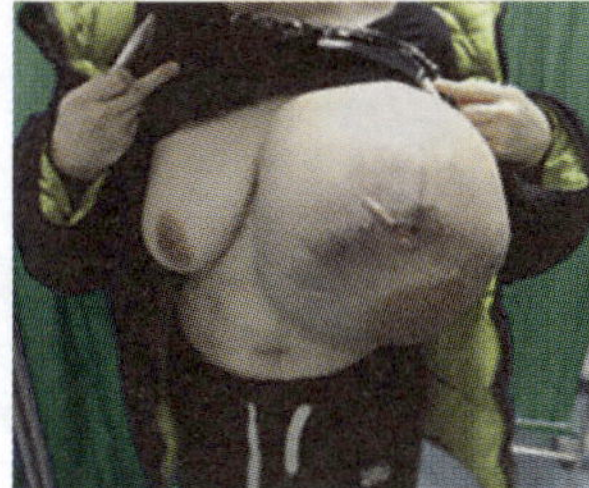
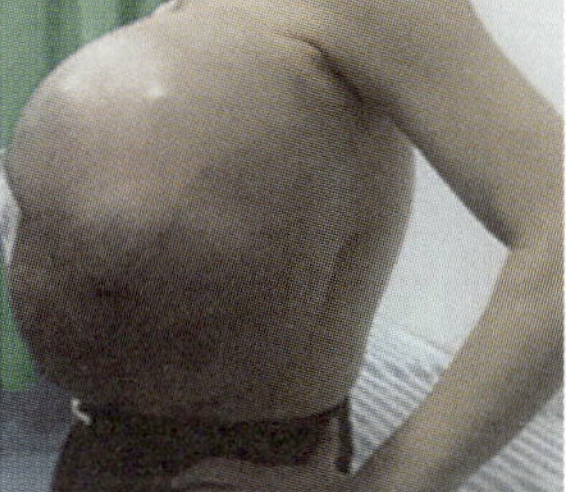

**Q37. A 40-year-old female presented to your OPD with this lesion in the left breast. What is the most probable diagnosis?**

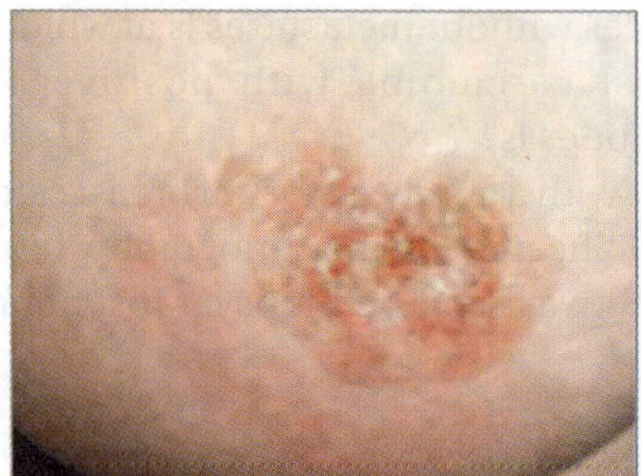
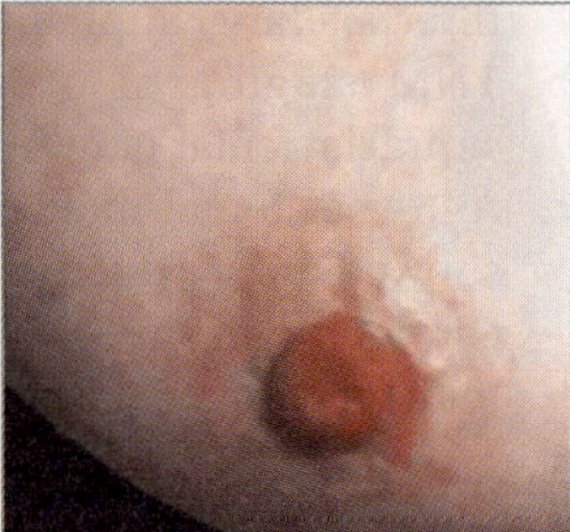

**Q38. Consider the following statements regarding Paget's disease of the breast:**

1. It is a malignant disease
2. Diagnosis can be established by scrape cytology
3. Lymph nodes involvement is an associated clinical feature
4. Treatment of choice is simple mastectomy

Which of the statements given above is/are correct?

**Q39. Answer the following:**

a. A lady primigravida developed fluctuant painful mass of breast and fever after 14 days of delivery. Preferred treatment option is:
b. Retromammary abscess arises from:
c. A breast abscess was seen on a nursing woman. The most frequent pathogen causing her mastitis and abscess development is

**Q40. Answer the following:**

a. An OPD visit from a young woman with bilateral breast O/E, mass was firm and mobile. What is the diagnosis on the basis of findings?

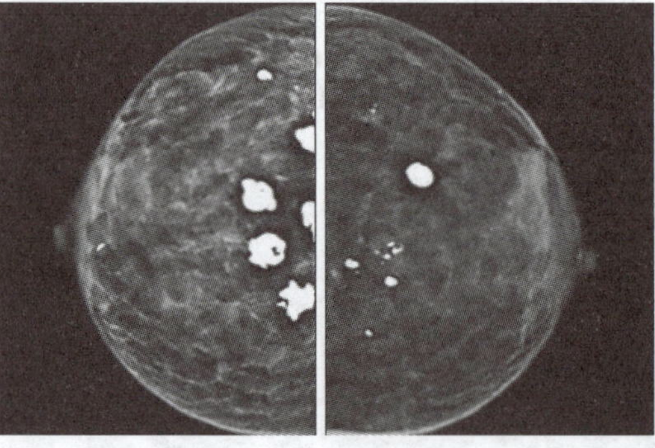

b. Van Nuys grading system is used for

**Q41. Answer the following:**

a. A 50-year-old lady presented with lump in the left breast, which has developed suddenly in weeks. Perimenstrual symptoms are present. No associated family history. On examination, the lump is well circumscribed, fluctuant, 1.5 cm oval in shape. Most likely diagnosis:

b. Since the commencement of puberty at the age of 12, the 14-year-old girl, who is healthy and of normal height and weight for her age, has complained that her right breast has grown to twice the size of her left breast. Both breasts have a similar consistency on palpation with normal nipples areolae. The most likely cause for these findings is:

## ANSWERS

**Ans. 1** a. The breast parenchyma made up of supportive tissue and ductolobular. TDLU is the term used to describe the combination of the lobule and the terminal ductule. The TDLU, or most active region of the breast tissue, responds to hormones such as growth hormone, progesterone, prolactin, and estrogen

b. 50% of the ductolobular tissue is located in the upper outer quadrant and about 20% in the central region.

**Ans. 2** a. Pectoral fascia

b. Premammary fascia

c. Suspensory ligament of Cooper

d. Subcutaneous fat

e. Pectoralis major muscle

f. Retromammary fat

**Ans. 3** a. Most of the breast's lymphatics empty into the internal mammary and axillary lymph nodes. The axillary nodes receive around 85% of the lymph that comes from the breast and are grouped into the subsequent categories:

- Lateral nodes along the lower border of the axillary vein lying lateral to the thoracodorsal vascular pedicle
- Anterior or pectoral nodes between the lateral borders of pectoralis major and pectoralis minor and the lateral thoracic vessels; these are the sentinel lymph nodes in most patients.
- Posterior along the subscapular and thoracodorsal vessels just anterior to the latissimus dorsi muscle
- A central or medial group of nodes embedded in fat in the center of the axilla

- Interpectoral or Rotter's nodes—a few nodes lying between the pectoralis major and minor muscles
- Apical nodes that lie above and medial to the pectoralis minor tendon and lateral to the first rib; the apical nodes receive the efferent lymphatic channels from all the axillary lymph nodes.

The apical nodes drain into the subclavian lymph trunk, which joins the supraclavicular nodes before entering the great veins, either directly or via the jugular trunk or thoracic duct.

b. Axillary lymph nodes are classified into three levels surgically.

| *Level* | |
|---|---|
| I | Below and lateral to the lateral border of the pectoralis minor muscle (the majority) |
| II | In front of and behind the pectoralis minor muscle (including the Rotter's nodes) |
| III | Above and medial to the medial border of pectoralis minor muscle |

The internal mammary nodes lie along the internal mammary vessels deep to the plane of the costal cartilages, superficial to the parietal pleura which drain the medial half of the breast.

**Ans. 4** a. Combination of clinical examination, radiological imaging, and tissue sampling taken for either cytological or histological analysis. This combined approach is called "triple assessment".

b. Dial of a clock method

**Ans. 5**
- *Image A:* Therapeutic aspiration of a complicated cyst. Ultrasonography shows needle aspiration of a sharply defined, anechoic cyst with internal echoes—the floating debris.
  - BI-RADS score 2 (Breast Imaging Reporting and Data System)
- *Image B:* Fibroadenoma. Ultrasonography shows a well-circumscribed, solid mass suggestive of fibroadenoma in a young woman.
  - BI-RADS score 3
- *Image C:* Imaging features of breast carcinoma on ultrasonography. This shows a solid, irregular-shaped mass, taller than wider, with angular irregular margins. BI-RADS score 5.

**Ans. 6** BI-RADS: Breast Imaging Reporting and Database System

| *Category* | *Assessment* | *Probability of malignancy* | *Recommendation of follow-up* |
|---|---|---|---|
| 0 | Incomplete assessment | Not applicable | Need additional imaging/prior mammogram for comparison |

*Contd...*

*Contd...*

| Category | Assessment | Probability of malignancy | Recommendation of follow-up |
|---|---|---|---|
| 1 | Negative | 0% | Routine annual screening mammogram (women over age 40) |
| 2 | Benign | 0% | Routine annual screening mammogram (women over age 40) |
| 3 | Probably benign | >0% but less than or equal to 2% | Initial short-term follow-up (usually 6 months) |
| 4 | Suspicious Abnormalities | | Biopsy should be consider |
| | 4a: Low suspicion of malignancy | >2% to less than or equal to 10% | |
| | 4b: Intermediate suspicion of malignancy | >10% to less than or equal to 50% | |
| | 4c: High suspicion of malignancy | >50 to <95% | |
| 5 | Highly suggestive of malignancy | More than or equal to 95% | Requires biopsy or surgical management |
| 6 | Known biopsy-proven malignancy | Not applicable | Category reserved for the lesions identified on imaging with biopsy proof of malignancy prior to definitive management |

**Ans. 7** a. Mediolateral oblique view; craniocaudal view.
b. The dose of radiation is approximately 1 mGy per film
c. Features of a normal mammogram—(A) mediolateral oblique view and (B) craniocaudal view.

**Ans. 8** Imaging features of breast cancer on mammography (Category BI-RADS 5):
- *Image A:* Irregular, spiculated mass
- *Image B:* Fine pleomorphic microcalcifications
- *Image C:* Architectural distortion

**Ans. 9** Magnetic resonance imaging showing carcinoma of the left breast (arrows).

- *Image A:* Precontrast
- *Image B:* Postgadolinium contrast
- *Image C:* Subtraction image

**Ans. 10** a. A condition known as Swiss cheese disease is juvenile papillomatosis.

- It affects young females with multiple firm palpable nodules.
- Under a microscope, many papillomas with or without atypia are present.
- Sclerosing adenosis, ductal hyperplasia, and apocrine cysts
- The lifetime risk of cancer is increased by a positive family history of breast cancer.

b. Costochondral junction pain without any radiological abnormalities and lateral chest wall pain in the anterior axillary line and over serratus anterior.

**Ans. 11**

| *Exclude cancer* | *Consider medication* |
|---|---|
| • Assurance and chart the intensity of your breast pain with the VAS<br>• Adequate support and during the day tight sports brassiere | • 30 g of flax seed or evening primrose oil every day—rich sources of omega-3 fatty acids and γ-linolenic acid, respectively<br>• Four times per day, apply a topical nonsteroidal anti-inflammatory cream (piroxicam or diclofenac) (helpful for mild to severe mastalgia) |

| *If your pain score is greater than three on a VAS of 0–10, you ought to consider about taking systemic medicine.* |
|---|
| • 10 mg/day of tamoxifen for 3–6 months<br>• Danazol 50-300 mg every day for 3–6 months<br>• Twice a week, 30 mg of ormeloxifene—used for 3–6 months to treat nodularity and both cyclical and noncyclical mastalgia<br>• LHRH agonist (Short duration: usage for 3 months for persistent pain not eased by the following drugs) alone or in combination with antiestrogen: Tamoxifen or ormeloxifene |

**Ans. 12** a. Created and verified is the Cardiff–Lucknow nodularity scale, an objective measurement of nodularity consisting of a five-point ordinal scale that ranks the nodularity on a scale of 0–4.

b. • Fibroadenoma
   • Ductal papilloma

- Phyllodes
- Hamartoma
- Galactocele
- Breast cyst
- Hematoma
- Traumatic fat necrosis

**Ans. 13** a. There are rare cases of giant fibroadenomas during puberty. They have a diameter of >5 cm, develop quickly, and can be enucleated by making a submammary incision.

b. A family history of complex fibroadenoma is associated with a 3.0–4.0 relative risk for cancer, especially lobular carcinoma.

c. Ages above 30, suspicious imaging characteristics (microlobulation, for example), atypia on histology, size >5 cm, a family history of breast cancer, and the patient's desire are all indications for surgical removal.

**Ans. 14** a. *Tumor of phyllodes in the left breast:* Previously identified as cystosarcoma phyllodes, these benign tumors typically affect women over thirty, however, they can also affect younger women. They manifest as a large, occasionally gigantic tumor with a surface that is unevenly bosselated.

b. Due to a high rate of local recurrence, treatment consists of WLE with a 2-cm margin, encompassing the underlying pectoralis major muscle and the skin above it. Mastectomy is necessary for large tumors, recurring tumors, and malignant tumors. Women with malignant or recurring phyllodes tumors may be eligible for postoperative radiation. Malignant phyllodes may be treated with systemic chemotherapy.

**Ans. 15** a. *Nipple erosion in early Paget's disease:* A distinct kind of DCIS that develops in the nipple is called Paget's disease. It appears as nipple erosion that gradually encroaches on the areola and destroys the nipple. It could spread to the axillary lymph nodes and become invasive.

b. A triple assessment is required to rule out underlying cancer. In the absence of any underlying cancer, Paget's illness is treated with central core excision, which involves radiotherapy after a cone-shaped removal of the major milk ducts, the nipple, the areola, and the pectoralis major muscle. For Paget's disease with underlying malignancy, the therapies are mastectomy and evaluation of the axillary nodal status.

**Ans. 16** a. Poland's syndrome with congenital lack of the pectoralis major muscle and left breast (A), as well as ipsilateral hand symbrachydactyly (B)

b. Lateral view of the right breast with Mondor's disease Thrombophilia affecting the anterior chest wall and breast superficial veins.

**Ans. 17** a. *Modifiable risk factor*:

- *Obesity:* BMI >30 RR = 1.29 indicates an elevated risk in postmenopausal women.
- Parity increased risk in nulliparous women or first pregnancy after 35 years of age
- Breastfeeding for longer than 12 months provides a higher preventive impact against breast cancer than shorter breastfeeding periods.
- *Age at first delivery Early:* Under 20 years old, decreased risk Late: increased risk, older than 35
- Using HRT, use after age 10 years elevated risk (RR = 1.2).
- Use of tobacco RR = 1.07 for smoking for 20 years or longer; RR = 1.14 for smoking 25 cigarettes or more per day.
- *Drinking patterns*: RR = 1.05 for moderate drinking (less than one drink per day), 1.32 for moderate drinking (three or more drinks per day), and 1.46 for heavy drinking (more than four drinks per day).
- Radiation exposure RR = 6

b. *Nonmodifiable risk factor*:

- *Age:* Aging is a contributing factor. The median age at presentation is approximately 48 years old in low- and middle-income countries like India, compared to 60 years in the West (the UK, USA).
- *Sex:* Only 0.5–1% of breast cancer cases in men are due to female sex, making it a risk factor.
- *Ethnic groupings:* Ashkenazi Jews, Parsis in India, African Americans under 45 years old, and White Americans
- Breast cancer in the family history—two first-degree relatives with breast cancer: RR = 3; one first-degree relative (mother, sister, or daughter) with breast cancer: RR = 2.
- Innate tendency hereditary breast cancer accounts for 5–10% of all cases; mutations in BRCA1 and BRCA2 can cause up to 70% of these cases.
- Menarche early (before age 12)—the risk of breast cancer rises by around 5% for every year that menstruation starts earlier: For ages under 11, RR is 1.19.

- *Late menopause (>55 years)*: Breast cancer risk increases by about 3% for each year later menopause begins: RR = 1.12 for menopause at 55 years versus menopause at 45 years
- *High-risk breast lesions*: Proliferative conditions without atypia: RR = 1.8–2 complex fibroadenoma: RR = 3 papillomatosis: RR = 3 proliferative diseases with atypia: Atypical ductal and lobular hyperplasia: RR = 4–5 Lobular carcinoma in situ: RR = 8–10

**Ans. 18**

| *Classification* | *Hormone receptor* | *HER2/neu* | *Others* |
|---|---|---|---|
| Luminal A | Positive (either or both ER/PR) | Negative | Ki-67 low |
| Luminal B | Positive (either or both ER/PR) | Negative | Ki-67 high |
| Basal type (triple negative) | Negative | Negative | Ki-67 usually high |
| HER2/neu enriched | Negative | Positive | Ki-67 high |
| Claudin low | Negative | Negative | Claudin low |

(ER: estrogen receptor; HER2/neu: human epidermal growth factor receptor 2/neu; PR: progesterone receptor)

**Ans. 19** a. Diffuse redness (erythema) and skin edema involving more than one-third of the breast, with an enlarged left breast—features of inflammatory carcinoma.

b. Peau d'orange refers to the orange peel appearance of the skin of the breast and is a sign of locally advanced disease. Note that in people with darker skins the erythema takes on a brownish hue.

**Ans. 20** a. *Cancer en cuirasse:* Advanced breast cancer with extensive tumor infiltration of the skin of the breast, upper limb, and abdomen.

b. Cancer en cuirasse is due to extensive tumor infiltration of the skin of the breast, chest (in cases of postmastectomy recurrence), upper limb, and abdomen.

**Ans. 21** Key points of the eighth edition of the AJCC TNM staging system:

- Lobular carcinoma in situ is a high-risk benign lesion not a cancer.
- The T categorization of multiple synchronous tumors is documented using the (m) modifier
- The prefix (y) is used to denote the post-neoadjuvant therapy status.
- Satellite nodules in the skin must be separate from the primary tumor for it to be categorized as T4b.

- Pathological complete response (pCR) denotes the absence of tumor cells in the breast and axillary nodes in surgical specimens
- Inflammatory carcinoma remains classified as inflammatory carcinoma after NACT, even after complete remission
- Microinvasive (T1mi) carcinomas are defined as invasive tumor foci ≤1.0 mm.
- Tumors >1 mm and <2 mm should be reported as rounded to 2 mm.
- Tumor size should be measured to the nearest millimeter.

**Ans. 22** a. The indications for NACT are as follows:
- In locally advanced breast cancer—T3, T4/N2, and N3 disease: To downsize the tumor.
- Select cases of early breast cancer:
  - To downsize the tumor to facilitate BCS
  - HER2/neu-positive tumors
  - Triple-negative breast cancer (TNBC)
  - Premenopausal women (age < 50 years)
  - Patients with axillary node metastasis

b. Response evaluation criteria in solid tumors are used for reporting the response to NAST. The four RECIST categories are:
- Complete response (CR) (lesion not detectable on clinical palpation and imaging)
- Partial response (PR) (≥30% reduction in the maximal diameter)
- Stable disease (SD) (<30% reduction in maximal diameter)
- Progressive disease (PD) (≥20% increase in the maximal diameter)

**Ans. 23** a. *Mastectomy + level I, II, III axillary lymph node dissection*: The Scanlon adjustments divide the pectoralis minor muscle but do not remove it; Auchincloss retracted it; Patey/Madden removed it.

b. To repair the defect left after WLE, the dermoglandular plane and the plane connecting the breast parenchyma to the pectoralis muscle are the two planes on which the breast parenchyma is mobilized in the volume displacement technique.

c. More intricate methods that allow for significant volume resection—typically >20% of the breast volume—by involving glandular mobilization and skin excision

d. Tumor removal with a 1-cm margin of normal tissue cleared in three dimensions

**Ans. 24** Biopsy of a sentinel lymph node employing:

a. *Fluorescein dye*: The blue light illuminates the fluorescent sentinel lymph node
b. *ICG*—with an infrared "spy camera", the fluorescent sentinel lymph node is visible through imaging
c. Blue dye (methylene blue)—In the axilla, blue sentinel lymph nodes, and lymphatics are visible. Sentinel lymph nodes have an arrow to identify them.

**Ans. 25** a. Biceps and coracobrachialis muscles
b. Pectoralis major
c. Pectoralis minor
d. Latissimus dorsi (L. dorsi) muscle
e. Subscapularis muscle
f. Thoracodorsal nerve
g. Long thoracic nerve

**Ans. 26** a. Reconstruction with latissimus dorsi fap
b. Transversus abdominus muscle fap

**Ans. 27** a. The indications include the following:

- Patients with the locally advanced breast cancers (T3, T4, N1, N2, and N3)
- Following BCS
- After mastectomy if tumor size ≥5 cm; skin or chest wall involvement; lymphovascular invasion (LVI), grade 3
- Positive axillary lymph node for metastases.

b. After BCS, the breast receives just 45–50.4 Gy of radiation (with or without a boost) given in 25 fractions, or 40–42.5 Gy given in 15 or 16 fractions (hypofractionation).

c. A radiotherapy modality called APBI is available to certain patients who satisfy certain requirements (American Society for Radiation Oncology ABPI guidelines, 2016):

- Women 50 years of age or older with invasive ductal carcinoma, T1 disease, negative resection margins with a margin width of <2 mm, no LVI, ER positive, BRCA negative, and negative sentinel node.
- Women 50 years of age or older with low-risk DCIS (tumor size ≤2.5 cm, negative resected margin widths ≥3 mm, screen identified, low/intermediate nuclear grade)

In order to prevent any potential negative effects on healthy tissue, radiation is applied to the tumor bed as well as a small rim of surrounding tissue. For 5 days, it is administered twice a day.

**Ans. 28** a. The following regimens are used:

| CMF<br>cyclophosphamide (C),<br>methotrexate (M) and<br>5-fluorouracil (F) | Anthracycline-based<br>regimens: CAF<br>A—Adriamycin (doxorubicin)<br>CEF (E—epirubicin) | Taxane-based regimen<br>Docetaxel<br>Paclitaxel |
|---|---|---|

b. Adjuvant treatment is recommended for all invasive carcinomas with a diameter >1 cm, as well as node-positive tumors and tumors >0.5 cm with unfavorable prognostic characteristics (high grade, HER2/neu positive, presence of LVI, and TNBC).

**Ans. 29** a. Scores for the risk of recurrence (ROR) include:

| Oncotype Dx® | 21-gene recurrence score | Most popular ROR score, which assesses the expression of five reference genes and 16 cancer-related genes in tumor tissue embedded in paraffin |
|---|---|---|
| Prosigna® PAM50 | Ca breast prognostic gene signature | |
| MammaPrint® | 70-gene Ca breast recurrence assay | |
| ROR score as<br>• Low (<18),<br>• Moderate (19–30) or<br>• High (>30)<br>In patients with a low ROR score, chemotherapy can be avoided. | | |

b. The monoclonal antibody trastuzumab, commonly referred to as Herceptin®, specifically targets the HER2/neu receptor. It is used in conjunction with chemotherapy to treat HER2/neu-positive malignancies in addition to pertuzumab. Emtansine, a chemotherapy drug, is conjugated to trastuzumab to enable targeted delivery of the chemotherapy to HER2-positive cells. The cytotoxic agent T-DM1 is used in HER2/neu-positive illness

c. Hormonal therapy for breast cancer uses aromatase inhibitors (anastrozole, letrozole, and exemestane) and the selective estrogen receptor modulator tamoxifen.

Only tamoxifen is administered in premenopausal patients for a maximum of 10 years in patients with a high risk of relapse (tumor >5 cm, node positive), and 5 years in people at low risk.

Aromatase inhibitors are prescribed to postmenopausal women; when taken as an adjuvant, they have demonstrated superior efficacy than tamoxifen in terms of overall and relapse-free survival. They cost more than tamoxifen, and using them increases the risk of fracture and loss of bone density.

**Ans. 30** a. *Indications for genetic risk evaluation*:
- Any person, regardless of age, whose family has a known or probable pathogenic variation in a gene linked to cancer susceptibility
- Age of breast cancer diagnosis: ≤50 years
- Age upon diagnosis of TNBC: ≤60 years
- Two breast cancer primaries
- Male breast cancer, invasive ovarian cancer, pancreatic cancer, high-grade or metastatic prostate cancer, breast cancer at any age if at least one relative has been diagnosed with the illness and is over 50.
- Ca breast with two or more afflicted relatives at any age
- Male Ca breast
- An individual with a personal or family history of three or more of the following:
  - Breast cancer, sarcoma, brain tumor, adrenocortical carcinoma, and leukemia
  - Macrocephaly, endometrial or colon cancer, thyroid or kidney cancer, dermatological symptoms, or hamartomatous polyps in the gastrointestinal tract
  - Breast cancer with lobular cells, diffuse gastric cancer
  - Testicular Sertoli cell tumors, Ca pancreas, ovarian sex chord tumors, gastrointestinal cancer or hamartomatous polyps, or infantile skin pigmentation

b. A young woman with breast angiosarcoma.

**Ans. 31** Carcinoma

| *Calcification pattern in breast disorders:* | |
|---|---|
| Carcinoma | Branched, punctate, and microcalcification |
| Fibroadenoma | Popcorn (crushed stone that is coarse and granular) |
| Fat necrosis | Curvilinear |
| Fibrocystic disease | Powdery |

**Ans. 32** a. IIIC

b. Nipple retraction

c. T3N3M0

d. T2N3M0

TNM staging for breast cancer: 8th AJCC (2017)
- T: Primary tumor
- T1: Tumor ≤2 cm
- T2: Tumor >2 cm and ≤5 cm
- T3: Tumor >5 cm

- T4a: Extension to chest wall, not including pectoralis muscle
- T4b: Edema (including peau d'orange) or ulceration of skin, or satellite skin nodules confined to the same breast
- T4c: Both T4a and T4b
- T4d: Inflammatory carcinoma

*Note*:
- Invasion of dermis alone does not qualify as T4.
- Chest wall includes ribs, intercostal muscles and serratus anterior but not the pectoral muscles.
- Dimpling of the skin, nipple retraction, or other skin changes, except those in T4b and T4d, may occur in T1, T2, or T3 without affecting the classification.
  - N: Regional lymph nodes
  - N1: Metastasis to movable ipsilateral level I, II axillary LNsQ
  - N2a: Metastasis in ipsilateral level I, II axillary LNs fixed or matted
  - N2b: Metastasis only in clinically apparent ipsilateral internal mammary LNs and in the absence of clinically evident axillary LNs metastasis
  - N3a: Metastasis in ipsilateral infraclavicular LNsQ N3b: Metastasis in ipsilateral internal mammary LNs and axillary LNs
  - N3c: Metastasis in ipsilateral supraclavicular LNs
  - M: Distant metastases
  - M0: No distant metastasis
  - M1: Distant metastasis

**Ans. 33** a. T1cN1bM0
b. M1
c. Simple mastectomy

**Ans. 34** a. Routine clinical examination 3 monthly in first year with annual mammogram ("follow-up of breast cancer: Patients with breast cancer used to be followed for life to detect recurrence and dissemination. This led to large clinics with little value for either patient or doctor. It is current practice to arrange yearly or 2-yearly mammography of the treated and contralateral breast. There is a move to return the patient early to the care of the general practitioner with fast-track access back to the breast clinic if suspicious symptoms appear. There is currently no routine role for repeated measurements of tumor markers or imaging other than mammography.")

Breast cancer follow-up recommended for routine surveillance

- *History/physical examination*: Every 3–6 months for the first 3 years, every 6–12 months, 4 and 5 years, annually there after
- *Mammography*: Annually, beginning no earlier than 6 months after radiation therapy
- *Breast self-examination*: All women should be counseled to perform monthly.
- *Pelvic examination*: Annually
- *Coordination of care*: Continuity of care with breast cancer specialist and appropriate other health care providers.

*Not recommended for routine surveillance*:

- *Routine blood test:* Complete blood count and LFT are not recommended.
- *Imaging studies:* CXR, bone scans, liver USG, CT scans, FDG-PET scans, and breast MRI are not recommended for routine breast cancer surveillance
- *Tumor markers*: Cancer antigen 15.3, 27.29 and CEA are not recommended

b. Adjuvant radiotherapy: In this case, patient is 45-year-old (score 2) with size 5 cm (score 3), margin of 4 mm (score 2), necrotic features without high grade (score 2), the total score is 9. Usually for score 7–9, if local excision is done radiotherapy should be given. If simple mastectomy is done, there is no need of adjuvant treatment. In this patient next best step would be adjuvant radiotherapy.

c. Completion axillary lymph node dissection, chemotherapy, and radiotherapy

**Ans. 35** a. Hadfield's operation

b. Microdochectomy ("a lacrimal probe or length of stiff nylon suture is inserted into the duct from which the discharge is emerging. A tennis racquet incision can be made to encompass the entire duct or a periareolar incision used and the nipple flap dissected to reach the duct. The duct is then excised.")

**Ans. 36** On the basis of clinical findings, patient is having malignant cystosarcoma phyllodes, which is best treated by simple mastectomy.

**Ans. 37** Paget's disease of nipple

**Ans. 38** 1, 2, 3 and 4

**Ans. 39** A. Incision and drainage

B. It can be a worsening of a breast abscess, empyema thoracis, or rib osteomyelitis. There is no need to drain the retromammary abscess—conservative care suffices.

C. *S. aureus*

**Ans. 40** a. Fibroadenoma—Popcorn calcification (coarse, granular, and crushed stone)

b. DCIS

The Van Nuys criteria were developed by Silverstein and associates, from a series of DCIS patient's wide excision both with and without radiation therapy, and they suggested an approach for patient identification, who do not need radiation therapy based on:

*Van Nuys grading system*

- Width of the surgical margin
- DCIS nuclear grade and presence of microcalcification
- Size of the lesion
- Patient's age

**Ans. 41** a. *Breast cyst:*

- Mostly occur in last decade of reproductive life, as a result of nonintegrated involution of stroma and epithelium.
- *Clinical features:* Often multiple, may be bilateral and can mimic malignancy; typically present suddenly
- *Diagnosis:* Diagnosis can be confirmed by aspiration and/or ultrasound.
- *Treatment:* Aspiration—In cases of solitary cyst or cyst with small collection (reaspiration in cases of recurrence)

b. *Virginal hypertrophy:*

- Substantial augmentation, typically of both breasts
- It may also be unilateral.
- Usually results from a change in the breast's typical sensitivity to estrogenic hormones.
- Reduction mammoplasty is the treatment.

9

SECTION

# Cardiothoracic

CHAPTER

# 39 Cardiothoracic

## QUESTIONS

**Q1. Answer the following:**

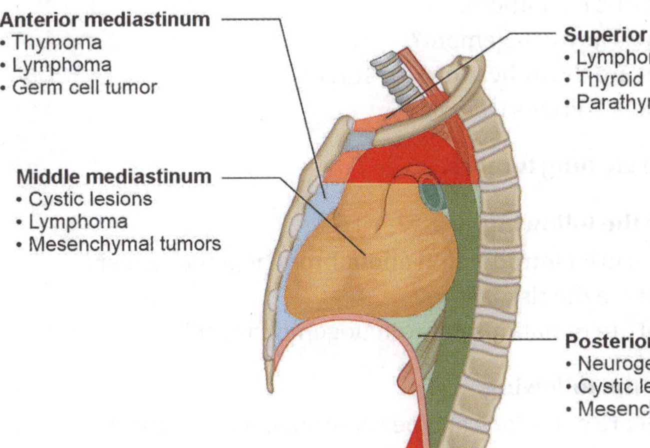


*Source:* Bailey and Love, 28th edition, page 992.

a. Describe the mediastinum parts.
b. Describe mediastinal mass in details.

**Q2. Answer the following:**

a. Describe thymoma.
b. What are the types of thymoma?
c. Describe clinical features of thymoma.

**Q3. Answer the following:**

a. Describe paraneoplastic syndrome (PNS) in thymoma.
b. What is investigation in thymoma?

**Q4. Answer the following:**

a. What is Masaoka staging system?
b. What is the management of thymoma?

**Q5. Answer the following:**

a. What is bronchogenic cyst?
b. Where can it arise from?
c. What are its complications?
d. What is the treatment?

**Q6. Answer the following:**

a. What is lung sequestration?
b. What is its most common location?
c. Describe its types.

**Q7. Answer the following:**

a. Describe chylothorax.
b. What is its management?
c. What are the indications for surgery?
d. What is Poirier's triangle?

**Q8. Enumerate lung tumors.**

**Q9. Answer the following:**

a. Give a brief introduction about bronchogenic cancer.
b. What are the risk factors?
c. What are mutations in bronchogenic cancer?

**Q10. Answer the following:**

a. What are pathological types of bronchogenic cancer?
b. What is the most common location?
c. What are its clinical features?
d. Describe pancoast tumor.

**Q11. Answer the following:**

a. Describe squamous cell carcinoma (SCC) of lung.
b. Describe adeno cancer of lung.
c. Describe small cell/oat cell cancer of lung.

**Q12. Describe paraneoplastic syndrome (nonmetastatic complication) associated with lung cancer?**

**Q13. Answer the following:**

a. Describe T staging of bronchogenic cancer.
b. Describe investigation for cancer lung.
c. Describe surgical method of taking biopsy.

**Q14. Answer the following:**

a. Describe the management of lung cancer.
b. What is the prognosis of lung cancer?

**Q15. Answer the following:**

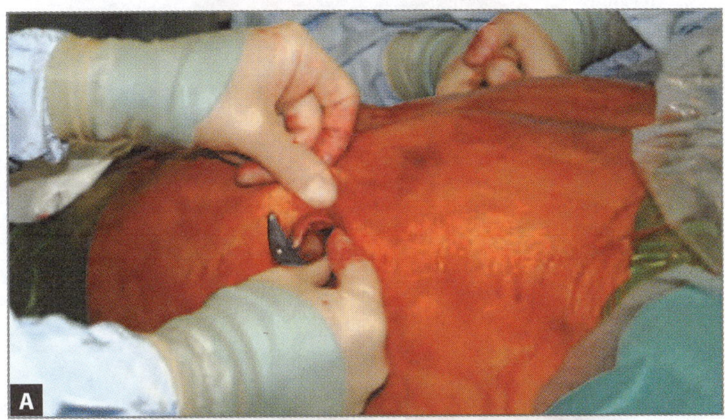


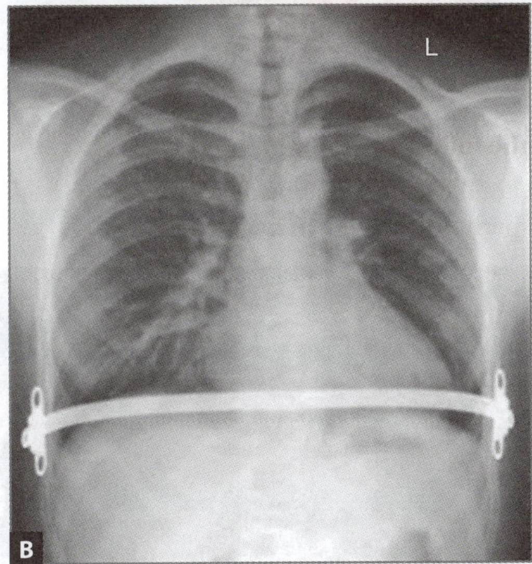


*Source:* Bailey and Love, 28th edition, page 996.

a. Describe the procedure performed in image A and X-ray finding in image B
b. Describe chest wall abnormalities.
c. Describe thoracoscore.

**Q16. Congenital diaphragmatic hernia: Describe 1, 2, 3, and 4 in given figure.**

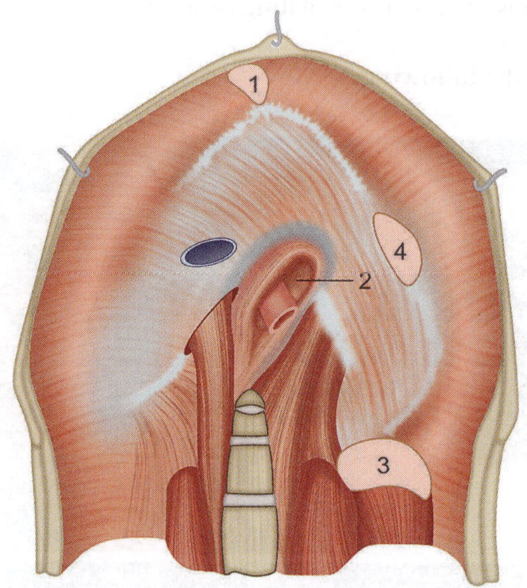


*Source:* Bailey and Love, 28th edition, page 995.

**Q17. Answer the following:**

a. What are the causes of lung abscess?
b. What pathology is shown in given figure?

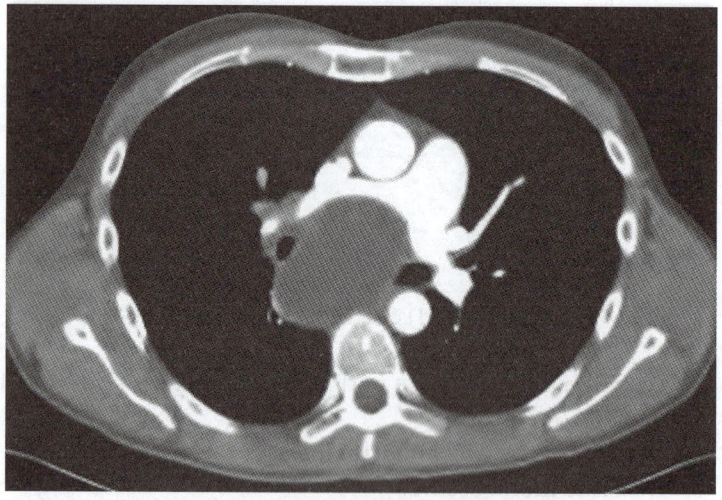

*Source:* Bailey and Love, 28th edition, page 993.

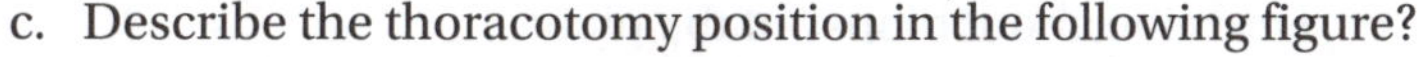

c. Describe the thoracotomy position in the following figure?

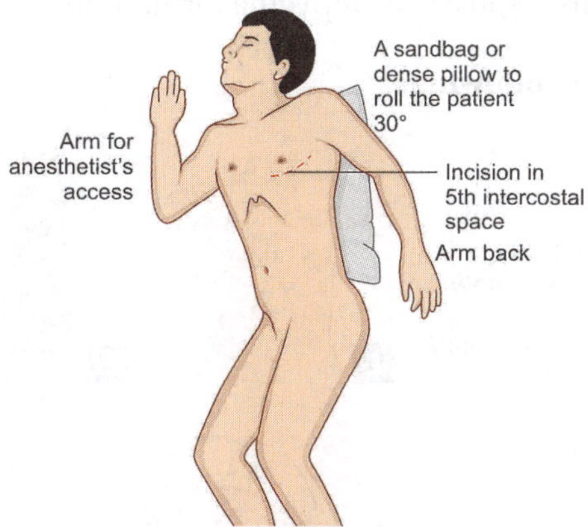


*Source:* Bailey and Love, 28th edition, page 988.

d. When is this condition seen?

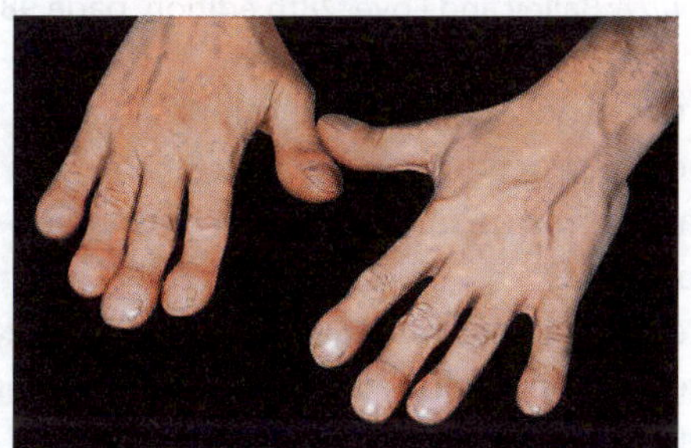

*Source:* Bailey and Love, 27th edition, page 926.

## Q18. Answer the following:

a. What are the uses of bronchoscopy?
b. What is depicted in the given figure?

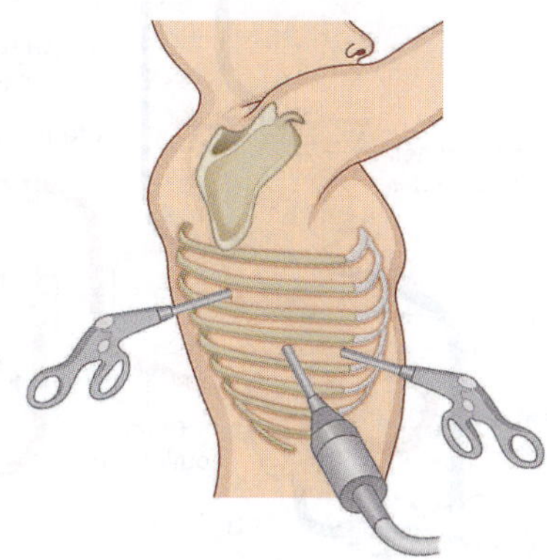

*Source:* Bailey and Love, 28th edition, page 982.

c. Describe about biopsy of the pleura.
d. What predisposes to empyema formation?

## Q19. Answer the following:

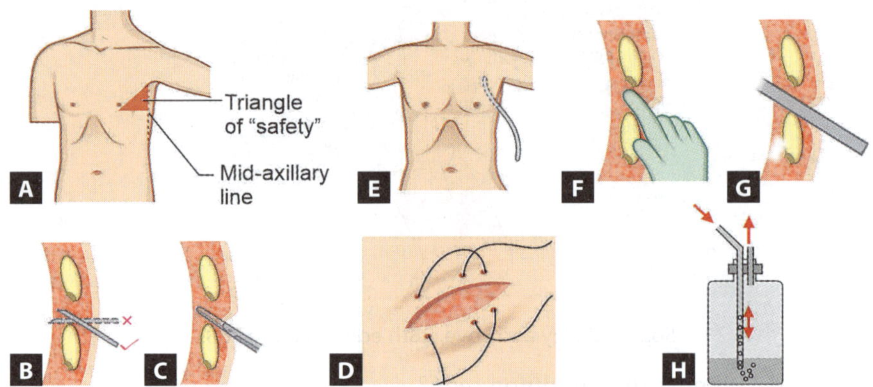


*Source:* Bailey and Love, 28th edition, page 981.

a. What is the procedure depicted here?
b. Describe the procedure in detail.
c. What are the indications for surgical intervention for pneumothorax?
d. What are the normal values of arterial blood gas (ABG)?
e. What are the spirometry values in obstructive and restrictive lung diseases?

## 20. Answer the following:

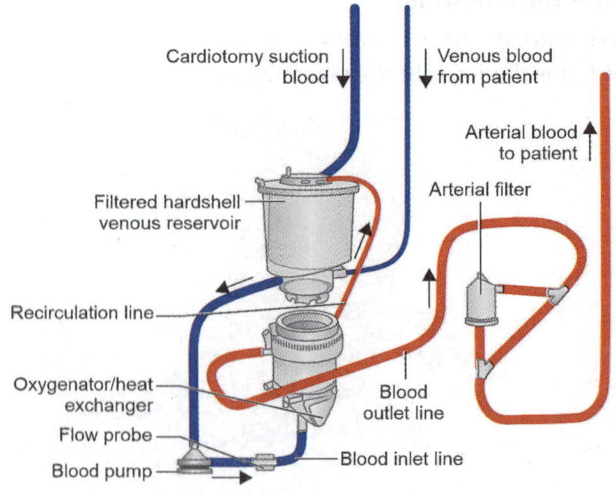


*Source:* Bailey and Love, 27th edition, page 885.

a. What is depicted in the given image?
b. What is the function of that machine?
c. What are the alternative uses of cardiopulmonary bypass (CPB)?
d. What is the procedure to connect cardiopulmonary bypass machine?
e. What are complications of CPB?

**Q21. Answer the following:**

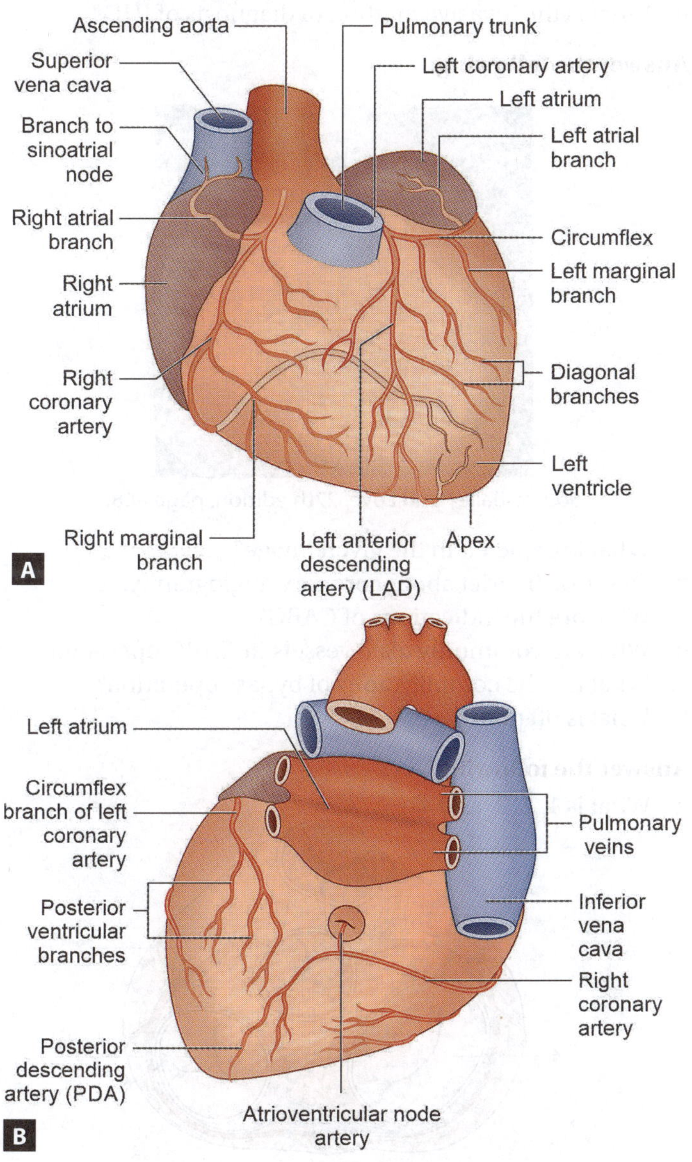


*Source:* Bailey and Love, 27th edition, page 887.

a. What is the blood supply of heart?
b. What are the three main vessels which supply the heart?
c. What is IOC for coronary occlusion?

**Q22. What is ischemic heart disease (IHD)?**

a. What is the pathophysiology of ischemic heart disease?
b. What are the risk factors for ischemic heart disease (IHD)?
c. What are investigations for IHD?
d. What is the invasive method of diagnosis of IHD?

**Q23. Answer the following:**

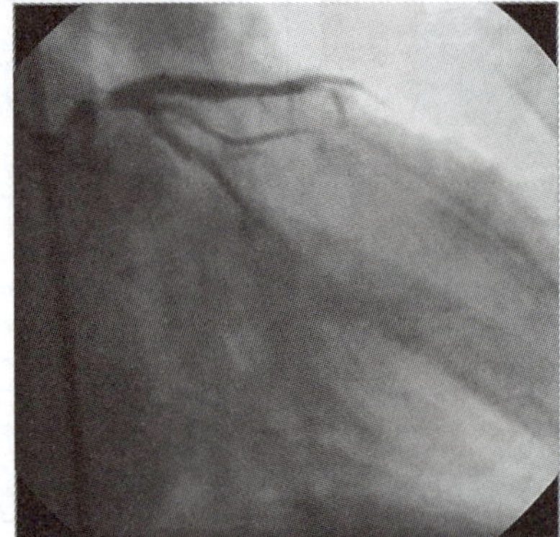

*Source:* Bailey and Love, 27th edition, page 888.

a. What is depicted in the given image?
b. Describe in brief about coronary angiography.
c. What are the indications of CABG?
d. What are commonly used vessels in CABG operation?
e. What are the complications of bypass operation?
f. What is off pump?

**Q24. Answer the following:**

a. What is 1, 2, 3, and 4?

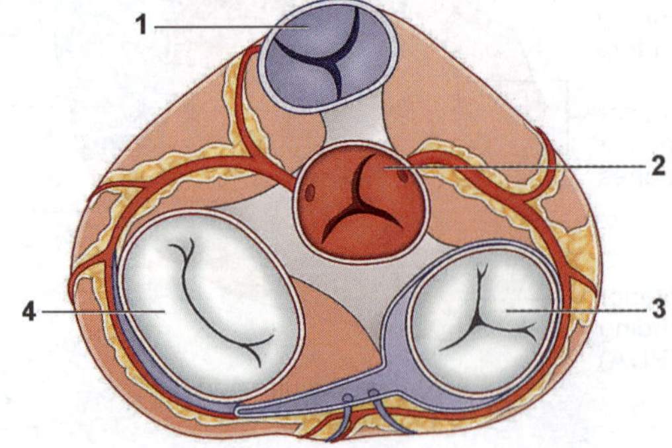


*Source:* Bailey and Love, 28th edition, page 954.

b. What are the various options for heart valve surgery?
c. What is shown in the given image?

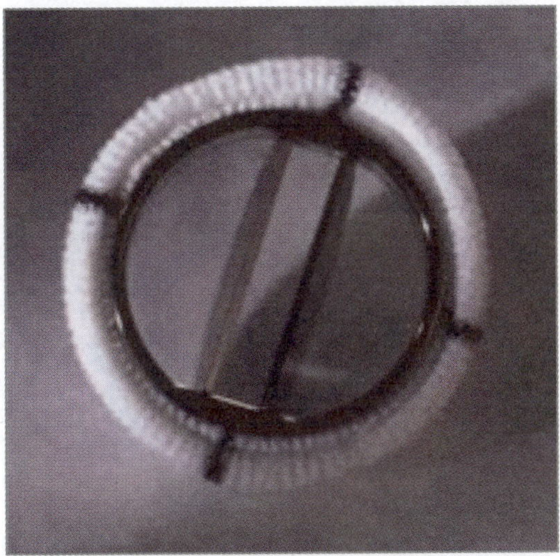

*Source:* Bailey and Love, 28th edition, page 955.

d. What is shown in the given image?

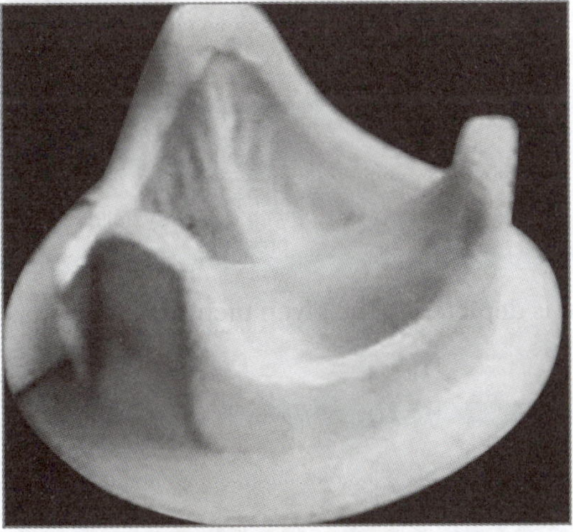

*Source:* Bailey and Love, 27th edition, page 900.

**Q25. Answer the following:**

a. What is the etiopathogenesis of mitral valve regurgitation?
b. What are the causes of mitral valve disease?

**Q26. Answer the following:**

a. What is depicted in the given picture?

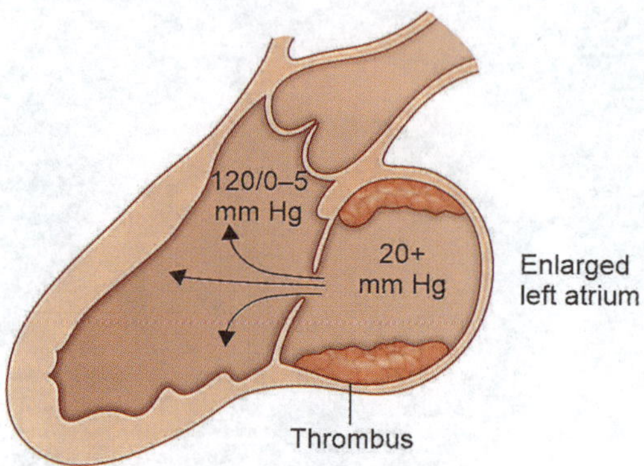


b. What is depicted in the given picture?

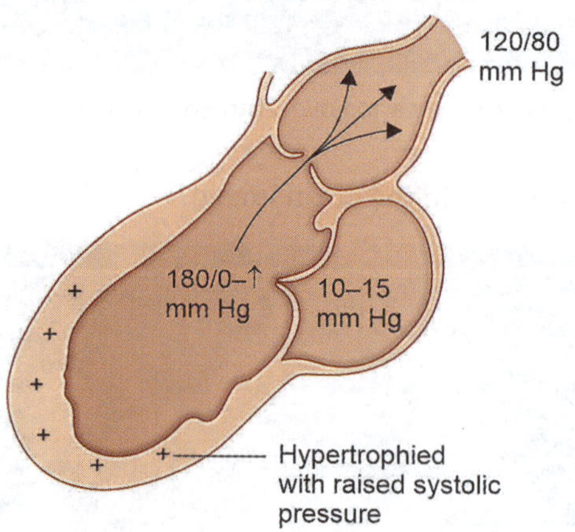


c. What is depicted in the given picture?

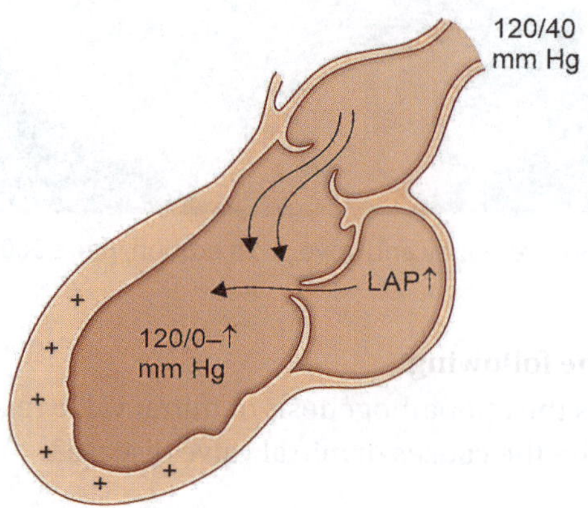

**Q27. Answer the following:**

a. What are the causes of aortic regurgitation?
b. What are the causes of aortic valve disease?
c. What are types of valves?
d. What are the complications of using valves?

**Q28. Describe the image?**

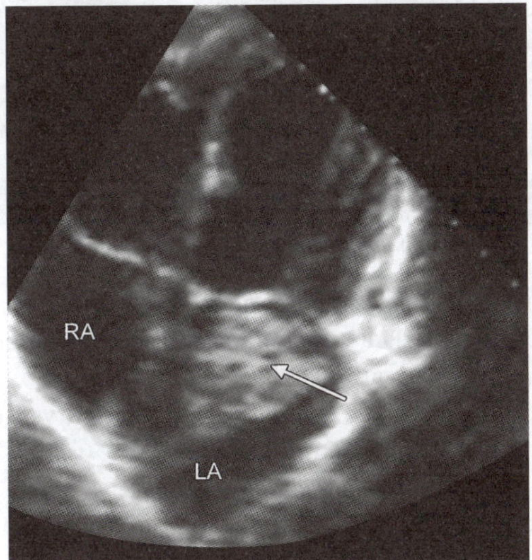


*Source:* Bailey and Love, 28th edition, page 972.

**Q29. Describe Images A and B. Answer the following regarding this condition.**

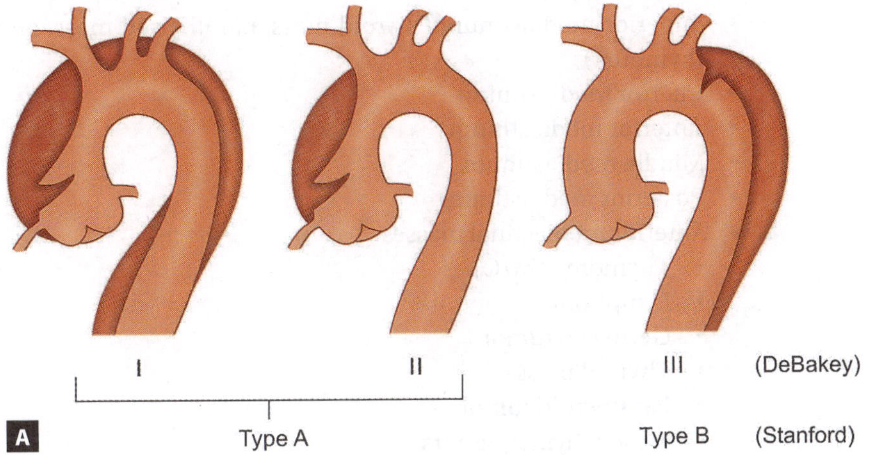

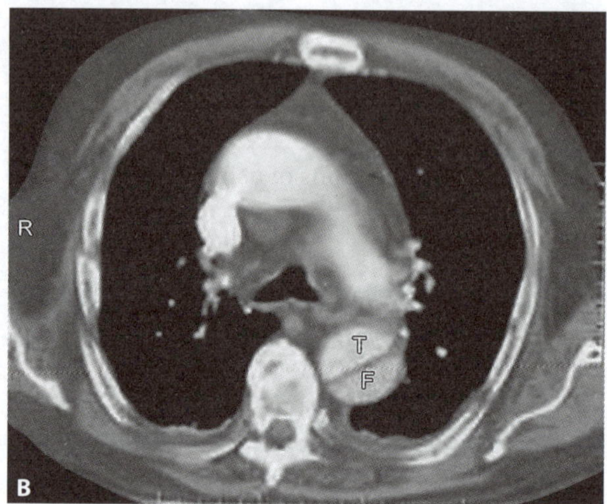


*Source:* Bailey and Love, 28th edition, page 971.

a. Describe aortic dissecting aneurysm.
b. What are the risk factors for aortic dissecting aneurysm?
c. What are investigations?
d. What is the classification of dissection aneurysm?
e. What are its clinical features?
f. What is the treatment ?
g. What is Crawford classification of thoracoabdominal aortic aneurysm?

## ANSWERS

**Ans. 1** a. Mediastinum parts

- Superior mediastinum (thyroid mass, parathyroid mass, and thymoma)
- Inferior mediastinum
- Anterior mediastinum
- Middle mediastinum
- Posterior mediastinum

b. • Anterior mediastinal masses
  - Thymoma (M/C)
  - Lymphoma
  - Germ cell tumor
  - Thyroid mass
  - Parathyroid tumor
  - Mesenchymal tumors

- Middle mediastinum masses
  - M/C lesion cyst (pericardial cyst, bronchogenic cyst)
  - Aneurysms
  - Lymph node masses
  - Ectopic pheochromocytoma
- Posterior mediastinum masses
  - Neurogenic tumors (M/C)
  - Meningocele
  - Mesenchymal tumors
  - Pheochromocytoma
  - Lymphoma

**Ans. 2** a. Thymoma
- M/C neoplasm of thymus
- *M/C location:* Anterior mediastinum
- Seen in 40–60 years age group
- It is surrounded by well-defined fibrous capsule

b. Types of thymoma
- Lymphocytic
- Epithelial
- Mixed (M/C)

c. Clinical features of thymoma
- Usually asymptomatic, usually detected on X-ray chest as an incidental finding
- Dysplasia
- Dyspnea
- Superior vena cava (SVC) syndrome
- Paraneoplastic syndrome (M/C: Myasthenia gravis)

**Ans. 3** a.
- Muscle-related PNS
  - Myasthenia gravis
  - Neuromuscular dystrophy
  - Myotonic dystrophy
- Blood-related PNS
  - Cytopenia
  - Red cell aplasia
  - Hypogammaglobulinemia
  - Erythrocytosis
- Orthopedic-related PNS
  - Rheumatoid arthritis (RA)
  - Systemic lupus erythematosus (SLE)
  - Polymyositis
  - Sarcoidosis

b. • *Investigations:*
  - Tissue biopsy is needed to confirm thymoma (Differential diagnosis: Lymphoma)
  - Elevated cytokeratin is the best marker.
- *Infraorbital canal (IOC)*: Computed tomography (CT) scan
  - *On CT:* Lymphoma—Associated lymph node enlargement is present along with the mass.
  - *On CT:* Thymoma—Well-defined solitary lesion.

**Ans. 4** a. Masaoka staging system
- *I:* Macroscopic well-encapsulated lesion, no microscopic invasion
- *II:* Well-defined capsule, infiltrated into fat and pleura, microscopic invasion present
- *III:* Macroscopic invasion into lungs, pericardium, and great vessels
- *IV a:* Pleural and pericardial metastases
- *IV b:* Lympho/hematogenous metastases present

b. Management
- Total thymectomy performed through sternotomy for symptomatic cases.
- Large thymoma >5 cm thymectomy + chemo
- *Myasthenia gravis:* Thymectomy + anticholinesterase drugs
- Video-assisted thoracoscopic (VATS) thymectomy (Recent)

**Ans. 5** a. Bronchogenic cyst
- Congenital lung lesion due to anomalous development of foregut or trachea bronchial tree

b. • It can arise in two places.
- Mediastinum (M/C 85%)
  - No trachea bronchial communication.
- Pulmonary parenchyma (15%)
  - Tracheobronchial communication +
  - M/C location right lung lower lobe

c. • It can rupture resulting in pneumothorax.
- It can compress the lung tissue atelectasis.
- It can go for infection.
- Risk of malignant transformation
- Hemoptysis is seen, if communicates with tracheobronchial tree.

d. Treatment
- Excision of cyst with VATS method.

**Ans. 6** a. It is a normally developed lung tissue containing bronchioles, alveoli, and receiving blood supply from aorta.

b. M/C in lower lobes, left more common than right.

c. *Two types:*

1. Intralobar sequestration
    - Sequestration within the lung parenchyma
    - 75% (M/C)
    - Has communication with tracheobronchial tree
    - It can get infection.
    - Abscess
    - Hemoptysis
    - M/C in left lung
    - Drains 100% of its blood into pulmonary vein
2. Extralobar sequestration
    - Sequestration outside the lung parenchyma
    - 25%
    - Also known as Rokitansky lobe
    - No communication with tracheobronchial tree
    - Associated with congenital diaphragmatic hernia
    - Drains blood into:
        - Azygous vein 80%
        - Pulmonary vein 20%

**Ans. 7** a. Chylothorax:

a. Triglyceride (TG) level in fluid >110 mg/dL (1.2 mmol/L)

b. It is a complication of surgery or malignancy.

b. *Management*:

- Initially managed by conservative means
- Fat-free diet
- Medium chain TG
- Protein diet
- Fat-free TPN

c. *Indication for surgery*:

- No improvement after 5 days of conservative management
- Chyle loss >1,500 mL
- Nonheeling for >2 weeks
- *Surgery*: Ligation of thoracic duct in Poirier triangle

d. *Boundaries of Poirier's triangle*:

- Vertebral column
- Arch of aorta

  Left subclavian artery

In this triangle the thoracic duct drain into the junction of left Lt subclavian vein + Lt internal jugular vein.

**Ans. 8**

- Benign
  - *M/C:* Pulmonary hamartoma
  - Pulmonary hamartoma
  - M/C in males
  - *X-ray:* Popcorn calcification
  - M/C located peripherally
- Malignant
  - Bronchogenic cancers
  - Malignant mesothelioma (it arises from pleura)

**Ans. 9**

a. *Bronchogenic cancer*:
  - M/C primary malignant tumor in mediastinum
  - M/C seen in lung hilum
  - M/C visceral cancer
  - M/C cause of death due to cancer

b. *Risk factors*:
  - Smoking
  - Air pollution
  - Asbestos, nickel exposure
  - Scars in lungs—can lead to adeno cancer
  - Radiation

c. *Mutations*:
  - KRAS (M/C in adeno cancer)
  - BCL2
  - Cmyc

**Ans. 10**

a. *Small cell cancer (oat cell):*
  - High risk of metastasis present
  - Poor prognosis
  - Response to chemotherapy is excellent
    - Increased paraneoplastic syndromes are present
    - Usually centrally located
    - High chances of metastasis
  - Brain
  - Bone
  - Liver
  - Adrenal

*Nonsmall cell cancer:*
  - Adeno cancer
  - SCC
  - Large cell cancer

- Bronchoalveolar cancer (it spreads by air, satellite lesions are present)
- Less risk of metastasis
- Good prognosis
- No response to chemotherapy
- M/C type adenocarcinoma
- M/C type among smokers is SCC
- Undifferentiated type is large cell cancer
  - Low risk of producing paraneoplastic syndromes
  - Peripherally located (SCC is centrally located)
  - Less risk of metastasis

b. M/C location of tumor is right lung upper lobe

c. C/F of lung cancer:
- M/C is cough
- Dyspnea
- Chest pain
- Hemoptysis (source of hemoptysis is bronchial artery)
- Malignant pleural effusion
- Clubbing is present (resolves after tumor excision)
- Hoarseness + [recurrent laryngeal nerve (RLN) involvement]
- SVC obstruction (SCC)
- Eaton—Lambert syndrome seen in small cell tumors

d. Pancoast tumor
- A tumor located at the apex of lung
- Causes destruction of first and second ribs
- Causes atrophy of hand muscles
- Causes Horner's syndrome
  - Ptosis
  - Miosis
  - Anhidrosis
- It is usually SCC

**Ans. 11** a. Squamous cell cancer of lung
- M/C cancer in India: SCC
- *M/C among smoking males:* SCC
- Pancoast tumor is SCC
- Usually centrally located
- It can form cavity inside the tumor
- It has the best prognosis
- *PNS:* It produces ectopic PTH—hypercalcemia, hypophosphatemia, and clubbing
- *Treatment*: Surgical excision of tumor

b. Adeno cancer:
- M/C type worldwide
- M/C in females
- M/C peripherally located
- It produces lung to lung metastases
- Good prognosis (not as good as SCC)
- Noguchi classification is used in olden days (now TNM is used)
- *PNS:* Pulmonary disseminated intravascular coagulation (DIC), hypertrophic osteoarthropathy, and migratory thrombophlebitis (Trousseau's syndrome)

c. Small cell/oat cell cancer
- Most aggressive cancer
- Worst prognosis
- Responds to CT and RT
- M/C type causing extrathoracic metastasis
- PNS M/C—produces
- Ectopic ADH—syndrome of inappropriate antidiuretic hormone secretion (SIADH)—Hyponatremia
- Ectopic ACTH—Hypocalcemia and Cushing's syndrome
- Myasthenic Eaton-Lamber syndrome
- Cerebellar degeneration
  - ♦ Extra edge
    - Large cell cancer
      - » *PNS:* Galactorrhea in females and gynecomastia in males

**Ans. 12** Paraneoplastic syndrome (nonmetastatic complication)

| *Small cell cancer* | *Squamous cell cancer* | *Large cell cancer* | *Adenocarcinoma* |
|---|---|---|---|
| • Excess ADH secretion causes SIADH and hyponatremia<br>• Ectopic ACTH causes hypokalemia and Cushing syndrome<br>• Retinal blindness<br>• Myasthenic Eaton—Lambert syndrome<br>• Cerebellar degeneration | • *Ectopic PTH produc-tion causes*: Hypercalcemia and hypophos-phatemia<br>• Clubbing in all nonsmall cell cancer | • Galactorrhea in females<br>• Gynecomastia in males | • Hypertrophic pulmonary osteoarthropathy<br>• DIC<br>• Migratory thrombophlebitis (Trousseau's syndrome) |

**Ans. 13** a. T staging of bronchogenic cancer

| | |
|---|---|
| T1 | Tumor size ≤3 cm<br>Involving lobar bronchus<br>Not involves main bronchus<br>• T1a: <1 cm<br>• T1b: 1–2 cm<br>• T1c: 2–3 cm |
| T2 | Tumor size 3–5 cm<br>• Main bronchus involved (but Carina not involved)<br>• Atelectasis, obstructive pneumonitis present<br>• It involves pleura (visceral) |
| T3 | Tumor size 5–7 cm<br>Carina not involved<br>*It involves:*<br>• Parietal pleura<br>• Chest wall<br>• Phrenic nerve<br>• Parietal pericardium |
| T4 | Tumor size >7 cm<br>• Satellite tumor nodules in IL lobe<br>• Infiltration into esophagus, trachea, heart, and vertebra<br>Carina is involved |

b.

| ***Noninvasive investigations for lung cancer*** | ***Invasive investigations*** |
|---|---|
| • Chest X-ray<br>• *CT thorax*: First investigation to be done for suspects<br>• Assess for lung resectability<br>• Any node >2 cm in mediastinum is metastatic node<br>• Positron emission tomography (PET)—CT<br>• Sputum cytology | • Bronchoscopy transbronchial needle biopsy<br>• Endobronchial ultrasonography (USG) and biopsy<br>• CT guided biopsy<br>• Chances of pneumothorax<br>• Done for peripherally located tumors |

c. Surgical methods of taking biopsy

| *Mediastinoscopy*: | *Mediastinotomy:* | *VATS:* |
|---|---|---|
| • Under GA a transverse incision is made over supra sterna notch<br>• A scope is passed through the incision<br>• Biopsy is taken from subcarinal nodes and paratracheal nodes<br>• Pneumothorax and bleeding can happen in this procedure | • Incision is made in 2nd intercostal space (ICS)<br>• Mediastinal nodes biopsy can be taken (Lt Para aortic nodes biopsy can be taken) | • Latest<br>• Staging is done based on VATS |

**Ans. 14** a. Management of lung cancer

- Surgical excision (best)
- Chemotherapy given only for small cell cancer (90% regression is seen)
- *N2 cases*: Neoadjuvant CT is advised
- *Adeno cancer*: Oral tyrosin kinase inhibitor: Geftinib

*Types of resection:*

*Segmentectomy and Wedge resection:*
- For small tumors
- If each segment is removed anatomically ligating the segmental pulmonary artery and vein and bronchus, it is segmental resection.
- Nonanatomical resection is wedge resection.

*Lobectomy*:
- Treatment of choice in early stage lung cancer
- Can be performed via thoracotomy or VATS.
- Bronchus is stapled or sewn.
- One or two ICD drain left and removed later.

*Pneumonectomy:*
- Removal of whole lung and has highest mortality—5–8%
- Procedure reserved for centrally placed tumor or tumors involving Main bronchus.
- Fixation of tumor to aorta, heart, or esophagus means unresectable.
- Ligate the main pulmonary artery, superior and inferior pulmonary veins and main bronchus divided without stump.
- Drainage of space is important—No suction is applied. Only ICD drain kept and leave it unclamped or unclamp it for 1 minute for every 1 hour, slowly the fluid level within the space rises and fills the pneumonectomy space.

b. *Prognosis*: 5 years survival

- *SCC*: 35–50%
- *Adeno cancer*: 25–45%
- *Small cell*: 5%

**Ans. 15**

a. *Image A:* Insertion of preformed bar placed thoracoscopically beneath the pectus excavatum. (The Nuss procedure)
*Image B:* Chest X-ray showing insertion of a metal bar bracing the sternum forward

b.

| Pectus excavatum | Pectus carinatum |
|---|---|
| Disk-shaped deformity | Pigeon-shaped deformity @ Pigeon chest |
| *Open operation:* Ravitch procedure<br>Minimally invasive surgery: NUSS procedure | |

c. Thoracoscore:
   - It is the most widely used model to assess risk of operative mortality in thoracic surgery.
   - It is done preoperatively.

   It is based on nine variables.

   Mnemonic "ASAP—Plan Doctor CME"
   1. Age
   2. Sex
   3. American Society of Anesthesiologist Score
   4. Performance status
   5. Priority of surgery
   6. Dyspnea score
   7. Comorbidity score
   8. Malignant diagnosis
   9. Extent or duration of surgery

**Ans. 16** Diagram of sites of hernias. The usual sites of congenital diaphragmatic hernia: (1) Foramen of Morgagni; (2) Esophageal hiatus; (3) Foramen of Bochdalek (pleuroperitoneal hernia); and (4) Dome.

**Ans. 17** a. Causes of lung abscess.
   - Specific pneumonia streptococcal
     - Staphylococcal
     - Pneumococcal
     - *Klebsiella* spp.
     - Anaerobic
   - Bronchial obstruction
     - Carcinoma
     - Carcinoid
     - Foreign body
     - Postoperative atelectasis
   - Chronic respiratory
     - Sepsis
     - Sinusitis
     - Tonsillitis
     - Dental infection
   - Septicemia
   - Penetrating lung injury

b. Computed tomography scan of the chest showing a bronchogenic cyst splaying the carina.

c. Emergency left anterior thoracotomy for access to the heart. This requires no special support or devices.

d. Finger clubbing is seen in a patient with bronchogenic carcinoma.

**Ans. 18** a. Uses of bronchoscopy
- *Diagnostic:* Confirmation of disease: carcinoma of the bronchus; inflammatory or infective processes
- *Investigative:* Tissue biopsy
- *Preoperative assessment*
  - Before lung resection
  - Before esophageal resection
  - Persistent hemoptysis
- Therapeutic
  - Removal of secretions
  - Removal of foreign bodies
  - Stent placement, endobronchial resection, etc.

b. Video-assisted thoracoscopic surgery (VATS) utilizes modern thoracoscopic instruments and digital technology and avoids large incisions.

c. Biopsy of the pleura
- Cytological examination of the pleural fluid (low yield)
- Abrams' needle (low yield in malignancy)
- Computed tomography (CT)-guided needle biopsy of a suspicious area
- VATS biopsy
- Open surgical biopsy

d. Pulmonary infection
- Unresolved pneumonia
- Bronchiectasis
- Tuberculosis
- Fungal infections
- Lung abscess
- Aspiration of pleural effusion—Any etiology
- Trauma—Penetrating injury
- Surgery
- Esophageal perforation

Extrapulmonary sources—Subphrenic abscess

Bone infections—Osteomyelitis of ribs or vertebra

**Ans. 19** a. Insertion of chest drain

b. • Triangle of safety
- Penetration of the skin, muscle, and pleura
- Blunt dissection of the parietal pleura
- Suture placement
- gauging the distance of insertion
- Digital examination along the tract into the pleural space

- Withdrawal of central trochar and positioning of drain
- Underwater seal chest drain bottle.

c. Second ipsilateral pneumothorax
- First contralateral pneumothorax
- Bilateral spontaneous pneumothorax
- Pneumothorax fails to settle despite chest drainage
- *Spontaneous hemothorax:* Professions at risk (e.g., pilots, divers)
- Pregnancy

d. • pH 7.35–7.45
- $PaCO_2$ 4.5–6 kPa (35–50 mm Hg)
- $PaO_2$ 11–14 kPa (83–105 mm Hg)
- Standard bicarbonate 22–28 mmol/L
- Anion gap 10–16 mmol/L
- Chloride 98–107 mmol/L

e. Spirometry values in obstructive and restrictive lung diseases.

| | ***Obstructive pattern*** | ***Restrictive pattern*** |
|---|---|---|
| PEFR | ↓↓ | Normal or ↓ |
| FEV1 | ↓↓ | Normal or ↓ |
| FVC | Normal or ↓ | ↓↓ |
| FEV1/FVC | <70 | >80 |

(FEV1: forced expiratory volume in 1 second; FVC: forced vital capacity; PEFR: peak expiratory flow rate)

**Ans. 20** a. The components of the cardiopulmonary bypass (CPB) circuit.

b. It oxygenates blood, removes particles, maintains temperature, and circulation (except to heart).

c. The alternative uses of cardiopulmonary bypass (CPB) are:
- Rewarming from profound hypothermia
- Resuscitation in severe respiratory failure
- As an adjunct in pulmonary embolectomy
- In single- and double-lung transplantation
- In cardiopulmonary trauma
- In certain noncardiac surgical procedures (e.g., resection of highly vascular tumors and tumors invading large blood vessels)

d. Procedure to connect cardio pulmonary bypass machine
- Sternotomy
- Expose
- *Arterial cannulation*: Ascending aorta

- *Venous cannulation*: Purse string in right (Rt) atrium
  Extra edge—Machine is going to take care of entire circulation of body except myocardium.

*To prevent myocardial damage:*

- Infuse cardioplegic solution into coronary artery (potassium containing fluid) it arrests the heart in diastole and hence commonly used
- Intermittent cross clamping is performed usually heart develops ventricular fibrillation
- In pediatric cases total circulatory arrest—myocardium can with stand ischemia for 15–20 minutes.

e. *CPB working complications:*
- Bleeding disorders
- Infections
- Air embolism
- *GIT:* Mesenteric ischemia
- Myocardial ischemia
- Neurologic dysfunction
- Pancreatitis
- Vascular injury
- MODS

**Ans. 21** a. Blood supply of heart:
- *Left (Lt) coronary artery (LCA)*: It gives two branches Lt anterior descending artery that runs in the anterior interventricular groove and Lt circumflex artery that runs in atrioventricular (AV) septum.
- *Right (Rt) coronary artery*: It gives Rt circumflex artery that ends as posterior descending coronary artery in 90% and in 10% LCA gives posterior descending artery.

b. Three vessels that supply heart:
- Lt anterior descending artery (LAD)
- Lt circumflex artery
- Posterior descending coronary artery

Extra edge
- M/C diseased artery—Lt anterior descending artery
- M/C bypassed artery—Lt anterior descending artery

c. *IOC for coronary occlusion*: Selective coronary angiography

**Ans. 22** a. Ischemic heart disease (IHD) is a major cause of morbidity and mortality in resource-rich countries. The underlying pathology is mainly atherosclerosis of the coronary arteries.

Pathophysiology

Atherosclerosis is the process underlying the formation of focal obstructions or plaques in large- and medium-sized arteries. It is accepted that atherosclerosis is a chronic inflammatory process resulting from interactions between plasma lipoproteins, leukocytes (monocyte/macrophages, T lymphocytes), vascular endothelial cells, and smooth muscle cells. Atherosclerotic lesions can histologically be found at different stages in blood vessels including:

- The fatty streak
- Fibrous plaque
- Complicated lesion

b. Risk factors for ischemic heart disease (IHD)
- Advancing age
- Male gender
- Hyperlipidemia
- Diabetes mellitus
- Hypertension
- Smoking
- Family history of IHD
- Obesity
- Reduced physical activity

c. Noninvasive methods of diagnosis
- Resting electrocardiography
- Troponin and cardiac isoenzymes
- Exercise tolerance testing
- Echocardiography
- Radionuclide studies and cardiac magnetic resonance imaging—MRI is also very useful in assessing cardiac tumors, pericarditis and other structural heart disease.
- Positron emission tomography
- Computed tomography

d. Invasive methods of diagnosis—Coronary angiography

**Ans. 23** a. Coronary angiogram demonstrating severe stenosis in the left main stem prior to bifurcation of the left anterior descending and circumflex arteries.

b. Coronary angiography
- "Gold standard" for imaging of anatomy
- Demonstrates extent, severity, and location of stenoses
- Reduction in diameter of >70% is considered severe (90% reduction in cross-sectional area)
- Demonstrates quality and size of distal arterial tree
- Aids diagnosis of ischemia

- Evaluates suitability for surgery
- Aids in prognostic assessment

c. Indication for surgery (CABG)
- >50% stenosis of the left main stem (critical left main stem disease)
- >50% stenosis of the proximal left anterior interventricular artery
- Two or three main coronary arteries diseased (triple-vessel disease)
- Poor ventricular function associated with multivessel disease

Extra edge—

*Chronic stable angina:* Percutaneous transluminal coronary angioplasty (PTCA) > CABG

*Acute coronary syndrome:*
- *Unstable angina*: Becomes asymptomatic with antianginal drugs if recurrent unstable angina PTCA/thrombolysis.
- CABG done after 6 weeks.

*Other indications of CABG—*

Myocyte necrosis [ventricular septal defect (VSD)]:
- Patient presents in 3–7 days with pulmonary edema + pansystolic murmur + hypotension.
- *Treatment*: Patch closure

Papillary muscle necrosis (Mitral regurgitation)
- Presents with pulmonary edema + pansystolic murmur.
- *Treatment*: Mitral valve replacement

Ventricular aneurysm:
- Can happen due to necrosis, wall of ventricle bulges out.
- Repaired after connecting the heart to Bypass machine.

d. Commonly used vessels
- Long saphenous vein
- Lt internal mammary artery (LIMA)

| Long saphenous vein | Lt internal mammary artery (LIMA) |
|---|---|
| M/C used vein | For left coronary artery (LCA) and left circumflex artery (LAD) bypass we use only LIMA |
| 10 years patency 60% | 10 years patency is 90% |
| *Other veins:*<br>• Short saphenous vein<br>• Cephalic vein | *Other arteries:*<br>• Rt internal mammary artery<br>• Radial artery (Allen test is done before taking radial artery) |
| | Wound infection in diabetic patients |

e. *Complications of bypass operation:*
   - Bleeding
   - Arrhythmia (M/C sinus tachycardia)
   - Neurological dysfunction
   - Poor cardiac output
   - Mortality 2–3%
   - Wound infection

f. *Off pump coronary artery surgery:* Octopus device is used without bypass machine usage.

   Extra edge—

   *Prognosis of CABG operation:*
   - 95% living at 1 year after operation
   - 90% after 5 years
   - 75% after 10 years

**Ans. 24** a. Four valves of the heart:
   1. Pulmonary valve
   2. Aortic valve
   3. Tricuspid valve
   4. Mitral valve

b. *Options for heart valve surgery:*
   - Valve repair
   - Valve replacement—Mechanical, biological, stented, stentless, and homograft

c. Bileaflet mechanical valve

d. Porcine heterograft stented valve

**Ans. 25** a. *Degenerative:*
   - Myxomatous degeneration of the valve and subvalvular apparatus (Barlow's disease)
   - Fibroelastic deficiency (in elderly patients)
   - *Senile calcification*: Calcified annulus
   - *Connective tissue disorders (e.g., Marfan syndrome, Ehlers-Danlos syndrome)*: Disruption of mitral valve apparatus

   *Ischemic*:
   - Papillary muscle rupture—following myocardial infarction
   - Dynamic mitral regurgitation—as a result of transient ischemia
   - Poor left ventricular function—most common 'functional' cause secondary to myocardial ischemia

   *Rheumatic*:
   - *Previous acute rheumatic fever:* Stiffened leaflets unable to coaptation

   *Infective*:
   - *Endocarditis:* Leaflet destruction and perforation

b. *Causes of mitral valve disease*:
   - Stenosis
     - Rheumatic heart disease (common)
     - Calcification of valve or chordae
     - Congenital (rare)
   - Regurgitation
     - Rheumatic heart disease
     - Valve prolapse
     - Left ventricular dilatation or hypertrophy
     - Ischemia
     - Bacterial endocarditis

**Ans. 26** a. Features and pathophysiology of mitral stenosis. The aorta and left ventricle are relatively small because of chronically reduced cardiac output. The atrium is enlarged and may fibrillate, become stagnant and contain a thrombus. The ventricle fills with a turbulent jet that may be detected as a diastolic murmur or a thrill at the apex

b. Features and pathophysiology of aortic stenosis. Hemodynamic changes in aortic stenosis. Aorta with poststenotic dilatation.

c. Hemodynamic consequences of aortic regurgitation. The left ventricle dilates and hypertrophies and there is a diastolic murmur. (LAP: left atrial pressure)

**Ans. 27** a. Causes of aortic regurgitation according to predominant anatomical location of pathology:
   - Valve leaflet disease
     - Congenital, e.g., bicuspid valve leading to degenerative changes, occasionally with ventricular septal defect
     - Rheumatic heart disease
     - Infective endocarditis
   - Aortic wall pathology
     - Inflammatory, e.g., connective tissue disorders such as ankylosing spondylitis, systemic lupus erythematosus, rheumatoid arthritis
     - Systemic disease, e.g., tertiary syphilis
     - Degenerative, e.g., Marfan syndrome, aortic root dissection, senile aortopathy, leading to aortic root/annular dilatation

b. 
   - Stenosis
     - Congenital
     - Rheumatic heart disease
     - Acquired calcification and fibrosis of valve or chordae tendineae with age

- Regurgitation
  - Rheumatic heart disease
  - Infective endocarditis
  - Congenital
- *Inflammatory:*
  - Systemic lupus erythematosus
  - Rheumatic ankylosing spondylitis
- *Dilatation of aortic root:*
  - Marfan syndrome
  - Dissection
- *Systemic disease:*
  - Syphilis
  - Ulcerative colitis

c. Types of valves:

| ***Mechanical valve*** | ***Biological valve*** |
|---|---|
| Can be used in any age group for any valve available in many sizes | • Allograft from Cadavers<br>• Autograft from same person<br>• Hetero (xeno) graft: M/C used porcine valves |
| *Advantage:* Long durability | *Advantage:* Turbulence is less no anticoagulant needed |
| *Disadvantage:* Thrombogenic, hence lifelong anticoagulants needed | *Disadvantage:* Less life expectancy |

d. • M/C complication using a valve is thrombus formation
- Thrombus formation M/C in mechanical valve
- Thrombus formation M/C in mitral valve
- Valve leaks
- Prosthetic valve endocarditis—(MC organism—Staph epidermidis)—Mortality 50%

**Ans. 28** Transthoracic echocardiography view of left atrial (LA) myoma (arrow) atrial myxoma: It is common in 3rd to 6th decade among females. This is the most common benign cardiac mass in adult. Myxomas are neoplasm of endocardial origin and often appear as an ovid pedunculated mass most commonly seen in the left atrium (75%) or the right atrium (20%), and rarely, in the ventricles.

| ***Sporadic*** | ***Familial*** |
|---|---|
| | As a part of Carney's complex |
| M/C in left (Lt) atrium | M/C found in ventricle |
| Usually solitary | Usually multiple |

- Clinical feature is most commonly such as MS or MR
- Ventricular forms present as obstructive features
- Tumor plop sound heard mid-diastolic

*Complication:* Emboli like manifestation can happen if it is disconnected.

*Investigation:* 2D echo or [Transesophageal Echo (TEE)]

*Treatment:* Surgical excision of myxoma

**Ans. 29**
- *Image A:* Stanford classification of aortic dissections according to whether the ascending aorta is involved (type A) or not (type B). This is simpler than the DeBakey classification (types I, II, and III).
- *Image B:* Computed tomography scan showing acute dissection of the descending thoracic aorta. (F: false lumen; T: true lumen)
  a. *Aortic dissecting aneurysm:*
    - Aortic dissection is caused by a circumferential or less frequently, transverse tear of the intima.
    - *Most common site:* Right lateral wall of the ascending aorta
    - *Another common site:* Descending thoracic aorta (just below the ligamentum arteriosum)
    - *Peak incidence:* Sixth and seventh decades
    - Men are more commonly affected.

  b. • *Most common risk factor:* Hypertension (HTN)
    - *Other risk factors:*
      - Marfan's syndrome
      - Ehlers–Danlos syndromes (EDS)
      - Takayasu arteritis
      - Coarctation of aorta

  c. *Investigation of choice*
    - *Stable patients:* CECT thorax
    - *Unstable patient:* Transesophageal echo (TEE)

  d.

| DeBakey classification | Stanford classification |
|---|---|
| • *Type I:* Ascending, arch and descending aorta involved<br>• *Type II:* Ascending aorta alone involved<br>• *Type III:* Descending aorta alone involved | • *Stanford A:* DeBakey I and II (A—Ascending aorta)<br>• *Stanford B:* DeBakey III |

  e. *Clinical features*
    - Pain
    - Shock

- *Blood pressure (BP):* Disproportionate BP between upper limbs or disproportionate BP between upper limb (UL) and lower limb (LL) presentation: Severe pain; hypotension; myocardial infarction (MI) (if coronary ostium is involved in dissection)
- *X-ray chest:* Widened mediastinum

f. *Treatment:* Emergency Dacron graft repair

g.
- *Type I:* From Lt subclavian artery up to renal artery.
- *Type II*: From Lt subclavian artery up to bifurcation of aorta (largest)
- *Type III:* From middle of descending aorta up to bifurcation of aorta.
- *Type IV:* It involves supra renal aorta ± renal artery (not present inside thorax)

10

SECTION

# Vascular

# CHAPTER 40 Arterial Disorder

## QUESTIONS

**Q1. Answer the following:**

a. Identify the mode of imaging and associated condition.

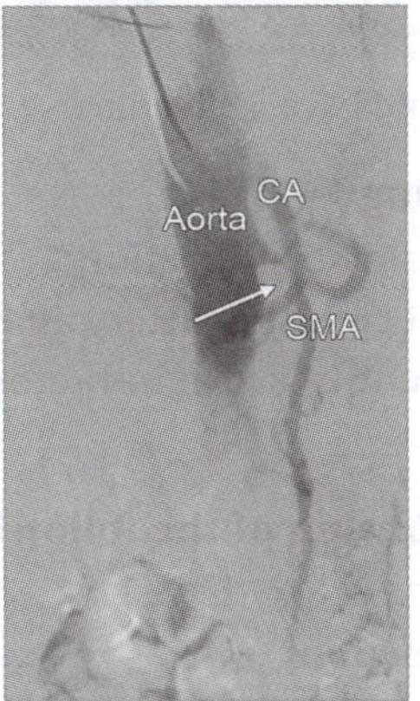


*Source:* Bailey and Love, 28th edition, page 997.

b. Identify the mode of imaging and associated condition.

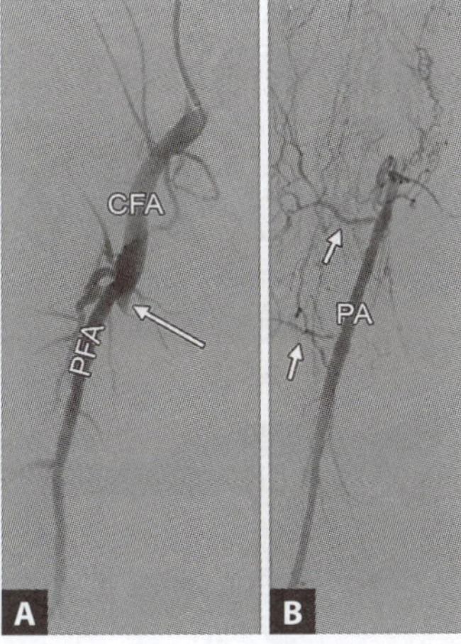


*Source:* Bailey and Love, 28th edition, page 998.

c.

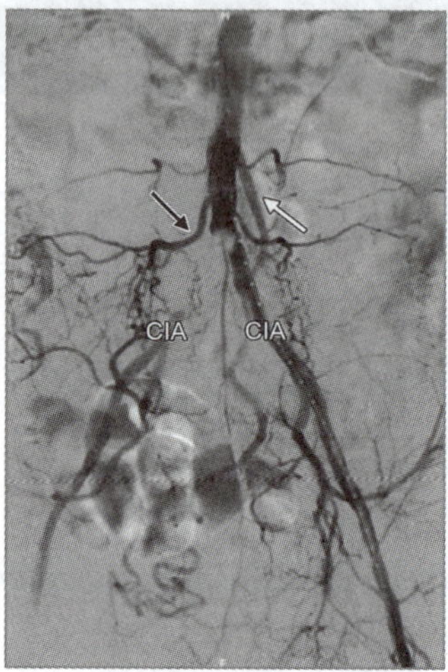


*Source:* Bailey and Love, 28th edition, page 998.

**Q2. Answer the following:**

a. What is intermittent claudication?

b. What is the most common artery affected in it?

c. What are the features of characteristical lower limb arterial stenosis?

**Q3. What is the relationship of the following condition to the site of disease?**

a. Aortoiliac obstruction

b. Iliac obstruction

c. Femoropopliteal obstruction

d. Distal obstruction

**Q4. Answer the following:**

a. Name the procedure shown in the given image.

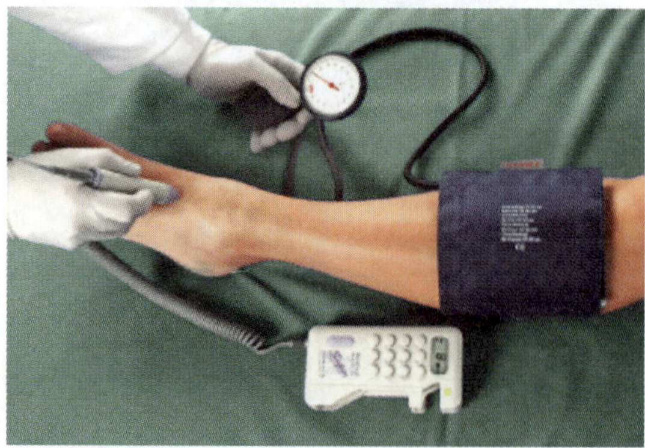

*Source:* Bailey and Love, 28th edition, page 1001.

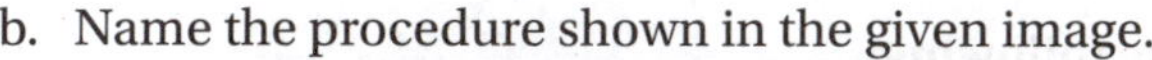

b. Name the procedure shown in the given image.

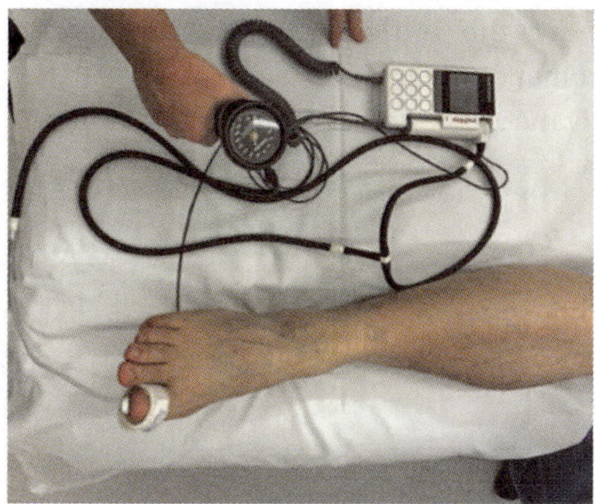

*Source:* Bailey and Love, 28th edition, page 1001.

**Q5. Answer the following:**

a. What is ABPI and its significance?
b. What is toe brachial pressure index (BPI)?

**Q6. Answer the following:**

a. What is the mode used by duplex Doppler ultrasound to provide image of vessel?
b. What is the marry boot?
c. Identify the graft shown in image.

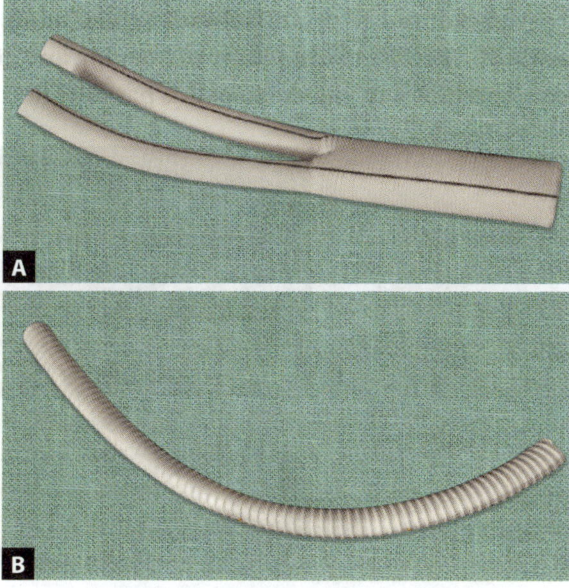


*Source:* Bailey and Love, 28th edition, page 1007.

**Q7. Answer the following:**

a. What are the indications for carotid endarterectomy in symptomatic patients?

b. Identify the image and associated condition.

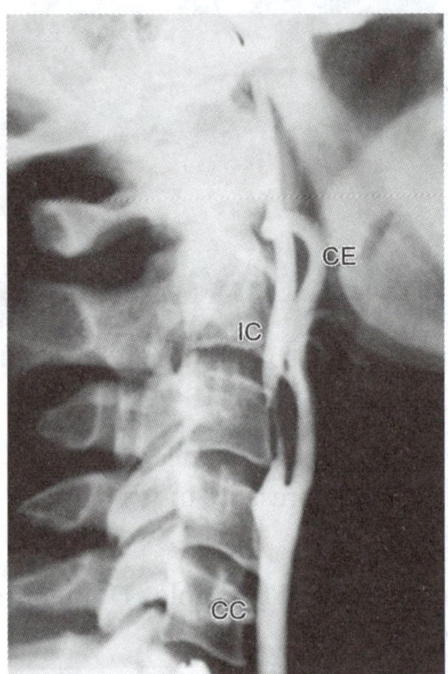


*Source:* Bailey and Love, 28th edition, page 1008.

**Q8. A patient presented with an ischemic right hand. Imaging is shown, kindly identify the modality of imaging and give probable diagnosis and how will you manage this patient?**

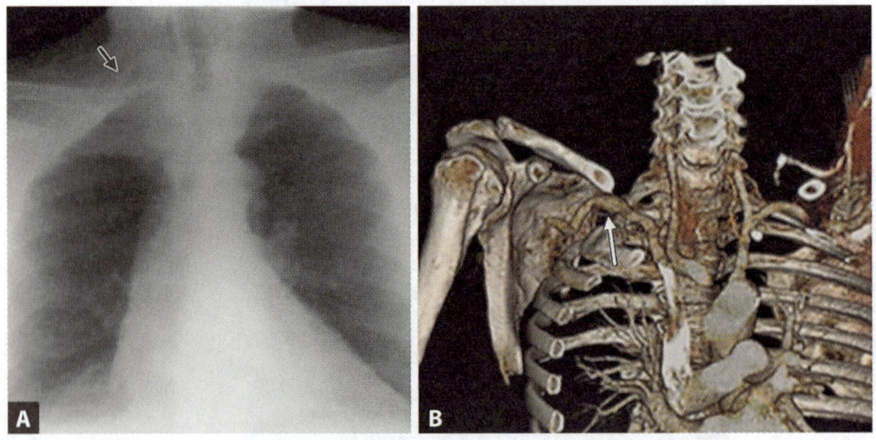


*Source:* Bailey and Love, 28th edition, page 1009.

**Q9. Identify the clinical image and explain the associated condition.**

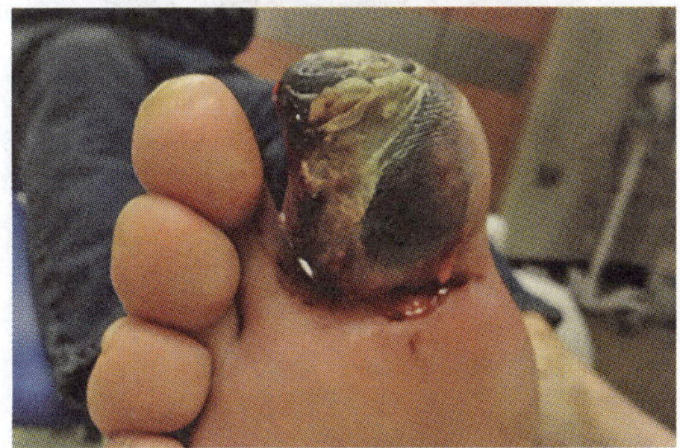

*Source:* Bailey and Love, 28th edition, page 1009.

**Q10. Answer the following:**

a. What are the five Ps of acute limb ischemia (ALI)?
b. What is the use of Rutherford's classification?
c. Enumerate grades of Rutherford's classification.

**Q11. Answer the following:**

a. What are the classical clinical feature of compartment syndrome and its treatment?
b. What are the indications of amputation?

**Q12. Classify aneurysm according to the following:**

a. Wall
b. Etiology
c. Morphology

**Q13. Answer the following:**

a. Identify the imaging modality and the associated condition.

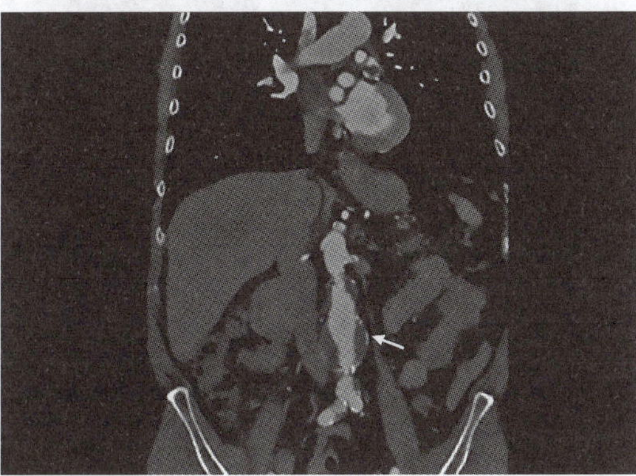

*Source:* Bailey and Love, 28th edition, page 1018.

b. Identify the intraoperative finding.

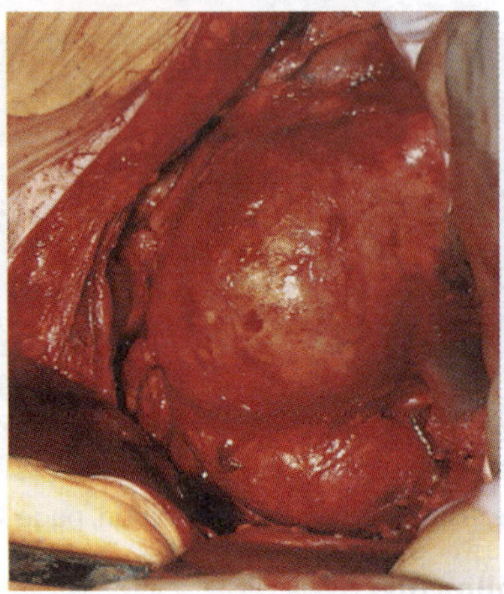

*Source:* Bailey and Love, 28th edition, page 1019.

**Q14. Answer the following:**

a. Identify the image and prosthesis.

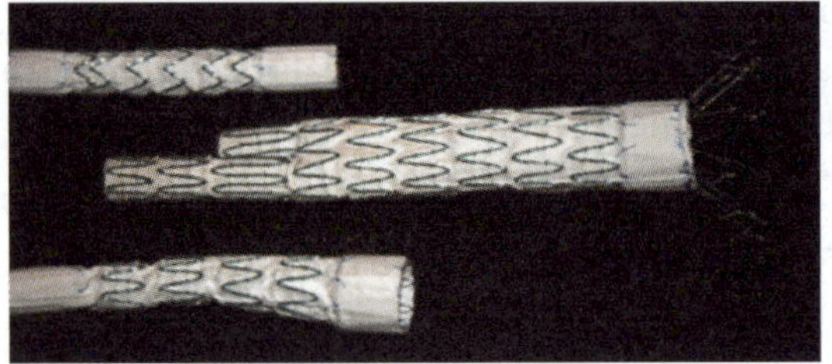

*Source:* Bailey and Love, 28th edition, page 1020.

b. Identify the image and type of endoleak.

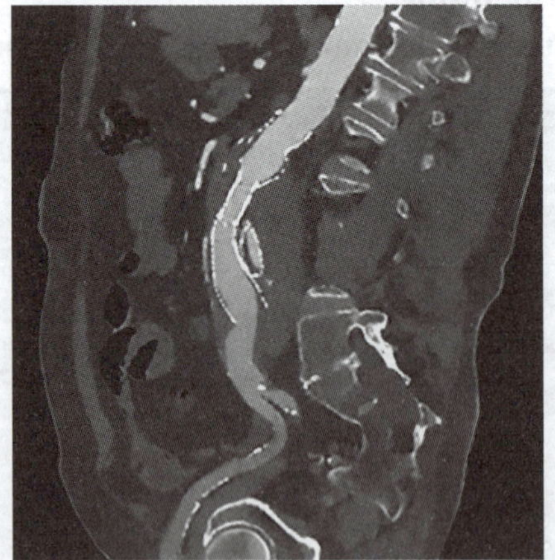

*Source:* Bailey and Love, 28th edition, page 1021.

**Q15. Enumerate types of endoleak following endovascular aneurysm repair and their definition.**

**Q16. Answer the following:**

a. Identify the image and the associated condition.

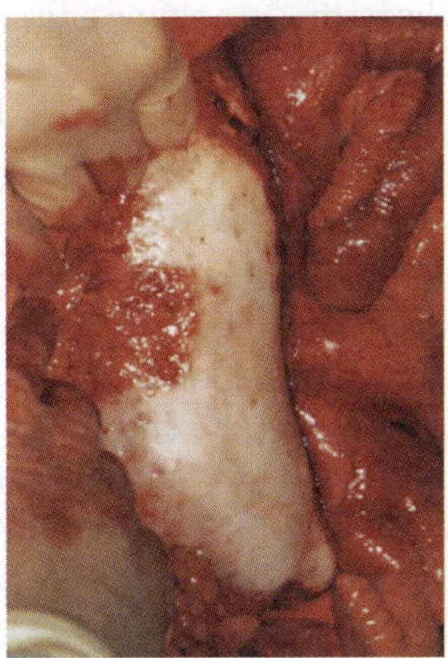

*Source:* Bailey and Love, 28th edition, page 1022.

b. How is a ruptured abdominal aortic aneurysm managed?

**Q17. Answer the following:**

a. Thromboangiitis obliterans (Buerger's disease) and its treatment.
b. Raynaud's syndrome and its treatment
c. What is the sequence of color changes in finger in Raynaud's disease (INISS/NEET SS 2022)?
d. Describe cystic myxomatous degeneration and its management.

## ANSWERS

**Ans. 1** a. Antegrade aortogram via retrograde brachial artery access demonstrating superior mesenteric artery stenosis (arrow). (CA: celiac artery; SMA: superior mesenteric artery)

b. (A) Digital subtraction angiogram from the common femoral artery (CFA) demonstrating a flush right superficial femoral artery occlusion (arrow). (B) Reconstitution of the popliteal artery (PA)

c. Aortoiliac bifurcation disease with an occluded right common iliac artery (CIA) and critically stenosed left CIA. Collateralization has occurred via the lumbar arteries (black arrow) and the inferior mesenteric artery (white arrow).

**Ans. 2** a. It is typically defined as crippling cramp-like discomfort experienced in the muscles and is the outcome of anaerobic muscle metabolism, i.e.,
- Resulting by walking;
- Absent when making the initial move (unlike osteoarthritis);
- Alleviated by resting in a sitting and standing position (usually within 5 minutes).

*Note:* Nerve compression can be brought on by osteoarthritis, lumbar intervertebral disc prolapse, or spinal stenosis. It normally only goes away after resting in a seated position for more than 5 minutes.

The claudication distance—the distance a patient can walk without stopping—varies very little day-to-day is first, by the work demands and hence oxygen requirements of the muscles affected, e.g., walking up hill, increasing the speed of walking and/or carrying heavy weights, and second, by general health conditions that reduce oxygen delivery capacity of the arterial system, e.g., anemia or cardiorespiratory disease.

b. Superficial femoral artery (70% of cases).

c. Features of chronic lower limb arterial stenosis or occlusion
- Dependent rubor or sunset foot
- Arterial pulsation decreased or nonexistent
- Slow capillary refilling
- Arterial bruit
- Intermittent claudication
- Rest pain
- Ulceration
- Gangrene

**Ans. 3** a. Claudication in the buttocks, thighs, and calves, femoral and distal pulses (both limbs) bruit over the aortoiliac region, impotence (Leriche)

b. Unilateral claudication involving the calf, thigh, and occasionally the buttocks bruise over the iliac area, distal and femoral pulses on one side only—Absent

c. Unilateral claudication in the calf, femoral pulse palpable with unilateral distal pulses—Absent

d. Femoral and popliteal pulses palpable, ankle pulses + Claudication in the calf and foot

**Ans. 4** a. This portable Doppler probe and sphygmomanometer measure the dorsalis pedis artery's (DPA) systolic pressure, as part of assessing the ankle brachial pressure (ABP) index.

b. Toe pressures being performed from the hallux. An absolute pressure from the hallux of <50 mm Hg indicates severe ischemia that is likely to prevent healing of ulceration.

**Ans. 5.** a. It is the proportion of the systolic pressure at the ankle to that of the ipsilateral arm. The greatest brachial systolic pressure is the denominator, and the greatest pressure in the dorsalis pedis, posterior tibial, or peroneal artery is the numerator.

| | | |
|---|---|---|
| • Normal resting ABI is 0.9–1.4<br>• ABI below 0.9 indicates a hemodynamically significant arterial lesion<br>• ABI <0.4 suggests chronic limb threatening ischemia (CLTI) | It can be helpful to retest following exercise until pain starts to appear; a decline in the resting ABI of >20% following exercise is suggestive of flow-limiting artery disease | Artificially high ABI readings (>1.4) can be caused by media sclerosis and calcification of the arterial wall, causing noncompressibility of vessel and a falsely elevated ABI; this pattern of disease typically occurs in patients with diabetes mellitus |

b. Since sclerosis seldom affects the toe (digital) arteries, a combination of the ABI and toe-brachial pressure index (TBI) is recommended as a more accurate diagnostic method for identifying patients with diabetes mellitus (DM) who have severe large-vessel steno-occlusive disease.

A TBI <0.6 suggests a significant arterial lesion that may have been overlooked if ABI was used in isolation.

**Ans. 6** a. B mode

b. Miller cuf or St. Mary's boot construction of the lower anastomosis using a small collar of vein between the polytetrafluoroethylene (PTFE) and the recipient artery, which may improve patency.

c. (A) A Dacron bifurcation graft; (B) polytetrafluoroethylene (PTFT) graft.

**Ans. 7** a. Carotid endarterectomy indicated in symptomatic patients 50% or greater carotid stenosis, and the following:

- Ipsilateral amaurosis fugax or monocular blindness
- Paresthesia or contralateral facial paralysis
- Paralysis of the arm or leg or paresthesia, If the dominant hemisphere is affected
- Hemianopia
- Dysphasia
- Neglect or inattention to senses.

b. Carotid stenosis. A unilateral localized stenosis suitable for operation. (CC: common carotid; EC: external carotid; IC: internal carotid)

**Ans. 8**
- *Image A:* A right cervical rib was seen on a chest X-ray (CXR) (black arrow).
- *Image B:* A computed tomography (CT) angiogram showed stenosis of the subclavian artery (SCA) with poststenotic dilatation (lined with thrombus) (white arrow) caused by the cervical rib.

The patient had been ejecting material into the hand from the SCA.

Distal thromboembolectomy, cervical rib excision, and SCA repair were all successful treatments for the patient.

**Ans. 9.** *Diabetic gangrene.*

Three factors commonly combined to induce diabetic gangrene are:

1. Ischemia secondary to macrovascular disease
2. Microvascular dysfunction
3. Peripheral sensorimotor neuropathy (PSN)

Which causes the skin to become trophic; and immunosuppression brought on by too much sugar in the tissues, which makes the body more vulnerable to infection.

**Ans. 10** a. Pain, pallor, paresthesia, paralysis, and pulselessness

b. Acute limb ischemia

c.

| Grade | Category | Sensory loss | Motor deficit | Doppler signals | | Prognosis |
|---|---|---|---|---|---|---|
| | | | | Arterial | Venous | |
| I | Viable | None | None | Audible | Audible | No immediate threat |
| IIA | Marginally threatened | None or minimal (toes) | None | Inaudible | Audible | Salvageable if promptly treated |
| IIB | Immediately threatened | More than toes | Mild/moderate | Inaudible | Audible | Salvageable with immediate revascularization |
| III | Irreversible | Profound or insensate | Paralyzed | Inaudible | Inaudible | Limb irreversibly damaged, major tissue loss, amputation |

**Ans. 11** a. Extreme pain that is out of proportion to clinical findings and that gets worse over time even with the right analgesics. The patient frequently reports feeling paresthesia or numbness along

the nerves that run through the compartment (hypoxia is most susceptible to nonmyelinated type C sensory fibers).

*Treatment*—Immediate fasciotomy of the compartment to relieve the compression. The calf, particularly the anterior tibial compartment, is the site of fasciotomy; however, compartment syndrome can also occasionally affect the thigh, arm, and foot.

b. *Indications for amputation:*

| ***Dead limb*** | ***Deadly limb*** | ***"Dead loss" limb*** |
|---|---|---|
| Gangrene | • Spreading cellulitis<br>• Wet gangrene<br>• Arteriovenous (AV) fistula<br>• Other (e.g., malignancy) | • Paralysis<br>• Severe rest pain with unreconstructible critical leg ischemia<br>• Other (e.g., contracture, trauma) |

**Ans. 12** a to c. *Classification:*

| ***Wall*** | ***Morphology*** | ***Etiology*** |
|---|---|---|
| • True (all three layers involved :intima, media, and adventitia)<br>• False (single layer of fibrous tissue) | • Fusiform<br>• Saccular | • Atheromatous<br>• Mycotic (bacterial rather than fungal)<br>• Collagen disease<br>• Traumatic |

**Ans. 13** a. An infrarenal aortic aneurysm in the coronal plane is visible on an abdominal CT scan (arrow). Blood flowing through the thrombus-containing sac is enhanced with a contrast agent and appears white.

b. Thrombus removed from an abdominal aortic aneurysm (AAA); this thrombus is the reason an angiogram may give a false impression of aneurysm diameter on digital subtraction angiography (DSA).

**Ans. 14** a. Endovascular prosthesis

b. A stent-graft retracted into the aneurysm sac, creating a type Ib endoleak.

**Ans. 15**
- Type I persistent filling of the aneurysm sac owing to an ineffective seal at the proximal (Ia) or distal (Ib) end of the stent-graft.
- Type II persistent filling of the aneurysm sac owing to retrograde flow of blood from aortic collaterals, e.g., inferior mesenteric artery (IMA) and lumbar arteries
- Type III persistent filling of the aneurysm sac owing to structural failure of the stent-graft as a result of component disconnection (IIIa) or stent fabric tear (IIIb).

- Type IV persistent filling of the aneurysm sac owing to stent-graft fabric porosity.
- Type V (endotension) persistent filling of the aneurysm sac without evidence of types I–IV endoleak.

**Ans. 16** a. Inflammatory abdominal aortic aneurysm (white "icing" effect). It can be technically challenging to treat these lesions.

b. *Management:*

I. Early diagnosis (abdominal/back pain, pulsatile mass, and shock)
II. Immediate resuscitation (oxygen, intravenous replacement therapy, and central line)
III. Maintain systolic pressure, but not >100 mm Hg
IV. Urinary catheter
V. Cross-match blood
VI. Rapid transfer to the operating room

**Ans. 17** a. *Thromboangiitis obliterans (Buerger's disease/TAO)*—Thrombophlebitis of superficial or deep veins, disease of occlusive small and medium-sized limb arteries, and Raynaud's syndrome; It typically affects young, male smokers.

- *Histopathological examination (HPE):* Thrombosis is caused by inflammatory alterations in the artery and vein walls.
- *Treatment:* Complete cessation of smoking, which only delays the illness's progression.
- Amputations may eventually be necessary for established artery occlusions, but treatment is similar to that for atheromatous disease.

b. *Raynaud's syndrome:* Peripheral artery sign of a collagen illness, such as rheumatoid arthritis (RA) or systemic lupus erythematosus (SLE).

*Clinical features:* For Raynaud's disease but they may be much more aggressive.

Raynaud's syndrome may also follow the use of vibrating tools. In this context, it is a recognized industrial disease and is known as "vibration white finger".

*Treatment:* Primarily at the underlying problem, even though the aforementioned conservative measures frequently prove beneficial. Multiple amputations and digit necrosis are common outcomes of the syndrome when it is due to collagen disease. Since sympathectomy yields unsatisfactory results, it is not recommended. Steroids, nifedipine, and vasospastic antagonists are possible treatment choices. Patients who have vibration white finger should avoid using vibrating instruments.

c. Characteristic sequence of blanching, dusky cyanosis followed by red engorgement, often accompanied by pain.
d. Accumulation of transparent fluid in a main artery's outer layers, resembling a synovial ganglion, especially the popliteal artery. The lesion may narrow the vessel, causing claudication.
   *IOC:* Duplex scan.
   *Management:* Decompression, by removal of the myxomatous material, may be successful but in some cases excision of the diseased artery with interposition vein graft repair is required.

CHAPTER

# 41 Venous Disorder

## QUESTIONS

**Q1. Answer the following:**

a. How much percent of the total blood volume is contained in venous system?
b. Identify the graph and describe what light blue line and dark blue line depicts.

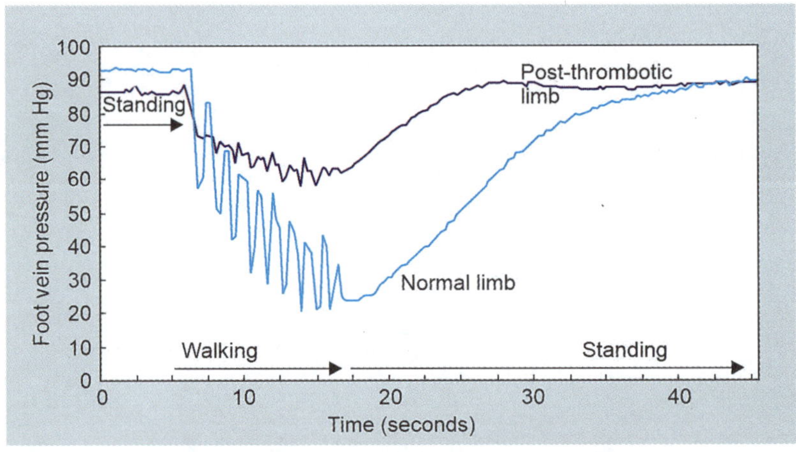


*Source:* Bailey and Love, 28th edition, page 1027.

**Q2. Answer the following:**

a. What are the factors causing venous hypertension?
b. Describe CEAP [Clinical (C), Etiological (E), Anatomical (A), and Pathophysiological (P)] classification for chronic venous disorder.

**Q3. Answer the following:**

a. Write compression hosiery classification according to THR pressure it exerts.
b. Identify the image.

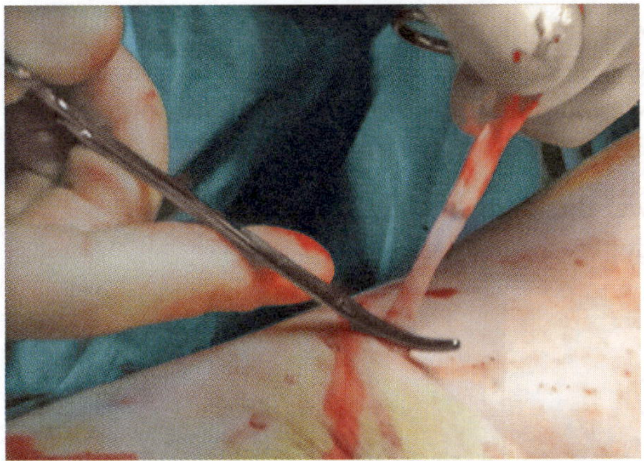

*Source:* Bailey and Love, 28th edition, page 1035.

**Q4. Answer the following:**

a. Identify the image.

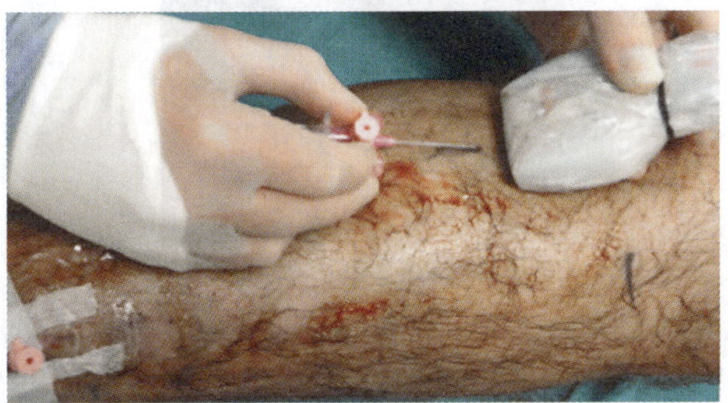

*Source:* Bailey and Love, 28th edition, page 1035.

b. Identify the image.

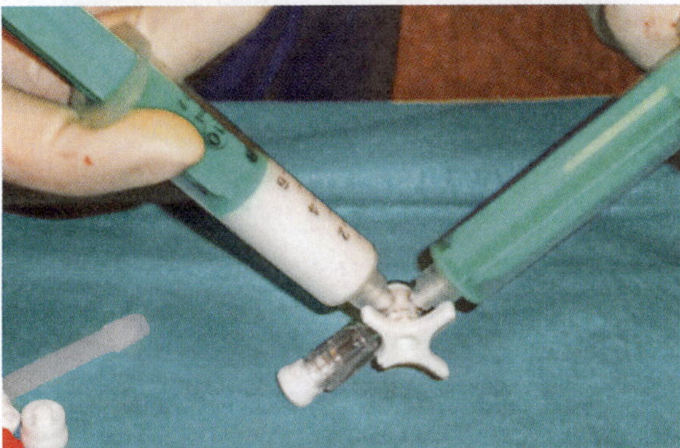

*Source:* Bailey and Love, 28th edition, page 1036.

c. What are the advantages of UGFS?

**Q5. Answer the following:**

a. What are the risk factors for venous thromboembolism?

b. What anomalies in fibrinolysis and thrombosis contribute to a higher risk of venous thrombosis?

**Q6. Answer the following:**

a. Identify the image.

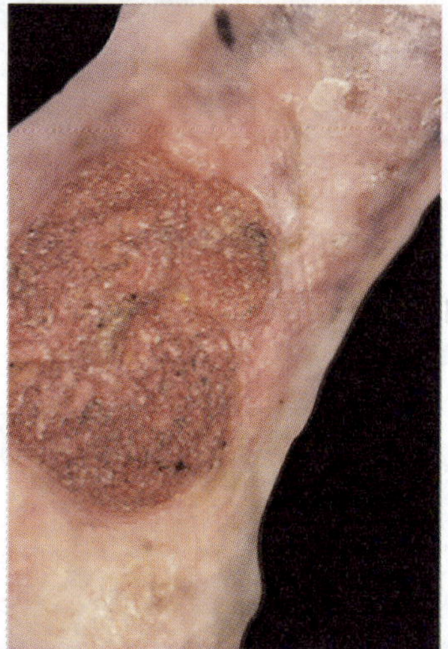

*Source:* Bailey and Love, 28th edition, page 1040.

b. A 64-year-old gentleman presented with swelling over left lower limb associated with raised local temperature and tenderness over calf region. Identify the pathological feature depicted in image.

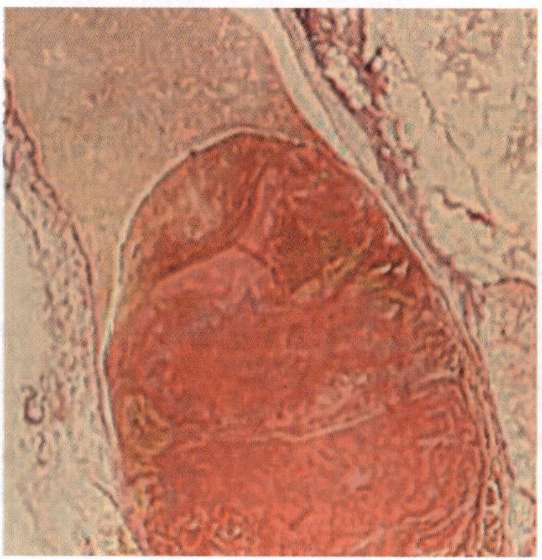

*Source:* Bailey and Love, 28th edition, page 1043.

**Q7. Answer the following:**

a. What is modified Wells criteria for predicting deep vein thrombosis (DVT)?

b. Identify the image.

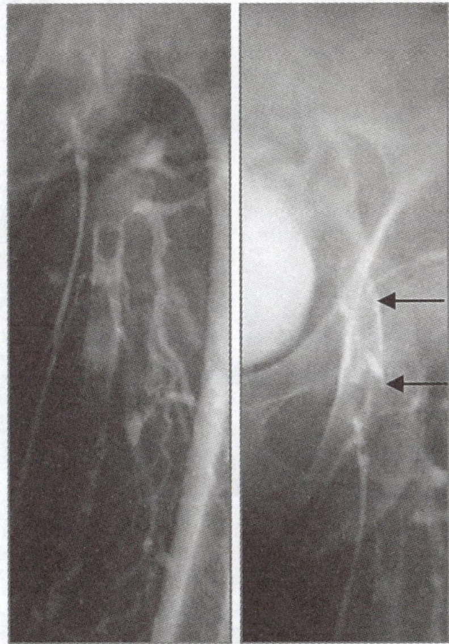

*Source:* Bailey and Love, 28th edition, page 1045.

c. Identify the image.

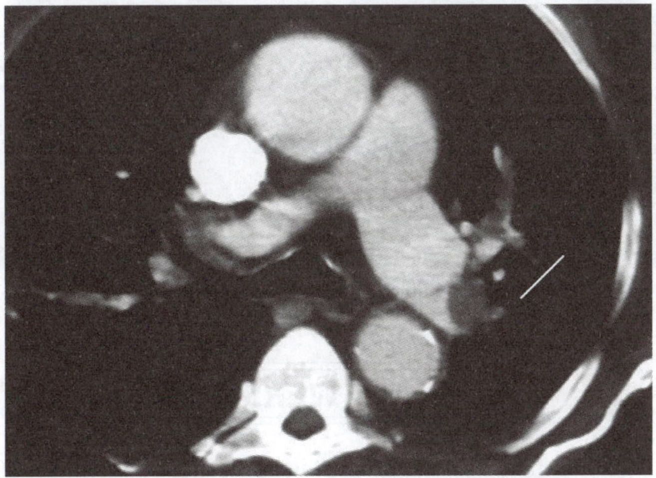

*Source:* Bailey and Love, 28th edition, page 1045.

**Q8. Which patient groups are at low, medium, and high risk for venous thromboembolism?**

**Q9. Answer the following:**

a. Identify the image and associated condition.

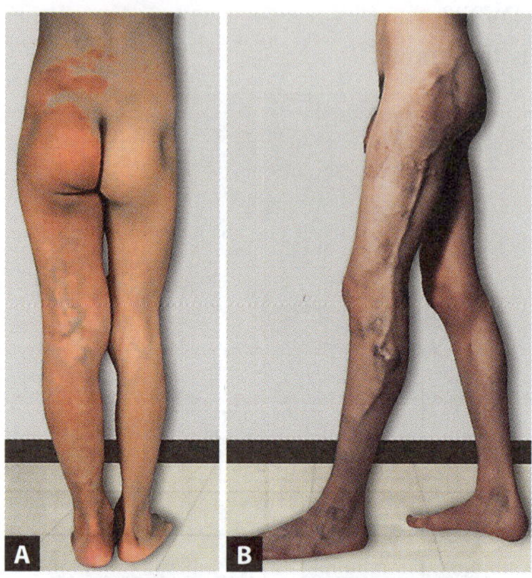


*Source:* Bailey and Love, 28th edition, page 1047.

b. Identify the image and associated condition.

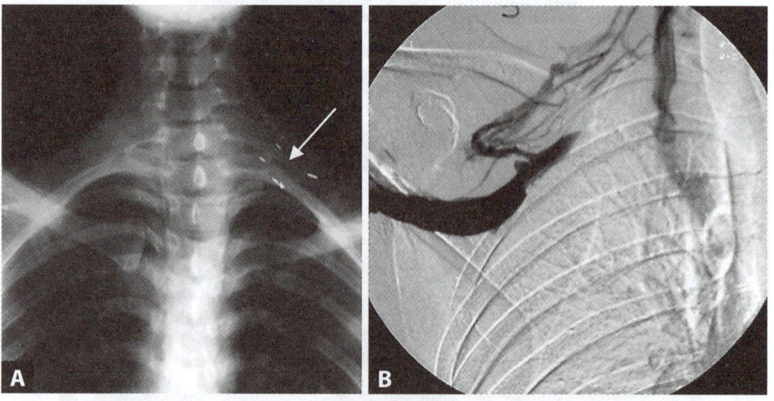


*Source:* Bailey and Love, 28th edition, page 1047.

## ANSWERS

**Ans. 1** a. 60% of the TBV, with an average pressure of around 5–10 mm Hg.

b. Graph illustrating how exercise affects superficial venous pressure in both healthy and sick conditions.

- *The light blue line*—shows the reduction in pressure primarily related to the action of the calf muscle pump.

- *The dark blue line*—shows how venous dysfunction is associated with (a/w) reduced net antegrade flow during exercise, resulting in a relative ↑ in venous pressure when compared with normal (venous hypertension).

**Ans. 2** a.

| ***Pressure gradient dysfunction*** | ***Dysfunction of the venous system*** |
|---|---|
| *↑ abdominal or thoracic pressure:*<br>• COPD<br>• Pregnancy<br>• Obesity<br>• Large tumor<br>• Constipation<br>*Decreased calf muscle pump function:*<br>• Immobility<br>• Ankle joint fusion<br>• Paralysis | *Venous structural deficit:*<br>• Valvular agenesis<br>• Valvular incompetence<br>• Venous dilatation<br>• Venous tortuosity<br>• Vein wall noncompliance<br>• Reduction in venous tone<br>• Arteriovenous (AV) fistula<br>*Venous occlusion:*<br>• Agenesis<br>• Thrombosis<br>• Iatrogenic/trauma<br>*Venous compression:*<br>• May–Thurner syndrome<br>• Pelvic/abdominal tumor<br>• Pelvic/radiation to the abdomen |

b. The CEAP chronic venous diseases are classified as:

| *For clinical classification:* | *For etiological classification:* | *For anatomical classification:* | *For pathophysiological classification:* |
|---|---|---|---|
| • C0: No signs of venous disease<br>• C1: Telangiectasia or reticular veins<br>• C2: Varicose veins<br>• C3: Edema<br>• C4a: Pigmentation or eczema<br>• C4b: LDS or atrophie blanche<br>• C4c: Corona phlebectatica<br>• C5: Healed venous ulcer<br>• C6: Active venous ulcer | • Ec: Congenital<br>• Ep: Primary<br>• Es: Secondary (post-thrombotic)<br>• En: No venous cause identified | • As: Superficial veins<br>• Ap: Perforator veins<br>• Ad: Deep veins<br>• An: No venous location identified | • Pr: Reflux<br>• Po: Obstruction<br>• Pr,o: Reflux and obstruction<br>• Pn: No venous pathophysiology identifiable |

Clinical class can be further characterized as symptomatic (s), asymptomatic (a) or recurrent following previous successful treatment or healing (r), e.g., C2a, C2s, and C6r.

**Ans. 3** a. *Class 1:* 14–17 mm Hg;
*Class 2:* 18–24 mm Hg; and
*Class 3:* 25–35 mm Hg.

b. Phlebectomy after endothermal ablation carried out under tumescent anesthesia.

**Ans. 4** a. Figure illustrating cannulation of veins during ultrasound-guided foam sclerotherapy.

b. Foam sclerotherapy or Tessari method of foam sclerosant preparation.
- Two syringes connected using a three-way tap.
- A 1:3 or 1:4 mixture of sclerosant and air is drawn into one syringe, and it is then forcefully oscillated between the two syringes ten or twenty times.
- This method produces foam that is stable for around 2 minutes, thus it is best to inject it right away.
- After elevating the leg to remove blood from the veins, foam is injected, starting with superficial varicosities and concluding with the great saphenous vein (GSV) or small saphenous vein (SSV).
- 1–2 mL of foam should only be injected at a time, and the ultrasonic probe should be used to monitor and massage the foam's distribution.
- No more foam should be injected once the junctional incompetence site has been seen with foam.
- Because the number of foam injections strongly correlates with the incidence of problems, the maximum volume of foam that should be injected in a single session should not exceed 10–12 mL. Compression is then applied as following endothermal ablation.

c. *Advantages:*
- It is a less unpleasant surgery because it does not require tumescent anesthesia, yet postoperative pain is likely to be similar.
- No vein, either axial or tributary, is too twisted.
- It also allows the treatment of calf veins with overlying skin damage or ulceration without the need to pierce through damaged skin.
- The cost of consumable therapy is quite inexpensive.

**Ans. 5** a. Risk factors for venous thromboembolism.

| Patient factors | Disease or surgical procedure |
|---|---|
| • Age<br>• Obesity<br>• Varicose veins<br>• Immobility<br>• Pregnancy<br>• Puerperium<br>• High-dose estrogen therapy<br>• Previous deep vein thrombosis or pulmonary embolism<br>• Thrombophilia | • Trauma or surgery, especially of pelvis, hip and lower limb<br>• Cancer, particularly metastatic to the abdomen and pelvis<br>• Heart failure<br>• Recent myocardial infarction<br>• Paralysis of lower limb(s)<br>• Infection<br>• Inflammatory bowel disease (IBD)<br>• Nephrotic syndrome<br>• Polycythemia<br>• Paraproteinemia<br>• Paroxysmal nocturnal hemoglobinuria (PNH) antibody or lupus anticoagulant<br>• Behçet's disease<br>• Homocystinemia |

b. A higher risk of venous thrombosis is caused by abnormalities of thrombosis and fibrinolysis (thrombophilia).

| Congenital | Acquired |
|---|---|
| • Protein C, protein S, or antithrombin III deficiency<br>• Antiphospholipid (Ab) or lupus anticoagulant<br>• Dysfibrinogenemias<br>• Activated protein C resistance or factor V Leiden gene deficiency | Antiphospholipid antibody or lupus anticoagulant |

**Ans. 6** a. Marjolin's ulcer (a squamous cell cancer arising in a chronic venous ulcer).

b. Organized thrombus.

**Ans. 7** a. Modified Wells criteria for DVT

| Variable | Score |
|---|---|
| Lower limb trauma or surgery or immobilization in a plaster cast | 1 |
| Bedridden for >3 days or surgery in last 4 weeks | 1 |
| Tenderness along the line of femoral or popliteal veins | 1 |
| Entire limb swollen | 1 |
| Calf >3 cm larger circumference than other side 10 cm below tibial tuberosity | 1 |
| Pitting edema | 1 |

*Contd...*

*Contd...*

| *Variable* | *Score* |
|---|---|
| Dilated collateral superficial veins (not varicose veins) | 1 |
| Previous DVT | 1 |
| Malignancy (including treatment up to 6 months ago) | 1 |
| Intravenous drug abuse | 3 |
| Alternative diagnosis more likely than deep vein thrombosis (DVT) | -2 |
| Low probability (5%) of DVT (score -2–0); moderate probability (17%) of DVT (score 1 or 2); high probability (17–53%) of DVT (score >2). | |

b. An ascending venogram of a deep vein thrombosis seen as filling defects (arrows) with contrast passing around the thrombus.
c. A computed tomography (CT) pulmonary angio showing pulmonary emboli as filling defects (arrows) in the pulmonary artery.

**Ans. 8** Patients at low, medium, and high risk for venous thromboembolism.

| *Low* | *Medium* | *High* |
|---|---|---|
| • No risk factors; any age; minor sx <30 minutes<br>• Age <40; no additional risk factors; major sx >30 minutes<br>• Minor trauma or medical illness | • Major surgery; risk factors such as age 40 or older<br>• Major medical illness: heart/lung disease, cancer, inflammatory bowel disease (IBD)<br>• Major burns/trauma<br>• Mild disease, trauma, or surgery in a patient with a history of pulmonary embolism (PE), thrombophilia, or DVT | • Significant orthopedic surgery or a hip, pelvic, or lower limb fracture. Major cancer surgery in the abdomen and pelvis<br>• Significant trauma, illness, or surgery in a patient with DVT, PE, or thrombophilia<br>• Paralysis of the lower limbs (e.g., stroke, paraplegia)<br>• Major amputation of a lower limb |

**Ans. 9.** a. Klippel-Trénaunay syndrome.
- *Image A:* This patient's leg is longer and has a capillary nevus
- *Image B:* In this instance, there is a substantial lateral anomalous axial vein.

b. Thoracic outlet syndrome:
- *Image A:* Cervical ribs on plain X-ray
- *Image B:* Occlusion of the axillary vein and its collaterals occur when the arm is elevated. The patient's left side was previously decompressed during surgery [arrow in (A)]

11

SECTION

# Abdominal

# CHAPTER 42 Bariatric Surgery

## QUESTIONS

**Q1. Definitions of overweight and obesity.**

**Q2. What are the conditions that are associated with severe and complex obesity?**

**Q3. According to International Federation for the Surgery of Obesity and Metabolic Disorders (IFSO) 2018 registry, which of the following surgery is most commonly done?**

a. Sleeve gastrectomy
b. One anastomosis gastric bypass
c. Roux-en-Y gastric bypass (RYGB)
d. Lap adjustable gastric banding

**Q4. The false statement regarding mini gastric bypass:**

a. Retrocolic one anastomosis bypass done
b. Longer gastric pouch than in standard gastric bypass
c. Increased risk of Barret esophagus seen
d. Difficult to manage the anastomotic leak

**Q5. Name the surgery shown below.**

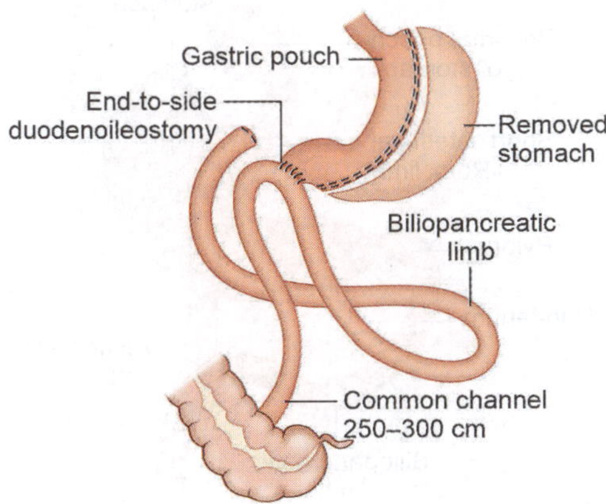


*Source:* Bailey and Love, 28th edition, page 1188.

**Q6. Why bariatric surgery is important for weight loss?**

**Q7. Describe metabolic surgery.**

**Q8. What are NICE accredited guidance on the make-up of the medical and surgical bariatric multidisciplinary team?**

**Q9. What are the criteria of NICE guidance on bariatric surgery, 2014?**

**Q10. What is OS-MRS scores (Obesity Surgery-Mortality Risk Score)?**

**Q11. What are the types of bariatric surgery?**

**Q12. Answer the following:**

a. What is this depicted image?

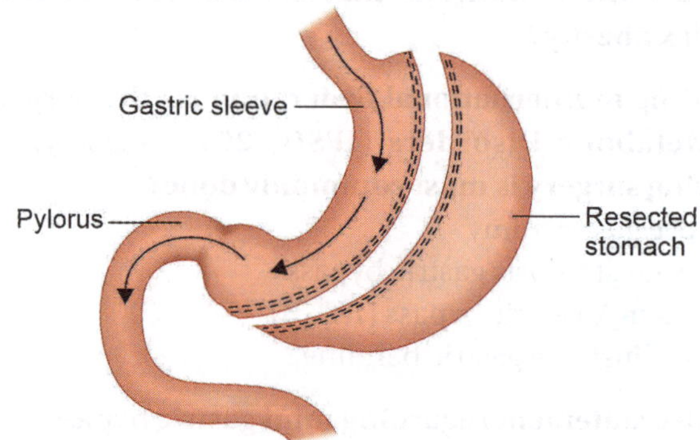


*Source:* Bailey and Love, 28th edition, page 1186.

b. What is this depicted image?

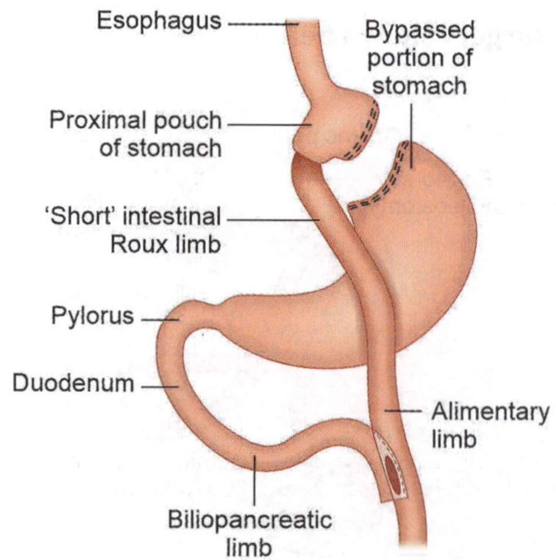


*Source:* Bailey and Love, 28th edition, page 1186.

**Q13. What is in depicted image A and B?**

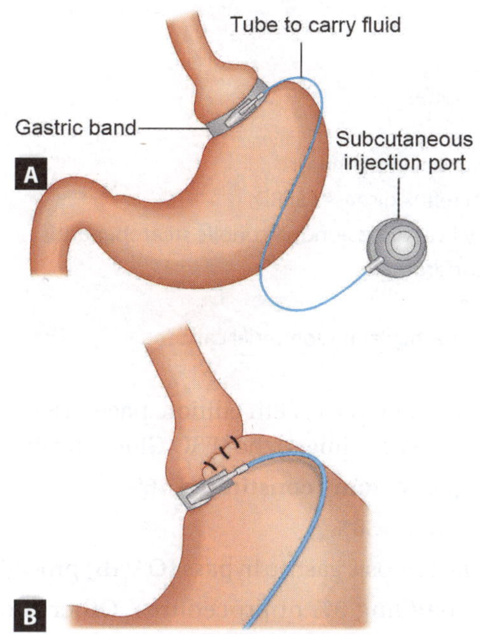


*Source:* Bailey and Love, 28th edition, page 1187.

**Q14. What are the complications of bariatric surgery?**

**Q15. What are the postoperative supplements in bariatric surgery?**

## ANSWERS

**Ans. 1**

| *Adult weight status* | *BMI (kg/m²)* |
|---|---|
| Normal | 18.5–24.9 |
| Overweight | 25.0–29.9 |
| Class 1 obesity | 30.0–34.9 |
| Class 2 obesity | 35.0–39.9 |
| Class 3 obesity | ≥40.0 |

Body mass index (BMI) = weight (kg)/height ($m^2$)

- Obesity in children is defined as BMI at or above the 95th centile.
- "Superobesity" is a term commonly used to describe BMI ≥49.9 kg/$m^2$.

**Ans. 2**

- Hypertension
- Type II diabetes
- Obstructive sleep apnea
- Dyslipidemia
- Arthritis and functional impairment
- Gastroesophageal reflux disease (GERD)
- Nonalcoholic fatty liver disease/nonalcoholic steatohepatitis
- Polycystic ovary syndrome
- Clinical depression
- Various cancers, in particular endometrial cancer

**Ans. 3** a. (*Ref:* Bailey and Love, 28th edition, page 1185)
*IFSO Registry:* According to the IFSO Global Registry, in 2018

- **Sleeve gastrectomy constituted 46%**
- Gastric bypass 38%
- One-anastomosis gastric bypass (OAGB) procedures 7.6%
- Gastric banding 5% of procedures. Other procedures include the biliopancreatic diversion (BPD) procedure and its duodenal switch variant (BPD/DS).
- Sleeve gastrectomy is the most common operation and has gained rapid popularity at the expense of gastric banding and to a lesser extent gastric bypass.

**Ans. 4** a. (*Ref:* Bailey and Love, 28th edition, page 1187)

- One-anastomosis gastric bypass, previously known as a mini-gastric bypass, was first described by Rutledge. The goal was to create a less technically demanding procedure than traditional gastric bypass, using a larger gastric pouch and only one anastomosis (antecolic loop gastrojejunostomy without a Roux-en-Y configuration).
- Although weight loss results have been documented, complications such as marginal ulcers, symptomatic biliary reflux leading to gastritis or esophagitis, and managing anastomotic leaks might result in a potentially large volume of pancreatic and biliary secretions.
- With the Roux-en-Y historically being the standard in surgery of the stomach for ulcer disease and cancer, there is further concern owing to possibly ↑ risk of Barrett's and gastric cancer or esophageal cancer associated with biliary reflux.

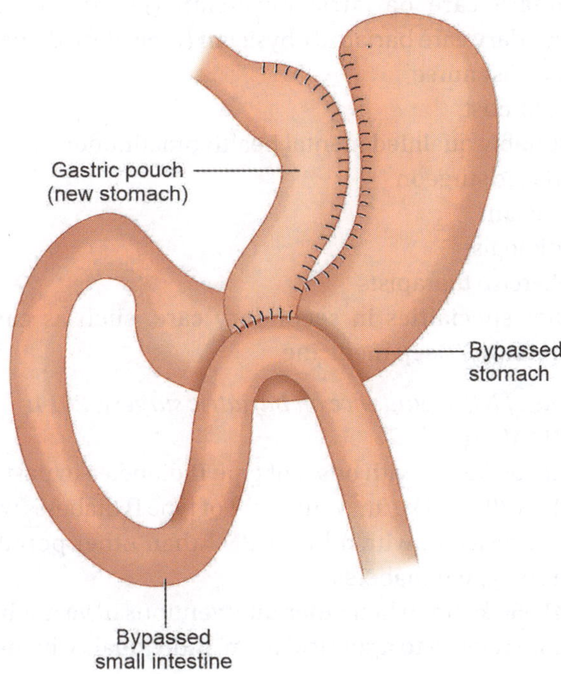


**Ans. 5** *Single-anastomosis duodeno-ileal bypass with sleeve gastrectomy (SADI-S):*

- This procedure is based on the BPD/DS.
- Sleeve gastrectomy F/B an end to side duodeno-ileal anastomosis
- Length of the alimentary limb (common channel) is 250–300 cm.
- *Advantages:* Preservation of the pylorus, elimination of one anastomosis compared with the duodenal switch, and reducing operating time and risk of perioperative complications.

**Ans. 6** *Rationale for surgery:*

- Because of the tendency for basal metabolic rate (BMR) to ↓ with diet modification, most people will regain weight, returning to the previous homeostatic set point
- Bariatric surgery appears to alter this and "reset" this point, with 15–25% weight loss.
- Procedure leads to long-term survival benefit and improves obesity-related disease and quality of life.

**Ans. 7** *Metabolic surgery:* Significant impacts of surgery on metabolic syndrome and diabetes, which might have a greater influence than weight loss alone. Weight loss alone may not be enough to improve type II diabetes. Surgery is incredibly economical.

**Ans. 8**
- Primary care bariatric physician (general practitioner) or secondary care bariatric physician (typically a diabetologist)
- Specialist nurse
- Anesthetist
- A suitably qualified mental health practitioner
- Bariatric surgeon
- Dietician
- Radiologist
- ± Exercise therapists
- Other specialties in secondary care, such as cardiology and respiratory/sleep medicine

**Ans. 9** *Criterias of NICE guidance on bariatric surgery, 2014:*
- BMI ≥40 kg/m$^2$
- BMI ≥35 kg/m$^2$ with onset of type II diabetes in past 10 years
- BMI of 30–34.9 kg/m$^2$ with onset of type II diabetes within 10 years
- Asian descent, with a lower BMI than other populations at the start of type II diabetes
- BMI >50 kg/m$^2$ when other interventions have not been effective.

Before referral to a surgical team, individuals who meet the aforementioned requirements must also be enrolled in or scheduled for evaluation in a weight-management program.

**Ans. 10** *To add one point for each of the below factors:*
- Age >45 year
- BMI >50
- Male
- Hypertension (HTN)
- ↑ risk of deep vein thrombosis (DVT) or pulmonary embolism (PE)

The more the points, there is increased risk of mortality.

**Ans. 11** *Types of bariatric surgery:*

| ***Restrictive:*** | ***Mostly restrictive (and partly malabsorptive):*** | ***Mostly malabsorptive:*** |
|---|---|---|
| • Adjustable silicone gastric banding<br>• Sleeve gastrectomy<br>• Vertical banded gastroplasty | • Short-limb (50–100 cm) Roux-en-Y gastric bypass<br>• Long-limb (150 cm) Roux-en-Y gastric bypass | • BPD +/– DS |

**Ans. 12** a. *Sleeve gastrectomy:*
- Most commonly performed operation in India
- The smaller curve-based gastric tube is built to fit a 32–36 Fr Bougie size.

- The Achilles heel of this operation is risk of staple leak at angle of HIS
- Reduces the intake of food and produces weight loss
- Least complicated surgery, malabsorption is not seen.

b. Roux-en-Y jejunojejunostomy restoration with a short vertical gastric pouch based on the smaller curvature following a gastric bypass.

*Roux-en-Y gastric bypass:*

- Mostly restrictive and partly malabsorptive
- Stomach is made into a small pouch of 50 mL capacity
- Roux limb made and brought to anastomose to the pouch. The length of Roux Limb varies here from 100 to 150 cm. Y limb will be around 100 cm.
- Most commonly done surgery done now is this operation.

**Ans. 13** *Adjustable gastric band:* Figure showing

- *Image A:* A small 'virtual' pouch of stomach below the GE junction and
- *Image B:* Gastro-gastric tunnelling sutures.

*Lap adjustable gastric banding:*

- Band wrapped at upper part of fundus with adjustable subcutaneous port.
- Lesser curve approached by pars flaccida technique
- The access port is sutured to rectus in upper abdomen for ease of access by a noncoring, Huber needle used for band adjustment.
- Type of pure restrictive surgery, early satiety occurs.

**Ans. 14** *MC cause of death in bariatric surgery:*

- Immediate postoperative—anastomotic leak and peritonitis
- within 30 days—DVT/PE
- Overall—DVT/PE

*Gastric banding:*

- Early complication—port site infection
- Late complication—slippage of band and necrosis, perforation, and weight regain

*Sleeve gastrectomy:*

- Early complication—leak from angle of HIS, bleeding, DVT, and PE
- Late complication—GERD and weight gain

*RYGB:*

- Early complication—anastomotic leakage, bleeding, obstruction, and DVT/PE

- Late complication—Peterson hernia, adhesive colicky, and weight regain

*Biliopancreatic diversion operations:*

- Early complication—anastomotic leakage and DVT/PE
- Late complication—severe malabsorption

**Ans. 15** *After gastric banding:*

- Multivitamin
- Minerals
- Thiamine if vomiting
- Vitamin D
- Iron

*All other surgeries (RYGB, BPD, and sleeve gastrectomy):*

- Same as above
- Selenium
- Copper
- Zinc
- Folic acid
- Vitamin $B_{12}$
- Vitamin A, D, E, and K

CHAPTER

# 43 Esophagus

## QUESTIONS

**Q1. Answer the following:**

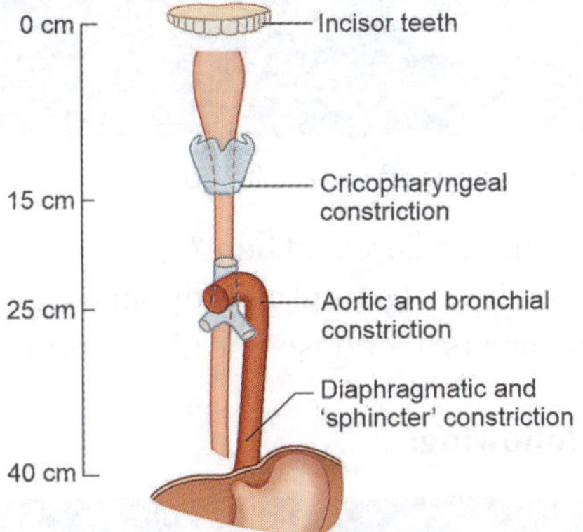


*Source:* Bailey and Love, 28th edition, page 1107.

a. Describe surgical anatomy of esophagus.
b. Which is narrowest parts in esophagus (natural constrictions)?

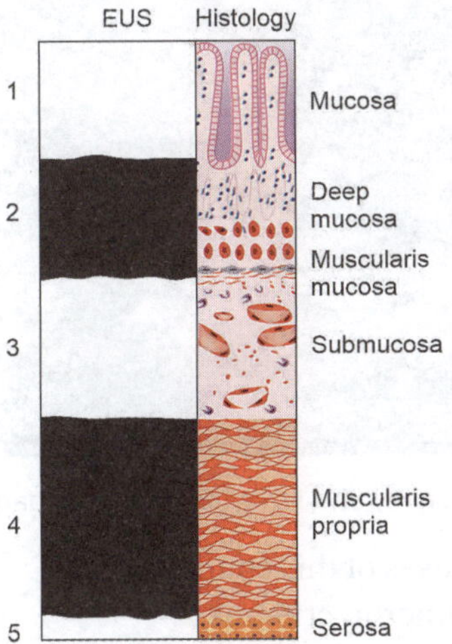


*Source:* Bailey and Love, 27th edition, page 1070.

## Q2. Answer the following:

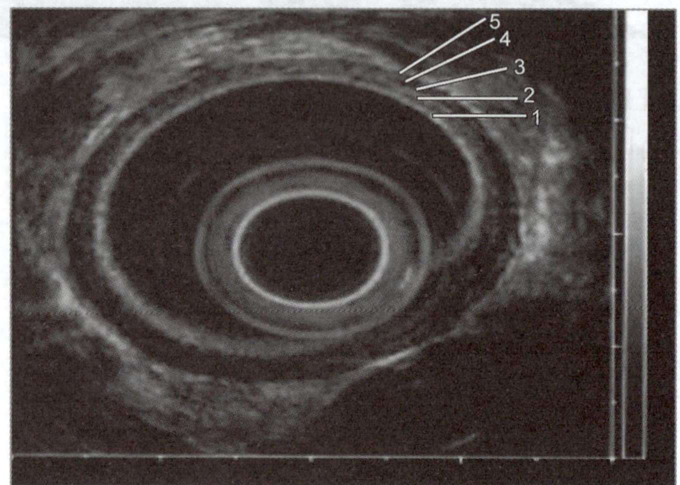


*Source:* Bailey and Love, 27th edition, page 1070.

a. What is the image depicted here?
b. What are the investigations in esophagus?
c. How many layers in endoscopic ultrasound?

## Q3. Answer the following:

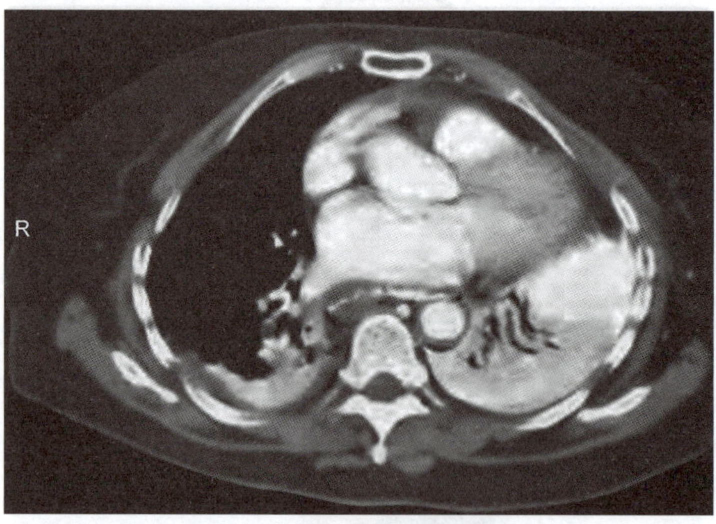


*Source:* Bailey and Love, 27th edition, page 1073.

a. What are the causes of this condition?
b. What are the Cameron criteria?
c. What are the investigations for esophageal perforation?

**Q4. Describe difference between alkali poisoning and acid poisoning.**

**Q5. Answer the following:**

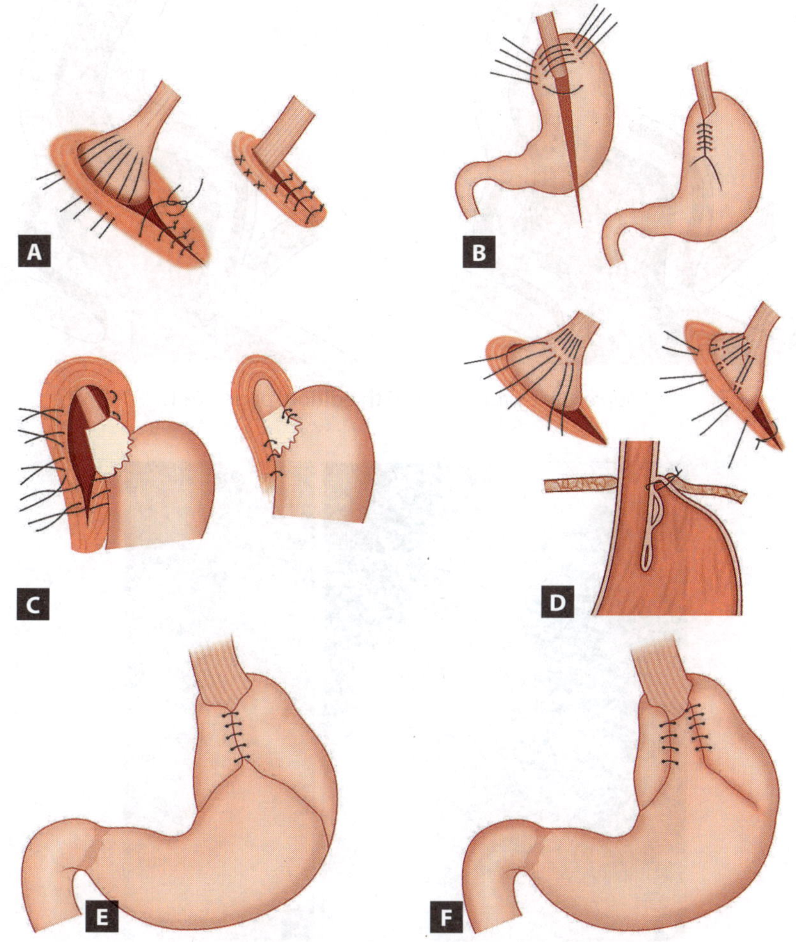


*Source:* Bailey and Love, 27th edition, page 1079.

a. What is this operation done for?
b. What is Pathophysiology for this condition?
c. What are the clinical features?
d. What are the investigations?
e. What are the complications of gastroesophageal reflux disease (GERD)?
f. What is the surgical treatment?
g. What are the newer devices used for GERD by endoscopic method?

## Q6. Answer the following:

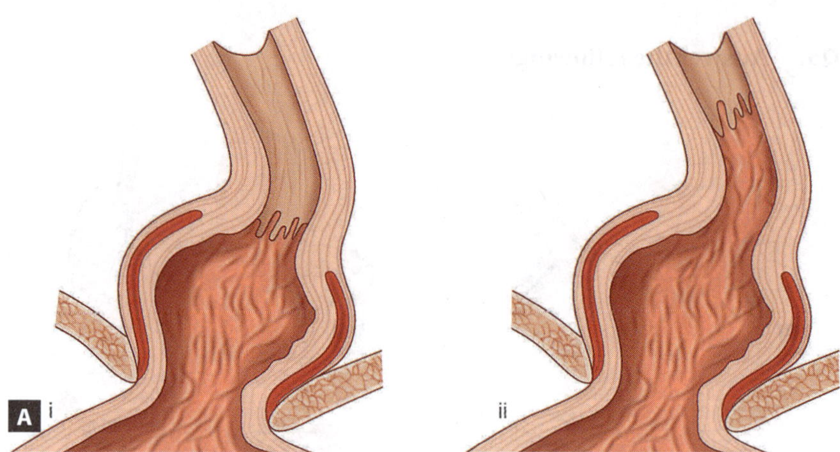


*Source:* Bailey and Love, 27th edition, page 1081.

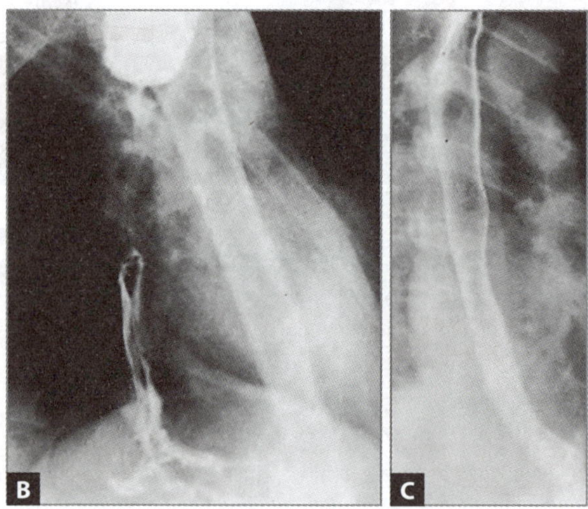


*Source:* Bailey and Love, 27th edition, page 1082.

a. What is the depicted image here?
b. What are the types of hiatal hernias?
c. In which of these hernias, angle of HIS is not disturbed?
d. Describe salient points of these hernias.

## Q7. Answer the following:

a. Describe Images shown below in context of esophageal tumors.
b. What are the predisposing factors of esophageal tumors?
c. What are the clinical features of esophageal tumors?

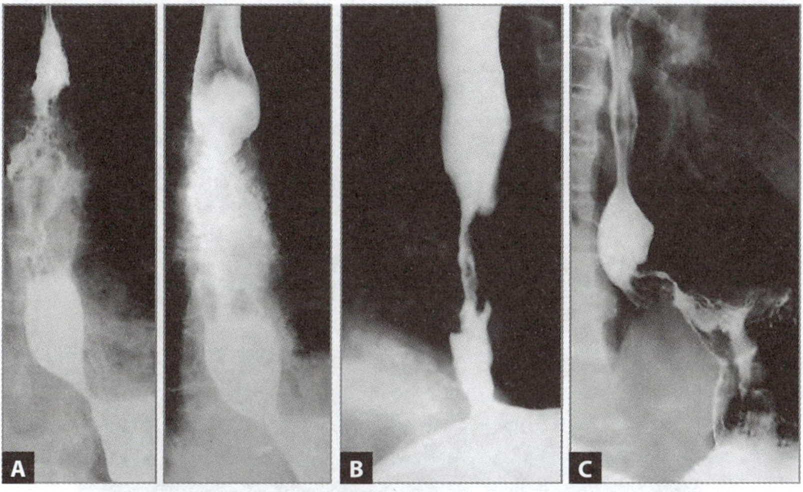


*Source:* Bailey and Love, 27th edition, page 1085.

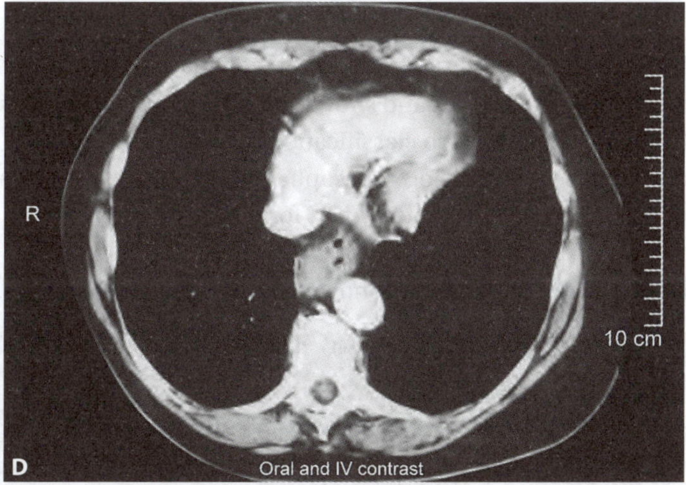


*Source:* Bailey and Love, 27th edition, page 1086.

**Q8. Answer the following:**

a. TNM staging of cancer esophagus
b. Investigations for cancer esophagus

**Q9. Describe management of cancer esophagus.**

**Q10. Answer the following:**

a. What is Orringer operation?
b. What are the conduits for cancer esophagus surgery?
c. What are the routes of taking up the conduit?
d. What are the parts of esophagus on the basis of cancer?

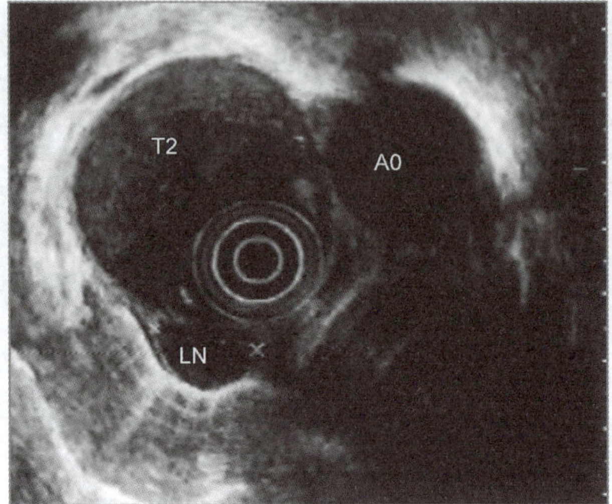


*Source:* Bailey and Love, 27th edition, page 1091.

**Q11.** Describe endoscopic appearance of malignant nodes.

a. Identify the images and shown condition in given images
b. What is the Chicago classification of motility disorders?
c. What is the physiology of esophagus and motility disorders?
d. What is the gold standard IOC for motility disorder?

**Q12.** a. Identify the images and shown condition in given images.

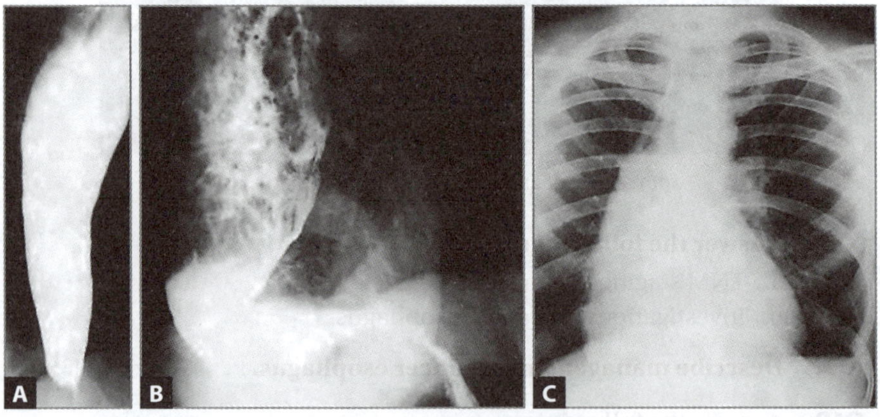


*Source:* Bailey and Love, 27th edition, page 1097.

b. What is the Chicago classification of motility disorders?
c. What is the physiology of esophagus and motility disorders?
d. What is the gold standard IOC for motility disorder?

**Q13. Answer the following:**

a. What are the clinical features of achalasia cardia?
b. What are the investigations of achalasia cardia?
c. What are the complications of achalasia cardia?
d. What is Eckhardt score?

**Q14. What is the difference between diffuse esophageal spasm (DES) and nutcracker esophagus (NCE)?**

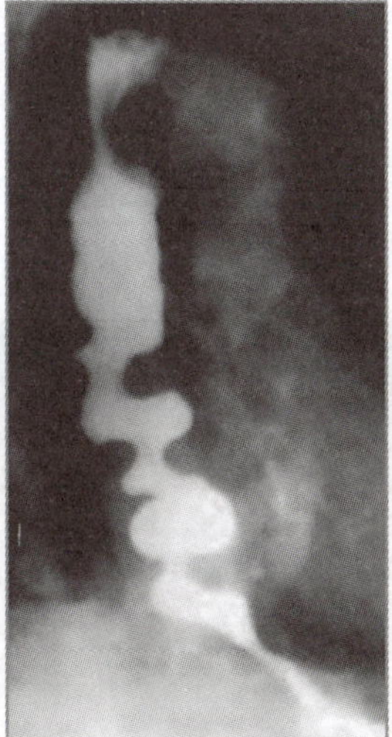

*Source:* Bailey and Love, 27th edition, page 1099.

**Q15.**

a. What is this?

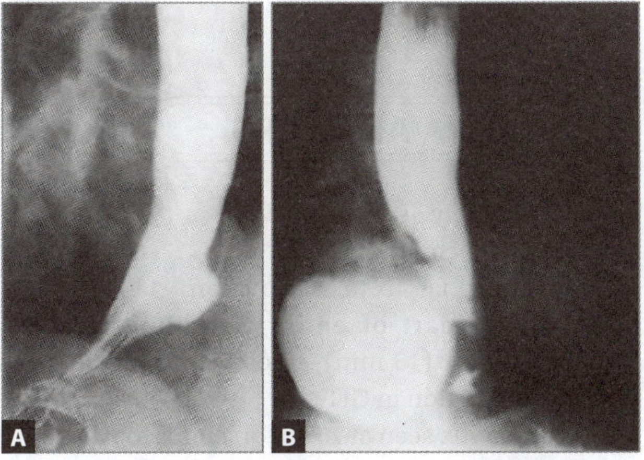


*Source:* Bailey and Love, 27th edition, page 1100.

b. What is this?

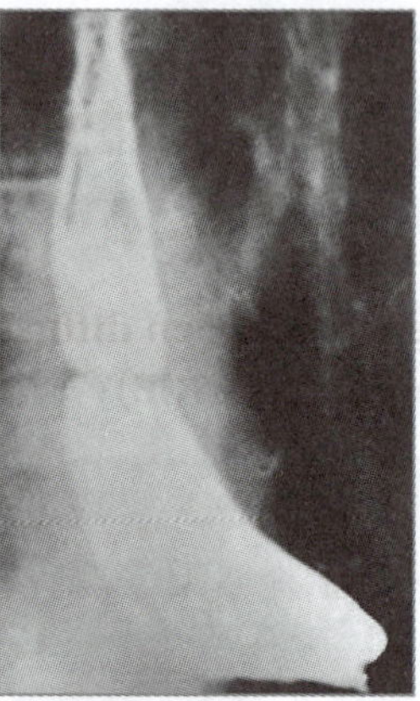

c. What is this?

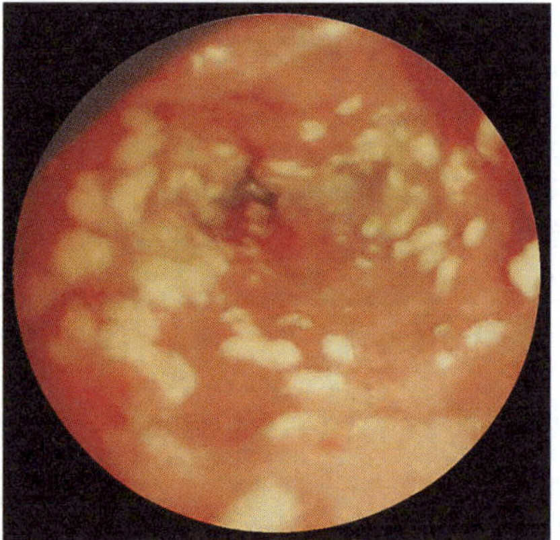

*Source:* Bailey and Love, 27th edition, page 1104.

## ANSWERS

**Ans. 1** a. *Surgical anatomy of esophagus:*
- Length—25 cm
- From cricopharynx to OG junction
- Narrowest part of entire gastrointestinal tract (GIT)—cricopharynx (13 mm)—most common site of foreign body (FB) obstruction in GIT
- Cricopharynx seen at 15 cm on endoscopy.
- Esophagus has no serosa (GB has no submucosa).

- Esophagus—10th vertebra level enters diaphragm (VOA—inferior vena cava, esophagus, and aorta)
- Normal IAP = 5–8 mm Hg, thoracic pressure = –4 mm Hg
- This increased intra-abdominal pressure is the most important mechanism to prevent GERD.
- Minimum length of esophagus needed to prevent GERD—1 cm
- Angle of His—esophagogastric angle

b. *Narrowest parts in esophagus—natural constrictions:*
   - 15 cm—cricopharynx
   - 25 cm—arch of aorta
   - 27 cm—left bronchus
   - 40 cm—OG junction

**Ans. 2** a. Radial endosonography indicating wall layers as alternating hyper- and hypoechoic band

b. *Investigations in esophagus:*
   - Upper GI endoscopy—best to study the esophagus. Length of tube = 100 cm.
   - Upper GI endoscopy can pass up to D4.
   - Most common site of esophageal injury—cervical esophagus by endoscopy
   - *Endoscopy ultrasonography (USG):* IOC for T and N staging of esophageal cancer

c. There are five layers seen in endoscopy:
   1. Layer 1—mucosa (hyperechoic)
   2. Layer 2—muscularis mucosa (hypoechoic)
   3. Layer 3—submucosa (hyperechoic)
   4. Layer 4—muscularis propria (hypoechoic)
   5. Layer 5—adventitial layer

**Ans. 3** Computed tomography (CT) scan showing the site of perforation in the lower esophagus.

a. *Causes:*
   - Iatrogenic—MC cause (MC site—cervical esophagus)
   - Barotrauma (Boerhaave syndrome)
   - Corrosive—alkali ingestion
   - Trauma

b. *Cameron criteria: Nonoperative treatment of esophageal perforation:*
   - Endoscopy perforation
   - Small septic foci
   - Draining collection in mediastinum
   - Cervical esophagus perforation

c. *Investigations for esophageal perforation:*
- First done investigation—chest X-ray shows mediastinal air known as Naclerio V sign.
- Early and suspected esophageal perforation IOC–CT thorax with oral GI contrasts

**Ans. 4**

| ***Alkali poisoning*** | ***Acid poisoning*** |
|---|---|
| Consumed in large amounts | Only few sips only they swallow due to severe pain in mouth |
| Liquefactive necrosis | Coagulative necrosis |
| Destroy all the layers and can cause esophageal perforation | Forms eschar and limited to superficial layers and no perforation |
| Esophagus more damaged than stomach | Stomach is more damaged than esophagus |
| • Long-term damage continues<br>• Develops corrosive stricture for 3–6 months | Long-term damage is rare, only gastric antral stricture can develop |

**Ans. 5** a. Various operations for the surgical correction of GERD (MC disease of GIT).
- The original Allison repair of hiatus hernia (this is ineffective and is no longer done)
- Nissen fundoplication
- Hill procedure
- Belsey mark IV operation

b. *Pathophysiology:*
- Normal pressure of LES = 10–26 mm Hg
- Pressure <10 mm Hg results in GERD.
- Decreased intra-abdominal length <1 cm is the most important mechanism for GERD.

*Causes of GERD:*

| | |
|---|---|
| • Tea<br>• Coffee<br>• Alcohol<br>• Smoking<br>• Pregnancy<br>• Obesity<br>• High-fat diet | *Drugs:*<br>• Anticholinergics<br>• Barbiturates<br>• Calcium channel blocker (CCB)<br>• Diazepam<br>• Prostaglandin E1 (PGE1) analogs |

c. *Clinical features:*
- MC symptom—heart burn
- MC complication—reflux esophagitis—MC presentation is retrosternal discomfort.

- Nocturnal asthma/paroxysmal nocturnal cough—laryngopharyngeal reflux (LPR)

d. *Investigations:*
- Gold standard—24-hours ambulatory pH monitoring
- Sensor kept 5 cm above OG junction
- Reflux of acid at pH <4 is counted every time.
- *Prerequisites to do this test:*
    - Stop PPI for 7 days before test.
    - Patient comes in empty stomach and after catheter kept inside, she is sent back to do routine activities.
    - Every time pH <4 strikes the sensor will get a count.
- With all the values, we calculate a score known as DeMeester score >14.7 is diagnostic of GERD.
- LPR is detected by 24 hours double probe pH monitoring keeping two sensors one at above OG junction and another at cricopharynx level.

e. *Complications of GERD:*
- MC reflux esophagitis, IOC to find is by endoscopy, has two classifications—Los Angels and Savary Miller classifications.
- LPR causing—nocturnal asthma
- Peptic stricture—MC in lower end of esophagus, thick stricture involving all layers and hence needs surgical excision and keep jejunal conduit interposition.
- Schatzki's ring, MC in squamocolumnar junction (biopsy above the ring is squamous epithelium and below is columnar epithelium), thin submucosal ring, and hence can be easily treated by dilatation + fundoplication.
- Barret's esophagus—conversion of squamous epithelium to columnar epithelium. The type of columnar epithelium is intestinal columnar epithelium with biopsy showing goblet cells. To confirm the dysplasia we must take biopsy at all four quadrant at every 1 cm of Barret's esophagus—known as Seattle biopsy protocol.
- Adenocarcinoma—40 times risk in Barret's esophagus. Incidence = 0.5–1%/year. Hence keep Barret's cases under surveillance.

f. *Surgical treatment: Basics in fundoplication operations:*
- Pull the esophagus into peritoneal cavity at least 3 cm.
- Narrow the hiatus.
- Wrap the lower end of esophagus using the fundus.
- Keep 52 Fr Bougie while wrapping.

*Techniques in surgery:*

- Five ports used.
- Pars flaccida technique—opening the lesser sac along the lesser curvature.
- Before wrap ensure the wrap is free by doing "shoeshine maneuver".

*Named surgeries*:

- Nissen fundoplication, 360° posterior wrap, can cause gas-bloat syndrome
- Toupet—270° posterior wrap
- Dor—180° anterior wrap
- Watson—90° anterior wrap
- Belsey Mark IV repair—thoracoscopic approach. If there dense abdominal adhesions, we do this surgery.

MC complication of fundoplication—Paralytic ileus > pneumothorax

g. *Newer devices used for GERD by endoscopic method*:

- Radiofrequency ablation device—STRETTA procedure.
- *Transoral Incisionless Fundoplication (TIF) EsophyX:* A special device EsophyX is kept at OG junction by endoscopy.
- *Enteryx procedure*: Endoscopic injection of synthetic implants to enhance LES strength.
- LINX is a new device made up of magnets kept at OG junction to prevent reflux delivered laparoscopically.
- For patients who have shortened esophagus, Collis gastroplasty is done.

**Ans. 6** a. (i) The interrelationship of the lower esophageal sphincter, the squamocolumnar junction and the diaphragm in sliding hiatus hernia; (ii) Barrett's esophagus and sliding hernia.

A paraesophageal hernia showing the gastroesophageal junction just above the diaphragm and the fundus alongside the esophagus, compressing the lumen.

b. *Four types:*

1. *Type 1:* Sliding
2. *Type 2:* Paraesophageal/Rolling
3. *Type 3:* Mixed
4. *Type 4:* Massive (along with stomach-small bowel, colon, etc., will go up)

c. Type 2 rolling/PE hiatus hernia

d. *Salient points:*

- MC presentation of sliding hiatus hernia—GERD
- Sliding hiatus hernia can be electively planned for surgery—fundoplication

- Rolling hiatus hernia is an emergency—it can bleed or perforate—immediate gastropexy must be done.

**Ans. 7** *The classic appearances of a midesophageal proliferative squamous cell carcinoma:*

- *Image A:* Squamous cell carcinoma of the esophagus producing an irregular stricture with shouldered margins
- *Image B:* Adenocarcinoma of the lower esophagus, spreading upward from the cardia
- *Image C:* CT scan showing a primary tumor of the lower esophagus

a. *Benign tumors:*
- MC is leiomyoma
- MC in lower third esophagus
- On contrast-enhanced CT (CECT), hypodense lesion seen.
- Endoscopic ultrasound (EUS)—this appears in 4th layer and rarely second layer (NEET SS).
- Treatment—enucleation

*Malignant tumor:*
- MC site—middle third in world level and in India
- MC type is SCC in world/India.
- MC type in western countries—adenocarcinoma

b.

| ***Squamous cell cancer*** | ***Adenocarcinoma*** |
|---|---|
| • Hot tea<br>• Smoking<br>• Alcohol<br>• Achalasia—8%<br>• Plummer–Vinson syndrome<br>• Corrosive ingestion—1000 times<br>• Mb deficiency<br>• Tylosis palmaris et plantaris<br>• Low SE status | • GERD<br>• Barret's<br>• Scleroderma<br>• Obesity<br>• High SE status<br>• *Deficiency of antioxidants:*<br>– Alcohol is not a risk factor for adenocancer<br>– Smoking is a risk factor for both. |

*H. pylori CAG-A toxin:*
- Causes distal gastric cancer
- Protects esophageal adenocarcinoma
- No relation with squamous cell cancer

c. *Clinical features:*
- Rapidly progressive dysphagia in 6 months
- More of solids > liquids
- To get dysphagia—60% lumen or two-thirds circumference must be involved.
- Tracheoesophageal fistula—aspiration + lung infection
- 90% inoperable on presentation

**Ans. 8** a. *TNM staging of cancer esophagus:*

| *T staging* | *N staging* | *M staging* |
|---|---|---|
| • T1a—muscularis mucosa<br>• T1b—submucosa<br>• T2—up to muscularis propria<br>• T3—invades adventitia<br>• T4a—resectable adjacent structures such as pleura, pericardium, and diaphragm<br>• T4b—unresectable structures such as trachea, bronchus, aorta, and vertebra | • N1—1–2 nodes<br>• N2—3–6 nodes<br>• N3—>7 nodes | • M1—distant mets<br>• MC site—lungs |

b. *Investigations:*
- IOC to diagnose endoscopic biopsy
- IOC for T and N stagings—EUS
- IOC for M staging—positron emission tomography (PET)-CT
- Overall staging of cancer esophagus—CECT thorax

**Ans. 9** *Inoperable cases:*
- Palliative self-expanding metallic stent through the growth
- Laser luminization
- Feeding jejunostomy

*Operable cancers:*
- The tumor spreads submucosally for long distance, hence a clearance of 10 cm proximal and 5 cm distal is needed for cancer esophagus.
- Three level nodes may be involved: (1) Abdominal; (2) Thoracic; (3) Neck nodes.
- *Types of esophagectomy:*
    - Transthoracic
    - Transhiatal

| *Ivor Lewis two-stage procedure* | *McKeown three-stage procedure* |
|---|---|
| • Subtotal esophagectomy<br>• Two-stage lymphadenectomy (abdominal and thoracic nodes)<br>• Two Incisions: (1) Abdominal and (2) thoracic (two regional nodes removed)<br>• Intrathoracic anastomosis<br>• Leak percentage is less<br>• Mortality if leaks is high | • Total esophagectomy<br>• Three stage LN dissection (all three)<br>• *Three incisions:* (1) Abdominal, (2) thoracic, and (3) Cervical (three regional nodes removed)<br>• Neck anastomosis<br>• Leak percentage is more<br>• Mortality is less as the contamination into the mediastinum never happens and secretions can be drained out |

**Ans. 10** a. *Transhiatal esophagectomy (THE): Orringer operation:*
- Two incisions—neck and abdominal
- Neck anastomosis
- Mortality is less as thorax is not opened.
- Nodal clearance is less.
- Postoperative radiotherapy is given after THE.

b. *Conduits for surgery:*
- Best conduit for esophageal replacement, stomach as it is highly vascular and less chances of necrosis.
- Best conduit in cases of corrosive injury to stomach and esophagus and for long segment replacement—colon
- Best conduit for short segment replacement of esophagus—jejunum, especially in peptic stricture cases.
- Gastric conduit is based on the right gastroepiploic artery and right gastric artery.

c. *Routes of taking up the conduit:*
- Posterior mediastinal—shortest and most dependent route. 28 cm only
- Substernal route—second option, if posterior mediastinal route not available as in corrosive ingestions. 30 cm length
- Subcutaneous route—less commonly used. Cosmetically ugly, least dependent route

d. *Parts of esophagus on basis of cancer:*
- Cervical esophagus—15–20 cm (cricopharynx to sternal notch)
- Upper thoracic—20–25 cm (sternal notch to azygous vein)
- Mid thoracic—25–30 cm (azygous vein and inferior pulmonary vein)
- Lower thoracic—30–40 cm (IPV to OG junction)

**Ans. 11** Endosonography demonstrates malignant nodes. These are usually large, hypoechoic, and round compared with normal nodes.

**Ans. 12** a. *Achalasia of the esophagus:* (A) Barium swallow showing the smooth outline of the stricture, which narrows to a point at its lower end; (B) Tortuosity and sigmoid appearance of the lower esophagus; (C) Mediastinal shadow due to a large, fluid-filled esophagus.

b. *Chicago classification*:

| *Hypomotility disorders* | *Hypermotility disorders* |
|---|---|
| Achalasia (most common overall)<br>• Type 1—most common<br>• Type 2—best prognosis<br>• Type 3—rare type | • DES<br>• NCE—most common hypermotility disorder |

c. *Achalasia and esophagogastric junction disorders:*

| | |
|---|---|
| Type 1 achalasia (classic) | • Mean integrated relaxation pressure (IRP) >15 mm Hg<br>• 100% failed peristalsis.<br>• Distal contractile integral (DCI) <100 mm Hg cm/s |
| Type 2 achalasia with esophageal compression | • Mean IRP >15 mm Hg<br>• 100% failed peristalsis<br>• Panesophageal pressurization<br>• DCI is difficult to measure<br>• In manometry, isobaric contraction seen at 30 mm Hg |
| Type 3 (spastic achalasia) | • Mean IRP >15 mm Hg<br>• No normal peristalsis<br>• Segmental increased DCI seen<br>• Spastic contractions with DCI >450 mm Hg cm/s<br>• Rarely panesophageal pressurization seen |
| Achalasia in evolution (esophagogastric outlet obstruction) | • IRP >15 mm Hg<br>• Peristalsis and DCI look normal |

*Major disorders of peristalsis:*

| | |
|---|---|
| Distal esophageal spasm | • Mean IRP—Normal<br>• DCI >450 mm Hg cm/s<br>• >20 premature contractions |
| Jackhammer esophagus (hypercontractile esophagus) | • DCI >8,000 for at least two swallows<br>• IRP is normal |

d. High-resolution manometry (uses 32 sensors)

**Ans. 13** a. *Clinical features:*

- *MC in young females:*
  - MC symptom—dysphagia (both solids and liquids—more for liquids); slow progressive type
- Triad of achalasia—dysphagia + weight loss + reflux
- Nocturnal asthma (also seen in GERD cases)

b. *Investigations:*

- Barium swallow—bird-beak appearance, pencil tip, and abrupt cut-off
- Hurst phenomenon—flow of contrast beyond bird beak due to contrast load and weight

Please note: Rat tail is a feature of cancer esophagus (irregular narrowing in esophagus).

- *X-ray chest:* Presence of mediastinal gas fluid level behind heart shadow

- *X-ray abdomen:* Absent fundus gas shadow
- *IOC:* High-resolution manometry

c. *Complications of achalasia cardia:*
- MC complication—reflux esophagitis
- Aspiration
- MC tumor—SCC (8%)
- Adenocarcinoma—below air fluid level
- Sigmoid mega esophagus

d. *Eckardt Score:* Post-treatment score of achalasia to assess the response

**Ans. 14** *Difference between DES and NCE:*

| *Diffuse esophageal spasm* | *Nutcracker esophagus* |
|---|---|
| • Middle-aged female<br>• C/F—dysphagia + chest pain<br>• Aggravated by cold fluids and stress<br>• Treatment is medical—CCB<br>• Surgery can be done—long esophagomyotomy is advised up to carina<br>• Barium swallow—Corkscrew esophagus | • MC hypermotility disorder<br>• M = F<br>• C/F—mimics such as MI and usually admitted in ICU<br>• No surgery advised<br>• Only medical treatment with CCB<br>• Barium swallow—pulsion or epiphrenic diverticulum |

**Ans. 15** a. Epiphrenic diverticulum proximal to the gastroesophageal sphincter. (A) Small and asymptomatic; (B) large, symptomatic, and appearing as a gas-filled bubble on the chest radiograph.

b. Schatzki's ring, a thin submucosal web completely encircling the whole of the lumen, usually situated at the squamocolumnar junction.

c. Endoscopic appearance of esophageal candidiasis.

# 44 CHAPTER

# Gallbladder and Bile Ducts

## QUESTIONS

**Q1. Answer the following:**

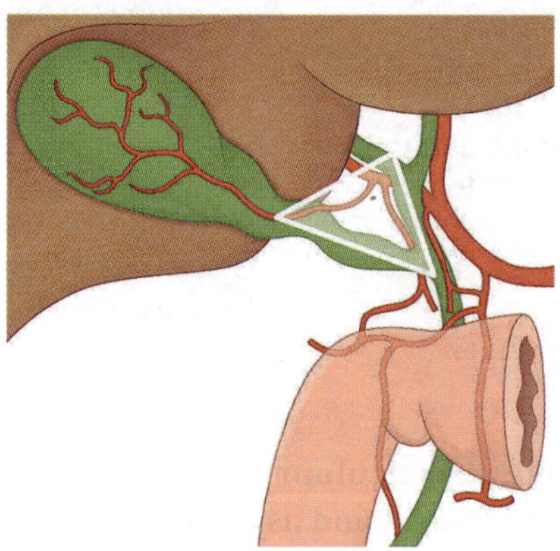

*Source:* Bailey and Love, 28th edition, page 1233.

a. Which triangle is shown in this image?
b. What are the boundaries of that triangle?

**Q2. Answer the following:**

a.

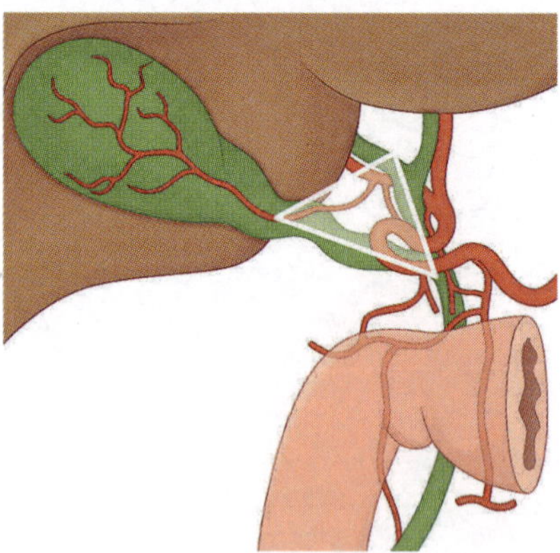

*Source:* Bailey and Love, 28th edition, page 1233.

b.

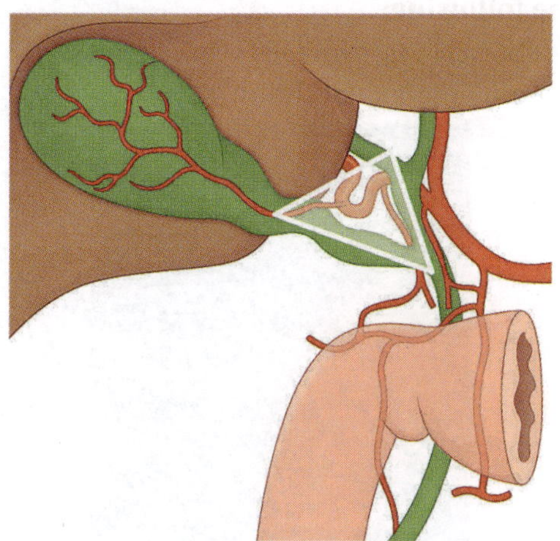

*Source:* Bailey and Love, 28th edition, page 1233.

What is depicted in "a" and "b"

**Q3. Regarding the anatomy of biliary system—false statement is:**

a. Cystic plate is fibrous sheet continuous with liver capsule of segments IV and V.
b. Cystic plate must be exposed to achieve critical view of safety.
c. Rouviere's sulcus marks the right anterior sectoral vein.
d. R4U line is very important during laparoscopic cholecystectomy—all dissection performed ventral to the line.

**Q4. What is depicted in this plain radiograph?**

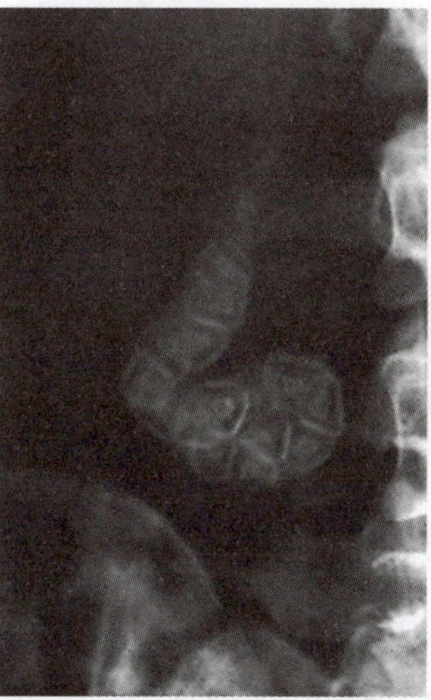

*Source:* Bailey and Love, 28th edition, page 1234.

**Q5. Answer the following:**

a. What is shown in this image?
b. Is that premalignant condition?

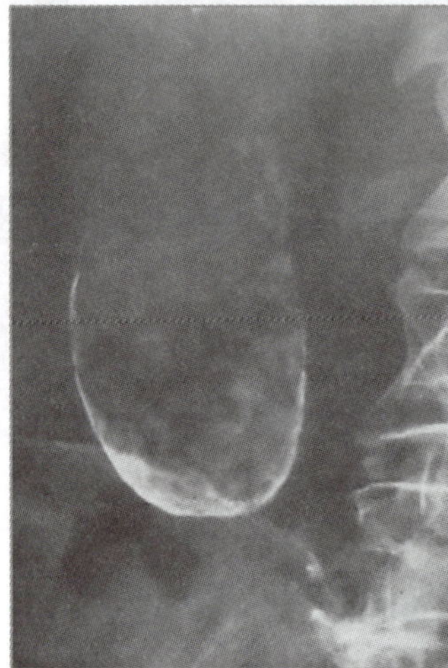

*Source:* Bailey and Love, 28th edition, page 1233.

**Q6. The following are the findings of acute cholecystitis in ultrasonography (USG), except:**

a. USG is the initial imaging modality of choice
b. 90–95% sensitive
c. Gallbladder (GB) wall thickened >3 mm
d. USG showing murphy sign
e. None

**Q7. What anomaly is shown in that image?**

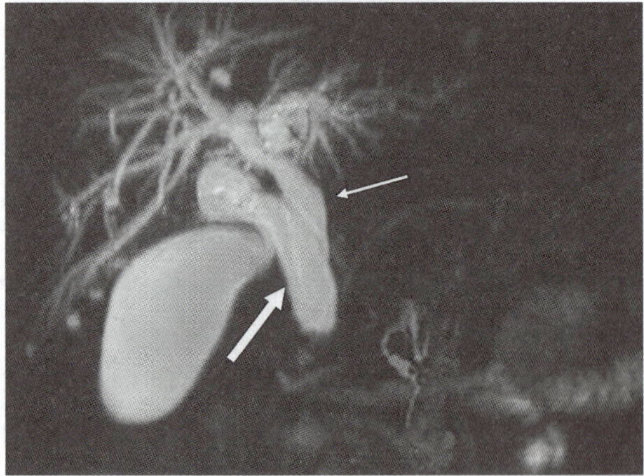

*Source:* Bailey and Love, 28th edition, page 1240.

## Q8. Answer the following:

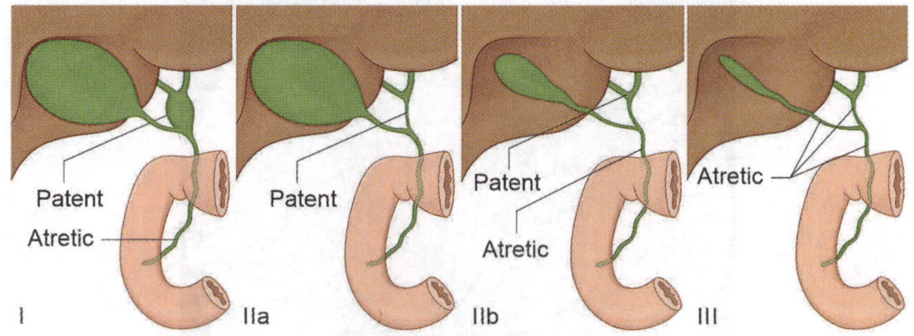


*Source:* Bailey and Love, 28th edition, page 1241.

a. What is that anomaly?
b. What is the classification for this condition?
c. What are the differential diagnosis for this condition?

## Q9. Answer the following:

a. What is shown in that image?
b. What is 1, 2, 3, and 4?
c. What hormone is work here and what is its action here?
d. What stimulates this hormone?

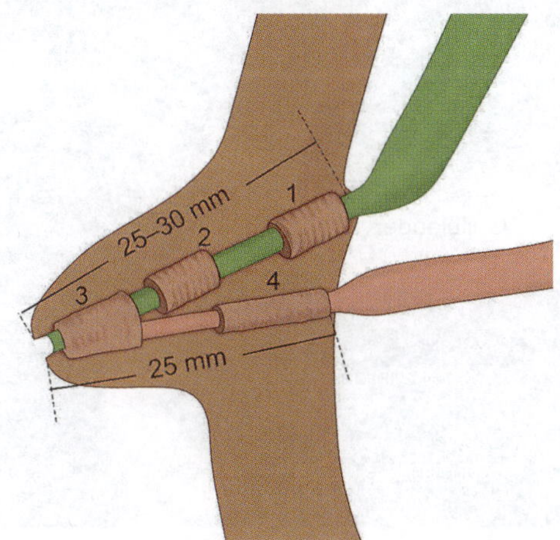


*Source:* Bailey and Love, 28th edition, page 1262.

## Q10. Answer the following:

a. What is this investigation?
b. What are the indications of this investigation?
c. What are the complications of this investigation?

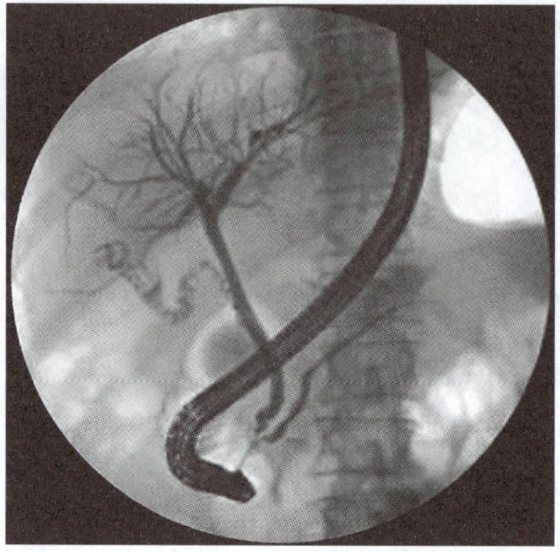

**Q11. Answer the following:**

a. What is that investigation?
b. What is the contrast material used for this investigation?
c. What are the advantages of this investigation?

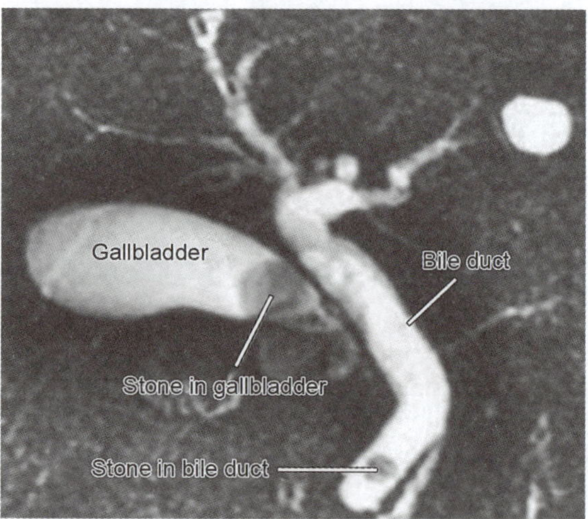


*Source:* Bailey and Love, 28th edition, page 1264.

**Q12. Answer the following:**

a. What investigation is shown in this image?

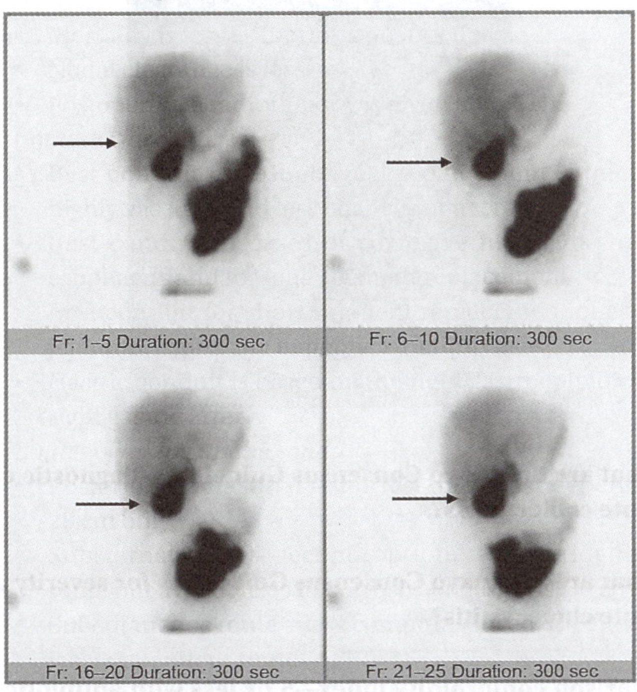


b. What is that sign shown in arrow?

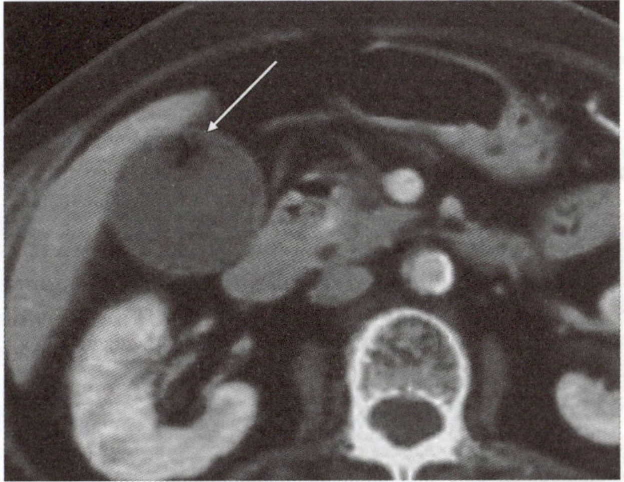

c. What is that sign shown in arrow?

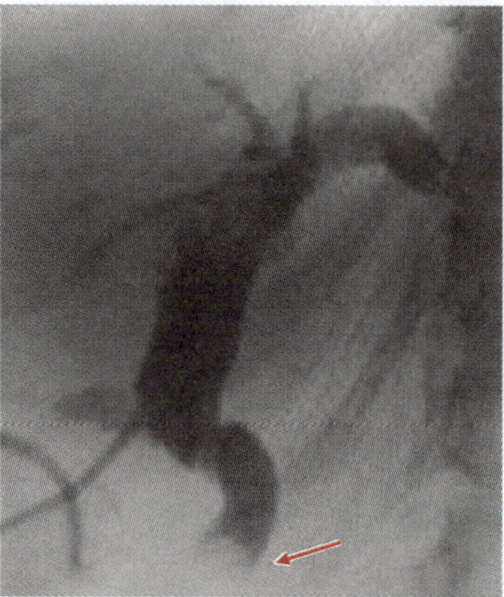

**Q13. What are the Tokyo Consensus Guidelines diagnostic criteria for acute cholecystitis?**

**Q14. What are the Tokyo Consensus Guidelines for severity grading of acute cholecystitis?**

**Q15. Charlson comorbidity index—5 or less with antibiotics controls the inflammation—what will you do as per Tokyo guidelines?**

a. Early cholecystectomy
b. Delayed LC
a. Observation
b. GB drainage

**Q16. What is a, b, and c?**

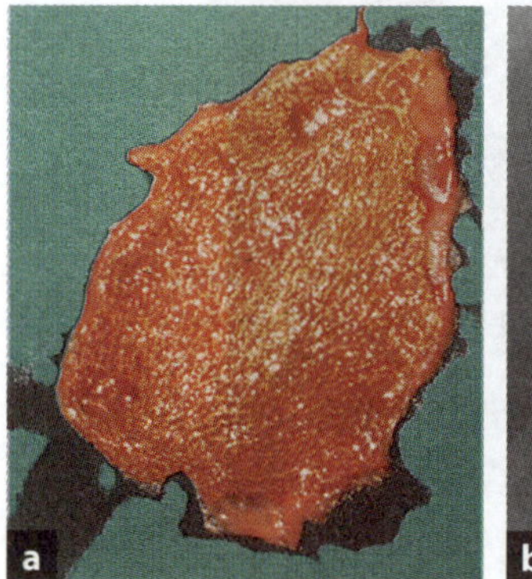


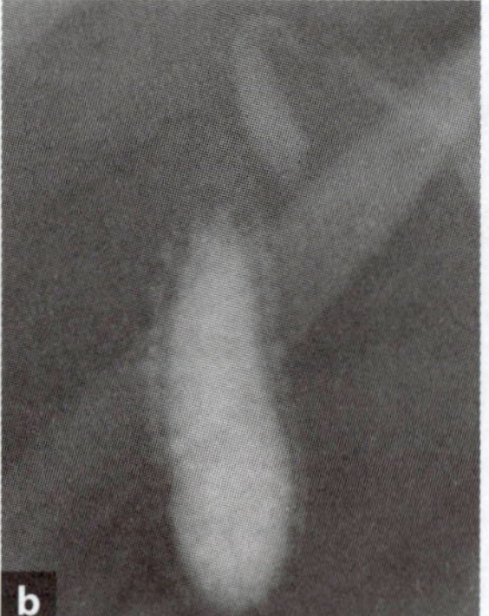


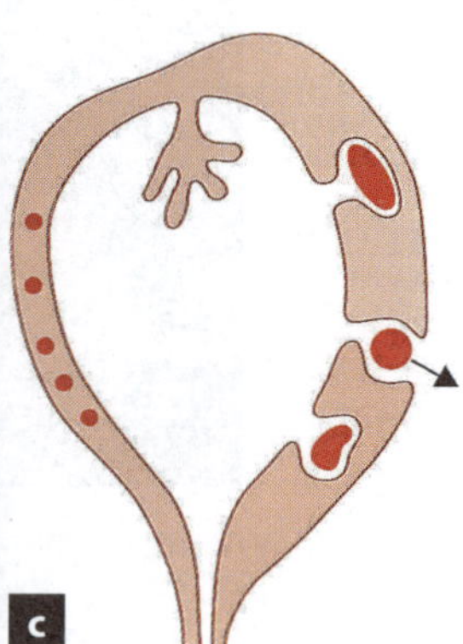


*Source:* Bailey and Love, 28th edition, page 1247.

## Q17. Answer the following:

a. What procedure is shown in that image?
b. What are the important operative steps?

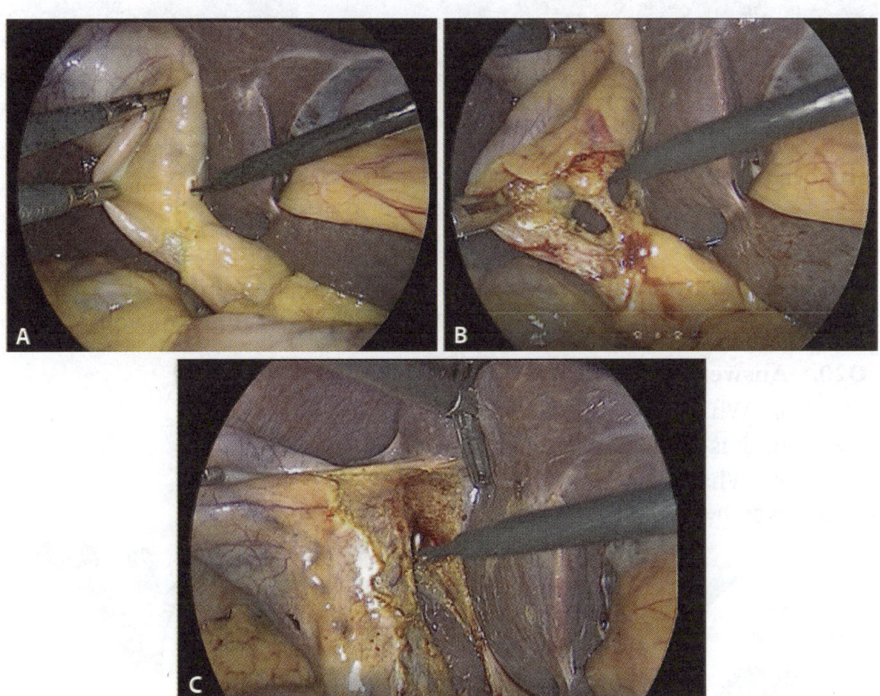


*Source:* Bailey and Love, 28th edition, page 1250.

## Q18. What is this classification?

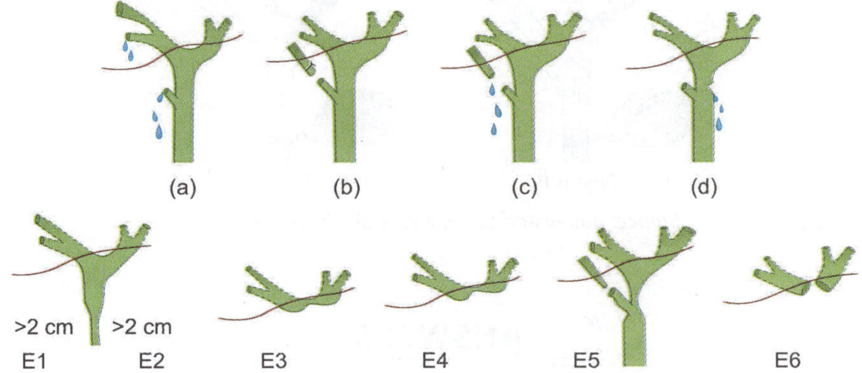


*Source:* Bailey and Love, 28th edition, page 1252.

**Q19. What is that technique?**

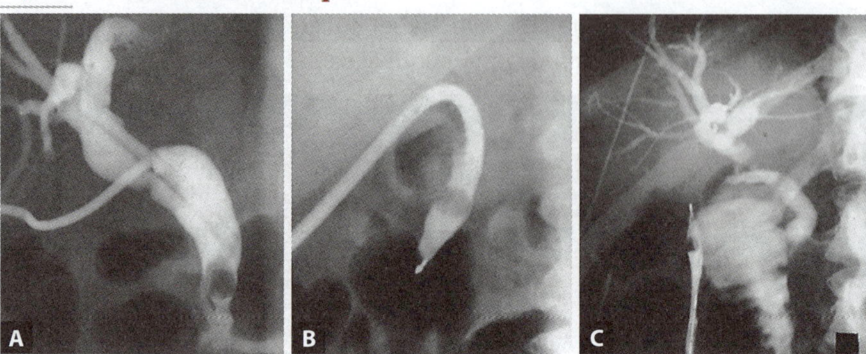


*Source:* Bailey and Love, 28th edition, page 1254.

**Q20. Answer the following:**

a. What is that classification?
b. It is done for which condition?
c. What are the risk factors for it?

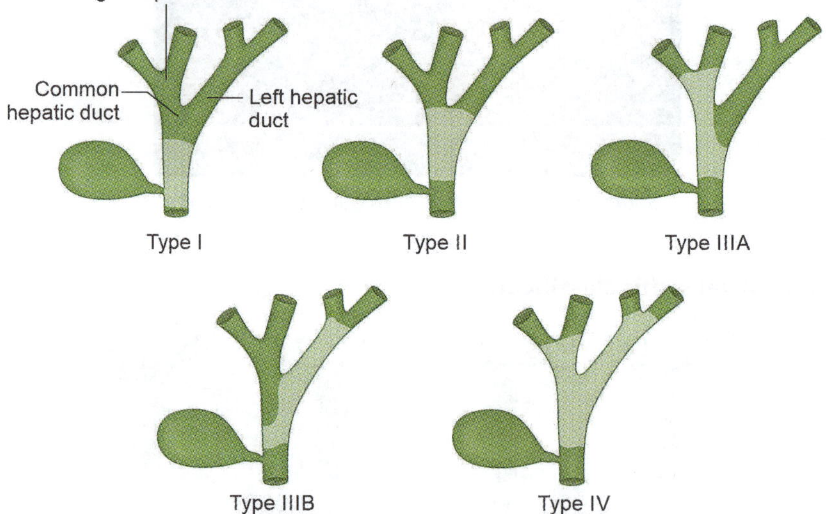


*Source:* Bailey and Love, 28th edition, page 1257.

## ANSWERS

**Ans. 1** a. Hepatocystic triangle

b. **Calot's triangle, also called as the hepatobiliary triangle**, it was described by Calot as the space bordered by the cystic duct inferiorly, the common bile duct (CBD) medially and the superior border of the cystic artery.

**Ans. 2** a. Tortuous common hepatic artery

b. Tortuous right hepatic artery with a short cystic artery
Both are the examples of the "caterpillar turn" or "Moynihan's hump", which can lead to inadvertent arterial injury or bleeding during cholecystectomy.

**Ans. 3** c. (*Ref:* Bailey and Love, 28th edition, page 1234)

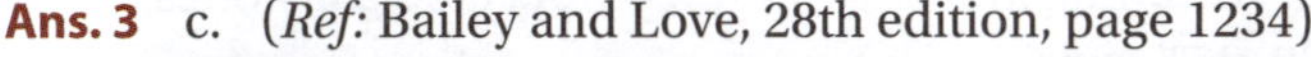

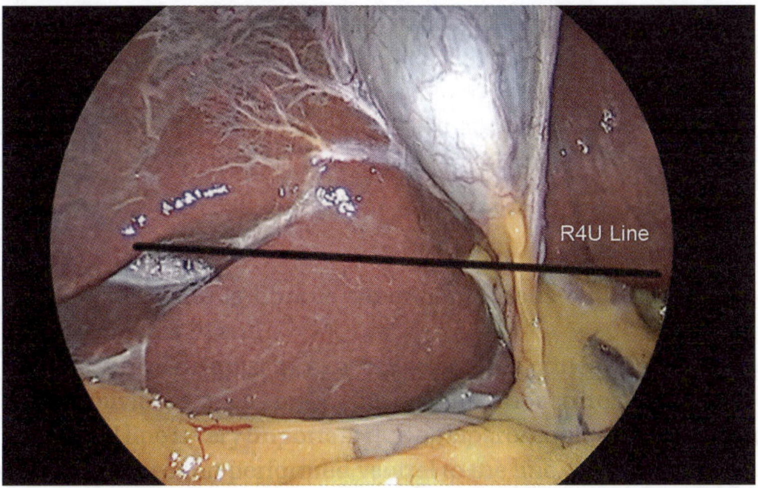


*Explanation—Rouviere's sulcus and R4U line:*

- The cystic plate is a fat ovoid fibrous sheet continuous with the liver capsule of segments IV (medially) and V (laterally).
- It is located in the GB bed and needs to be exposed to achieve the critical view of safety (CVS) during cholecystectomy.
- Rouviere's sulcus on the under surface of the right lobe of the liver running to the right of the hepatic hilum marks the position of the right posterior sectoral pedicle.
- The advantage of identifying Rouviere's sulcus and the line joining the roof of the sulcus to the base of segment IV (R4U line) (Rouviere's sulcus → segment IV → umbilical fissure) is that the cystic duct and the cystic artery lie ventral (anterosuperior) to the line and the CBD lies below the line.
- CBD injury can be minimized by maintaining the dissection ventral to the line during cholecystectomy.
- In the case of difficulty, all dissection during laparoscopic cholecystectomy should be performed ventral to the R4U line.

**Ans. 4** Plain radiograph showing radio-opaque stones with the center containing radiolucent gas in a triradiate or biradiate fissure **("Mercedes-Benz" or "seagull" sign)**.

**Ans. 5** a. Porcelain GB (calcification of the GB) (rare condition)
b. Yes, so we should do prophylactic cholecystectomy in this case.

**Ans. 6** e. (*Ref:* Bailey and Love, 28th edition, page 1235)

- Only 75% of GB stones are identified by CT imaging and it is not used as a screening modality for uncomplicated gallstones.
- USG is 90–95% sensitive.
- Acute calculous cholecystitis is diagnosed radiologically (by USG) (sensitivity 90–95%) by thickening of the GB wall (>3 mm), presence of pericholecystic fluid or direct tenderness when the probe is pushed against the GB (ultrasonographic Murphy's sign).

**Ans. 7** Magnetic resonance (MR) cholangiopancreatography demonstrating low insertion of the cystic duct (thick arrow) into the CBD (thin arrow).
Complete dissection of the low insertion of cystic duct should be avoided because there is a potential to compromise the vascular supply of the CBD, which leads to stricture formation.

**Ans. 8** a. Extrahepatic biliary atresia
b. The Japanese and Anglo-Saxon classification describes three main types (Kasai):
   1. *Type I:* Atresia restricted to the CBD
   2. *Type II:* Atresia of the common hepatic duct:
      - *Type IIa:* A patent GB and a patent CBD are present.
      - *Type IIb:* The GB, cystic duct, and CBD are also obliterated.
   3. *TYPE III:* Atresia of the right and left hepatic ducts and the entire extrahepatic biliary tree.

c. The most common differential diagnoses are Alagille syndrome (biliary atresia, congenital heart disease, and skeletal and other abnormalities), progressive familial intrahepatic cholestasis, and cystic fibrosis.
   - Neonatal hepatitis is the most difficult to differentiate.
   - Liver biopsy and radionuclide excretion scans are helpful.

**Ans. 9** a. Sphincter of Oddi dysfunction (SOD)—made of four sphincters as a complex
b. • Superior choledochal sphincter
   • Inferior choledochal sphincter

- Sphincter ampulla
- Sphincter pancreaticus

c. Hormone that acts here and opens it—cholecystokinin (CCK)
   - CCK contracts GB and opens the SOD.

d. CCK is stimulated by fatty chime.

**Ans. 10** a. *Endoscopic retrograde cholangiopancreatography (ERCP):*
   - Done with side viewing scopy.
   - Sphincterotomy done at 11'o clock or 1'o clock position
   - SOD pressure falls down and SOD will be always relaxed and opened.
   - Contrast passed inside the biliary and pancreatic system.
   - Keep a stent inside the bile duct known as double pig tail or DJ stent.

b. *Indications for ERCP:*
   - Sphincterotomy—SOD dyskinesia
   - *Stone removal:*
     - Stenting (obstructive jaundice)—self-expanding metallic stent (SEMS) for growth in bile duct
   - Biopsy
   - Pancreas divisum—minor duct papillotomy
   - Gall stone pancreatitis

c. *Complications:*
   - ERCP-induced pancreatitis (M/C)
   - Cholangitis
   - Bleeding
   - Perforation of duodenum
   - Mortality—0.1%

**Ans. 11** a. Magnetic resonance cholangiopancreatography (MRCP)

b. No contrast is used (bile and pancreatic juice acts as contrast).

c. *Advantages:*
   - Noninvasive
   - Has replaced ERCP in diagnostic purposes.
   - IOC for BD stones, BD malignancy, and pancreatic duct pathologies

**Ans. 12** a. *Hydroxy iminodiacetic acid (HIDA scan):*
   - It is a radiotracer substance injected into blood stream—taken up by liver and excreted into bile duct without metabolization. On the way, it gets concentrated in GB.

- *Applications:*
  - Detects physiology of bile flow
  - Detects bile leak
  - Gold standard for acute cholecystitis—nonvisualization of GB.

b. Mercedes Benz sign seen in GB stones
c. Meniscus sign in CBD stone

**Ans. 13**

| ***A. Local signs of inflammation*** | ***B. Systemic signs of inflammation*** | ***C. Imaging findings*** |
|---|---|---|
| 1. Murphy's sign<br>2. Right upper quadrant pain/tenderness/mass | 1. Fever<br>2. Elevated CRP<br>3. Elevated WBC count | Imaging findings characteristic of acute cholecystitis |

*Source:* Bailey and Love, 28th edition, page 1244.

*Suspected diagnosis:* 1 item in A + 1 item in B
*Definite diagnosis:* 1 item in A + 1 item in B + C

**Ans. 14** Tokyo consensus guidelines for severity grading of acute cholecystitis.

| ***Grade III (severe) acute cholecystitis*** | |
|---|---|
| *Associated with dysfunction of any one of the following organs/systems:* | |
| • Cardiovascular dysfunction | Hypotension requiring treatment with dopamine ≥5 μg/kg/min, or any dose of epinephrine |
| • Neurological dysfunction | Decreased level of consciousness |
| • Respiratory dysfunction | $PaO_2/F1O_2$ ratio <300 |
| • Renal dysfunction | Oliguria; creatinine >2.0 mg/dL |
| • Hepatic dysfunction | Prothrombin time (PT-INR) >1.5 |
| • Hematological dysfunction | Platelet count <100,000/$mm^3$ |
| ***Grade II (moderate) acute cholecystitis*** | |
| *Associated with any one of the following conditions:*<br>• Elevated white cell count (>18,000/$mm^3$)<br>• Palpable tender mass in the right upper abdominal quadrant<br>• Duration of complaint >72 hours<br>• Marked local inflammation (gangrenous cholecystitis, pericholecystic abscess, hepatic abscess, biliary peritonitis, and emphysematous cholecystitis)<br>***Grade I (mild) acute cholecystitis*** does not meet the criteria of grade II or grade III acute cholecystitis. Grade I can also be defined as acute cholecystitis in a healthy person with no organ dysfunction and mild inflammatory changes in the gallbladder, making cholecystectomy a safe and low-risk operative procedure | |

*Source:* Bailey and Love, 28th edition, page 1245.

**Ans. 15** a. (*Ref:* Bailey and Love, 28th edition, page 1246)

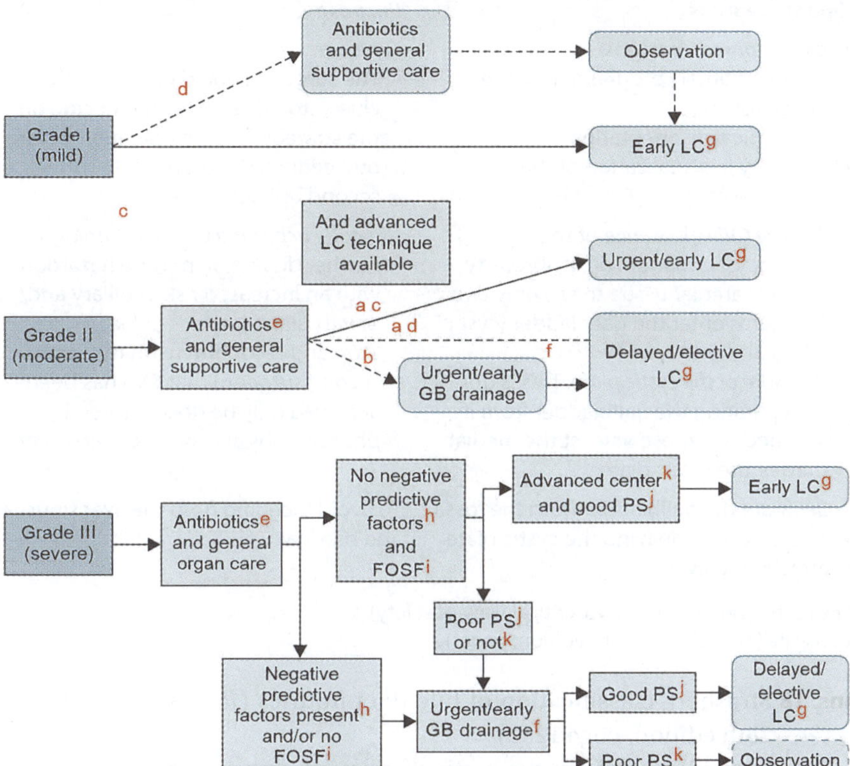


**Ans. 16** a. Cholesterolosis ("strawberry GB")

b. Diverticulosis of GB with dots of contrast medium in the GB wall.

c. Types of cholecystitis glandularis proliferans (polyps, intramural or diverticular stones, and fistula)

**Ans. 17** a. Laparoscopic cholecystectomy

b. Important operative steps during cholecystectomy

| ***Operative steps*** | ***Purpose*** |
|---|---|
| *Retraction*<br>*Proper retraction in the correct direction:*<br>• The fundus is retracted towards the patient's right shoulder and the infundibulum is retracted inferolaterally toward the patient's right side | • Opens the hepatocystic triangle<br>• Increases the angle between the cystic duct and the CBD<br>• Limits the dissection above Rouvière's sulcus<br>• Mental and spatial orientation of the anatomy, variation, and landmarks |

*Contd...*

*Contd...*

| *Operative steps* | *Purpose* |
|---|---|
| *Look out for red flag signs:*<br>• Failure of timely progression of the dissection<br>• Anatomical disorientation<br>• Difficulty in visualization of the operative field | *Time out:*<br>• The surgeon should recognize these clues, stop dissection and decide on the strategy for safe operation before proceeding. Do not hesitate to seek a second opinion |
| • *Achieve CVS:* Clearance of the hepatocystic triangle of all fibrofatty and soft areolar tissue to see only two structures enter the gallbladder (cystic artery and duct)<br>• *Exposure of the cystic plate:* This is done by separating the gallbladder from its liver bed to expose at least the medial third of the cystic plate | *Difficulty achieving CVS is a warning:*<br>• Further dissection may be hazardous, with an increased risk of biliary and/ or vascular injury<br>• Stop and reconfirm (with the team/ second surgeon) that CVS has been achieved may be documented by photographs and/or video recordings |
| • Separate the gallbladder from the fossa<br>• This is done by leaving the cystic plate attached to liver | To avoid bleeding from the liver sinuses and bile leak |

(CBD: common bile duct; CVS: critical view of safety)
*Source:* Bailey and Love, 28th edition, page 1250.

**Ans. 18** Strasberg classification of bile duct injuries (*Ref:* Bailey and Love, 28th edition, page 1252)

a. A bile leak from the cystic duct stump or minor biliary radical in the GB fossa.
b. An occluded right posterior sectoral duct
c. A bile leak from the divided right posterior sectoral duct
d. A bile leak from the main bile duct without any major tissue loss
    - E1, transected main bile duct with a stricture >2 cm from the hilus
    - E2, transected main bile duct with a stricture <2 cm from the hilus
    - E3, stricture of the hilus with the right and left ducts in communication
    - E4, stricture of the hilus with separation of the right and left hepatic ducts
    - E5, stricture involving the right aberrant sectoral duct and the main bile duct
    - E6, complete excision of the extrahepatic ducts involving the confluence (this injury is not described in Strasberg's classification)

**Ans. 19** *Burhenne technique:* Extraction of a stone from the CBD

*Steps:*

a. T-tube in situ with a stone in the bile duct
b. Steerable catheter is manipulated into the duct and a basket placed around the stone.
c. The stone is extracted from the duct along the T-tube track.

**Ans. 20** a. Bismuth–Corlette classification
b. Done for cholangiocarcinoma
c. Risk factors for cholangiocarcinoma

| | |
|---|---|
| *Chronic inflammatory conditions* | • PSC<br>• Oriental cholangiohepatitis<br>• Hepatitis C infection |
| Parasitic infections | • *Opisthorchis viverrini*<br>• *Clonorchis sinensis* |
| Congenital | • Choledochal cysts<br>• Caroli's disease |
| Chemical agents | • Thorium dioxide (Thorotrast)<br>• Vinyl chloride<br>• Dioxin<br>• Asbestos |
| Postsurgical | • Biliary–enteric anastomosis |
| Nonalcoholic fatty liver disease | |

*Source:* Bailey and Love, 28th edition, page 1256.

# CHAPTER 45 Liver

## QUESTIONS

**Q1.** **What are the main functions of the liver?**

**Q2.** **What are the routinely available blood tests for the assessment of liver function?**

**Q3.** **What are the King's College selection criteria for liver transplantation in acute liver failure: Paracetamol (acetaminophen) and nonparacetamol induced?**

**Q4.** **What are the features of chronic liver disease?**

**Q5.** **What is the Child–Turcotte–Pugh (CTP) classification of hepatocellular function in cirrhosis?**

**Q6.** **What are the modalities employed for imaging of the liver?**

**Q7.** **Enumerate the grading of liver injuries according to American Association for the Surgery of Trauma (AAST)?**

**Q8.** **What is the procedure shown here?**

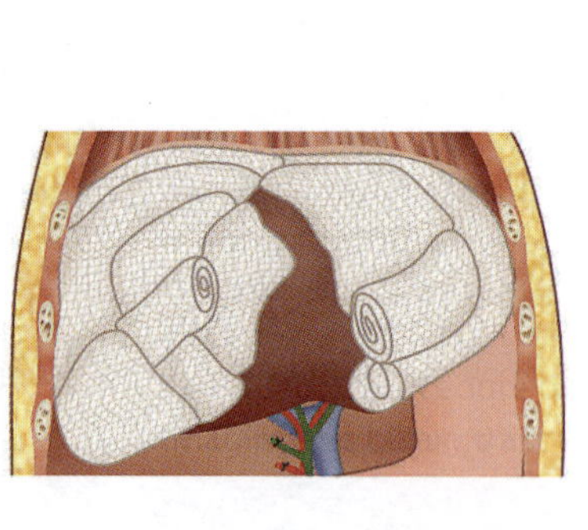
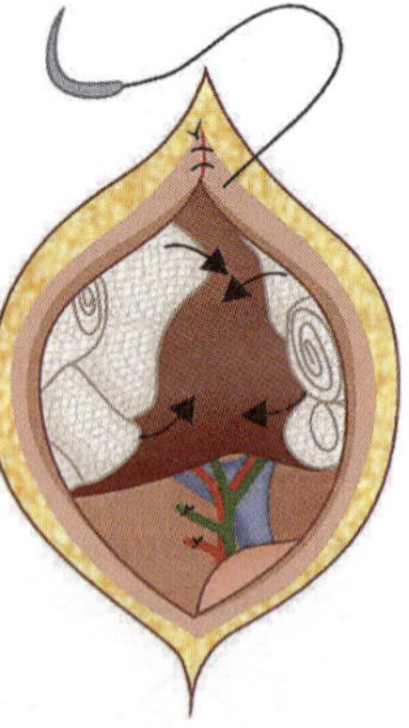

*Source:* Bailey and Love, 28th edition, page 1201.

**Q9.** **What is the procedure shown here?**

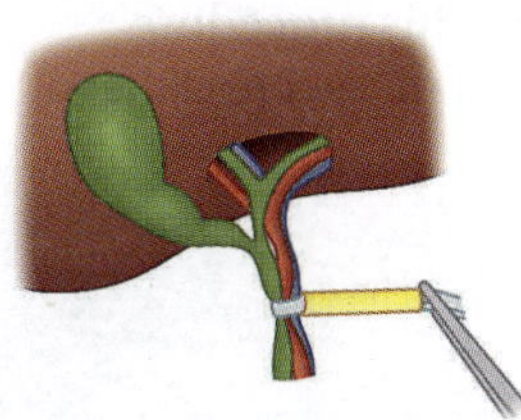

*Source:* Bailey and Love, 28th edition, page 1201.

**Q10.** **What are the management protocol for complications of portal hypertension (PHT)?**

**Q11.** **What is the management protocol of variceal bleeding?**

**Q12.** **Based on the diagram, answer the following:**

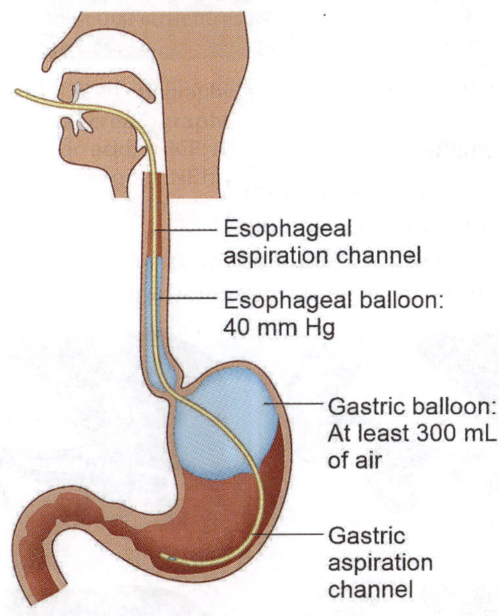


*Source:* Bailey and Love, 28th edition, page 1205.

a. Enumerate the tube which is shown here.
b. This tube is used for which condition?
c. What are the causes of portal hypertension?

**Q13. Based on the diagram, answer the following:**

a. Enumerate the procedure shown here.
b. Complications of this procedure
c. Contraindications for this procedure

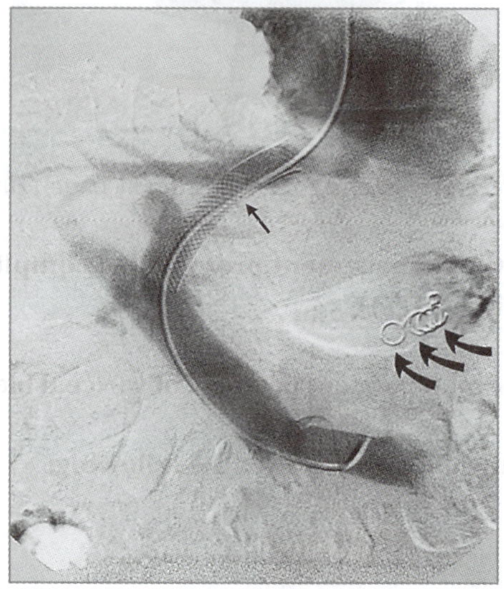

*Source:* Bailey and Love, 28th edition, page 1205.

**Q14. NEET-SS 2023:**

a. What shunts are shown here?
b. It is done for what pathology?
c. Enumerate various shunt operations.
d. Contraindications of shunt operations

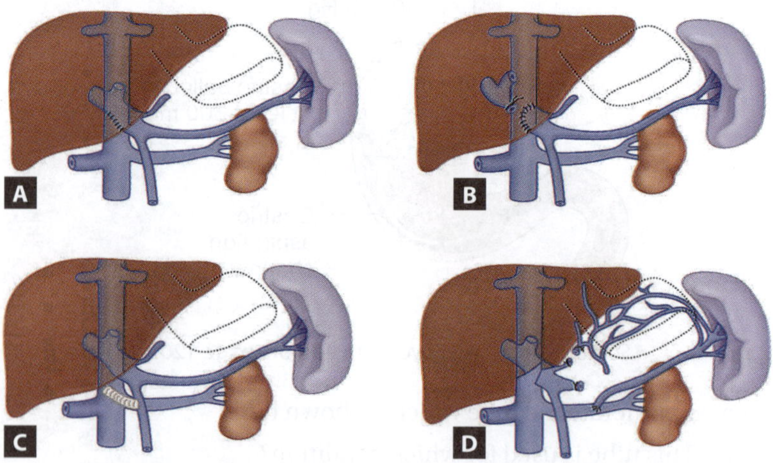


*Source:* Bailey and Love, 28th edition, page 1206.

**Q15. Answer the following:**

a. Management of bleeding esophageal varices
b. Treatment of ascites in chronic liver disease
c. Enumerate the important chronic liver conditions.

**Q16. Enumerate the procedure shown here.**

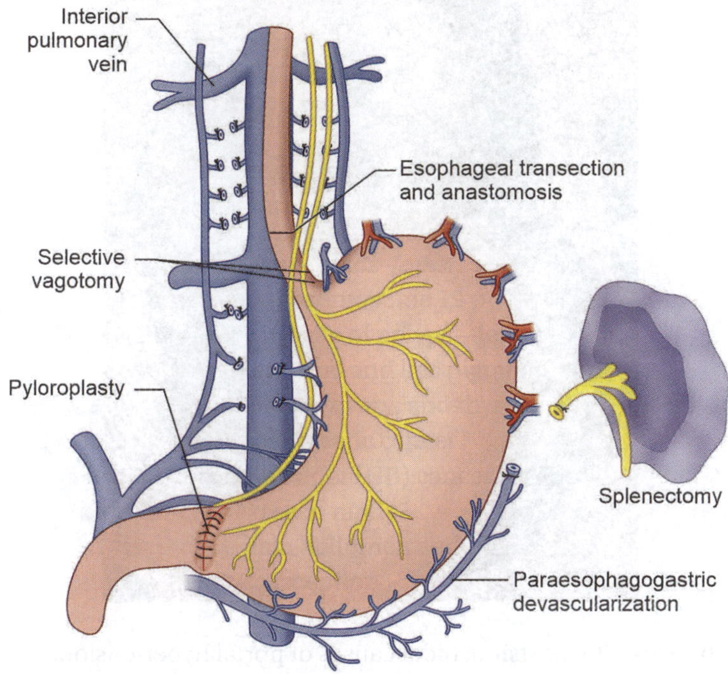


**Q17. Based on the diagram, answer the following:**

a. What procedure is shown here?
b. It is done for what pathology?
c. Describe various causes of portal hypertension.

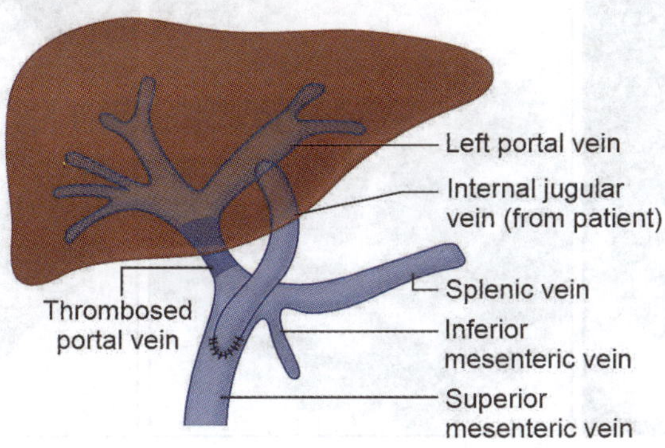

**Q18. Answer the following:**

a. Spot diagnosis.

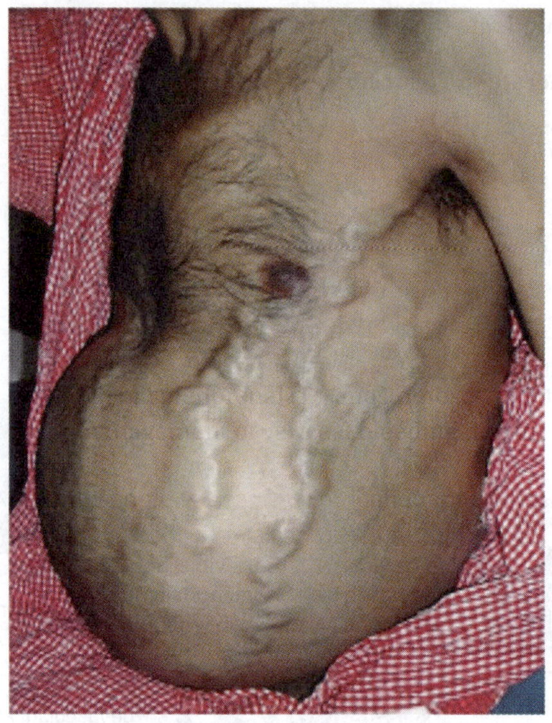

b. Describe postsinusoidal causes of portal hypertension.

**Q19. Describe differences between pyogenic and amoebic liver abscess.**

**Q20. Describe the classification for this pathology.**

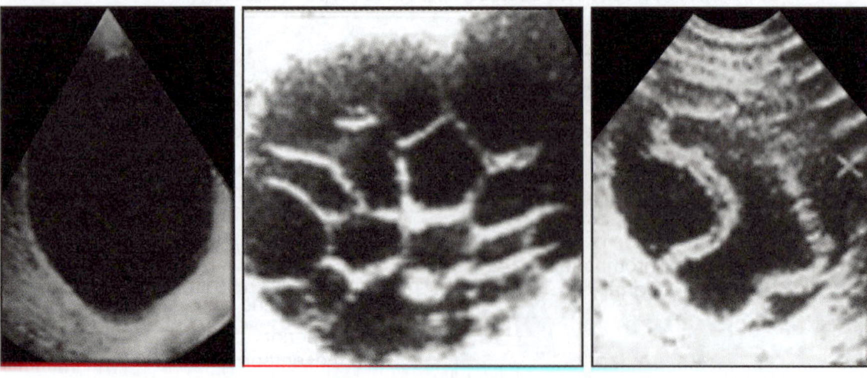

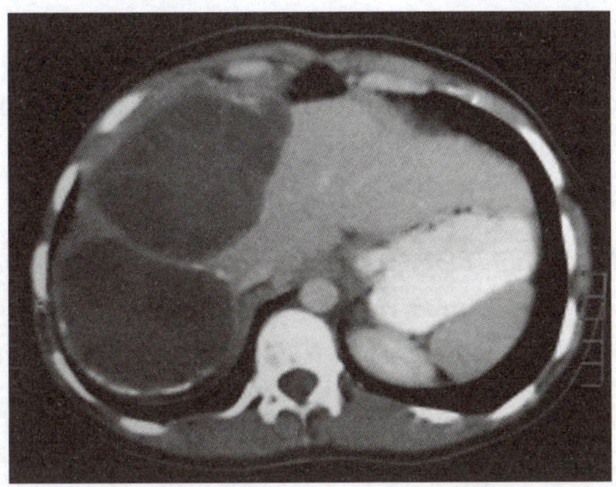

**Q21. Answer the following:**

a. What is percutaneous aspiration, infusion of scolicidal agents, and reaspiraion (PAIR) for hydatid cyst?

b, Contraindications for PAIR.

**Q22. Answer the following:**

a. What are the etiological factors for hepatocellular cancers?

b. Clinical features

c. Investigations

d. Treatment

e. What are Milan criteria of liver transplant in cirrhotic liver?

## ANSWERS

**Ans. 1**

- Maintaining core body temperature
- pH balance and correction of lactic acidosis
- Synthesis of clotting factors
- Glucose metabolism, glycolysis, and gluconeogenesis
- Urea formation from protein catabolism
- Bilirubin formation from hemoglobin after breakdown of effete red cells in the spleen
- Drug and hormone metabolism and excretion
- Removal of gut endotoxins and foreign antigens
- Vitamin and mineral storage, including A, D, E, K, and $B_{12}$
- Immunological function as part of the mononuclear phagocyte system
- Albumin production for transport of fatty acids, steroids, and waste products

- Angiotensin synthesis
- Body temperature through heat production
- Cytochrome P450 detoxifies contaminants and pollutants, insecticides, food additives, and alcohol

**Ans 2.**

**Routinely available blood tests for the assessment of liver function.**

| Test | Normal range | Significance |
|---|---|---|
| Bilirubin | 5–17 µmol/L (0.3–1.2 mg/dL) | Bilirubin is synthesized in the liver and excreted in bile. Increased levels may be associated with increased hemoglobin breakdown, hepatocellular dysfunction resulting in impaired bilirubin transport and excretion or mechanical biliary obstruction. In patients with known parenchymal liver disease, progressive elevation of bilirubin in the absence of a secondary complication suggests deterioration in liver function |
| Alkaline phosphatase (ALP) | 30–140 IU/L | The serum ALP is particularly elevated with cholestatic liver disease or biliary obstruction. It is important to note that routine laboratory analysis of ALP is not isoform specific and so ALP from a skeletal source may also lead to elevation, particularly Paget's disease and prostate cancer |
| Aspartate transaminase (AST) | 5–40 IU/L | Although significant liver injury does occur in the presence of normal liver blood tests, levels of the transaminase (AST, ALT, and GGT) usually reflect acute hepatocellular damage and GGT is a useful marker of alcohol intake |
| Alanine transaminase (ALT) | 5–40 IU/L | |
| Gamma-glutamyltranspeptidase (GGT) | 10–48 IU/L | |
| Albumin | 35–50 g/L (3.5–5 g/dL) | The synthetic functions of the liver are indicated by the ability to synthesize proteins (albumin level) and clotting factors (PT) and the standard method of monitoring liver function in patients with chronic liver disease is serial measurement of bilirubin, albumin, and PT |
| Total protein | 60–85 g/L (6–8.5 g/dL) | |
| Prothrombin time (PT) | 12–16 s | |

*Source:* Bailey and Love, 28th edition, page 1194.

**Ans. 3**

| *King's College selection criteria for liver transplantation in acute liver failure: Paracetamol (acetaminophen) and nonparacetamol induced* | |
|---|---|
| ***Paracetamol toxicity*** | ***Nonparacetamol toxicity*** |
| Criteria met if arterial pH <7.30 or/and all three of the following present:<br>1. INR >6.5 (PT >100 s)<br>2. Serum creatinine 3.4 mg/dL (301 μmol/L)<br>3. Grade III or IV encephalopathy[a]<br>Additionally,[b]<br>• Hyperlactatemia or hyperphosphatemia are strong predictors of poor prognosis for survival without transplantation | Criteria met if INR >6.5 (PT >100 s) or/and Three out of five of the following present:<br>1. Age <10 or >40<br>2. Etiology non-A, non-B hepatitis, idiosyncratic drug reactions<br>3. Duration of jaundice before development of encephalopathy >7 days<br>4. PT >50 s (approximate INR >3.5)<br>5. Serum bilirubin >18 mg/dL (300 μmol/L) |

[a]Hepatic encephalopathy grades can be described as:
- Grade 1: Inverted sleep pattern, agitation, forgetfulness, irritability, and apraxia
- Grade 2: Lethargy, time and/or place disorientation, personality change, and ataxia
- Grade 3: Somnolence to semistupor but responds to verbal stimuli, place disorientation, asterixis, and hyperactive reflexes
- Grade 4: Coma

[b]The addition of lactate or phosphate thresholds to the criteria may improve sensitivity and negative predictive value.
(INR: international normalized ratio; PT: prothrombin time)
*Source:* Bailey and Love, 28th edition, page 1195.

**Ans. 4**
- Lethargy
- Fever
- Jaundice
- Protein catabolism (wasting)
- Coagulopathy (bruising)
- Cardiac (hyperdynamic circulation)
- Neurological (hepatic encephalopathy)
- PHT
- Ascites
- Esophageal varices
- Splenomegaly and hypersplenism
- Cutaneous
- Spider naevi
- Palmar erythema

**Ans. 5**

| *Child-Turcotte-Pugh (CTP) classification of hepatocellular function in cirrhosis* | | | |
|---|---|---|---|
| ***Points*** | ***1 point each*** | ***2 points each*** | ***3 points each*** |
| Bilirubin (pmol/L) | <34 | 34–50 | >50 |
| Albumin (g/L) | >35 | 25–35 | <25 |
| Ascites | None | Easily controlled | Poorly controlled |
| Encephalopathy | None | Grade I or II | Grade III or IV |
| INR | <1.7 | 1.7–2.2 | >2.2 |

CTP-A: 5 or 6 points; CTP-B: 7–9 points; CTP-C: 10–15 points. (INR: international normalized ratio)

*Source:* Bailey and Love, 28th edition, page 1196.

Overall surgical mortality rates are increased by 10% in CTP-A disease, 30% in CTP-B, and 75–80% in CTP-C. MELD scores correlate with operative mortality: 1% increase for each MELD point up to 20 and a further 2% for each point above 20, with rates considerably higher following emergency presentation.

**Ans 6.**

| ***Modalities employed for imaging of the liver*** | |
|---|---|
| Imaging modality ultrasonography | *Principal indication:*<br>• Standard first-line investigation<br>• CEUS 90% accurate for focal lesions |
| Spiral CT | • Investigation of malignancy<br>• Cancer surveillance<br>• Anatomical planning for liver surgery |
| MRI<br>MRCP<br>ERCP | • Alternative to spiral CT<br>• Characterization of liver lesions<br>• Liver-specific contrast agents are taken up by hepatocytes, which are absent in malignant lesions, which consequently contrast with the enhanced background liver<br>• First-line noninvasive cholangiography<br>• Investigation and surveillance of parenchymal liver disease (sclerosing cholangitis and autoimmune cholangitis) for the development of malignancy<br>• Therapeutic procedure only<br>• Imaging the biliary tract when endoscopic intervention is required (stones, strictures, iatrogenic, and traumatic injury) |
| PTC | Biliary tract imaging when ERCP not possible or failed |

*Contd...*

*Contd...*

| | |
|---|---|
| EUS | • Generally for examination of the extrahepatic biliary tree and pancreas<br>• Caudate lobe, hilar nodes, and liver parenchyma can be assessed |
| Octreotide scanning | • Form of scintigraphy used to identify and localize NETs and carcinoid tumors<br>• Particularly useful to exclude metastatic disease |
| HIDA scanning | Determination of the patency of the intra- and extrahepatic biliary system and investigation of biliary atresia and jaundice following liver transplantation |
| Angiography | • To detect vascular involvement by tumor<br>• Treatment of vascular pathology (pseudotumors, hemobilia, iatrogenic injuries, and trauma) |
| PET scanning | • To quantify tumor spread<br>• Differentiate benign and malignant pathologies |
| Laparoscopy ± laparoscopic ultrasonography | • To detect peritoneal and serosal disease, assess the extent of tumors and spread<br>• Ultrasonography to determine the relationship of tumors to vascular structures and biopsy of liver tumors and superficial lesions |

(CPUS: contrast-enhanced ultrasonography; CT: computed tomography; ERCP: endoscopic retrograde cholangiopancreatography; EUS: endoscope ultrasonography; HIDA: hepatobiliary iminodiacetic acid; MRCP: magnetic resonance cholangiopancreatography; MRI: magnetic resonance imaging: NET: neuroendocrine tumor; PET: positron emission tomography; PTC: percutaneous transhepatic cholangiography)
*Source:* Bailey and Love, 28th edition, page 1197.

## Ans. 7

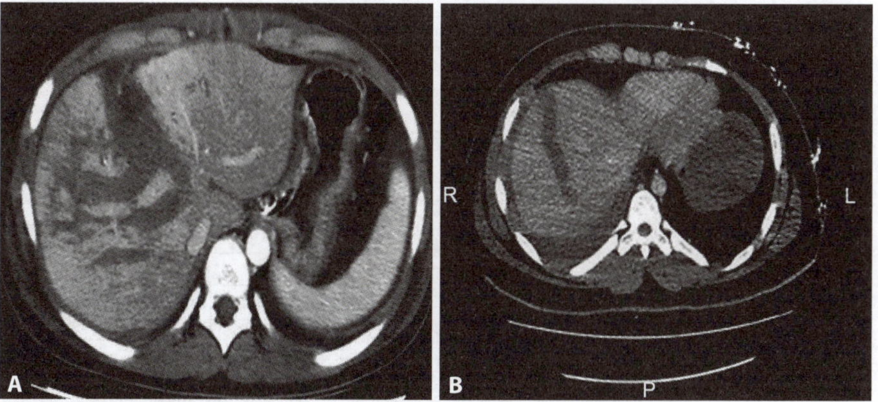


Computed tomography scans demonstrating the significant differences between blunt (A) and penetrating (B) trauma (assault with a kitchen knife).
*Source:* Bailey and Love, 28th edition, page 1200.

| *Grading of liver injuries according to American Association for the Surgery of Trauma* | |
|---|---|
| Grade 1 | • *Hematoma:* Subcapsular, <10% surface area<br>• *Laceration:* Capsular tear, <1 cm parenchymal depth |
| Grade 2 | • *Hematoma:* Subcapsular, 10–50% surface area<br>• *Hematoma:* Intraparenchymal, <10 cm diameter<br>• *Laceration:* Capsular tear 1–3 cm parenchymal depth, <10 cm length |
| Grade 3 | • *Hematoma:* Subcapsular, >50% surface area of ruptured subcapsular or parenchymal hematoma<br>• *Hematoma:* Intraparenchymal, >10 cm<br>• *Laceration:* Capsular tear, >3 cm parenchymal depth<br>• Vascular injury with active bleeding contained within liver parenchyma |
| Grade 4 | • *Laceration:* Parenchymal disruption involving 25–75% hepatic lobe or involves 1–3 Couinaud segments<br>• Vascular injury with active bleeding breaching the liver parenchyma into the peritoneum |
| Grade 5 | • *Laceration:* Parenchymal disruption involving >75% of hepatic lobe<br>• *Vascular:* Juxtahepatic venous injuries (retrohepatic vena cava/central major hepatic veins) |
| *Additional points:*<br>• Advance one grade for multiple injuries up to grade III<br>• "Vascular injury" (i.e., pseudoaneurysm or arteriovenous fistula) appears as a focal collection of vascular contrast that decreases in attenuation on delayed images.<br>• *"Active bleeding":* Focal or diffuse collection of vascular contrast that increases in size or attenuation on a delayed phase. | |

*Source:* Bailey and Love, 28th edition, page 1200.

**Ans. 8** Packing the liver to achieve hemostasis. The abdomen can then be closed and the patient transferred to critical care for stabilization prior to relook laparotomy 24–48 hours later.

**Ans. 9** Pringle maneuver

**Ans. 10**

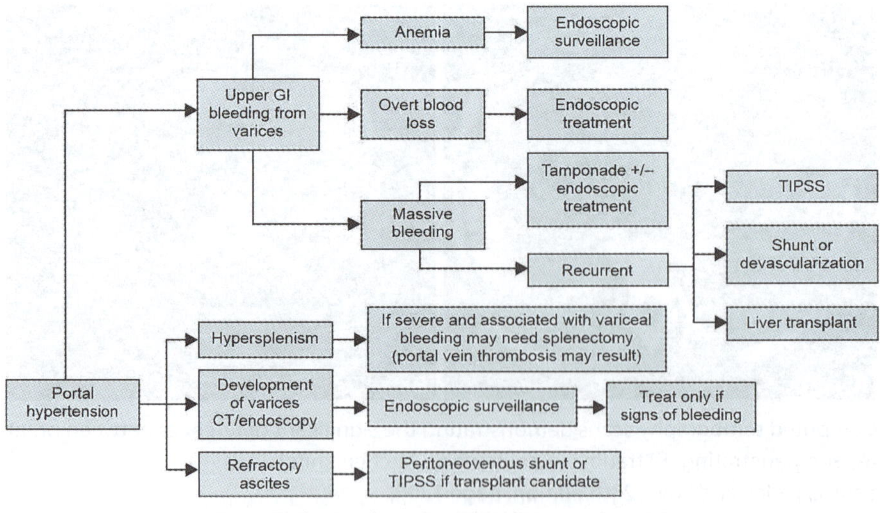


*Source:* Bailey and Love, 28th edition, page 1203.

**Ans. 11**

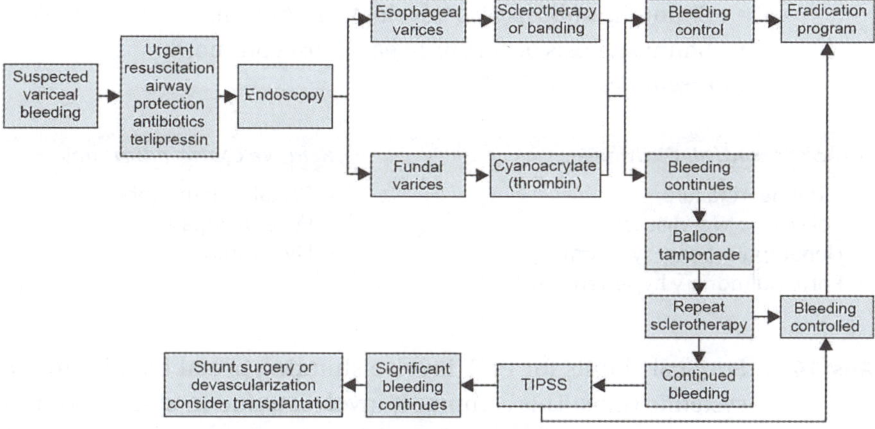


*Source:* Bailey and Love, 28th edition, page 1204.

**Ans. 12** a.
- Esophageal and gastric balloon tamponade with a Sengstaken–Blakemore or Minnesota tube
- *Esophageal balloon:* 40 mm Hg pressure
- *Gastric balloon:* At least 300 mL of air

b. Used for variceal bleeding management

c. Causes of PHT
- *Presinusoidal:*
  - *Extrahepatic:* Portal vein thrombosis, splenic vein thrombosis (pancreatitis and pancreatic tumor), myelofibrosis, arterioportal shunt, and tropical splenomegaly
  - *Intrahepatic:* Schistosomiasis, congenital hepatic fibrosis and portal infiltration (sarcoidosis), drugs and toxins, and veno-occlusive disease (VOD)
- *Sinusoidal:* Cirrhosis
- *Postsinusoidal:* Hepatic vein (HV) occlusion [Budd-Chiari syndrome (BCS)], VOD, and congestive cardiac failure

**Ans. 13** a. Angiogram following insertion of a transjugular intrahepatic portosystemic stent shunt (TIPSS) (open arrow). Contrast in the portal vein flows through the metallic stent and outlines the right HV. Pressure measurements are taken from within the portal vein before and after insertion. Solid arrows indicate coils placed at the site of previous embolization.
Stent is made up of polytetrafluoroethylene (PTFE)

b. *Complications of TIPS:*
- *Early complication:* Capsule rupture (NEET SS/PG) with intraperitoneal hemorrhage

- Within 1 month—encephalopathy can happen.
- Shunt thrombosis also develops in 1 month.
- Shunt stenosis occurs in 1 year (most common).

c. *Contraindications for TIPS:*

| *Absolute contraindications* | *Relative contraindications* |
|---|---|
| • Right heart failure<br>• Poly cystic liver disease<br>• Hepatopulmonary syndrome<br>• Porto pulmonary hypertension | • Portal vein thrombosis<br>• Encephalopathy<br>• Liver tumors |

**Ans. 14** a. Surgical shunts for PHT involve shunting portal blood into the systemic veins. This commonly involves a side-to-side portocaval anastomosis (A) or end-to-side portocaval, (B) mesocaval "H graft", (C) or splenorenal (D) anastomoses.

b. Done for management of variceal bleeding due to PHT

c.

| *Nonselective shunts* | *Selective shunts* |
|---|---|
| Entire portal blood is diverted into systemic circulation and hence encephalopathy develops | Only splenic blood diverted; portal blood is flowing into liver and metabolized and hence no encephalopathy; but there is ascites formed |
| *Types:*<br>• End-to-side portocaval<br>• Side-to-side portocaval<br>• 16-mm interposition portocaval<br>• TIPS also nonselective<br>• LINTON= Conventional= Proximal splenorenal shunt: Splenectomy is done and proximal splenic vein anastomosed to left renal vein | *Types:*<br>• End-to-side portocaval<br>• Side-to-side portocaval<br>• 16-mm interposition portocaval<br>• TIPS also nonselective<br>• LINTON= Conventional= Proximal splenorenal shunt: Splenectomy is done and proximal splenic vein anastomosed to left renal vein |

d. *Contraindications of shunt operations:*

- Splenic vein thrombosis
- Superior mesenteric vein (SMV) thrombosis
- Splanchnic vein thrombosis

**Ans. 15** a.

- Blood transfusion
- Correct coagulopathy
- Esophageal balloon tamponade (Sengstaken–Blakemore or Minnesota tube)

- Drug therapy (terlipressin)
- Endoscopic sclerotherapy or banding
- Assess portal vein patency (Doppler ultrasonography or CT)
- TIPSS
- Surgery
- Portosystemic shunts
- Splenectomy and gastric devascularization
- Sugiura procedure

b.
- Salt restriction
- Diuretics
- Abdominal paracentesis
- Peritoneovenous shunts
- TIPSS
- Liver transplantation

c.

| ***Important chronic liver conditions*** | |
|---|---|
| ***Condition*** | ***Common presentations*** |
| Primary sclerosing cholangitis | Abnormal liver function tests (LFTs), pruritus, or jaundice |
| Primary biliary cirrhosis | Malaise, lethargy, pruritus, and abnormal LFTs |
| Budd-Chiari syndrome | Ascites, pain, and abdominal distension |
| Caroli's disease | Abdominal pain, sepsis, and biliary obstruction |
| Simple liver cysts | Coincidental finding, pain, and palpable mass |
| Polycystic liver disease | Hepatomegaly and pain |

*Source:* Bailey and Love, 28th edition, page 1207.

**Ans. 16** *Sugiura operation:* Devascularization operation (it is done in case where shunt operations not possible):

- Ligation of veins near esophagus.
- Vagotomy
- Pyloroplasty
- Esophageal transection and anastomosis
- Splenectomy

**Ans. 17** a. REX shunt—most physiological shunt done for extrahepatic portal vein obstruction (EHPVO) between SMV to left portal vein using internal jugular vein (IJV) of the baby.

b. For EHPVO

c. Sinistral/left PHT

- There is a splenic vein thrombosis due to chronic pancreatitis.
- Hence short gastric vessels dilate and develop only left side PHT with isolated gastric varices + splenomegaly
- Treatment of choice—splenectomy

| ***Noncirrhotic portal fibrosis (NCPF)*** | ***EHPVO (extrahepatic PV obstruction)*** |
|---|---|
| Second and third order of PV branches are fibrosed | Main or first order portal vein obstructed |
| MC in age 20–40 years | MC in <10 years<br>Hence stunted growth seen |
| *Common features:*<br>• Esophagogastric varices rupture and hematemesis (MC presentation)<br>• Splenomegaly (more bigger in NCPF)<br>• Liver histology is normal<br>• LFT is normal<br>• No ascites | |
| *Treatment:*<br>• Splenectomy + proximal splenorenal shunt (LINTON)<br>• They do not develop encephalopathy as their liver is normal<br>• REX shunt—most physiological shunt done for EHPVO between SMV to Left portal vein using IJV of the baby | |

**Ans. 18** a. Inferior vena cava (IVC) web causing BCS and liver failure

b. *VOD versus BCS:*

- *VOD:*
  - Sublobular venules gets thrombosis
  - *MC etiology:* Follows bone marrow transplant
  - *Others:* Pyrazolidone alkaloids and azathioprine
  - *Drug of choice:* Defibrotide
  - Venography shows HV and IVC normal; Wedge HV pressure is increased
- *BCS:*
  - *Two causes:* HV thrombosis and IVC occlusion by congenital membranous webs
  - BCS—MC cause in western is HV thrombosis. The thrombosis mc due to polycythemia rubra vera.
  - BCS—MC cause in Asians/Indians is IVC webs
  - IOC to diagnose—hepatic venography is gold standard—SPIDER WEB appearance
  - Contrast-enhanced computed tomography (CECT) abdomen shows enlarged caudate lobe—hot spot of caudate lobe seen

*Management*:

- No role of thrombolytic agents as it is a well-formed thrombus.
- Liver is normal. Shunt operations are planned as shown below:
  - Liver failure cases: Liver transplant is treatment of choice
  - *Shunt operations:*
    - *HV thrombosis:* Side-to-side portocaval shunt (SSPCS) done
    - *IVC webs:* Double shunt operation done (SSPCS + cavoatrial shunt) or SSPCS with IVC stenting

Clinical method to find—HV thrombosis alone or IVC web: Yes we can find out seeing the multiple collaterals running from below upwards in IVC obstruction cases.

**Ans. 19**

| ***Pyogenic abscess*** | ***Amoebic liver abscess*** |
|---|---|
| • Sick patient with fever, chills and rigors with hepatomegaly<br>• Severe right hypochondrial tenderness++ | Hepatomegaly + pain (MC symptom—pain) |
| M:F = 1.5:1 | • Male >>>> Female, in menstruating females it is never seen<br>• Iron deficiency anemia is protective |
| *Predisposing factors:*<br>• MC in immunocompromised cases<br>• Diabetes mellitus<br>• Predisposing factor | • Alcohol |
| *Lab values:* Increased AST, ALT, Alk. po4, Bilirubin | *Lab values*:<br>• All values normal<br>• Only PT may be elevated (NEET SS) |
| *Serology:* Negative for Amoeba<br>Blood culture is positive | *Serology:* Amoebic antigen+<br>Blood culture is negative |
| *CECT abdomen:*<br>• Clustered abscess seen with peripheral rim enhancement<br>• They may be 50:50 single or multiple (see below image) | *CECT abdomen:*<br>• Well defined abscess with no peripheral enhancement but there may be peripheral wall edema++<br>• Trophozoites are present in the wall<br>• Mostly they are solitary<br>• MC in segment 7 (see below image) |

*Contd...*

*Contd...*

| ***Pyogenic abscess*** | ***Amoebic liver abscess*** |
|---|---|
| 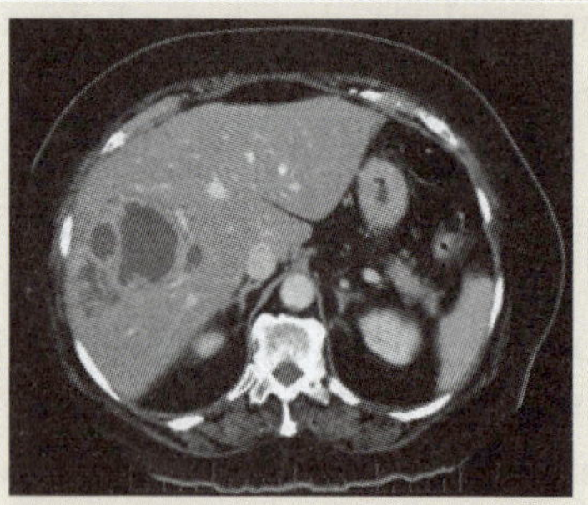 | 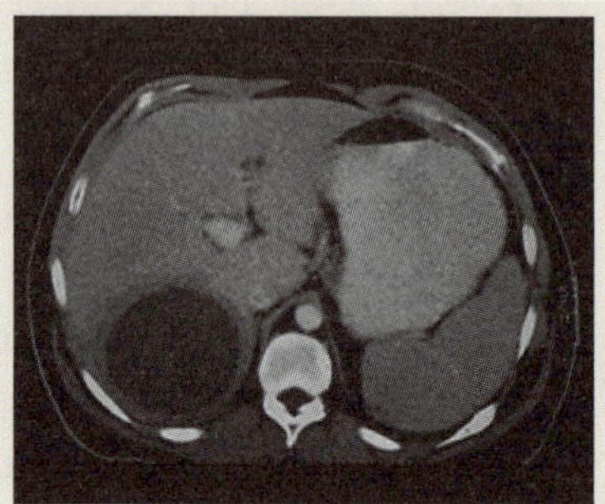 |
| *Complications:*<br>• Sepsis<br>• Endogenous endophthalmitis (MC in diabetes—3% of patients will develop due to *Klebsiella*)<br>• Osteomyelitis<br>• Infective endocarditis | *Complications:* Color of pus-Anchovy sauce colour odorless.<br>• MC complication is reactive pleural effusion in right side (not rupture)<br>• MC site of rupture into peritoneal cavity<br>• Rupture into pleura—put an ICD<br>• Rupture in bronchus (broncho pleural fistula)—cough shows anchovy sauce sputum. Treated by lying in prone position and bronchodilators+ chest physiotherapy. Pus drained via sputum<br>• Rupture into mediastinum |
| *Treatment:*<br>• Immediate treatment of choice is aspiration of abscess<br>• Based on Pus C/S and blood C/S higher antibiotics are given | *Treatment:* One-third of patients has H/o amoebic dysentery two-thirds develops from subclinical infection<br>• TOC—injection metronidazole 750 mg TDS for 2 weeks and convert to oral<br>• Luminal amebicide diloxanide furoate, emetine, etc., × 10 days<br>• Aspiration—indications: Doubtful diagnosis<br>  – >5 cm-sized abscess<br>  – Located on left lobe<br>  – Superficial located abscess<br>  – Not responding for >3 days<br>*Surgical treatment:*<br>• DP stent under USG guidance. Stent left for 2 weeks to 1 month.<br>• Even after complete drainage of abscess-the residual cavity remains up to 6–9 months |

(ALT: alanine transaminase; AST: aspartate transaminase; CECT: contrast-enhanced computed tomography; USG: ultrasonography )

**Ans. 20** Gharbi et al. classification of hydatid cysts is old classification

*In the image, it is WHO classification:*

- CE 1—unilocular cyst
- CE 2—multiseptated (honeycomb/Rosette like)
- CE 3—floating membrane (water lily sign)
- CE 4—heterogenous cysts with partial calcification
- CE 5—calcified wall

Types 1, 2, and 3 are active cysts.

Types 4 and 5 are Inactive and dead cysts.

*Risk of biliary-cyst communication (for NEET SS):*

- Male patients
- Abnormal preoperative serum alkaline phosphatase and γ-glutamyltransferase (GGT)
- Multiple cysts, multilocular, and degenerated cysts
- Cysts near the biliary bifurcation
- Presence of bile-stained or purulent cyst
- Cyst diameter >10 cm was an independent clinical predictor for the presence of intrabiliary rupture

**Ans. 21** a. PAIR

- Given with prophylactic cover of albendazole
- Scolicidal agents—20% hypertonic saline (best), 0.5% silver nitrate, 95% ethanol, absolute alcohol, mebendazole 2.4 μg/mL, 10% povidone Iodine

b. *Contraindications for PAIR:*

- Superficially located cyst (chance of rupture)
- Honey combing of cysts (multiple thick internal septae)—CE2
- Communication with biliary tree
- Dead or inactive cysts
- Lung/brain cysts—CE4 and 5
- Peritoneal rupture or pleural rupture

**Ans. 22** a. *Etiological factors:*

| *Infections* | *Cirrhosis* | *Environmental* | *Metabolic diseases* |
|---|---|---|---|
| • HBV<br>• HCV | • Alcohol<br>• Autoimmune<br>• Primary biliary | • Aflatoxins<br>• Pyrrolidone alkaloids<br>• Thorotrast<br>• Nitrosamines | • Hemochromatosis<br>• Alpha 1 AT deficiency<br>• Wilsons<br>• Glycogen storage diseases<br>• EHBA |

(EHBA: extrahepatic biliary atresia; HBV: hepatitis B virus; HCV: hepatitis C virus)

b. *Clinical features:*
- K/C/O cirrhosis sudden decompensation of liver with pain, mass, and weight loss all suggest malignancy
- *Paraneoplastic syndromes:*
  - MC is hypercholesterolemia > hypoglycemia
  - Hypercalcemia
  - Polycythemia (erythrocytosis) [MC paraneoplastic syndrome (PNS) in renal cell carcinoma (RCC)—increased erythrocyte sedimentation rate (ESR)]

c. *Investigations: Tumor markers:*
- Alpha-fetoprotein (AFP) >20 ng/mL—70% have elevation
- AFP >400 ng/mL—conclusive of HCC
- Glypical-3
- PIVKA—protein induced vitamin K absence—descarboxy prothrombin
- AFP-L3 lectin 3 fraction

Contrast-enhanced computed tomography abdomen with triple phase is gold standard:
- Rapid contrast enhancement of tumor in arterial phase
- Rapid wash out in portal venous phase
- Phases in Liver on CECT:
  - Early arterial
  - Late arterial
  - Portal venous phase
  - Delayed

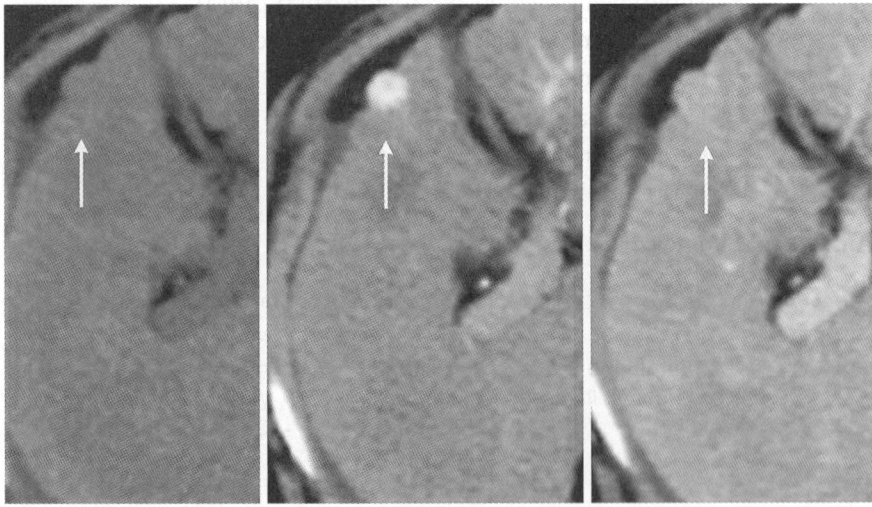

See the phases of HCC in CECT.

*Various staging systems in HCC:*

| ***OKUDA staging*** | ***CLIP—Cancer of Liver Italian Program*** | ***Chinese University Prognostic index (CUPI)*** |
|---|---|---|
| T—tumor size<br>A—albumin<br>A—ascites<br>B—bilirubin | | |

Latest staging system which helps in Diagnosis and treatment—Barcelona Clinic Liver Staging (BCLC Staging)

d. The Barcelona Clinic Liver Group staging system for the management of hepatocellular carcinoma (HCC). Patients with asymptomatic early tumors (stage 0-A) are candidates for curative therapies (resection, transplantation, or local ablation). Asymptomatic patients with multinodular HCC (stage B) are suitable for chemoembolization (TACE), whereas patients with advanced symptomatic tumors and/or an invasive tumoral pattern (stage C) are candidates for sorafenib. End-stage disease (stage D) includes patients with grim prognosis who should be treated by best supportive care.

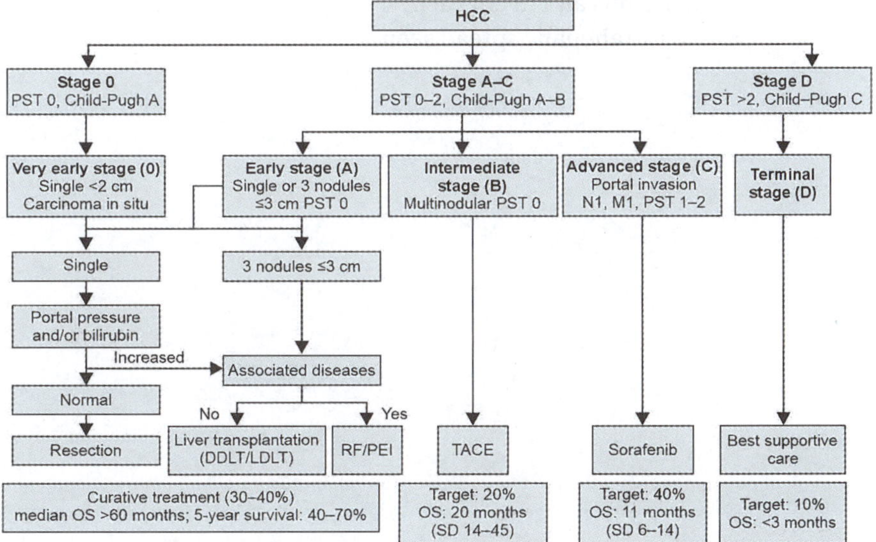


(DDLT: deceased donor liver transplantation; LDLT: living donor liver transplantation; OD: overall survival; PEI: percutaneous ethanol injection; PST: ECOG performance status; RF: radiofrequency ablation; SD: standard deviation; TACE: transcatheter arterial chemoembolization)

*Source:* Bailey and Love, 28th edition, page 1215.

- *Best is surgical resection:*
  - In a cirrhotic liver—future liver remnant (FLR) must be at least 40%
  - In a normal liver—FLR must be at least 25%
  - If above FLR is not possible—liver resection in contraindicated

  *Ablative therapies:*
  - Percutaneous ethanol Injection (PEI)
  - Percutaneous acetic acid injection
  - Percutaneous thermal ablations—radiofrequency Ablation (RFA) and cryoablation
  - Heat sink effect is seen in patients who have tumors very close to blood vessels will have the thermal effect dissolved by running blood and less effective.

  *Interventional procedures:*
  - TACE—transarterial chemoembolization: into hepatic artery we can inject chemotherapy—loaded with lipoidal sodium, which carries chemotherapy to tumor
  - TARE—transarterial radioembolization

e. *Liver transplantation: Milan criteria of liver transplant in cirrhotic liver:*
   - <5 cm single lesion
   - <3 lesions all 1–3 cm each
   - No extrahepatic spread seen

# 46 CHAPTER Pancreas

## QUESTIONS

**Q1. Enumerate the causes of raised serum amylase level other than acute pancreatitis.**

**Q2. What are the steps in the early management of severe acute pancreatitis?**

**Q3. Based on the figure, answers the following questions:**

a. What is that anomaly?
b. What is the IOC for this condition?
c. What is the treatment?
d. What are the complications of this condition?

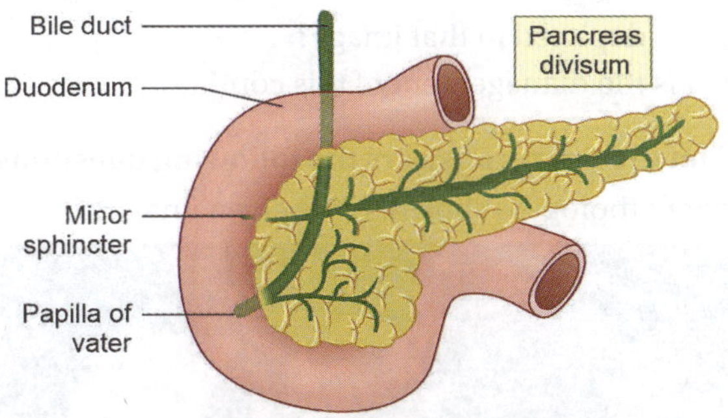


**Q4. Based on the figure, answers the following questions:**

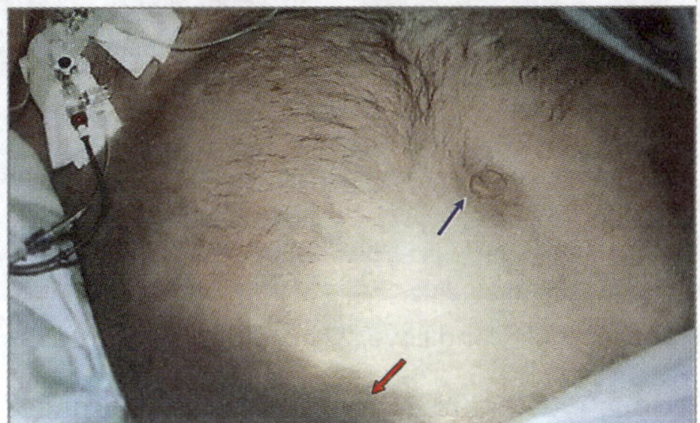

a. What is shown in red arrow and blue arrow?
b. In which condition these signs are seen?
c. What are the etiological factors for this condition?
d. What are the X-ray findings of this condition?

**Q5. Based on the figure, answers the following questions:**

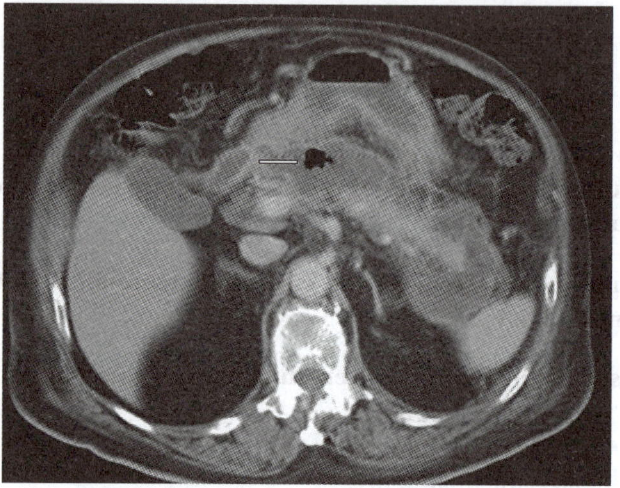

*Source:* Bailey and Love, 27th edition, page 1226.

a. What is depicted in that image?
b. What is the management of this condition?

**Q6. Based on the figure, answers the following questions:**

a. What pathology is shown in the given image?

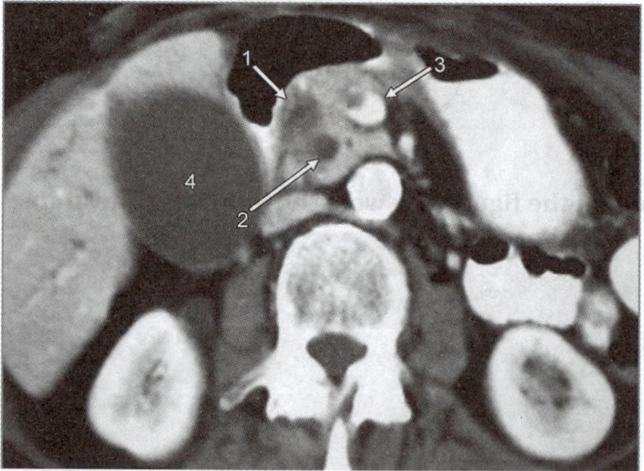


*Source:* Bailey and Love, 27th edition, page 1216.

b. What does 1, 2, 3, and 4 depict in the given image?

**Q7. What are the complications of acute pancreatitis?**

**Q8. Based on the figure, answers the following questions:**

a. What is shown in the given image?
b. What is the classification system for that?
c. What are its clinical features?
d. What is the investigation for this condition?
e. What is the management for this condition?

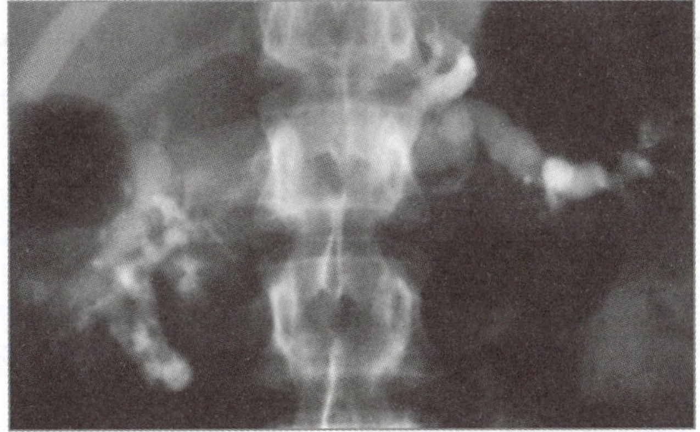

*Source:* Bailey and Love, 27th edition, page 1217.

**Q9. What are the scoring systems in acute pancreatitis?**

**Q10. Based on the diagram, answer the following questions:**

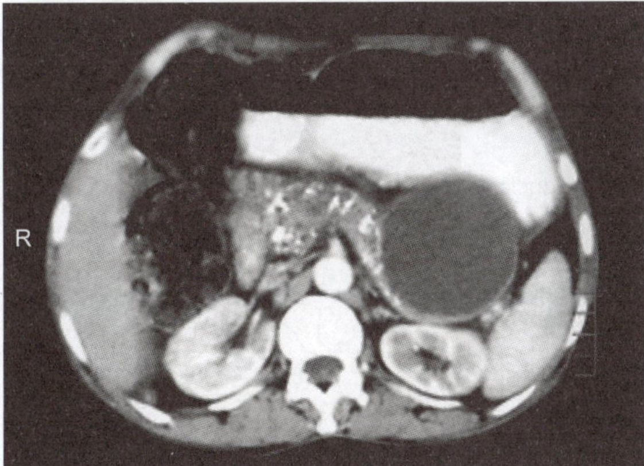


a. What pathology is shown in the given image?
b. What is the most common site for it?
c. Describe the classification for it.
d. What are clinical features and management of it?
e. What are complications of this condition?

**Q11. How will you differentiate pseudocyst from a cystic neoplasm?**

**Q12. What is Milwaukee classification of sphincter of Oddi (SOD) dysfunction?**

**Q13. What are the risk factors for the development of pancreatic cancer?**

**Q14. How will you manage the cystic neoplasms of the pancreas?**

**Q15. Based on the figures, answers the following questions:**

a. What procedure is it?
b. For what pathology it is done?
c. What procedure is modified in it?

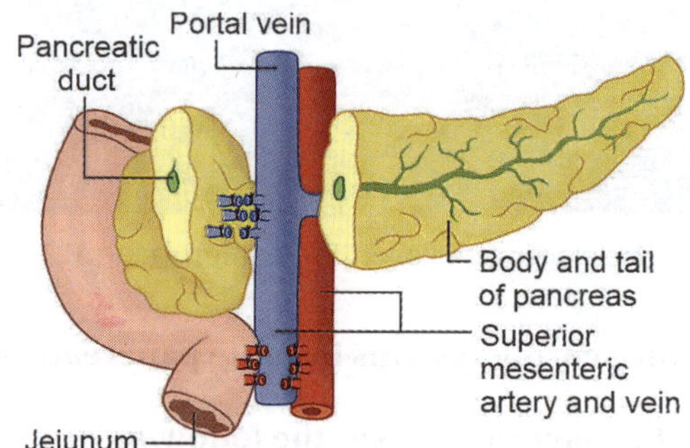


*Source:* Bailey and Love, 27th edition, page 1237.

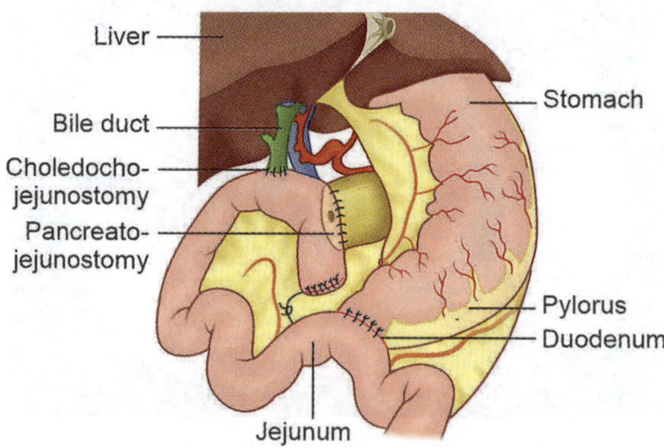


*Source:* Bailey and Love, 27th edition, page 1237.

# ANSWERS

**Ans. 1**
- Upper gastrointestinal tract perforation
- Mesenteric infarction
- Torsion of an intra-abdominal viscus
- Retroperitoneal hematoma
- Ectopic pregnancy
- Macroamylasemia
- Renal failure
- Salivary gland inflammation

**Ans. 2** Admission to **high dependency unit (HDU)/intensive care unit (ICU)**
- Analgesia
- Aggressive fluid rehydration
- Supplemental oxygen
- Invasive monitoring of vital signs, central venous pressure, urine output, and blood gases.
- Frequent monitoring of hematological and biochemical parameters (including liver and renal function, clotting, serum calcium, and blood glucose)
- Nasogastric drainage (only initially)
- Antibiotics, if cholangitis suspected; prophylactic antibiotics can be considered.
- CT scan essential if organ failure, clinical deterioration or signs of sepsis develop.
- ERCP within 72 hours for severe gallstone pancreatitis or signs of cholangitis.
- Supportive therapy for organ failure if it develops (inotropes ventilatory support, hemofiltration, etc.)
- **If nutritional support is required, consider enteral (nasogastric) feeding**.

**Ans. 3**
a. Pancreas divisum
b. Intraoperative cholangiography (IOC)—endoscopic retrograde cholangiopancreatography (ERCP) >magnetic resonance cholangiopancreatography (MRCP)
c. Treatment—Minor duct sphinterotomy
d. Recurrent pancreatitis.

**Ans. 4**
a. Red arrow—gray turner sign, blue arrow—Cullen sign
b. Seen in acute pancreatitis

c. Etiology of pancreatitis; (Get Smashed-I)
   - G—Gallstones [Molluscum contagiosum (MC) cause in adults]
   - E—Ethanol
   - T—Trauma (MC cause in children)
   - S—Steroids
   - M—mumps
   - A—autoimmune (PAN, systemic lupus erythematosus (SLE), etc.)
   - S—scorpion venom
   - H—Hyperlipidemia, Hypercalcemia, and hyperparathyroidism
   - E—ERCP, Emboli
   - D—Drugs (Azathioprine, thiazides, furosemide, tetracyclines, 6-mercaptopurine, etc.)
   - I—Infections [Coxsackie, cytomegalovirus (CMV), echovirus, ascaris lumbricoides, and clonorchis sinensis, etc.]

   *Drugs that cause acute pancreatitis are:*
   - Corticosteroids
   - Azathioprine
   - Asparaginase
   - Valproic acid
   - Thiazide diuretics
   - Estrogens

d. *X-ray abdomen erect findings:*
   - Gasless abdomen
   - Colon cutoff sign
   - Ground glass appearance
   - Sentinel loop sign
   - Renal halo sign

**Ans. 5** a. Infected pancreatic necrosis. Note the areas of reduced enhancement in the pancreas and the peripancreatic fluid collection with pockets of gas within it (arrow).

b. - Mostly the necrosis is sterile.
   - If it gets infected—there will be air, increased white blood cell (WBC) count and temperature.
   - In infected necrosis cases, we start antibiotics.
   - Under antibiotic coverage—we must remove the necrosis.
   - *Step up approach:* From minimally invasive to maximally invasive procedure. Ultrasonography (USG) guided percutaneous catheter drainage (PCD) done first, later as patient improves, minimally invasive method by laparoscopic

necrosectomy or video-assisted retroperitoneal debridement (VARD)-via a nephroscope introduced into the PCD tract.

**Ans. 6** a. Contrast-enhanced computed tomography scan of a patient with a carcinoma of the pancreatic head.

b. The dilated bile duct (1) and main pancreatic duct (2) can be seen, with tumor infiltration around them. There is a thrombus in the superior mesenteric vein (3). The gallbladder is distended (4).

**Ans. 7**

| Complications of acute pancreatitis. | |
|---|---|
| ***Systemic*** | ***Local*** |
| *(More common in the first week)* | *(Usually develop after the first week)* |
| *Cardiovascular:*<br>• Shock<br>• Arrhythmias<br>*Pulmonary:*<br>• ARDS<br>*Renal failure*<br>*Hematological*<br>• DIC<br>*Metabolic:*<br>• Hypocalcemia<br>• Hyperglycemia<br>• Hyperlipidemia<br>*Gastrointestinal:*<br>• Ileus<br>*Neurological:*<br>• Visual disturbances<br>• Confusion, irritability<br>• Encephalopathy<br>*Miscellaneous:*<br>• Subcutaneous fat necrosis<br>• Arthralgia | • Peripancreatic fluid collection<br>• Sterile pancreatic necrosis<br>• Infected pancreatic necrosis<br>• Pancreatic abscess<br>• Pseudocyst<br>• Pancreatic ascites<br>• Pleural effusion<br>• Portal/splenic vein thrombosis<br>• Pseudoaneurysm |

(ARDS: acute respiratory distress syndrome; DIC: disseminated intravascular coagulation)

**Ans. 8** a. *Endoscopic retrograde cholangiopancreatography:* Chronic pancreatitis. Most of the opacities lie within the duct system and are stones. Gross dilatation of ducts in the body and tail are due to obstruction by stones in the head of the pancreas.

b. ***TIGAR-O classification of etiology:***

- T—Toxic (Alcohol)—MC causes
- I—Idiopathic/tropical—Unknown cause; eating cassava root fibers in Kerala

- G—Genetic-*PRSS* gene mutation, SPINK-1 gene mutation, and CFTR gene mutation
- A—Autoimmune
- R—Recurrent acute pancreatitis (like in pancreas divisum)
- O—Obstructive

c. *Clinical features:*
- Pain abdomen; severe recurrent pain; addicted to opioids
- Diabetes—Responds only to insulin
- Steatorrhea

d. *Investigations:*
- Old tests not done now—Lundh meal test, pancreolauryl test
- *Latest for steatorrhea:*
  - *Fecal measurement of elastase:* <100—severe deficiency; >200 is normal
  - *Fecal fat excretion (on 100 g fat given):* > 7 g/day in stools is steatorrhea.
- *IOC to diagnose established chronic pancreatitis:* CECT abdomen-stricture, stones, and atrophy.
- *Gold standard to diagnose early cases of chronic pancreatitis:* ERCP—Chain of lakes appearance seen
- *Recent gold standard to diagnose early cases of chronic pancreatitis:* Endoscopic ultrasound (EUS)
- ERCP criteria—Known as Cambridge Criteria
- EUS criteria—Known as Rosemont Criteria

e. *Management*
- *Pain management:*
  - Analgesics is given initially.
  - Celiac plexus block using absolute alcohol—Laparoscopic or Contrast-enhanced computed tomography (CECT)-guided method.
  - Thoracoscopic splanchnicectomy also available.
- *Steatorrhea and weight loss:*
  - Pancreatic enzyme supplements—Creon, pancrelipase
  - The enzyme supplements must be given along with food
  - Acid reduction with PPI is needed while giving pancreatic enzyme tablets.
- Diabetes mellitus:
  - Best is by giving injection insulin

- *Surgical management:*

| Drainage procedures | Resection + Drainage procedures (hybrid procedures) | Resection procedure |
|---|---|---|
| • *Dilated duct:* >7 mm diameter. Modified Puestow procedure—Lateral pancreaticojejunostomy procedure<br>• For undilated duct—Izbicki procedure in which V-shaped excision of the duct done | • Frey's procedure—Head coring along with lateral pancreaticojejunostomy | • Distal pancreatectomy and splenectomy for problems in body and tail—child duval procedure<br>• Presence of head mass duodenum preserving pancreatic head resection (DPPHR)<br>– Beger's procedure<br>– Bem's modification<br>• *If suspicious of malignancy:* Whipple's procedure |

**Ans. 9**
- Ranson's scoring—Most widely used—3 is severe
- Apache 2—*Uses 12 factors:* >8 is severe
- Modified Glasgow score > 3
- Computed tomography (CT) severity index/Balthazar et al. scoring—best scoring
- C reactive protein—>150 mg/dL is severe
- BISAP score—Bed side index of severity of acute pancreatitis
- Revised Atlanta scoring system (RAS)
- Modified Marshall score
- q SOFA score used in sepsis

**Ans. 10** a. Pseudo cysts of pancreas (seen in acute and chronic pancreatitis)

b. MC near body and tail of pancreas

c. *D'egidio classification:*
   - Type 1—Follows acute pancreatitis; duct is normal
   - Type 2—Follows acute on chronic pancreatitis. Duct is abnormal with no stricture.
   - Type 3—Follows chronic pancreatitis; communication is seen with duct and duct has strictures.

d. C/F—Presents after 4 weeks with persistent pain and epigastric fullness and vomiting and early satiety.
   - Persistent elevation of serum amylase;
   - IOC—CECT abdomen;
   - EUS-guided fluid analysis shows increased amylase and normal carcinoembryonic antigen (CEA) (to differentiate from cystic neoplasm).

- *Management:*
    - Surgery advised for symptomatic pseudocysts only and for complication.
- *Surgical treatment:*
    - *Internal drainage:* Cystojejunostomy >Cystogastrostomy or cystoduodenostomy.
    - Cystogastrostomy done by open method, endoscopic method, or laparoscopic method
    - Infected pseudocyst—External drainage done.

e.

| **Possible complications of a pancreatic pseudocyst** | |
|---|---|
| ***Process*** | ***Outcomes*** |
| Infection | • Abscess<br>• Systemic sepsis |
| Rupture | |
| • Into the gut<br>• Into the peritoneum | • Gastrointestinal bleeding<br>• Internal fistula<br>• Peritonitis |
| Enlargement | |
| Pressure effects | • Obstructive jaundice from biliary compression<br>• Bowel obstruction |
| Pain | |
| Erosion into a vessel | • Hemorrhage into the cyst<br>• Hemoperitoneum |

**Ans. 11**
- History
- Appearance on CT and ultrasonography
- Fine needle aspiration (FNA) of fluid, preferably under endoscopic ultrasound guidance.
- CEA (high level in mucinous tumors)
- Amylase (level usually high in pseudocysts but occasionally in tumors)
- Cytology

**Ans. 12**

| ***Milwaukee classification of sphincter of Oddi (SOD) dysfunction*** |
|---|
| *Biliary-type SOD* |
| *Type I:*<br>• Typical biliary-type pain<br>• Liver enzymes (AST, ALT, or ALP) >2 times normal limit documented on at least two occasions during episodes of pain |

*Contd...*

*Contd...*

| ***Milwaukee classification of sphincter of Oddi (SOD) dysfunction.*** |
|---|
| • Dilated CBD >12 mm in diameter<br>• Prolonged biliary drainage time (>45 minutes)[a] |
| *Type II:*<br>• Biliary-type pain, and<br>• One or two of the above criteria |
| *Type III:* Biliary-type pain only |
| *Pancreatic-type SOD* |
| *Type I:*<br>• Pancreatic-type pain<br>• Amylase and/or lipase >2 times upper normal limit on at least two occasions during episodes of pain<br>• Dilated pancreatic duct (head >6 mm, body >5 mm)<br>• Prolonged pancreatic drainage time (>9 minutes)[a] |
| *Type II:* Pancreatic-type pain, and one or two of the above criteria |
| *Type III:* Pancreatic-type pain only |

[a]Difficult to measure and often eschewed in clinical practice

(AST: aspartate aminotransferase; ALT: alanine aminotransferase; ALP: alkaline phosphatase; CBD: common bile duct)

## Ans. 13

| ***Risk factors for the development of pancreatic cancer*** |
|---|
| Demographic factors |
| • Age (peak incidence 65–75 years)<br>• Male gender<br>• Black ethnicity |
| *Environment/lifestyle* |
| Cigarette smoking |
| *Genetic factors and medical conditions* |
| • *Family history*<br>• *Two first-degree relatives with pancreatic cancer:* Relative risk increases 18–57-fold<br>• Germline *BRCA2* mutations in some rare high-risk families<br>• Hereditary pancreatitis (50–70-fold increased risk)<br>• Chronic pancreatitis (5–15-fold increased risk)<br>• Lynch syndrome (HNPCC)<br>• Ataxia telangiectasia<br>• Peutz–Jeghers syndrome<br>• Familial breast-ovarian cancer syndrome<br>• Familial atypical multiple mole melanoma<br>• Familial adenomatous polyposis–risk of ampullary/duodenal carcinoma<br>• Diabetes mellitus<br>• Obesity<br>• HNPCC, hereditary nonpolyposis colorectal cancer |

**Ans. 14** Management algorithm for cystic neoplasms of the pancreas.

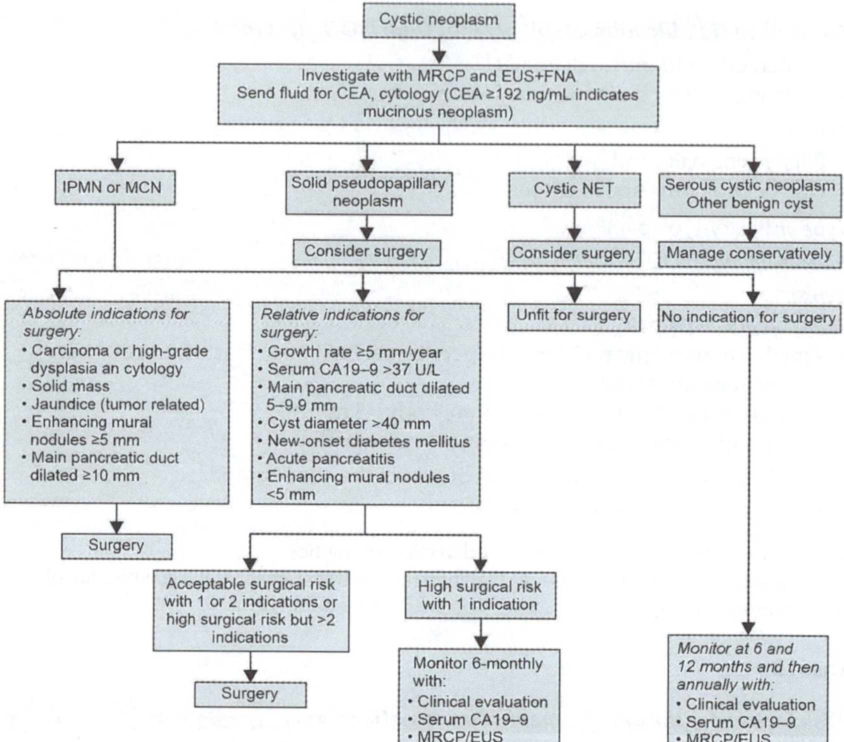


(CA19-9: carbohydrate antigen 19-9; CEA: carcinoembryonic antigen; EUS: endoscopic ultrasonography; FNA: fine-needle aspiration; IPMN: intraductal papillary mucinous neoplasm; MCN: mucinous cystic neoplasm; MRCP: magnetic resonance cholangiography and pancreatography; NET: neuroendocrine tumor)

*Source:* Adapted from European Study Group on Cystic Tumors of the Pancreas. European evidence-based guidelines on pancreatic cystic neoplasms. Gut. 2018;67:789-804.

**Ans. 15** a. Pylorus-preserving pancreatoduodenectomy.

b. It is done for pancreatic carcinoma

c. Whipple procedure

# CHAPTER 47 Spleen

## QUESTIONS

**Q1. What are the functions of the spleen?**

**Q2. Answer the following:**

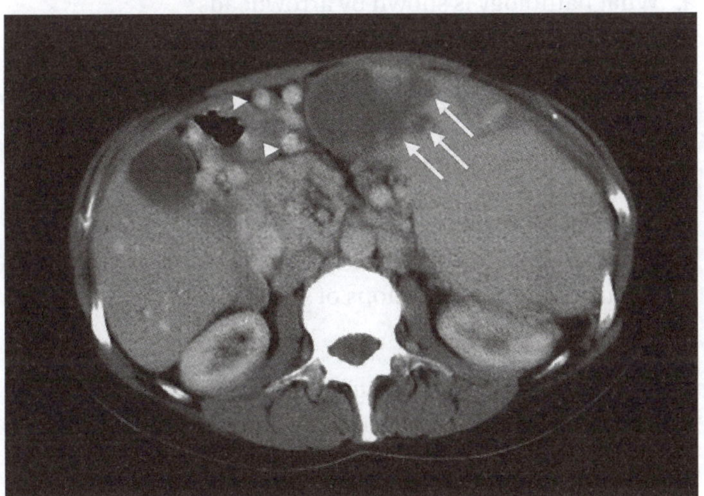

*Source:* Bailey and Love, 28th edition, page 1224.

a. What pathology is shown by arrows?
b. In which condition this pathology is seen?
c. What pathology is shown by arrowheads?

**Q3. What are the criteria for grading of splenic injury based on computed tomography?**

**Q4. Answer the following:**

a. What are the causes of splenic enlargement?
b. What is hypersplenism?

**Q5. Answer the following:**

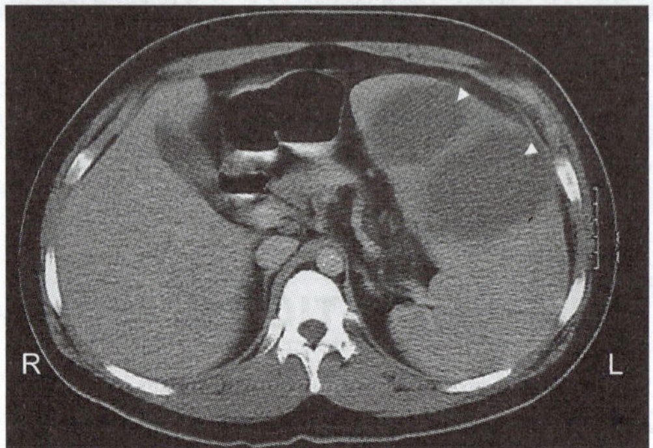


*Source:* Bailey and Love, 28th edition, page 1226.

a. What pathology is shown by arrowheads?
b. What are the risk factors for this pathology?
c. Which is the causative organism for it?
d. What is the management for it?

**Q6. Enumerate the vaccination protocol for splenectomy?**

**Q7. Answer the following:**

a. What are the indications of splenectomy?
b. What are the complications of splenectomy?

**Q8.**

a. What is opportunistic postsplenectomy infections?
b. How to prevent opportunistic postsplenectomy infections?

**Q9. Enumerate idiopathic thrombocytopenic purpura?**

## ANSWERS

**Ans. 1**
- Immune
- Filter function
- Pitting
- Reservoir
- Cytopoiesis

**Ans. 2**
a. Computed tomography scan showing a splenic infarct (arrows) in a patient with splenomegaly and hypersplenism.
b. Portal hypertension and portal vein thrombosis.
c. Varices are evident at the hilus and at the greater curvature of the stomach (arrowheads).

## Ans. 3

| Criteria for grading of splenic injury based on computed tomography | |
|---|---|
| Grade 1 | • Subcapsular hematoma <10% of surface area<br>• Parenchymal laceration <1 cm depth capsular tear |
| Grade 2 | • Subcapsular hematoma 10–50% of surface area<br>• Intraparenchymal hematoma <5 cm<br>• Parenchymal laceration 1–3 cm |
| Grade 3 | • Subcapsular hematoma >50% surface area; ruptured subcapsular or intraparenchymal hematoma ≥5 cm<br>• Parenchymal laceration >3 cm depth |
| Grade 4 | • Any injury in the presence of a splenic vascular injury or active bleeding confined within the splenic capsule<br>• Parenchymal laceration involving segmental or hilar vessels producing >25% devascularization |
| Grade 5 | Any injury in the presence of splenic vascular injury[a] with active bleeding extending beyond the spleen into the peritoneum–shattered spleen |

[a]Vascular injury is defined as a pseudoaneurysm or arteriovenous fistula and appears as a focal collection of vascular contrast that decreases in attenuation with delayed imaging. Active bleeding from a vascular injury presents as vascular contrast, focal or diffuse, that increases in size or attenuation in the delayed phase.

*Source:* Bailey and Love, 28th edition, page 1224.

## Ans. 4

| Causes of splenic enlargement | | |
|---|---|---|
| Infective | Bacterial | Typhoid and paratyphoid |
| | | Typhus |
| | | Tuberculosis |
| | | Psittacosis |
| | | Septicemia |
| | | Splenic abscess |
| | Spirochetal | Weil's disease |
| | | Syphilis |
| | Viral | Infectious mononucleosis |
| | | HIV-related thrombocytopenia |
| | Protozoal and parasitic | Malaria |
| | | Schistosomiasis |
| | | Trypanosomiasis |
| | | Kala-azar |
| | | Hydatid cyst |
| | | Tropical splenomegaly |

*Contd...*

*Contd...*

| ***Causes of splenic enlargement*** | | |
|---|---|---|
| Blood disease | Acute leukemia | Idiopathic thrombocytopenic purpura |
| | Chronic leukemia | Hereditary spherocytosis |
| | Pernicious anemia | Autoimmune hemolytic anemia |
| | Polycythemia vera | Thalassemia |
| | Erythroblastosis fetalis | Sickle cell disease |
| Metabolic | Rickets | |
| | Amyloid | |
| | Porphyria | |
| | Gaucher's disease | |
| Circulatory | Infarct | |
| | Portal hypertension | |
| | Segmental portal hypertension | Pancreatic carcinoma, splenic vein thrombosis |
| Collagen disease | Still's disease | |
| | Felty's syndrome | |
| Nonparasitic cysts | Congenital | |
| | Acquired | |
| Neoplastic | Angioma | |
| | Primary fibrosarcoma | |
| | Hodgkin's lymphoma | |
| | Other lymphomas | |
| | Myelofibrosis | |

(HIV: human immunodeficiency virus)
*Source:* Bailey and Love, 28th edition, page 1225.

b. Hypersplenism is an indefinite clinical syndrome that is characterized by splenic enlargement, any combination of anemia, leukopenia, or thrombocytopenia, compensatory bone marrow hyperplasia and improvement after splenectomy.

**Ans. 5** a. Computed tomography scan showing a multiloculated splenic abscess (arrowheads).

b. MC in immunocompromised, polycythemia, intravenous (IV) drug abusers, and trauma.
- MC route-hematogenous route

c. MC is *Staphylococcus* > *Streptococcus*
- Immunocompromised fellows may develop fungal abscess—*Candida*
- Sickle cell anemia—*Salmonella* causes abscess

d. • *IOC for diagnosis:* Hypodense lesion
   • *Unilocular abscess:* Percutaneous drainage
   • *Multiple abscess:* Splenectomy

**Ans. 6**

- If elective splenectomy is planned, consideration should be given to vaccinating against *Pneumococcus, Meningococcus* C (both repeated every 5 years) and *Haemophilus infuenzae* type b (Hib) (repeated every 10 years). The last two vaccines are commonly delivered as a combined preparation.
- Yearly influenza vaccination has been recommended, as there is some evidence that it may reduce the risk of secondary bacterial infection.
- Such vaccinations should be administered at least 2 weeks before elective surgery or as soon as possible after recovery from surgery but before discharge from hospital.
- Pneumococcal vaccination is recommended in those patients aged over 2 years.
- Hib vaccination is recommended irrespective of age.
- Overwhelming postsplenectomy infection (OPSI) due to *Capnocytophaga canimorsus* may result from dog, cat, or other animal bites.

| *Pneumococcal vaccine* | *Meningococcal vaccine* | *H. influenzae type B* |
|---|---|---|
| 13 valent–PCV 13<br>followed by<br>23 valent after 8 weeks | Quadrivalent meningococcal conjugate ACWY series<br>+<br>Monovalent Meningococcal serogroup B vaccine series | *H. influenzae* type B conjugate vaccine |

- All seasonal vaccines of influenza, measles, mumps, rubella, varicella, tetanus, diphtheria-tetanus-pertussis (DPT).
- *Ideal time for vaccination:* Ideal time–10–12 weeks prior to elective splenectomy or at least 14 days prior to surgery.
- Emergency settings after 14 days or upon discharge whichever comes first.
- *Autotransplant:* Into omental pouch (approximately 50% spleen) needed to prevent pneumococcal sepsis.
- *Booster doses:*
    - PPSV 23 vaccine every 5 years
    - Quadrivalent meningococcal ACWY (MPSV4)—every 5 years.
    - Monovalent serogroup B (Meningococcal B)—no booster
- *H. influenzae* B—no booster
- *Antibiotic prophylaxis:* Two approaches

| *Daily antibiotics* | *Emergency supply* |
|---|---|
| • Recommended by Australian Spleen Society<br>• Daily antibiotic prophylaxis for children up to 16 years or a minimum of up to 5 or 3 years after splenectomy<br>• In addition, they recommend lifelong prophylaxis for immune compromised patients and emergency (stand by antibiotics) for adults | • Oral amoxicillin or penicillin<br>• If allergic to above—Macrolide antibiotics<br>• Emergency supply we recommend Amoxicillin + Clavulanic acid or macrolide or quinolones (for penicillin allergic) |

**Ans. 7** a.

| *Emergency splenectomy* | *Elective splenectomy* |
|---|---|
| MC indication for splenectomy—blunt trauma | Idiopathic thrombocytopenic purpura is the MC elective indication |
| | *During some other surgery:*<br>• D2 lymphadenectomy<br>• Gastric cancer + spleen infiltration<br>• Pancreatic tail neoplasm |
| | *Hemolytic anemias:*<br>• Sickle cell<br>• Autoimmune hereditary spherocytosis |
| | Multiple abscess in spleen |
| | Tumors in spleen |

b. *Complications of splenectomy:*

| *Immediate complications* | *Intermediate complications* | *Delayed complications* |
|---|---|---|
| • Hemorrhage<br>• Gastric distension<br>• Hematemesis | • MC complication overall is left lung atelectasis<br>• Pancreatic fistula<br>• Gastric fistula<br>• Subphrenic abscess | • Thromboembolic manifests<br>• Overwhelming postsplenectomy infection (OPSI)<br>• Portal vein (PV) thrombosis |

**Ans. 8** a. *Opportunistic postsplenectomy infections:*

- MC after splenectomy for hematological causes > trauma causes.
- Bacterial infection-inability to remove capsulated bacterias—streptococcal and pneumonia
- *H. influenzae* and meningococcal
- Parasitic infection—Babesia and malaria
- Viral infection—not increased

- *Hematological effects:*
  - Increased platelet counts—can cause thrombotic manifests (if count >8 lakhs; antiplatelet drugs started)
  - Increased white blood cell (WBC) counts.

b. *Prevention of OPSI:*

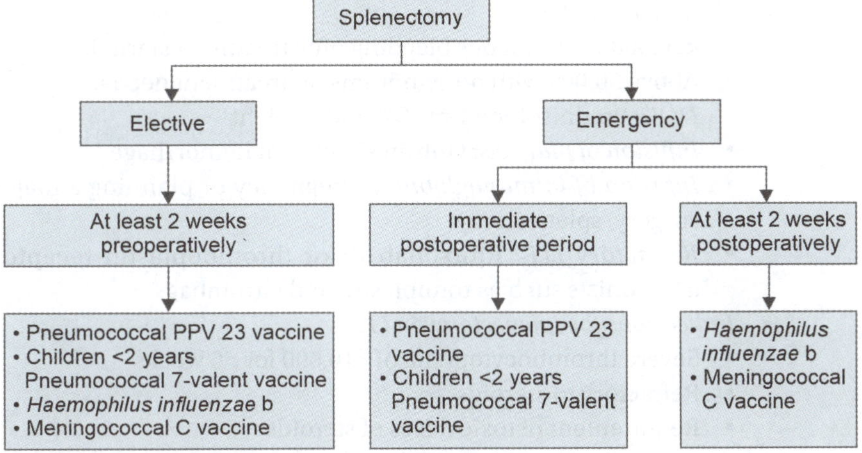


- *On discharge:* Postoperative antibiotics—
  - *Method 1:* Children are advised for next 2 years after splenectomy
  - *Method 2:* Some advocate for life-long prophylaxis
  - *Method 3:* Rational approach—to have antibiotics in hand and take when there is onset of febrile illness and rigors by patient himself and later come to hospital—MC followed.

**Ans. 9**
- Autoimmune disease
- Immunoglobulin G (IgG) antibodies are produced from spleen against the platelets and destroy the platelets.
- Hence, platelet count falls, mega thrombocytes seen.
- Bone marrow study is normal and all causes of thrombocytopenia ruled out before branding a patient as immune thrombocytopenia (ITP).
- *Clinical features:*
  - MC in young women
  - In children M = F
  - C/B—mucocutaneous bleeding, epistaxis, petechiae, and purpura.
  - Massive bleed or gastrointestinal (GI) bleed or hematuria or intracerebral bleed are very rare.

- *Management depends on platelet counts:*
    - *>50,000:* No need to worry, even major surgery can be done. Observation
    - *30,000–50,000:* Frequent follow-up is advised
    - *<20,000 + Mucous bleeding:* Hospitalize the patient
    - *<10,000:* Internal bleeding can happen
- *Treatment of ITP:*
    - <50,000 with mucous bleeding only treatment started.
    - Above 50,000 with no symptoms no treatment needed.
    - *DOC:* Prednisolone 1 mg/kg body weight
    - *Infusion of platelets:* Only in significant hemorrhage
    - *Infusion of immunoglobulin:* Pregnancy or planning a major surgery/splenectomy
    - *Refractory ITP:* Rituximab IV or thromboplastin receptor antagonists such as romiplastin and eltrombag.
- *Indications for splenectomy in ITP:*
    - Severe thrombocytopenia of <10,000 for >6 weeks
    - Refractory to steroids
    - Requirement of toxic doses of steroids
    - Incomplete response to steroids
    - Pregnant women in second trimester
    - Engagement in high-risk activities
- *During splenectomy:* Platelets are given only after ligating the splenic pedicle
- *Postoperative response:*
    - 72% complete response
    - Preoperative indium 111 scan shows splenic sequestration–Excellent response, liver sequestration will have bad response (NEET SS).
    - 15% cases relapses. MC cause of relapse is missed out ectopic spleen.

# CHAPTER 48 The Small Intestine

## QUESTIONS

**Q1. Why tumor is rare in small intestine?**

**Q2. Explain spot diagnosis.**

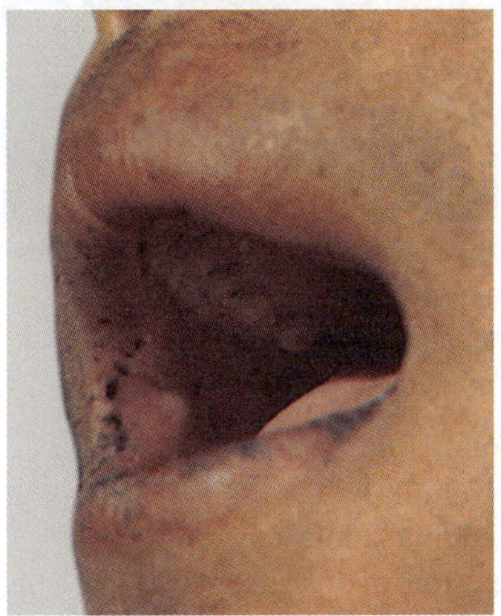

*Source:* Bailey and Love 28th edition, pages 1309.

**Q3. Describe opportunistic intestinal infections in patients with acquired immunodeficiency syndrome (AIDS).**

**Q4. Answer the following:**

a. Describe neuroendocrine tumors (NETs).
b. What are sites of NET?
c. Enumerate predominant hormone in NET in respect to their location.
d. What is the difference between primary carcinoids and secondary carcinoids?

**Q5. Describe features of carcinoid syndrome?**

**Q6. Answer the following**

a. Explain investigation in NET.
b. Explain management of NET.
c. What is SMART BOMBS?

**Q7. Answer the following:**

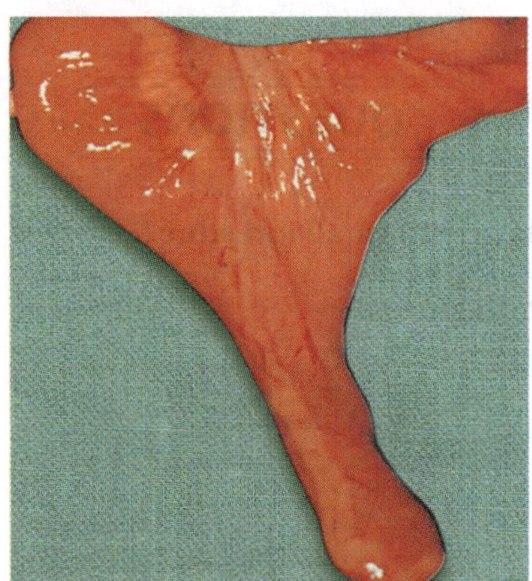

*Source:* Bailey and Love 28th edition, pages 1311.

a. What is spot diagnosis?
b. Enumerate the pathology in detail.
c. What are complications of this condition?

**Q8. Answer the following:**

a. Enumerate the stoma?
b. What are the complications of stoma?
c. How is end ileostomy constructed?

**Q9. Enumerate the common types of blind loop with diagram?**

**Q10. Answer the following:**

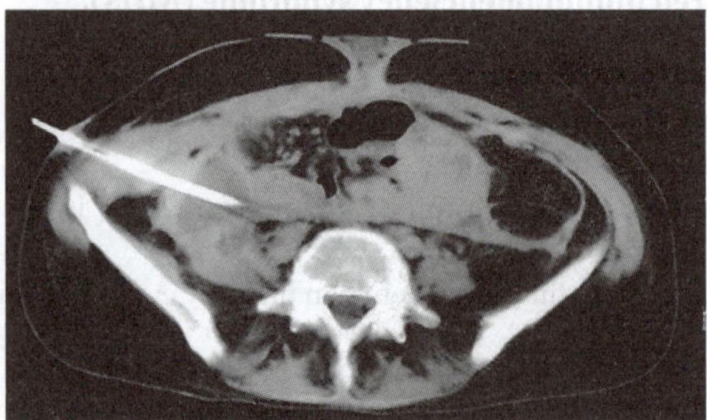

*Source:* Bailey and Love 28th edition, pages 1316

a. What is depicted in the image?
b. What are the principles in management of enterocutaneous fistula?
c. What are the factors preventing healing of fistula?

## ANSWERS

**Ans. 1** *Reasons why tumors are rare in small bowel (SB):*

- Rapid transit of food particles and hence carcinogens do not have exposure.
- Peyer's patches engulf the tumors.
- Rapid epithelial turn over in SB.

**Ans. 2** Melanin spot on the lips of *Peutz-Jeghers syndrome*

- STK 11 mutation—chromosome 19 p
- Most common (MC) site of polyps—jejunum
- Cutaneous marker—oral and lips pigmentation
- Other cancers—breast, ovary, and thyroid
- 100 times risk of pancreatic cancer
- Bile duct and gallbladder (GB) cancer
- Colon cancer also seen rarely
- MC symptom—pain abdomen and bleeding
- Pain due to intussusception

**Ans. 3**

| ***Bacterial*** | ***Viral*** | ***Protozoal*** | ***Fungal*** |
|---|---|---|---|
| • *Salmonella*<br>• *Shigella*<br>• *Yersinia*<br>• *Campylobacter*<br>• *Mycobacterium* avium-intracellulare (MAI) | *Cytomegalovirus* | • *Cryptosporidium*<br>• *Giardia* | *Candida albicans* |

**Ans. 4** a. • Also known as APUDomas (Amine precursor uptake and deuptake tumors)

• All these tumors have somatostatin receptors and exhibit function.

b. Sites of NET:

- Adrenal—pheochromocytoma
- Brain—medulloblastoma
- Thyroid—medullary cancer

- Pancreas—insulinoma, gastrinoma, etc. (insulinoma has no somatostatin receptor)
- Intestine—carcinoid

c.

| *Location* | *Site* | *Predominant hormone* |
|---|---|---|
| Foregut | Bronchus and thymus | 5-hydroxytryptophan and adrenocorticotropic hormone (ACTH) (low serotonin) |
| Midgut | Stomach, proximal duodenum, ileum, jejunum, right colon | Serotonin, histamine, bradykinin |
| Hindgut | Left colon and rectum | Somatostatin or peptide YY |

- MC in gastrointestinal tract (GIT)—appendix
- MC system affected is GIT system > Bronchus
- MC site— > Appendix > Ileum (Terminal) > Bronchus

d.

| *Primary carcinoids* | *Secondary carcinoids* |
|---|---|
| Primary neuroendocrine tumors (NETs) in gastrointestinal tract (GIT) with no metastasis in liver | NET in GIT + liver metastasis also |
| The carcinoid tumors produces substances which are detoxified into nontoxic products like 5-hydroxyindoleacetic acid (HIAA) in liver. Hence, they will not get any symptom MC symptom—pain abdomen > diarrhea | Presents with carcinoid syndrome as the active products are released into circulation |

**Ans. 5**
- Vasomotor symptoms (80%)—cutaneous flushing is the MC symptom. *Types of flushing:* Diffuse erythematous, violaceous, prolonged flushes, and bright red patchy.
  MC type of flushing seen in gastric carcinoids—bright red patchy
- GIT—explosive diarrhea. Due to serotonin.
- Cardiovascular—right heart problems are more common. The three most common cardiac lesions are pulmonary stenosis (90%), tricuspid insufficiency (47%), and tricuspid stenosis (42%).
- MC valve affected is tricuspid valve. Pulmonary regurgitation is not mentioned in books.
- Asthmatic attacks—bronchospasm
- Malabsorption and pellagra (dementia, diarrhea, and dermatitis) due to excessive diversion of tryptophan.

**Ans. 6** a. *Investigations:*
- 24 hours urinary 5-hydroxyindoleacetic acid (5HIAA) are highly specific.

- Neuroendocrine tumor marker—chromogranin A and synaptophysin
- Localization of tumor—somatostatin receptor scintigraphy with indium-111 labeled pentetreotide was used previously.
- Somatostatin receptor imaging with Gadolinium 68-DOTATATE computed tomography (CT) is the most sensitive to localize—95% cases.

*To look for metastasis:*

- MRI is helpful only to detect liver metastasis
- FDG is taken up only in high-grade NETs (e.g., high Ki-67 expression), whereas most NETs have low Ki-67 expression and are not apparent with this imaging modality—FDG.

PET-CT is only 38% helpful to detect metastasis.

- DOTATATE is used with sensitivity of around 97% for metastasis now (AIIMS 2019).

*Extra edge points:*

- Without liver metastasis—carcinoid syndrome is seen in retroperitoneal and ovarian carcinoids.
- Metastasis to liver depends on:
  - Size (<1 cm–10%; >1 cm: 90%)
  - Site (ileum has more chances, appendix lowest)
  - Ki 67 index and grade of tumor
- 2nd MC tumor in carcinoid—colorectal cancer
- Carcinoids may be multicentric nature.

b. *Management:*

- Treatment—surgical resection
  - R0—No microscopic margin
  - R1—Microscopic margin+
  - R2—Macroscopic margin+
- If there is liver metastasis—we must resect that also. Even with liver metastasis the NET have good prognosis followed by colorectal metastasis
- Carcinoid small intestine—10 cm margin resected with mesentery
- *Carcinoid appendix:*
  - *Tip, <1 cm, no invasion into mesoappendix:* Appendectomy is enough.
  - *More than >2 cm, infiltration to base, tumors in base:* Right hemicolectomy
  - 1–2 cm tumors in tip—appendectomy is enough if no mesoappendix involvement.

- *Postsurgical therapy:* If residual tumor or micro or macro metastasis—lanreotide is long acting somatostatin analogs. Pasireotide is latest.

c. *Smart bombs:* Radiolabeled somatostatin analogs that deliver radiation specifically to carcinoid cells.

**Ans. 7** a. Meckel's diverticulum

b. Classical points for Meckel's
- True diverticulum
- Antimesenteric border
- Incidentally detected resect

It is a congenital diverticulum (overall most common diverticulum)
- Persistent of proximal part of vitellointestinal duct (VID) is Meckel's (distal part of VID—is Raspberry tumor/umbilical adenoma)
- *Follows rule of 2: For adults—*
  - 2% individual
  - 2 inch in length
  - 2 feet proximal to ileocecal junction (IC) junction
- *Ectopic mucosa:*
  - Gastric mucosa (MC)
  - Pancreatic
  - Colonic
  - Brunner's glands
- Ectopic gastric mucosa disappears as the age advances.
  - *Children:*
    - Bleeding is the MC symptom.
    - Ectopic gastric mucosa seen in adjacent ileum and hence bleeds due to peptic ulcer.
    - IOC in children—Tc-99m pertechnenate scan
    - The sensitivity increases with cimetidine and glucagon
    - Hence, while resecting we must do resection and anastomosis as adjacent ileum contains ectopic mucosa.
  - *Adults:*
    - Obstruction is MC symptom
    - Ectopic mucosa is not there and hence bleeding is less common.
    - IOC—enteroclysis
    - Treatment—wedge resection can be done.

c. Complications of Meckel's diverticulum: Incidence—6.4%
- Bleeding
- Obstruction

- Hernia—Littre hernia
- MC tumor—carcinoid tumor
- Diverticulitis due to such huge list complications—resect the incidentally detected diverticulum.

*Direct line from Bailey:* Short, wide mouthed, and no nodularity—leave it; narrow mouth and nodularity advised resection.

**Ans. 8** a. *Stomas*

- May be colostomy or ileostomy
- May be temporary or permanent
- Temporary or defunctioning stomas are usually fashioned as loop stomas.
- An ileostomy is spouted; a colostomy is flush.
- Ileostomy effluent is usually liquid, whereas colostomy effluent is usually solid
- Ileostomy patients are more likely to develop fluid and electrolyte problems
- An ileostomy is usually sited in the right iliac fossa.
- End-colostomy is usually sited in the left iliac fossa
- Whenever possible, patients should be counseled and sited by a stoma care nurse before operation.

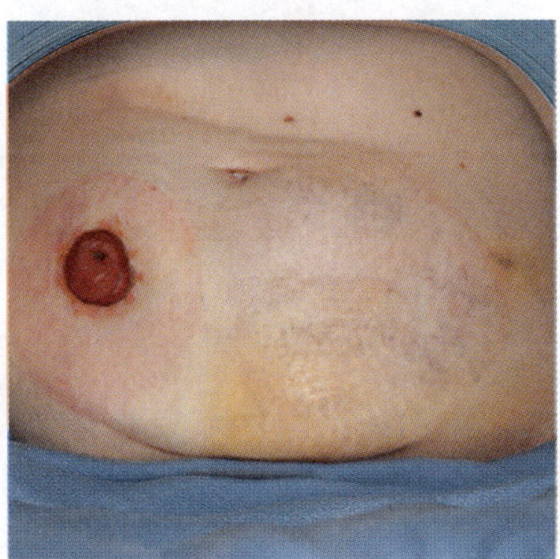

*Source:* Bailey and Love 28th edition, pages 1314.

b. *Stoma complications*

- Skin irritation
- Prolapse
- Retraction
- Ischemia
- Stenosis
- Parastomal hernia

- Bleeding
- Fistulation

c. Construction of an end ileostomy. The diagram is orientated such that the upper aspect of the stoma is to the right, thus when the sutures are tied the everted stoma is angled slightly inferiorly.

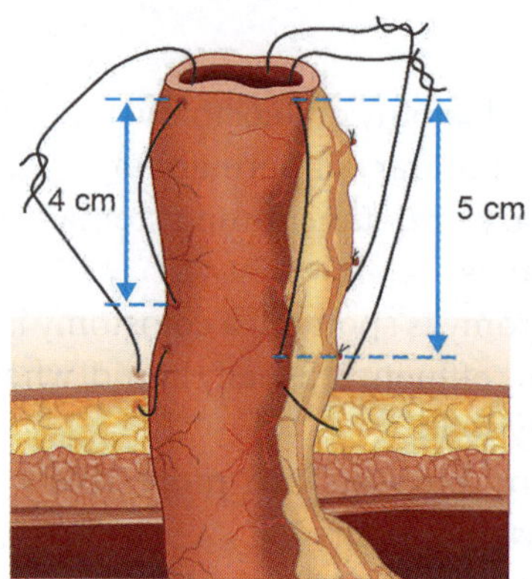


*Source:* Bailey and Love 28th edition, pages 1314.

**Ans. 9**

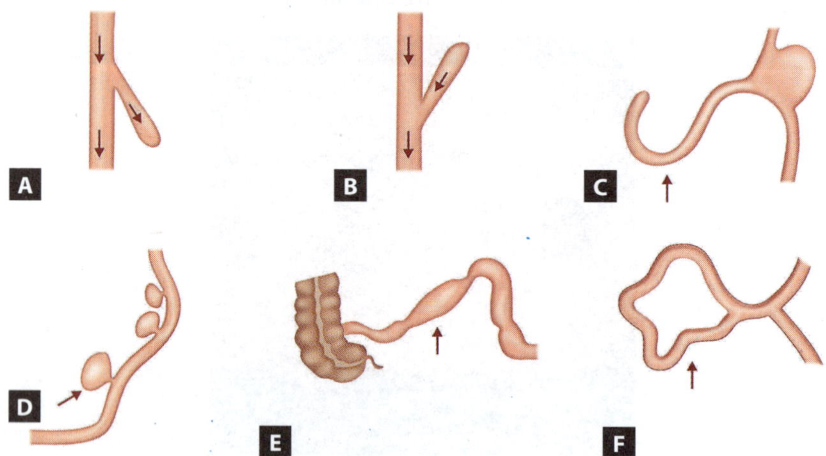


*Source:* Bailey and Love 28th edition, pages 1315.

*Common types of blind loop:*

- *Self-filling:* Deficiency occurs
- *Self-emptying:* No deficiency occurs
- Long afferent loop stasis in Pólya gastrectomy
- Jejunal diverticula
- Intestinal stricture causing stasis
- "Stenosis-anastomosis loop" syndrome.

**Ans. 10** a. Computed tomography (CT) scan in a patient with a complex enterocutaneous fistula and an intra-abdominal abscess being drained with a CT-guided catheter.

- MC cause—iatrogenic
- Types—high output (>500 mL/day); low output (<200 mL/day)
- MC complication of high output fistula—skin excoriation, fluid electrolyte imbalance, sepsis.
- Highest electrolyte imbalance—duodenal fistula

b. *Principles in management of enterocutaneous fistula: (SNAP)*

- S—Sepsis elimination
- N—Nutrition—a period of TPN
- A—Anatomical assessment
- P—Planned surgery after 6 weeks

c. *Factors preventing healing of fistula:*

- F—Foreign body in tract
- R—Radiation enteritis
- I—Inflammatory bowel disease
- E—Epithelialization of tract
- N—Neoplasm
- D—Distal obstruction
- S—Short tract (<2.5 cm tract)
- High output fistulas also

*Enteroatmospheric fistula:*

- Fistula is directly opening into the atmosphere and no intervening layers.
- Poor healing.

CHAPTER 49

# Inflammatory Bowel Disease

## QUESTIONS

**Q1. What are the differentiating features between Crohn's disease (CD) and ulcerative colitis (UC)?**

**Q2. What is the management of inflammatory bowel disease (IBD)?**

## ANSWERS

**Ans. 1**

| ***Crohn's disease*** | ***Ulcerative colitis*** |
|---|---|
| Incurable | Curable |
| Bimodal | Bimodal (one at young and another at old age) |
| IBD–1 [caspase activation and recruitment domains CARD or nucleotide binding and oligomerization (*NOD*) gene]–Chromosome 16q mutation (*Remember: BRCA*–1 12 q) | IBD–2–Chromosome 12 q mutation (*BRCA*–2: 13 q) |
| *Predisposing factors:* Smoking | *Preventive factors:*<br>• Smoking<br>• Appendectomy |
| *Involvement:*<br>• Mouth to anus<br>• Unaffected–rectum<br>• *MC involved:* Terminal ileum—known as terminal ileitis or regional enteritis | *Involvement:*<br>• MC involves rectum<br>• Spreads retrograde up to cecum<br>• Unaffected—anus<br>• Backwash Ileitis—terminal ileum involvement in 20% cases |
| *Vienna classification:*<br>24 types based on (A, B, C)<br>• Age—<40 or >40<br>• Behavior—Stricture/fistula, etc.<br>• Site—Location | *Types:*<br>• Proctitis<br>• Left colitis<br>• Pancolitis |

*Contd...*

*Contd...*

| ***Crohn's disease*** | ***Ulcerative colitis*** |
|---|---|
| *Clinical features:*<br>• MC symptom—pain abdomen<br>• Others—bleeding and diarrhea<br>• *Earliest feature:* Apthous ulcer<br>• Strictures+<br>• Fistulas±<br>• Intestinal obstruction+ | *Clinical features:*<br>• MC symptom—diarrhea<br>• Bleeding is MC here<br>• Rare feature—toxic megacolon<br>• Perforation |
| *Extraintestinal manifests:*<br>• MC—erythema nodosum<br>• Ankylosing spondylitis<br>• Peripheral arthritis<br>• Kidney stones<br>• Cholesterol gall stones | *Extraintestinal manifests:*<br>• MC—hepatic manifest (fatty liver)<br>• MC skin manifest—Pyoderma gangrenosum<br>• Primary sclerosing cholangitis (PSC)<br>• Uveitis<br>• Scleritis<br>All the extraintestinal manifests disappears on treatment—except PSC > Ankylosing spondylitis |
| *Pathological features:*<br>• Serpentine ulcer/bear claw ulcer<br>• Apthous ulcer<br>• Transmural involvement<br>• Skip lesions<br>• Fistula<br>• Noncaseating granuloma<br>• Mesenteric fat wrap<br>• Cobble stone appearance<br>• Death—MC due to malignancy<br>*Serpentine ulcer*<br>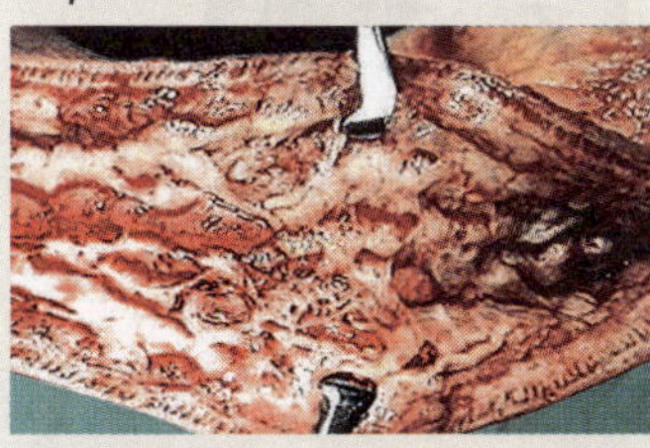<br>*Cobblestone*<br>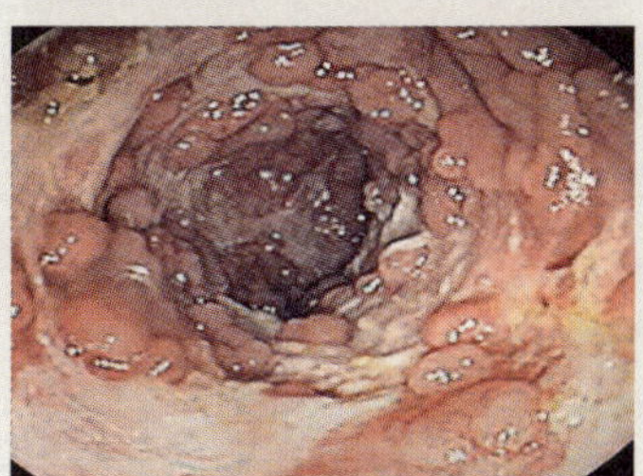 | *Pathological features:*<br>• Collar button ulcer<br>• Partial thickness only involved<br>• Continuous lesion<br>• No fistula, stricture, granuloma, or fat wrap<br>• Pseudopolyps appearance of uninvolved areas (they are not premalignant)<br>• Crypt abscess, cryptitis<br>• Toxic megacolon—full thickness involvement<br>*Pseudopolyps*<br>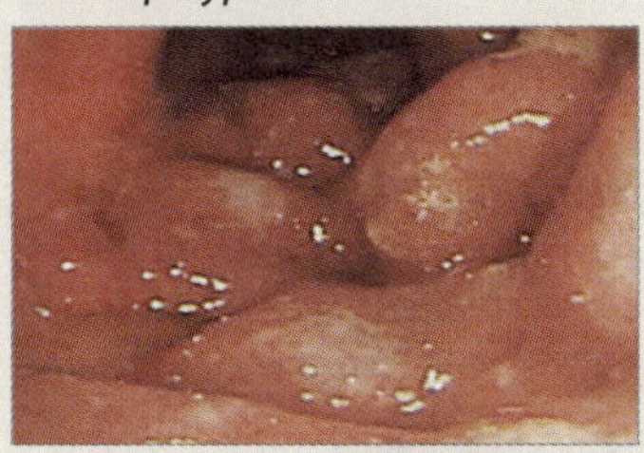 |

*Contd...*

*Contd...*

| ***Crohn's disease*** | ***Ulcerative colitis*** |
|---|---|
| *Investigations:*<br>• *IOC/Gold standard—Capsule endoscopy will show >ulcer in absence of nonsteroidal anti-inflammatory drugs (NSAIDs)*<br>*Biopsy:*<br>• *Push endoscopy (90–150 cm),*<br>• *Double balloon endoscopy (240–360 cm)*<br>• *Ileo colonoscopy (Terminal 50–80 cm can be entered) Stool for lactoferrin and calprotectin tests*<br>• *[Antisaccharomyces cereviciae antibody (ASCA)] + in 90%*<br>*Double balloon endoscopy*<br>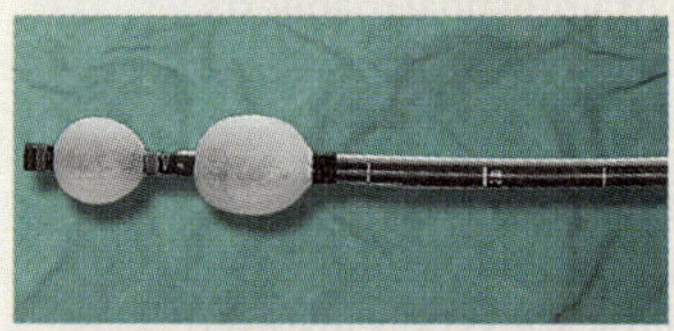 | *Investigations:*<br>• IOC—colonoscopic biopsy<br>• Every 5 cm—4 quadrant biopsy is taken<br>• Around 36 biopsies will be taken at surveillance to look for dysplasia<br>• *Antibody test:* P-antineutrophil cytoplasmic antibodies (ANCA) is positive<br>(Antineutrophilic cytoplasmic antibodies)<br>*Instead of barium enema—instant enema is used—with help of gastrografin and in an unprepared bowel* |
| *Barium investigations:*<br>• String sign<br>• Stierlin sign<br>• Garden hose pipe appearance (Bailey says lead pipe for Crohn's by mistake) | *Barium enema showing loss of haustration and known as pipe stem/lead pipe appearance*<br>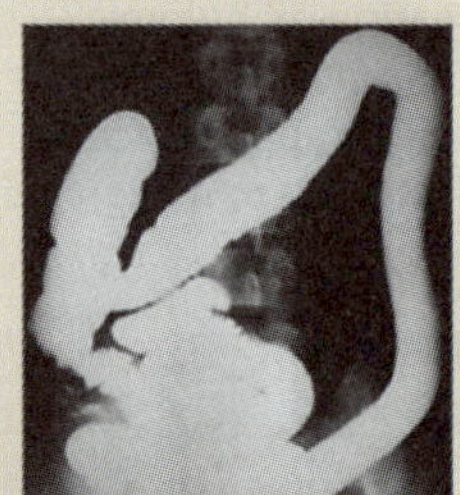 |
| • *Contrast-enhanced computed tomography (CECT) abdomen:*<br>• *Comb sign—increased vascularity to bowel shown as comb sign*<br>*Comb sign*<br>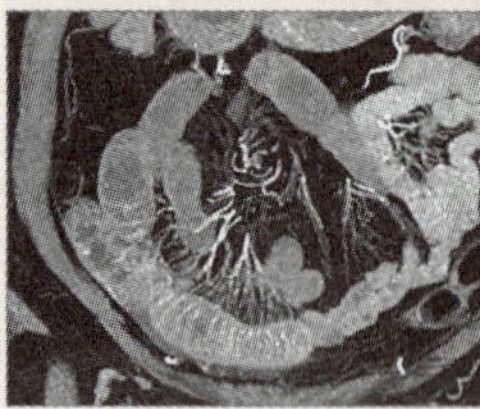 | |

*Contd...*

*Contd...*

| *Crohn's disease* | *Ulcerative colitis* |
|---|---|
| *Recto anal features:*<br>• MC affected area in colorectal and anal area—anus<br>• Fissures—multiple, lateral position are MC<br>• Fistulas—multiple and does not obey Goodsall's rule<br>• Treatment of Crohn's fistula—Setons and infliximab are used instead of surgery | *Recto anal features:*<br>• Not involves anus<br>• MC causes proctitis |
| *Complications:*<br>• Fistula<br>• Perforation<br>• Abscess<br>• Stricture<br>• Intestinal obstruction (MC due to stricture)<br>• Cancer (MC in terminal Ileum)<br>Same list stands for indications for surgery along with intractable pain<br>• MC indication for surgery is stricture causing obstruction | *Complications:*<br>• Intractability<br>• Toxic megacolon<br>• Perforation<br>• Bleeding PR<br>• Cancer—MC site—equally distributed<br>• In PSC + UC—cancer is MC in right colon<br>• Cancer risk increases after 8 years in pancolitis and 12 years in left colitis.<br>• Cancer risk in colon with CD and ulcerative colitis is same risk (Bailey mentions cancer risk in table +++ for Crohn's and ++ for ulcerative colitis)<br>• MC cause of death in both CD and UCC cancer |
| *Management of stricture:*<br>• Single stricture—resection<br>• Multiple short strictures strictureoplasty by Heineke Mikulicz type<br>• Multiple long strictures (>10 cm)—strictureoplasty by Finney's type | *Gold standard surgery:*<br>Total proctocolectomy + Ileal pouch anal anastomosis is advised after 8 years in pancolitis or 12 years in left colitis. If they are not willing they are advised to be in screening surveillance |

**Ans. 2**

| *Medical treatment* | |
|---|---|
| First-line drugs | • Amino salicylic acid compounds—sulfasalazine, balasalazine, olsalazine<br>• Mainly to maintain the remission<br>• Newer drug—mesalamine formulations releasing 5-ASA<br>– Timed release microgranules that release 5-ASA throughout the small intestine PENTASA |

*Contd...*

*Contd...*

| | |
|---|---|
| | – pH-sensitive resin that dissolve at pH 6–7 are Asacol, Lialda<br>– Rowasa–Enema formulation<br>– Canasa–Suppository |
| Immunosuppressants | • Azathioprine and mercaptopurine are second line drugs |
| Initiation of remission | • Deoxycorticosterone (DOC)—Steroids |
| Monoclonal antibodies | • Infliximab—TNF α inhibitor—heals fistulas<br>• Natalizumab—α-4 integrin antibody (causes progressive multifocal leukoencephalopathy and hence banned now—NEET SS)<br>• Vedolizumab—Monoclonal antibody against Mad CAM-1 (Mucosal address in cell adhesion molecule) |

| | |
|---|---|
| *Ileal pouch anastomosis*<br> 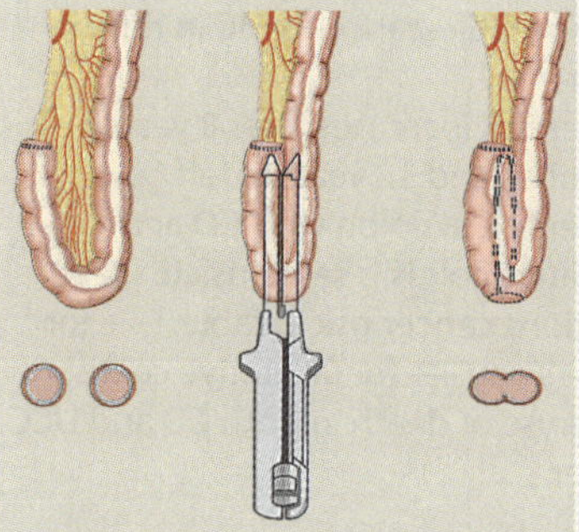<br>J pouch | • MC used pouch is J pouch made with last 30 cm ileum (two 15 cm limb folded) and anastomosed to ileum<br>• MC complication after this procedure—small bowel obstruction<br>• Second MC complication—pouchitis<br>• MC cause of pouchitis—altered colonic bacterial flora<br>• MC symptom of pouchitis—increased bowel movements<br>• First-line treatment for pouchitis—probiotics, second line—antibiotics, third line—ASA compounds. If they are not recovering with all the above—we do pouchectomy<br>• Nonresponsiveness may be due to missed Crohn's disease in which you made a pouch |
| Emergency cases | • Toxic megacolon<br>• Perforation<br>• Bleeding massive<br>• Fulminant colitis<br>In these cases we do not do total proctocolectomy (TPC) with ileal pouch anal anastomosis (IPAA)—we go with total colectomy with ileostomy and rectal closure and we reopen and remove the rectum after some time and do Ileal pouch anal anastomosis<br>*Types of pouch:*<br>• J, S, and W pouch<br>• Best is J pouch—Length is 10–15 cm |

*Indications of surgery in ulcerative colitis:*

- 20% of the patients will undergo colectomy.
- Most of them will undergo surgery in 1 year itself.

| Elective indications | Emergency indications |
|---|---|
| • Steroid related<br>– Resistant<br>– Dependency<br>– Complications<br>• Intractability<br>• Dysplasia in colon<br>• After 8 years in pancolitis and 12 years in left colitis | • Toxic megacolon<br>• Fulminant colitis<br>• Perforation<br>• Bleeding |

*Cancer and ulcerative colitis: High yield points:*

- Cancer is related to duration and extent directly proportional.
- UC related cancer arises from flat dysplasia or dysplasia associated mass lesions—But sporadic always follows adenoma carcinoma sequence.
- Evenly distributed in colon throughout (sporadic cancer MC in left side)
- Multiple synchronous lesions are seen in UC.
- Mucinous cancers are MC in UC, mucinous cancers very rare in sporadic type.
- Diagnosis is delayed because of symptoms overlap.
- Prognosis of cancer in UC related and sporadic is almost same.
- Think of malignancy in UC if they present with stricture with below features: More proximal to splenic flexure, increased duration and presents with obstruction (NEET SS question)

CHAPTER

# 50 Intestinal Obstruction

## QUESTIONS

**Q1. Enumerate causes of intestinal obstruction.**

**Q2. What is shown in the arrow?**

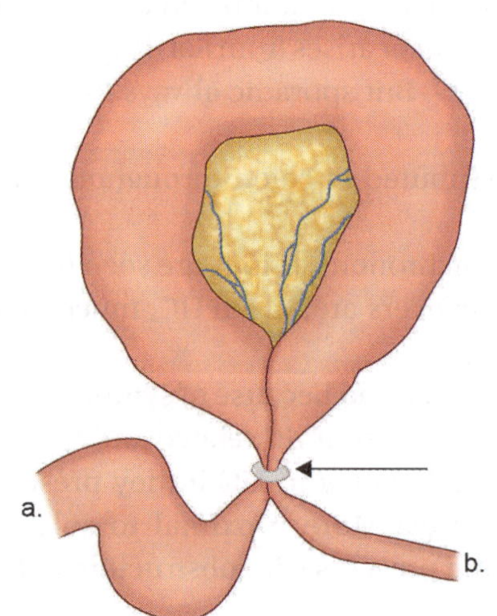


*Source:* Bailey and Love, 28th edition, page 1376.

**Q3. Enumerate potential sites of internal herniation.**

**Q4.** a. Enumerate the common causes of intra-abdominal adhesions.
b. What are the factors which cause prevention of adhesions?

**Q5. Answer the following:**

a. Enumerate classification of dynamic obstruction.
b. Four cardinal features of dynamic obstruction.
c. Causes of small bowel obstruction which produce no obstipation.
d. On opening the abdomen—bowel is distended massively: How to differentiate it is small bowel or large bowel obstruction by seeing one organ?

**Q6. Regarding intussusceptions, kindly answer the following:**

a. Most common age group
b. Most common cause
c. Brief anatomy
d. Most common variety
e. Clinical features in 6 months baby
f. Radiological features

**Q7. Answer the following:**

a. Midgut supplied by which artery?
b. What is Ladd's band?
c. Midgut volvulus and its management.
d. What is Ladd's procedure?

**Q8. Enumerate adult causes of small bowel obstruction.**

**Q9. Enumerate adult causes of large bowel obstruction.**

**Q10. Differentiation between viable and nonviable intestine.**

## ANSWERS

**Ans. 1**

| *Dynamic* | *Adynamic* |
|---|---|
| • Intraluminal<br>• Fecal impaction<br>• Foreign bodies<br>• Bezoars<br>• Gallstones | • Paralytic ileus<br>• Pseudo-obstruction |

**Ans. 2** Arrow: Closed-loop obstruction around a constricting band.

a. Impending strangulation, mild distension of the proximal limb and
b. Collapse of the distal limb of small bowel

**Ans. 3** The following are potential sites of internal herniation:

- The foramen of Winslow
- A defect in the mesentery
- A defect in the transverse mesocolon
- Defects in the broad ligament
- Congenital or acquired diaphragmatic hernia
- Duodenal retroperitoneal fossae

- Cecal/appendiceal retroperitoneal fossae
- Intersigmoid fossa

**Ans. 4** a. **Cause of intra-abdominal adhesions:**

| | |
|---|---|
| Acute inflammation | Anastomosis sites, raw areas reperitoneally sealed, trauma sites, and ischemia sites |
| Foreign material | Starch, gauze, silk, and talc |
| Infection | TB and peritonitis |
| Chronic inflammatory conditions | Chron's disease |
| Radiation enteritis | |

b. **Prevention of adhesions:** Factors that may limit adhesion formation include:

- Good surgical methods
- Applying saline to wash off clots from the peritoneal cavity
- Reducing the contact with the gauze
- Covering the raw peritoneal surfaces and anastomoses

**Ans. 5** a. *Classification of dynamic obstruction:*

| *Pediatric causes* | *Adult causes* |
|---|---|
| • *Newborn:*<br>– Duodenal atresia (most common cause)<br>– Ileal atresia<br>– Jejunal atresia<br>– Annular pancreas<br>– Midgut volvulus<br>• *Other children:*<br>– MC cause is intussusception<br>– Tumors<br>– Hernia<br>– Strictures | • *Small bowel causes*:<br>– Adhesions (most common cause)<br>– Congenital bands<br>– Hernia<br>– Tumors<br>– Stricture<br>• *Large bowel causes*:<br>– Cancer<br>– Volvulus |

b. *Four cardinal features of dynamic obstruction:*

- Colicky pain—if the bowel goes for gangrene it becomes dull aching continuous pain.
- Abdominal distension—MC by swallowed gas > gastrointestinal (GI) secretions
- Vomiting—projectile bilious vomiting
- Obstipation—Not pass motion + flatus

c. Causes of small bowel obstruction which produces no obstipation:
   - Richter's hernia (diarrhea seen)
   - Acute superior mesenteric artery (SMA) ischemia
   - Gallstone ileus

d. 
   - Cecum
   - Cecum distended is large bowel obstruction
   - Cecum is collapsed is small bowel obstruction
   - If ileocecal valve is not patent—cecum will not be dilated even in large bowel obstruction and entire small bowel also dilated.

**Ans. 6**

a. MC in age group 6 months–6 years
b. Rhinovirus infection causing hypertrophic Peyer's patches and that pulls the bowel and causes intussusception.
c. 
   - *Apex:* Lead point
   - *Innertube:* Intussusceptum
   - *Outer tube:* Intussuscipien

d. Ileocolic
e.

**Clinical features in 6 months baby**

- Red currant jelly stool
- Vomiting
- **Le Dance sign—empty right iliac fossa**
- Sausage-shaped mass towards umbilicus

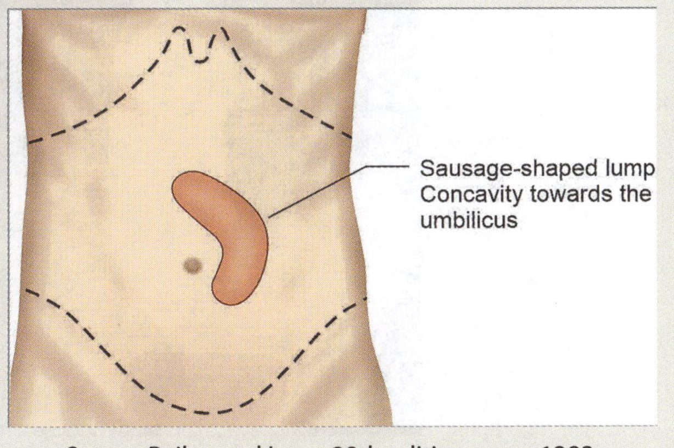


*Source:* Bailey and Love, 28th edition, page 1383.

f.

***Radiological features***

*USG features/CT features:*

- **Target sign**
- **Pseudokidney sign**
- **Bull's eye sign**

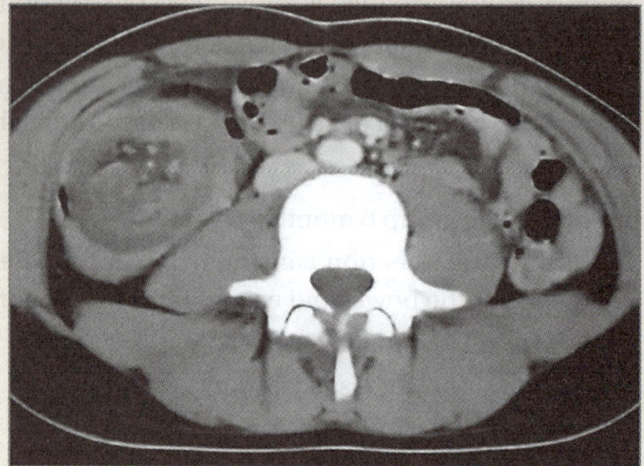

Abdominal CT s/o target sign of ileocolic intussusception
*Source:* Bailey and Love, 28th edition, page 1379.

*Barium enema:*

- **Claw sign/pincer sign**
- **Coiled spring sign**

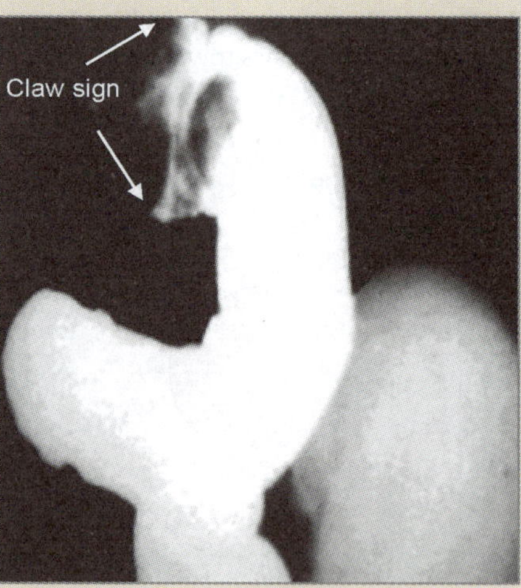


Claw sign

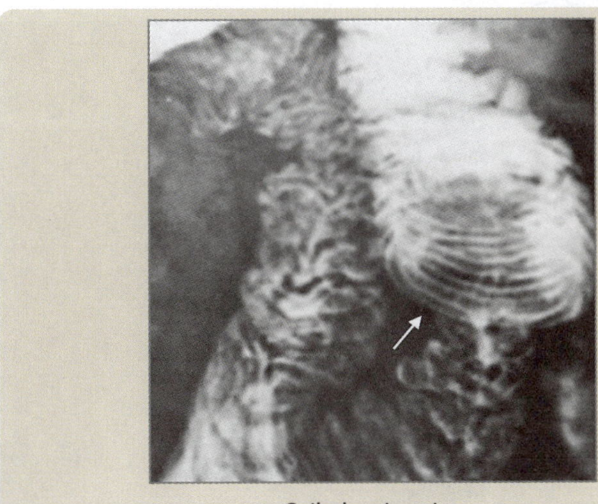

Coiled spring sign

**Ans. 7** a. *SMA:* 6th week of IUL, umbilicus is opened and the entire midgut comes out and goes back by 10th week and goes to normal anatomy.

b. Ladd's band fibrous stalks of peritoneal tissue that attach the cecum to the retroperitoneum in the right lower quadrant (RLQ). If present extends from duodenum to ascending colon. Ladd's band prevents rotation and normal fixation of bowel.

c. *Midgut volvulus:*
- Bilious vomiting + pain abdomen
- Intraoperative cholangiogram (IOC)–GI contrast study is done.
- Contrast-enhanced computed tomography (CECT) abdomen—Whirlpool sign
- Treatment for both no rotation or volvulus is Ladd's procedure.

d. *Ladd's procedure:*
- Untwist the volvulus
- Remove the Ladd band
- Keep all small bowel in right side and large bowel in left side
- Appendix also removed

**Ans. 8**

***Erect X-ray findings***

- Normal air fluid level: 3–5
- >5 air fluid level is pathological
- Air fluid level with vertical diameter: >2.5 cm it is pathological
- Step ladder pattern is seen
- String of pearls appearance is also seen if more of fluids present and less gas seen
- X-ray shows—no gas on colon and rectum

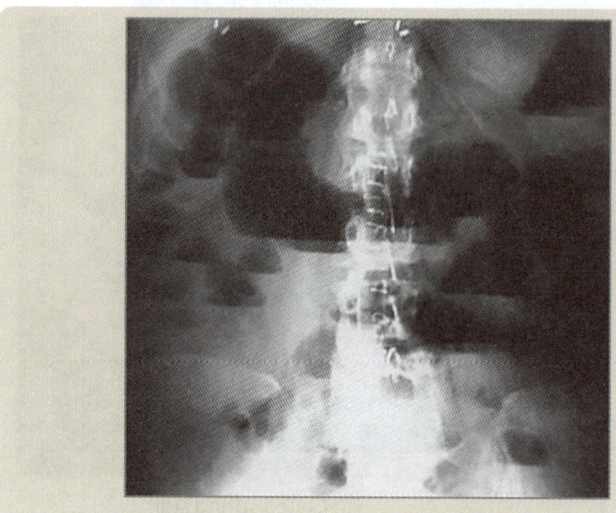
Step ladder pattern

| *Dynamic obstruction* | *Nondynamic obstruction (paralytic ileus)* |
|---|---|
| MC cause—adhesions | • MC cause—postoperative patient<br>• Electrolyte imbalance:<br>– MC hypokalemia<br>– Na, Mg, Cl disturbances<br>• Hypothyroidism<br>• Neurological causes |
| Four cardinal features are seen | Pain is absent |
| Bowel sounds +++ (Borborygmi) | Absent bowel sounds |
| *X-ray shows:*<br>• Multiple air fluid levels<br>• No gas in rectum | X-ray shows gas + in rectum and colon |
| *Management:*<br>• *Adhesive obstruction*:<br>– NPO and IVF<br>– For 24–48 hours<br>– >48 hours: Lap adhesiolysis<br>• *Other causes*: Surgery immediately done (sun should never set or raise) | *Management:*<br>• NPO<br>• IVF<br>• Electrolyte correction<br>• Wait for 48–72 hours<br>• If not resolved: CATCHPOLE REGIMEN—injection neostigmine |

**Ans. 9**
- Most common cause—cancer
- Second most common cause—volvulus

| *Cecal volvulus* | *Sigmoid volvulus* |
|---|---|
| • Misnomer—it is actually a cecocolic volvulus<br>• LC<br>• MC in young females<br>• Predisposed by repeated pregnancy | • MC type<br>• MC in old men<br>• Predisposed by High fiber diet |
| • MC in clockwise direction<br>• Please remember anteroposterior rotation of only cecum alone is known as cecal bascule | MC in anticlockwise > clockwise |
| • X-ray shows comma-shaped colon | • X-ray shows coffee bean shaped<br>• Barium enema—ace of spade or bird beak appearance 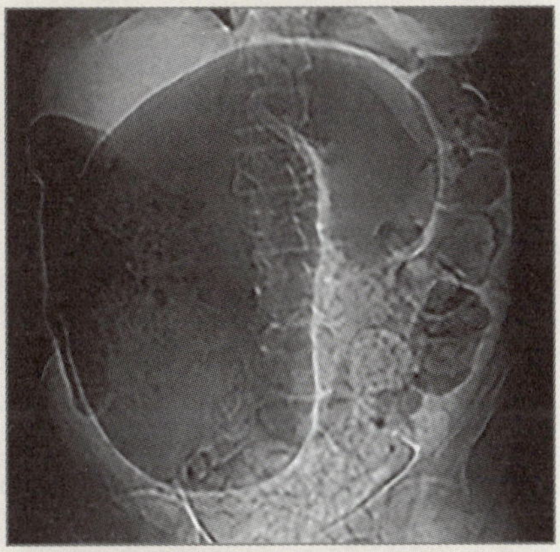<br>Coffee bean appearance |
| • *Treatment*: Right hemicolectomy<br>• Cecopexy is contraindicated | • *First line*: Sigmoidoscopic reduction<br>• *Definitive treatment*: Sigmoid colectomy |

*Pseudo-obstruction of colon:*

- Acute—Ogilvie syndrome
- Chronic-neurological causes, laxative abuse, and self-enema
- C/F: Abdominal distension, painless, and severe constipation
- Cecum if becomes distended >14 cm and not passing motion—colonoscopic decompression is done
- *Second-line treatment:* Injection neostigmine by making the patient sit in commode.

*Final treatment:* Subtotal colectomy

*Hartman's operation*:

- Composed of three components:
  - Resect the diseased colon
  - Proximal colostomy
  - Distal closure and leave inside
- Redo anastomosis done after 6 weeks

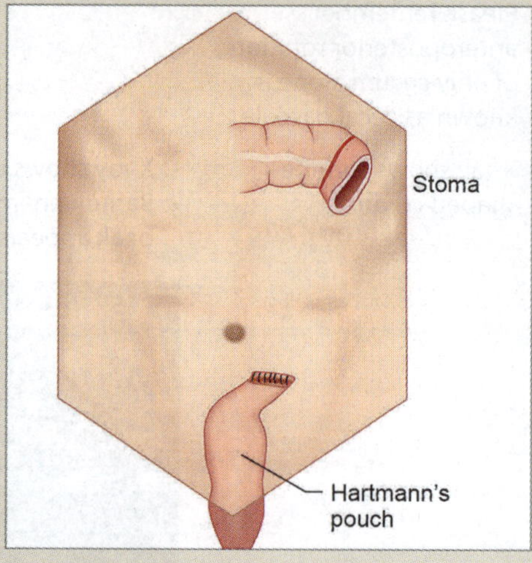


*Paul Mikulicz operation*:

- Patient very sick
- Bring the proximal colon as colostomy and leave the pathology there itself and bring the distal bowel as mucus fistula

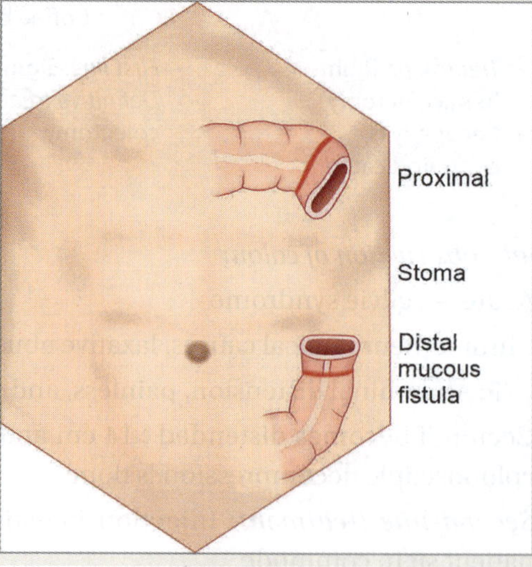

**Ans. 10**

| | ***Viable*** | ***Nonviable*** |
|---|---|---|
| Circulation | Dark color becomes lighter<br>Visible pulsation in mesenteric arteries | Dark color remains no detectable pulsation |
| General appearance | Shiny | Dull and lusterless |
| Intestinal musculature | Firm | Flabby, thin and friable |
| | Peristalsis may be observed | No peristalsis |

CHAPTER

# 51 Stomach and Duodenum

## QUESTIONS

**Q1. Make a line diagram and show blood supply of stomach.**

**Q2. Make a line diagram and show nerve supply of stomach.**

**Q3. Describe in brief the function and source of peptides and neuropeptides in the stomach.**

**Q4. Answer the following:**

a. What is depicted in the below figures?
b. Describe the investigation of gastric disorder.

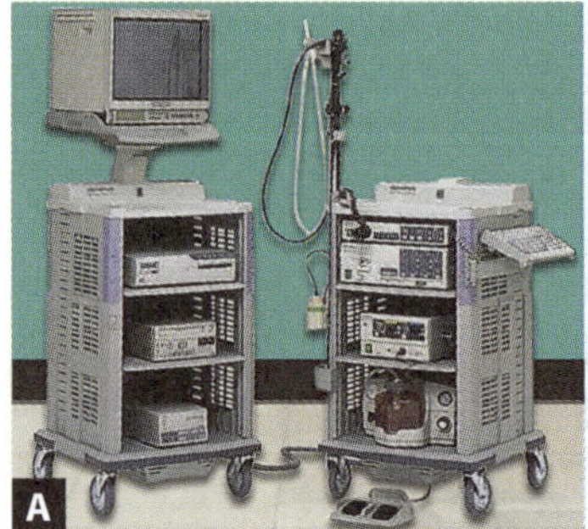


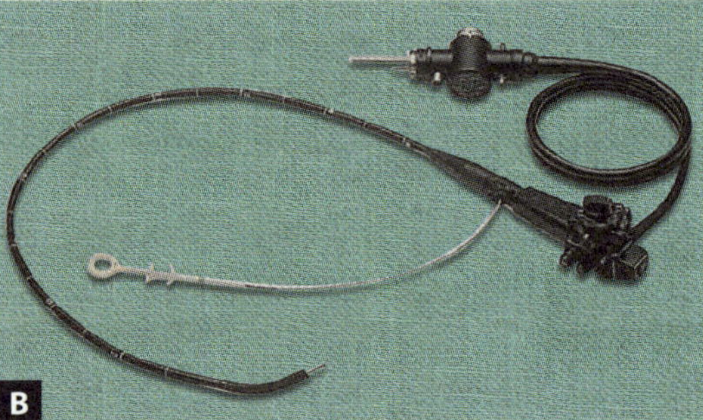


*Source:* Bailey and Love, 27th edition, page 1110.

**Q5. Answer the following:**

a. Most common type of peptic ulcer.
b. Difference between duodenal ulcer and gastric ulcer.

**Q6. What is the surgical management of gastric ulcer?**

**Q7. Answer the following:**

a. What is truncal vagotomy (TV)?
b. What is the complications of TV?

**Q8. Describe highly selective vagotomy.**

**Q9. Describe in brief the complications of peptic ulceration and management of them.**

**Q10. Based on the below figures, answers the following questions:**

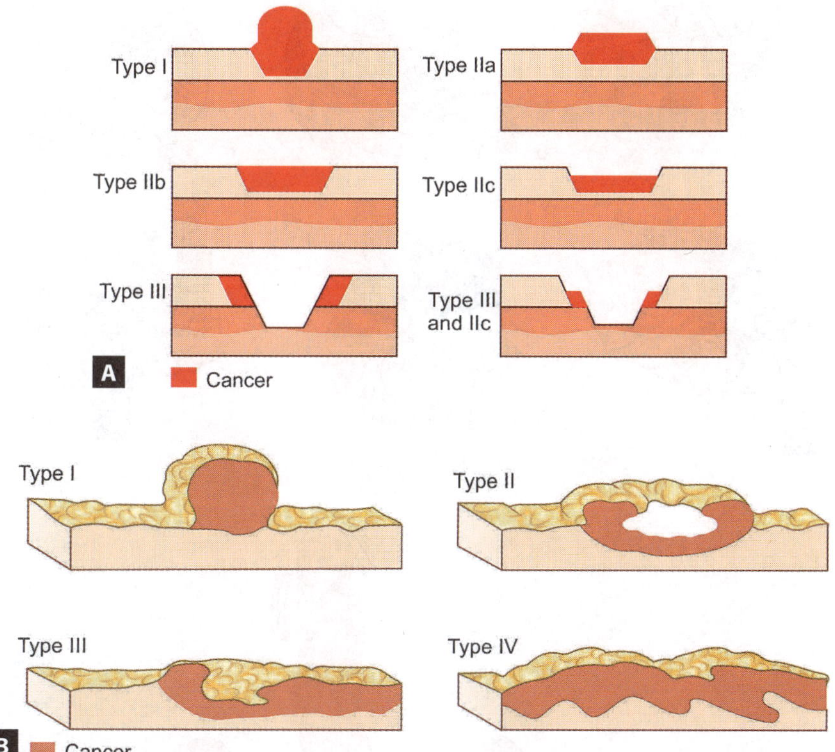


*Source:* Bailey and Love, 27th edition, pages 1132 and 1133.

a. Describe figures.
b. Risk factors for this condition
c. Clinical features
d. What are the clinical features to say the tumor is inoperable?
e. Union for International Cancer Control (UICC) staging of gastric cancer

**Q11. Answer the following:**

a. Describe early gastric cancer.
b. Minimum number of nodes removed.
c. Siewert classification of OG junction cancers.

**Q12.** **Identify the procedure in Figures A and B.**

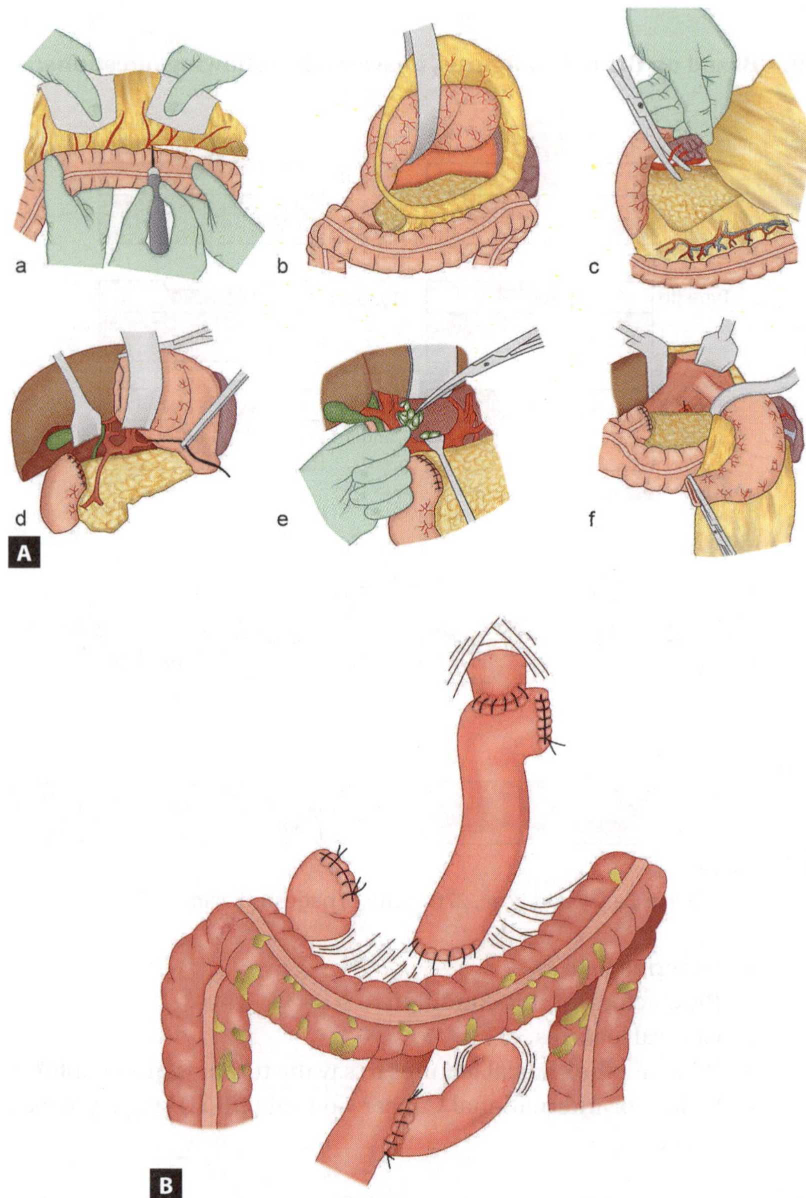


*Source:* Bailey and Love, 27th edition, page 1137.

**Q13.** **Answer the following:**

a. Investigation and management of gastric cancer
b. Palliative procedures for inoperable cancers

**Q14. Answer the following:**

a. Describe lymphatic drainage of the stomach.
b. Lymph node stations during resection in stomach.

**Q15. What is the difference between non-Hodgkin's lymphoma gastrointestinal stromal tumor (GIST)?**

**Q16. Answer the following:**

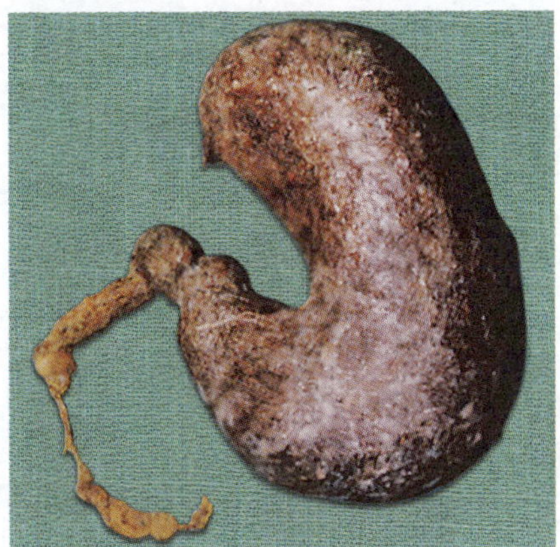

*Source:* Bailey and Love, 27th edition, page 1142.

a. Describe the depicted image in brief.
b. What is Rapunzel syndrome?
c. What is phytobezoars?

**Q17. Based on the figure, answers the following questions:**

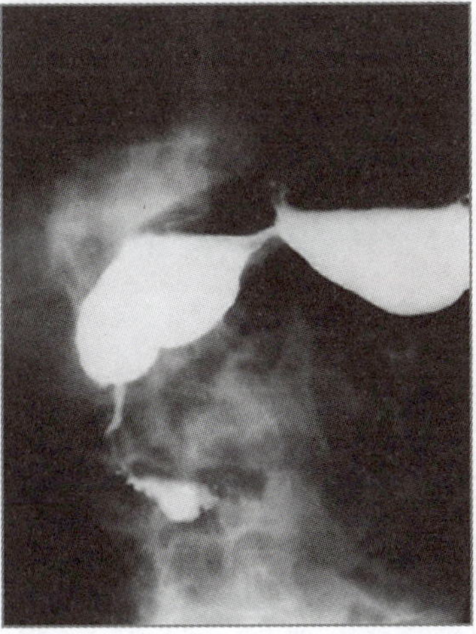

*Source:* Bailey and Love, 27th edition, page 1143.

a. Describe the depicted image in brief.
b. What is Borchardt's Triad?
c. Management

## ANSWERS

**Ans. 1**

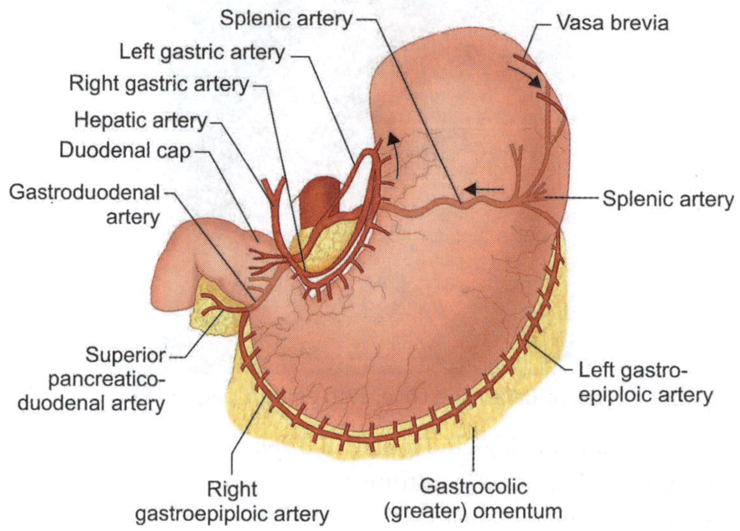


*Source:* Bailey and Love, 27th edition, page 1106.

**Ans. 2**

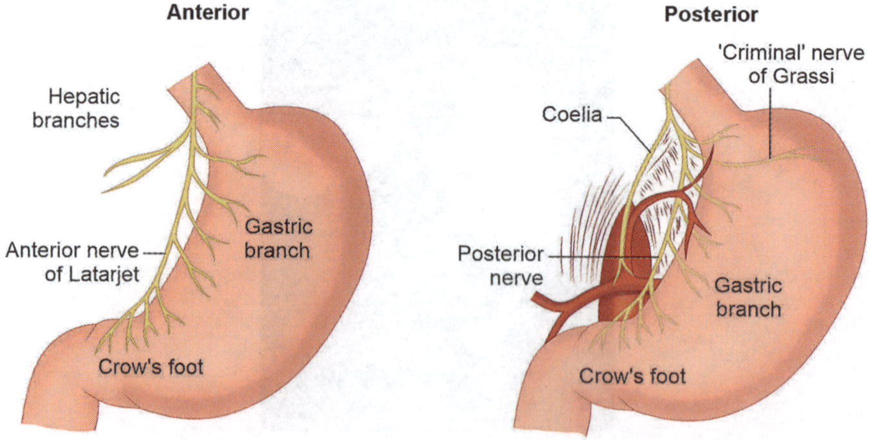


*Source:* Bailey and Love, 27th edition, page 1107.

*Vagus nerve branches:*

- Left vagus nerve is a thin nerve.
- Right vagus nerve is a thick nerve like a guitar string.

*Anterior gastric nerve (left):*

- Hepatic branch
- Gastric branches
- Crow's foot (nerve of Latarjet)

*Posterior gastric nerve (right):*

- *Criminal nerve of Grassi:*
  - Crow's foot
  - Celiac branch

**Ans. 3** *Function and source of peptides and neuropeptides in the stomach: (Ref: Bailey and Love, 27th edition, page 1110)*

| ***Function—stimulate secretion*** | ***Source*** |
|---|---|
| Gastrin | G-cells |
| Histamine | Enterochromaffin-like (ECL) cells |
| Acetylcholine | Neurons |
| Gastrin-releasing peptide | Neurons and mucosa |
| Cholecystokinin (CCK) | Duodenal endocrine cell |

| ***Function—inhibit secretion*** | ***Source*** |
|---|---|
| Somatostatin | D cells and neurons |
| Secretin | Duodenal endocrine cells |
| Enteroglucagon | Small intestinal endocrine cells |
| Prostaglandins | Mucosa |
| Neurotensin | Neurons |
| Glucose-dependent insulinotropic polypeptide (GIP) | Duodenal and jejunal endocrine cells |
| Peptide YY (PYY) | Small intestinal endocrine cells |

| ***Function—stimulate motility*** | ***Source*** |
|---|---|
| Acetylcholine | Neurons |
| 5-HT | Neurons |
| Histamine | ECL cell |
| Substance P | Neurons |
| Substance K | Neurons |
| Motilin | Neurons |
| Gastrin | G cells |

| ***Function—inhibit motility*** | ***Source*** |
|---|---|
| Somatostatin | D-cells and neurons |
| VIP | Neurons |
| Nitric oxide | Neurons and smooth muscle |
| Noradrenaline | Neurons |
| Encephalin | Neurons |
| Dopamine | Neurons |

**Ans. 4**

a. Videogastroscope
b. *The investigation of gastric disorders:*
   *(Ref: Bailey and Love, 27th edition, page 1110)*
   - Flexible endoscopy is the most commonly used and sensitive technique for investigating the stomach and duodenum.
   - Great care needs to be exercised in performing endoscopy to avoid complications and missing important pathology.
   - Axial imaging, particularly multislice CT, is useful in the staging of gastric cancer, although it may be less sensitive in the detection of liver metastases than other modalities.
   - Endoscopic ultrasound (EUS) is the most sensitive technique in the evaluation of the "T" stage of gastric cancer and in the assessment of duodenal tumors.
   - Laparoscopy is very sensitive in detecting peritoneal metastases, and laparoscopic ultrasound provides an accurate evaluation of lymph node and liver metastases.

**Ans 5.**

a. The most common type of Peptic Ulcer–Duodenal ulcer
b.

| ***Duodenal ulcer*** | ***Gastric ulcer*** |
|---|---|
| *MC site is first part of duodenum:*<br>• Anterior located—perforate<br>• Posterior located—bleed<br>• Bleeding is MC from gastroduodenal artery | *Modified Johnson Classification:*<br>• Type 1—MC–Incisura @Lesser curve<br>• Type 2—two ulcers—one in duodenum and another in stomach<br>• *Type 3:* Prepyloric ulcer<br>• *Type 4:* Proximal gastric ulcer in lesser curve side<br>• *Type 5:* Nonsteroidal anti-inflammatory drug (NSAID) induced ulcers |
| Unusual site of peptic ulcers—D2, D3 is seen in Zollinger–Ellison syndrome | |

*Contd...*

*Contd...*

| ***Duodenal ulcer*** | ***Gastric ulcer*** |
|---|---|
| *Etiopathology:* Increased acid production | *Etiopathology:*<br>• Due to loss of mucosal barrier<br>• Except type 2 and 3 ulcers are due to increased acid production |
| *Medical management:*<br>• Antiulcer drugs such as $H_2$ blockers, proton pump inhibitor (PPI) will be beneficial for duodenal ulcers<br>• Give them 6–8 weeks of PPI | *Medical management:*<br>• Type 1, four ulcers, heals very well with ulcer healing agents or coating agents like sucralfate and reduces the risk factors<br>• Type 2 and 3 ulcers may benefit from PPI |
| *Surgical treatment—Indications:*<br>• Intractable ulcer (when not healing with 8 weeks)<br>• Bleeding—MC indication of surgery<br>• Perforation<br>• Gastric outlet obstruction | *Surgical treatment—Indications:*<br>• Intractable ulcer (to rule of occult malignancy)<br>• Bleeding<br>• Perforation<br>• Obstruction |

**Ans. 6**

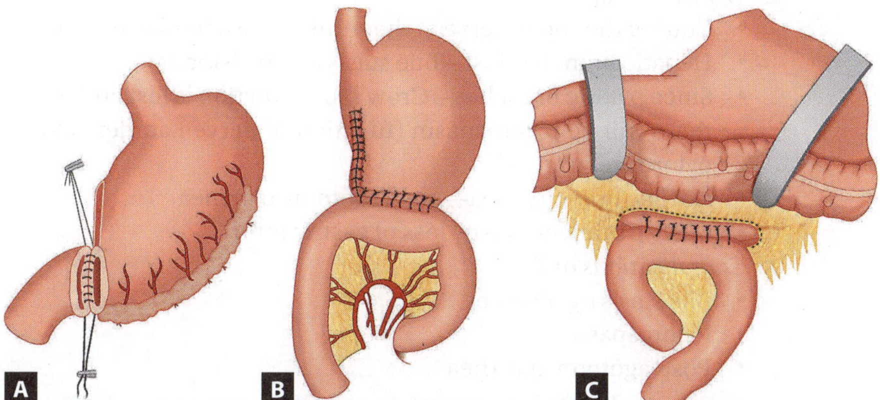


(A) Billroth I gastrectomy—the lower half of the stomach is removed and the cut stomach anastomosed to the first part of the duodenum; (B) Billroth II—two-thirds of the stomach is removed, the duodenal stump is closed and the stomach anastomosed to the jejunum; (C) Gastroenterostomy—the jejunum is anastomosed to the posterior, dependent, and wall of the stomach.
*Source:* Bailey and Love, 27th edition, pages 1120, 1121.

| Type 1 ulcer | Wedge resection |
|---|---|
| Type 4 ulcer | • Pouchet procedure<br>• Kelling–Madlener procedure<br>• Csendes procedure<br>• Followed by Billroth II reconstruction |
| Type 2/3 ulcer | Distal gastrectomy including gastric ulcer with Billroth II reconstruction along with above procedure, we also do—truncal vagotomy |

**Ans. 7**

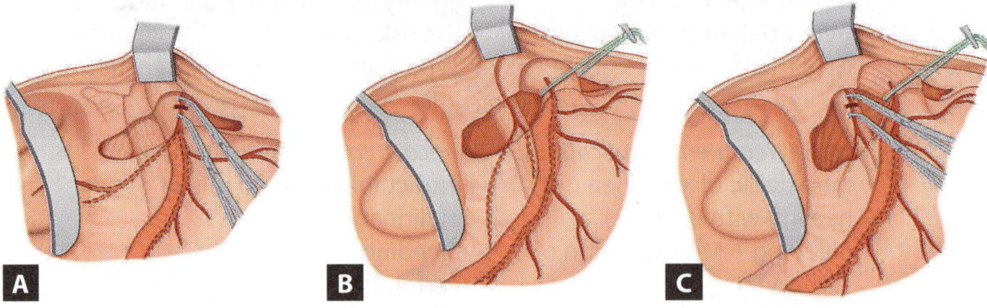


Truncal vagotomy: (A) Division of the anterior vagus; (B) Mobilization of the esophagus; (C) Division of the posterior vagus.
*Source:* Bailey and Love, 27th edition, page 1122.

a. *Truncal vagotomy (TV):*
   - Cutting the vagus nerve at the trunk at lower end of esophagus
   - Hepatic branch is lost—bile stasis and gallstones.
   - Since pyloric branches—Crow's foot function is lost and hence there will be pylorospasm (function of nerve Latarjet is to do pylorus relaxation).
   - Coeliac branch is lost—postvagotomy diarrhea
   - Gastric branches lost—loss of gastric tone
b. *Complications of TV:*
   - Bile stasis+ gallstones
   - Pylorospasm
   - Postvagotomy diarrhea

   *Since there is pylorospasm we must do—drainage procedures:*
   - Posterior gastrojejunostomy
   - Heineke-Mikulicz pyloroplasty

   These drainage procedures have their own list of complications.

   *Complications of TV with gastrojejunostomy (GJ):*
   - Complications of losing the vagus nerve—discussed already
   - *Problems due to GJ:*
     - Malabsorption syndromes
     - Afferent and efferent loop syndromes
     - Dumping syndromes

*Malabsorption:*

- Iron deficiency anemia (MC deficiency in gastric surgeries)
- Calcium deficiency—osteoporosis
- Vitamin $B_{12}$ deficiency

*Loop syndromes:*

| ***Afferent loop syndrome*** | ***Efferent loop syndrome*** |
|---|---|
| MC type due to kinking or adhesion of afferent limb | LC type |
| There will be bilious vomit only no food in vomit | There will be food + vomit<br>Emergency case |
| Self-limiting most of the time radionuclide study will show stagnation of contrast in afferent limb is the IOC | Urgent surgery needed |

*Dumping syndromes/postcibal syndrome:*

| ***Early dumping syndrome*** | ***Late dumping syndrome*** |
|---|---|
| Happens in half-hour massive fluid shift toward hypertonic food particle | • Happens in 2 hours<br>• This happens due to reactive hypoglycemia |
| C/F—Dehydration, thirsty, and giddiness | C/F—palpitation, tremors, and sweating |
| Diagnosis by PCV, there will be hemoconcentration | Diagnosis by PPBS value, hypoglycemia |

*Prevention of dumping syndromes:*

- Eat small split meals
- Dry meals
- High-fat diet
- Low-carbohydrate diet

*Treatment of dumping syndrome:*

- Conservative treatment
- DOC—octreotide
- Revisional surgeries—reverse Roux limb interposition

**Ans. 8**

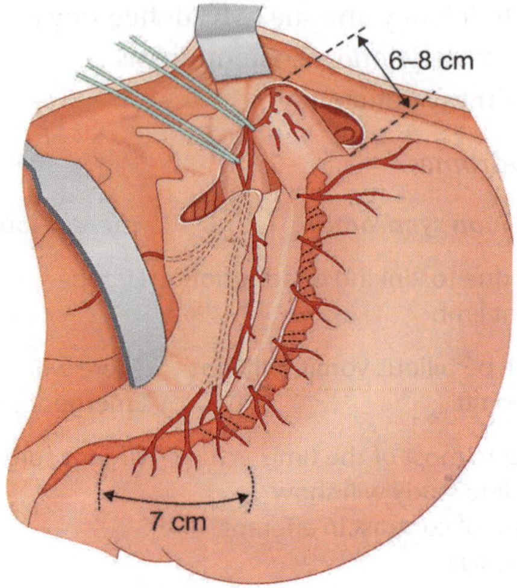


Highly selective vagotomy. The anterior and posterior vagus nerves are preserved but all branches to the fundus and body of the stomach are divided.
*Source:* Bailey and Love, 27th edition, page 1122.

*High selective vagotomy (parietal cell vagotomy):* The gastric branches are cut 7 cm proximal to pyloric orifice:
- Only the gastric branches are selectively cut
- No need of drainage procedure in this operation
- But the problem is we may miss few branches during surgery and hence risk of recurrence is more (5–10%).

**Ans. 9**

| *Complications* | *Duodenal ulcer* | *Gastric ulcer* |
|---|---|---|
| Intractable | HSV > TV/GJ | • Type 1—wedge resection<br>• Type 2/3—TV + distal gastrectomy + Billroth II<br>• Type 4—Pauchet, Kelling–Madlener and Csendes procedures |
| Bleeding | Three point U sutures +/–TV | Oversew the bleeding vessel or a wedge resection for unstable cases. MC vessel to bleed is left gastric artery—distal gastrectomy for stable cases |
| Perforation | <1 cm—closure<br>>1 cm—Graham patch<br>>3 cm—Jejunal patch and pyloric exclusion | • Omental patch if patient unstable<br>• Patient stable—distal gastrectomy |

**Ans. 10** Figure A—early gastric cancer, Japanese classification
Figure B—Bormann classification of advanced gastric cancer

a. *Early gastric cancer:*
- Tumor involving only mucosa and submucosa only
- With or without lymph nodes
- Diagnosed by confocal endoscopy and narrow band imaging scopy
- Japanese classification is used
- Treatment—EMR and ESD (endoscopic mucosal resection and submucosal dissection)

*Bormann's classification:* Based on gross examination:
- Polypoid
- Ulceroproliferative (fungating)
- Ulcerative
- Diffuse linitis plastica

*Lauren's classification:* Based on microscopic appearances:

| ***Histology*** | ***Intestinal*** | ***Diffuse*** |
|---|---|---|
| Epidemiology | MC in sporadic | MC in familial |
| Sex incidence | Males more common | Females more common |
| Age incidence | Elderly | Young |
| Risk factors | Environmental<br>*H. pylori* positive | • Genetic<br>• Family H/O<br>• Group A<br>• Pernicious anemia<br>• E-cadherin mutation—prophylactic gastrectomy in those patients |
| Metastasis | Hematogenous mets common | • Lymphatic mets MC<br>• Transcelomic spread is more common<br>• Peritoneal mets are MC |
| Hepatic metastasis | Nodular | Diffuse |
| Prognosis | Good | Bad |
| Pathology | Gland formation + MC in distal stomach | • Poor differentiated signet ring cells<br>• MC in proximal stomach |
| Genetics | • *APC* gene mutation<br>• P53 and P16 inactivation microsatellite instability | • Decreased E-cadherin<br>• P53 and P16 inactivation |

b. • MC site in India/World—incisura (antrum)
 • MC site in western—proximal stomach (Bailey gives western statistics only)
 • MC type is adenocarcinoma.

*Premalignant risk factors:*

| *6S* | *4A* |
|---|---|
| **S**—Smoking<br>**S**—Spirit<br>**S**—Spicy foods<br>**S**—Salted foods<br>**S**—Smoked foods<br>**S**—Stored foods | **A**—Adenomatous polyps<br>**A**—Atrophic gastritis<br>**A**—Anemia (pernicious anemia)<br>**A**—Blood group A |

*Others:*
- Menetrier's disease
- *H. pylori*—Cag A toxin—distal gastric cancer
- *H. pylori* is protective against OG junction adenocancers
- *H. pylori* is having no relation in proximal gastric cancer and SCC esophagus

*Genetic syndromes:*
- Li-Fraumeni syndrome
- Lynch syndrome
- Familial adenomatous polyposis (FAP)
- E-cadherin mutations

*Pernicious anemia:*
- Causes type A gastritis
- Antrum is not affected
- MC affects proximal stomach
- Premalignant and causes cancer in proximal stomach

c. *Clinical features:*

| ***STOMACH-features*** | |
|---|---|
| S—silent<br>T—tumor<br>O—Gastric outlet obstruction (GOO)<br>M—melena<br>A—anorexia<br>C—cachexia<br>H—hematemesis | *Krukenberg tumor:*<br>• Bilateral ovarian deposit<br>• Superficial deposit<br>• Seen in premenopausal women<br>  – Only<br>  – On C/S—inside ovary is normal<br>  – Transcelomic spread<br>• *Sister Mary-Joseph nodule:*<br>  – Transcelomic spread<br>  – Umbilical deposit |

*Contd...*

*Contd...*

| ***STOMACH-features*** | |
|---|---|
| | • *Blumer's shelf:*<br>– Per rectal deposit in POD<br>– Transcelomic spread<br>• *Virchow's node:*<br>– Left supraclavicular node (Troisier sign)<br>– Irish node—left axillary node<br>The two nodes are due to lymphatic spread |

d. Clinical features to say the tumor is inoperable:
- Liver mets+
- Ascites+
- Right sided above mentioned conditions are features of inoperability: In addition, if CECT shows peritoneal mets, pancreatic infiltration is also inoperable.

e.

| ***T staging*** | ***N staging*** | ***M staging*** |
|---|---|---|
| • T1—tumor involves mucosa and submucosa only<br>• T2—muscularis propria<br>• T3—penetrates subserosa<br>• T4—serosa and adjacent structures (adjacent structures does not include esophagus and duodenum) | • N1—1–2 nodes+<br>• N2—3–6 nodes+<br>• N3a—7–15 nodes+<br>• N3b—>16 nodes+ | • M1—Mets+ |

**Ans. 11** a. *Early gastric cancer:*
- Tumor involving only mucosa and submucosa only
- With or without lymph nodes
- Diagnosed by confocal endoscopy and narrow band imaging scopy
- Japanese classification is used.
- Treatment—EMR and ESD

b. Minimum number of nodes removed:
- Stomach—16 nodes
- Breast—10 nodes
- Esophagus—15 nodes
- Colon—12 nodes

c. *Siewert classification of OG junction cancers:*
- Type 1—tumors 1–5 cm above OG junction in distal esophagus
- Type 2—tumors at 1 cm above and up to 2 cm on the stomach side from OG junction
- Type 3—tumors from 2—5 cm below the OG junction

*Latest guidelines:*

- Types 1 and 2 are treated such as esophageal cancer by transhiatal esophagectomy.
- Type 3 is treated like gastric cancer by total gastrectomy.

**Ans. 12** Figure (A)—Radical total gastrectomy: (a) Dissection of omentum of the transverse colon; (b) Exposure of the lesser sac; (c) Splenectomy; (d) Division and oversewing of the duodenum; (e) Dissection of the left gastric artery nodes (group 17); (f) Mobilization of the esophagus. Figure B—esophagojejunostomy Roux-en-Y.

**Ans. 13** a.
- *Investigations:*
    - T and N staging—EUS
    - Diagnosis—endoscopic biopsy (6–8 biopsy taken from lesions)
    - Tumor market—CA 72-4
    - Mets—CECT abdomen
    - To diagnose peritoneal mets—most sensitive test—diagnostic laparoscopy (diagnostic of 30% time in planned surgery cases)
- *Treatment:*
    - *Surgical resection:*
        - Proximal margin—5 cm clearance proximal (NCCN guidelines says—4 cm margin proximal)
        - Distal up to duodenal first part
        - We either do subtotal gastrectomy or total gastrectomy
    - *Billroth II reconstruction:*
        - Gastrojejunal anastomosis after subtotal gastrectomy
        - No more gastroduodenal anastomosis (Billroth I done now)
        - Increased bile reflux is seen in this reconstruction.
    - *Duodenal stump blow out:*
        - Happens on 4th/5th POD
        - Bile and pancreatic juice leaks
        - No need of urgent surgery
        - USG-guided drainage is enough
- *Roux-en-Y reconstruction:*
    - Done after total gastrectomy
    - Two anastomosis—esophagojejunal and jejunojejunal anastomosis done
    - Herniation behind Roux limb is known as Peterson hernia.

b. *Palliative procedures: For inoperable cancers:*

- Gastric outlet obstruction (GOO) cases—palliative gastrojejunostomy or palliative gastrectomy

- for bleeding and GOO cases, palliative resection is done and has increased survival outcome than a palliative GJ.
- OG junction growth causing dysphagia—self-expandable metal stent (SEMS) can be done.

**Ans. 14**

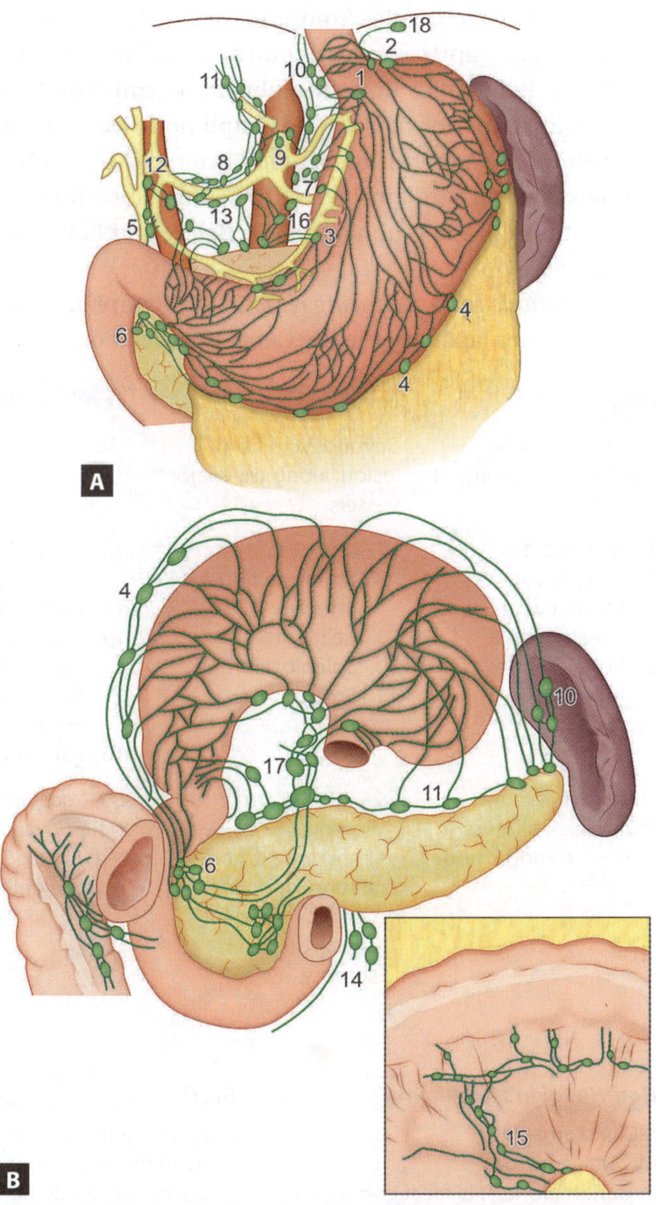


Lymphatic drainage of the stomach and nodal stations by the Japanese classification—(A) the anterior view of the stomach and (B) the posterior view.
*Source:* Bailey and Love, 27th edition, page 1136.

a. The lymphatics of the antrum drain into the right gastric lymph node superiorly, and right gastroepiploic and subpyloric lymph nodes inferiorly. The lymphatics of the pylorus drain into the right gastric suprapyloric nodes superiorly and the subpyloric lymph nodes situated around the gastroduodenal artery inferiorly. The efferent lymphatics from suprapyloric lymph nodes converge on the para-aortic nodes around the celiac axis, whereas the efferent lymphatics from the subpyloric lymph nodes pass up to the main superior mesenteric lymph nodes situated around the origin of the superior mesenteric artery. The lymphatic vessels related to the cardia orifice of the stomach communicate freely with those of the esophagus (*Ref:* Bailey and Love, 27th edition, page 1135)
b. *Lymph node stations during resection:* 16 lymph node stations are there as per Japanese Gastric Cancer Association.

| ***Level 1 nodes*** | ***Level 2 nodes*** | ***Level 3 nodes*** |
|---|---|---|
| Perigastric nodes (nodes <3 cm from tumor) | Beyond 3 cm from lesion, along the major vessels | |
| 1. Right cardiac<br>2. Left cardiac<br>3. Lesser curve<br>4. Greater curve<br>5. Suprapyloric<br>6. Infrapyloric | 7. Left gastric artery<br>8. Common hepatic artery<br>9. Celiac artery<br>10. Splenic hilum<br>11. Splenic artery | 12. Hepatoduodenal ligament<br>13. Retropancreatic<br>14. Superior mesenteric vessels<br>15. Middle colic vessel<br>16. Para-aortic |
| *D1—gastrectomy:*<br>Removal of all level 1 nodes+ station 7 node | *D2—gastrectomy:*<br>• Removal of all level 1 and level 2 nodes+ station 12 nodes<br>• Gold standard for cancer stomach surgery | *D3—gastrectomy:*<br>• Removal of all level 1, 2, 3 nodes<br>• Done only in Japan |

**Ans. 15**

| ***Non-Hodgkin's lymphoma*** | ***GIST*** |
|---|---|
| MC in stomach<br>MC site—antrum<br>In Burkitt alone, it is most common in fundus | • MC in stomach<br>• MC in proximal stomach in gastric curve side near fundus |

*Contd...*

*Contd...*

| ***Non-Hodgkin's lymphoma*** | ***GIST*** |
|---|---|
| *Types:*<br>• MC is diffuse large cell<br>• MALT (second MC)<br>• Mantle<br>• Burkitt | *Types:*<br>• Wild type—CD117 negative, CD 34 negative<br>• Normal GIST—both are positive |
| Origin—lymphatic tissues on gut wall | Origin—cells of Cajal or pacemaker cells |
| *Primary GI lymphoma (Dawson criteria):*<br>• No liver involvement<br>• No spleen involvement<br>• No bone marrow involvement<br>• No generalized lymphadenopathy<br>• Confined to one GI organ only | |

*Diagnosis: For both:*
- Endoscopy is difficult to diagnose due to normal mucosa
- Hence IOC—EUS-guided biopsy or CT-guided biopsy

| | |
|---|---|
| *Tumor markers:*<br>• Not mentioned in books<br>• There is a named staging for them known as Lugano staging | *Tumor markers:*<br>• CD 117—tyrosine kinase receptor mutation positive in 90%<br>• CD 37–40% positive |
| | PDGFRA—platelet-derived growth factor receptor antibody<br>Latest—DOG—discovered on GIST |
| *Management:*<br>• Maltoma early—*H. pylori* eradication alone is enough<br>• Advanced cases—R-CHOP regimen<br>– R—Rituximab<br>– C—Cyclophosphamide<br>– H—Hydroxy Adriamycin<br>– O—Oncovin<br>– P—Prednisolone<br>• DLC-R-CHOP<br>• For NHL of stomach—no need of surgery<br>*Indications of surgery in an NHL stomach:*<br>• Bleeding<br>• Perforation<br>• Obstruction<br>• Intractable pain<br>• Not responding to chemotherapy<br>Other GI lymphomas such as small intestine and large intestine—surgery advised first followed by R-CHOP | *Treatment:*<br>• Surgical resection with clear margin<br>• No lymph node dissection needed.<br>*Prognosis after surgery depends on Modified Joensuu criteria:*<br>• Size (>10 cm—Bad)<br>• Mitotic index (>5 mitotic index/50 HPF)<br>• Site (stomach—good)<br>*After surgery:*<br>For high-risk tumors will give imatinib mesylate or sunitinib |

**Ans. 16** a. Trichobezoars—hair balls in stomach, exclusively seen in psychiatric young, female patients. Hair balls can lead to perforation, obstruction, and GI bleeding. Diagnosis made on endoscopy. Treated by surgical removal of bezoars.

b. Rapunzel syndrome—long hair of trichobezoar extending from stomach up to Ileum

c. Phytobezoars—vegetable matter in stomach in patients who have gastroparesis like diabetes and in postgastric surgery patients, Also seen in surgical patients.

**Ans. 17** Barium meal showing organoaxial volvulus of the stomach associated with eventration of the diaphragm:

a. *It is gastric volvulus:*
   - Stomach can rotate and go for volvulus either in organoaxial (longitudinal axis) or mesentricoaxial (vertical axis)
   - MC type of volvulus is organoaxial volvulus and this associated with diaphragmatic hernia
   - Organoaxial volvulus associated with diaphragmatic hernia

b. *Borchardt's triad:*
   - Sudden onset of constant retching epigastric pain
   - Inability to vomit
   - Inability to pass the Ryle's tube (remember no vomiting)

c. Urgent surgery must be done—gastropexy and closure of diaphragm defects.

12

SECTION

# Genitourinary

# CHAPTER 52 Genitourinary

## QUESTIONS

**Q1. Answer the following:**

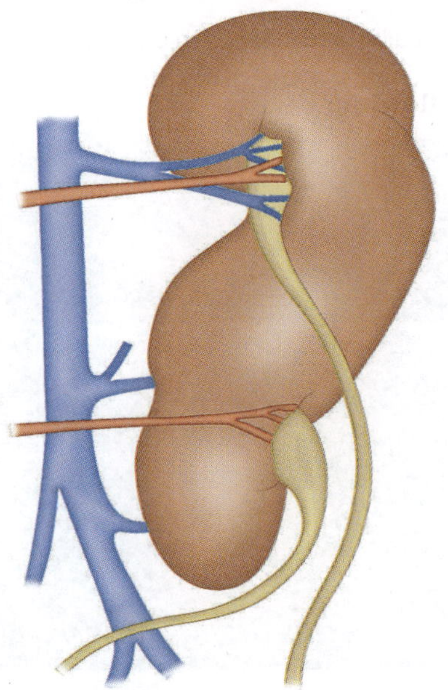

*Source:* Bailey and Love, 27th edition, page 1399.

a. What is the given condition?
b. What is the most common anomaly of this condition?
c. What is the position of ureters?

**Q2. Answer the following:**

a. What is the given condition?
b. What is the position of ureters?
c. What prevents the further ascent of the fused kidney?
d. What is the condition where isthmus is cut?
e. What are the intravenous pyelogram (IVP) findings?
f. What is the limit of lower pole fusion?

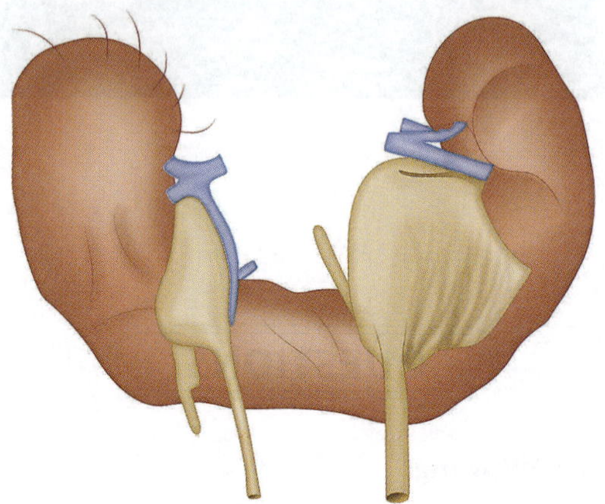

*Source:* Bailey and Love, 27th edition, page 1400.

**Q3. Answer the following:**

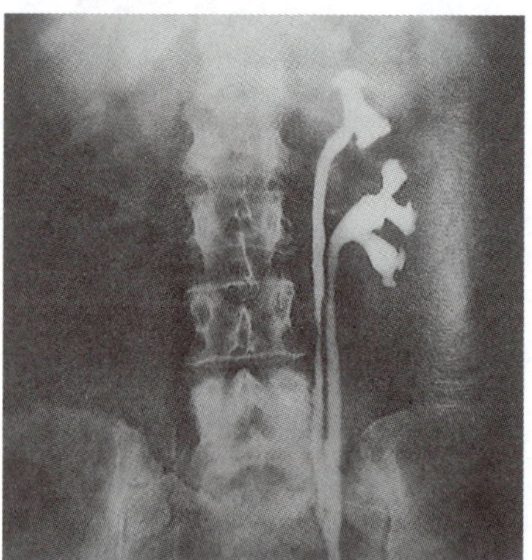

*Source:* Bailey and Love, 27th edition, page 1401.

a. What is shown in the diagram?
b. What is the association of upper pole moiety and lower pole moiety?
c. What is Weigert–Meyer rule?
d. What is opening of ectopic ureter in male and female?
e. Name the reflex associated with it.
f. What is the investigation done and what is the finding in it?

**Q4. Answer the following:**

a. What is the given image on IVP and what is the IVP finding?
b. What is the treatment of this condition?
c. In which condition nephrectomy is indicated?

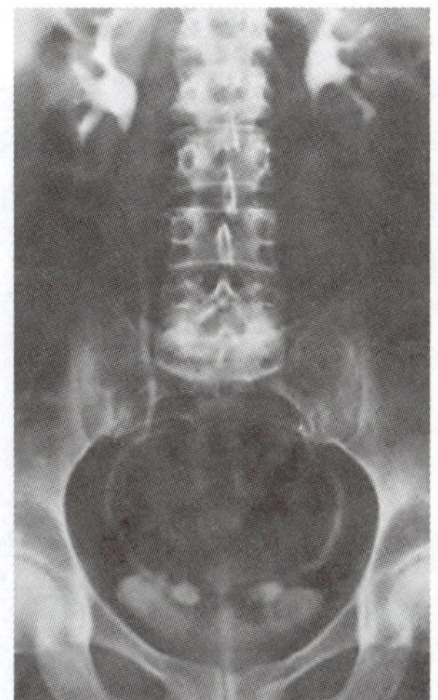

*Source:* Bailey and Love, 27th edition, page 1401.

**Q5. Answer the following:**

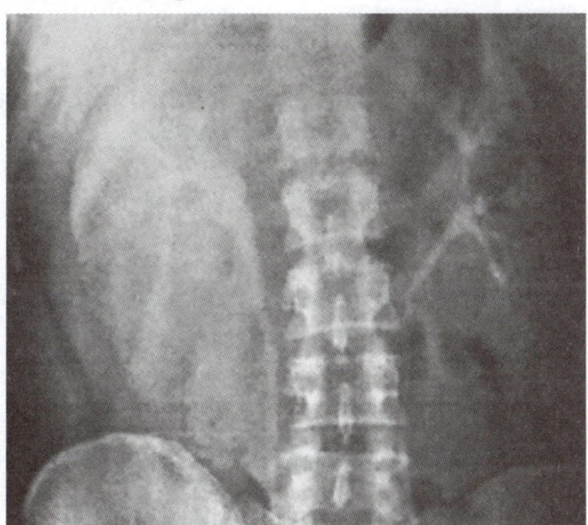

a. What is this given condition in IVP and what is the finding?
b. Name the gene and protein associated with this condition.
c. What are the criteria to diagnose this condition?
d. What is the most common presentation?
e. What is the most common type of renal stone associated with it?
f. What are the associated anomalies?
g. What are the treatment options?

**Q6. Answer the following:**

a. What is the most common organism for urinary tract infection (UTI)?
b. What is the Kass criteria?

## Q7. Answer the following:

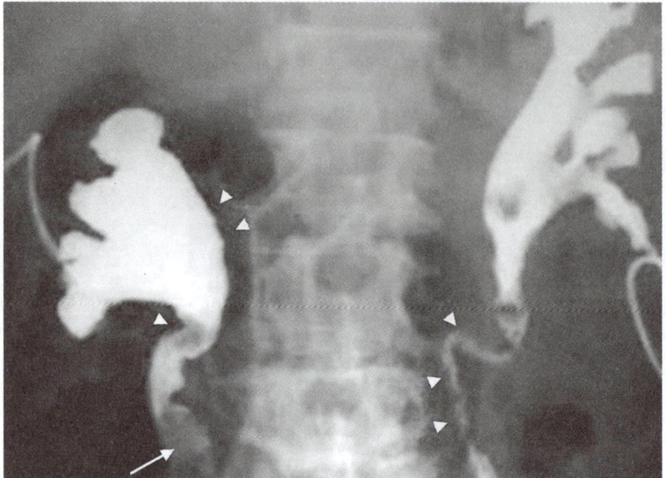

a. What is the condition and in which condition is it found?
b. What is the clinical presentation and what is the diagnostic modality?
c. What are the complications of this chronic condition?

## Q8. Answer the following:

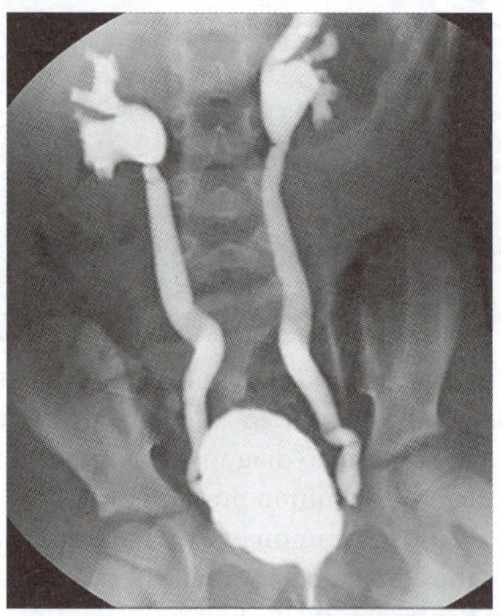

a. What is the given condition in micturating cysto-urethrogram (MCU)?
b. What is the cause of it?
c. What is the grading of this disease?
d. What is the treatment of this condition?

## Q9. Answer the following:

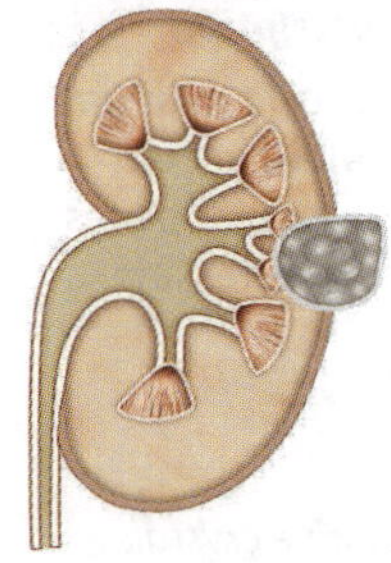

I – 0% are malignant

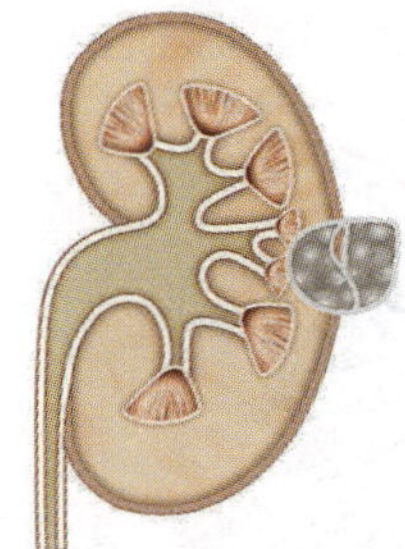

II – 0% are malignant

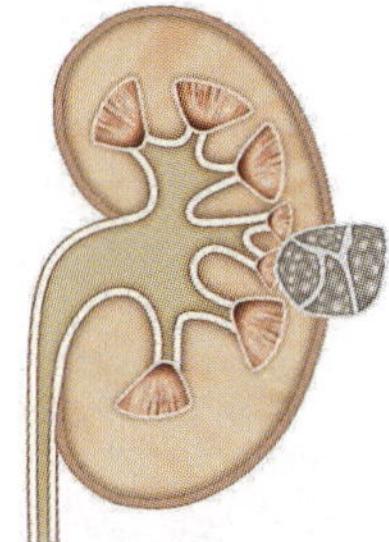

IIF – 5% are malignant

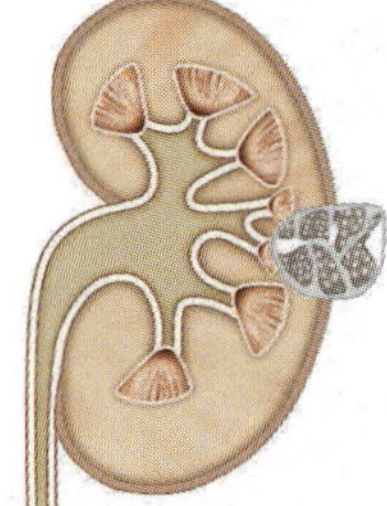

III – 50% are malignant

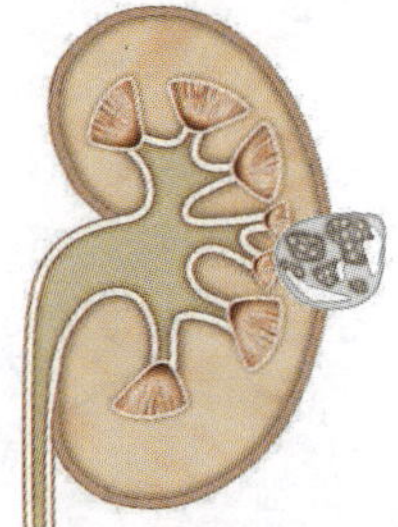

IV – 100% are malignant

*Source:* Bailey and Love, 27th edition, page 1390.

a. What is this condition?

b. Elaborate the classification used for it.

c. What is the management of this condition?

## Q10. Answer the following:

| ***Image*** | ***Description*** |
|---|---|
| 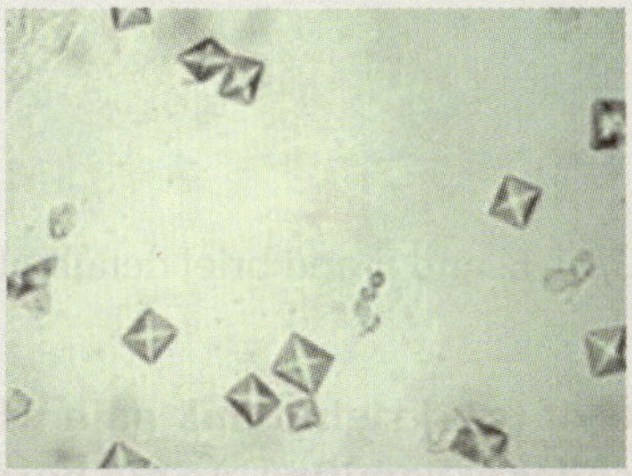 | *Calcium oxalate:*<br>• Bipyramidal shape/envelope shaped<br>• m/c type of crystals in urine |
| 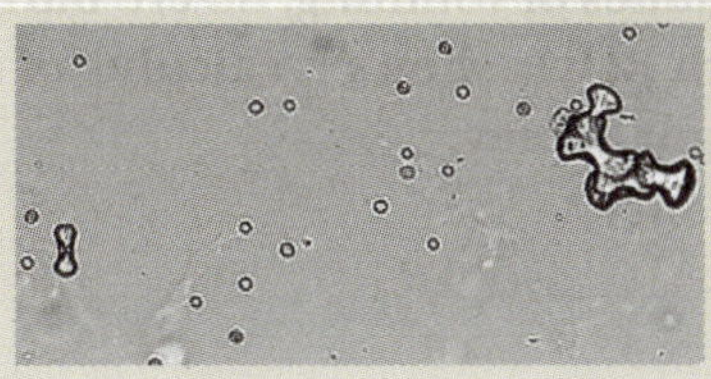 | *Calcium oxalate monohydrate:*<br>• Dumbbell shaped or Hour glass shaped crystals |

*Contd...*

*Contd...*

| Image | Description |
|---|---|
| 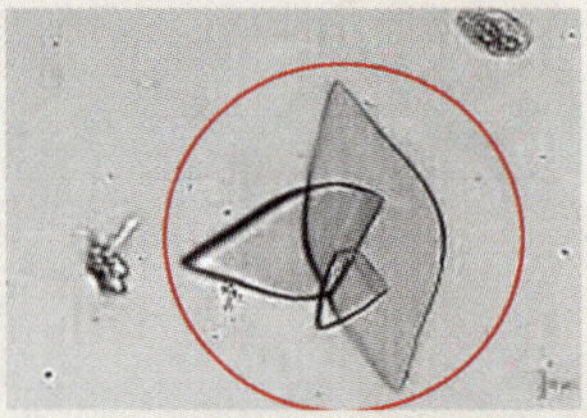 | *Uric acid crystals:*<br>• Multifaceted<br>• Irregular plates<br>• Rosettes line |
| 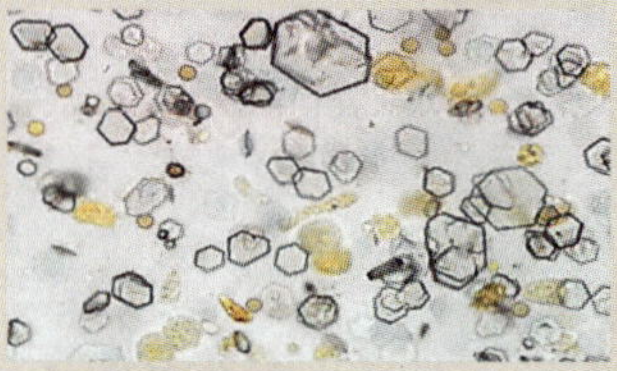 | *Cystine crystals:*<br>• Hexagonal<br>• Benzene ring like |
| 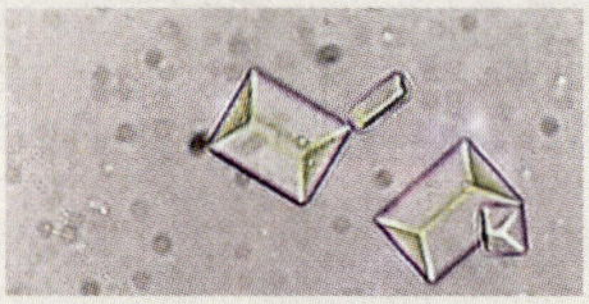 | *Struvite:*<br>• Coffin lid shape |
| 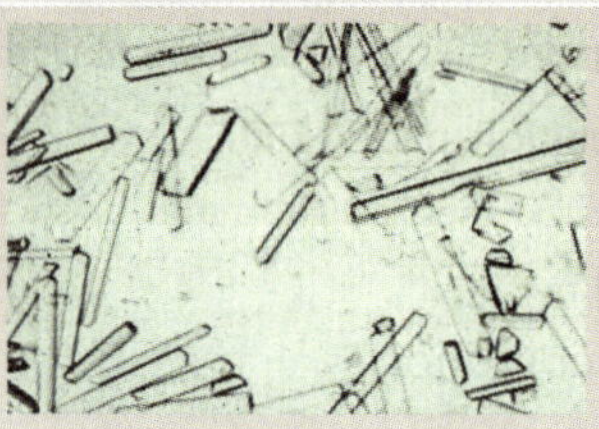 | *Brushite:*<br>• Needle shaped |

a. Ascending sequence of stone/crystal to break with difficulty by extracorporeal shockwave lithotripsy (ESWL)?
   1. D<F<B
   2. A<F<E
   3. B<F<D
   4. E<D<B

b. Name the crystal type of A, B, C, D, E, and F, and brief details about them.

**Q11. A patient came with complaints of (c/o) right flank pain which radiates to back, he has two episodes of vomiting, no c/o burning micturition. USG abdomen with pelvis shows a calculus of size 4.5 mm in the middle calyx of right kidney.**

a. What is the etiology of renal stone?
b. What is the mc kidney stone?
c. What is the treatment?
d. Name the drugs causing renal stones.

**Q12. What constriction in the ureter is shown. Identify 1, 2, 3, 4, and 5.**

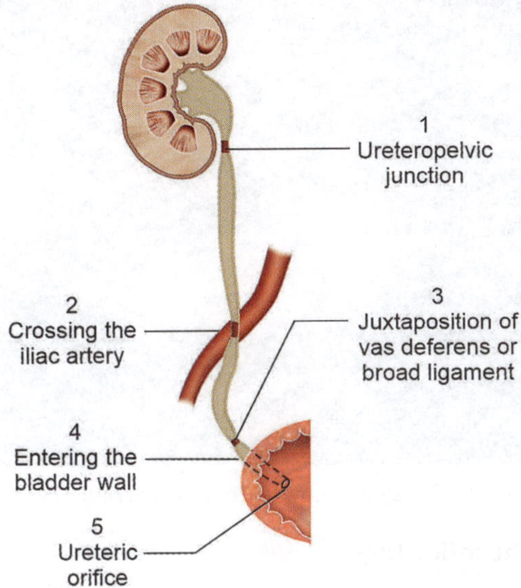


*Source:* Bailey and Love, 27th edition, page 1407.

**Q13. Answer the following:**

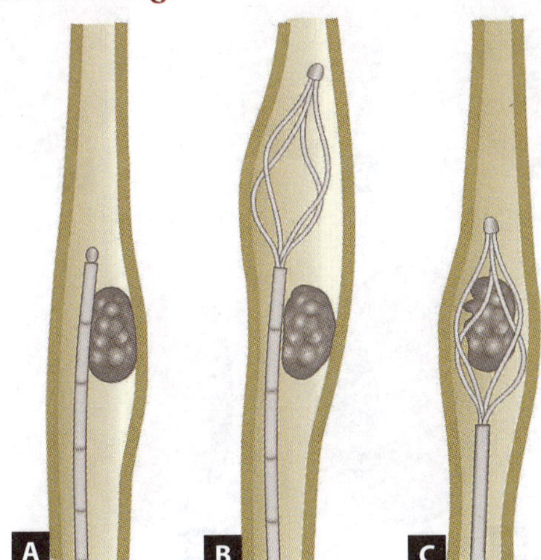


*Source:* Bailey and Love, 27th edition, page 1409.

a. What is the procedure depicted in the image?
b. What is it used for?
c. What is the other method?

**Q14. Answer the following:**

a. USG depicted is finding of which condition?
b. What does A, P, and C denote?

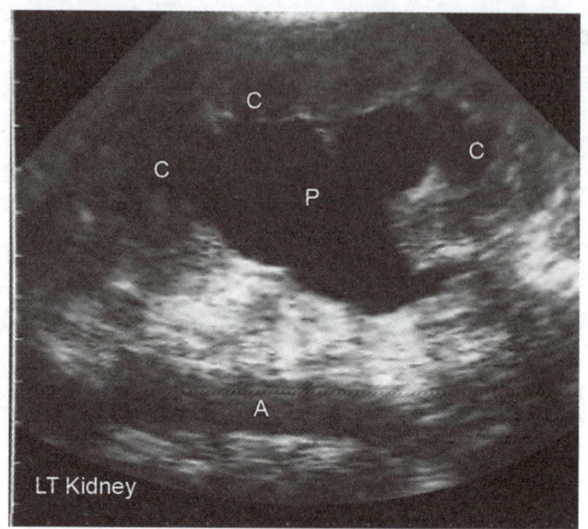


*Source:* Bailey and Love, 27th edition, page 1412.

**Q15. Answer the following:**

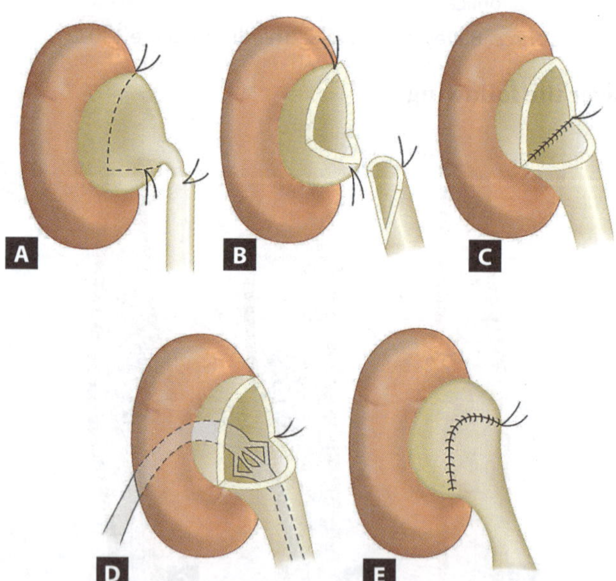


*Source:* Bailey and Love, 27th edition, page 1413.

a. What procedure is that?
b. What is it used for?

**Q16. Based on the figure, answer the following:**

a. Describe the image and a brief about grading?
b. What is the indication for radiological assessment of this condition?

c. Patient underwent abdominal trauma, laparotomy was planned by consultant doctor (Dr.) suspecting holo organ injury. During laparotomy renal trauma was encountered unexpectedly. What will be your next step?

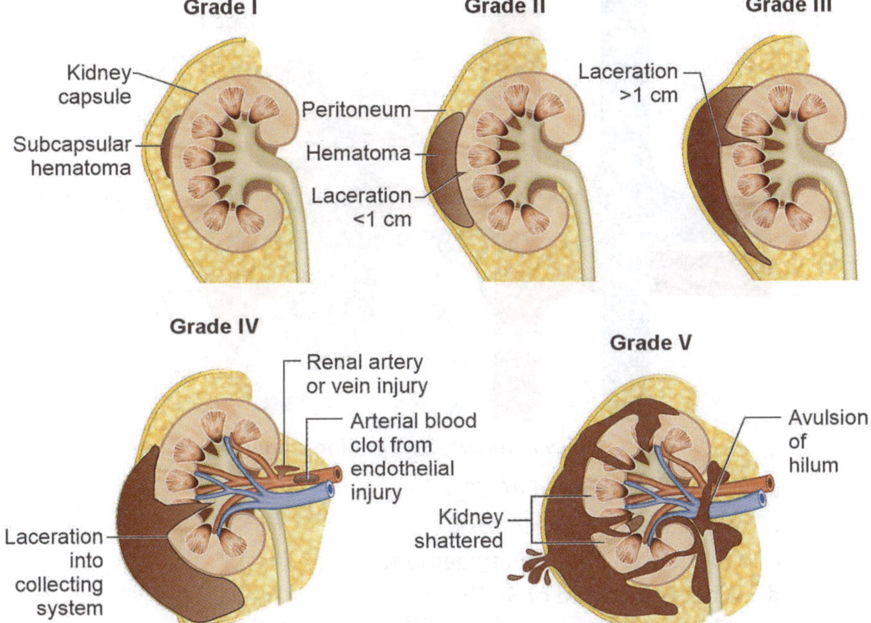


*Source:* Bailey and Love, 27th edition, page 1414.

**Q17. Based on the figure, answer the following:**

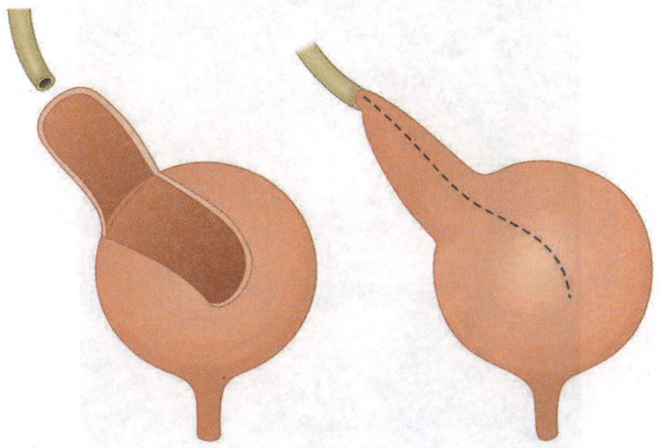

*Source:* Bailey and Love, 27th edition, page 1415.

a. What is this?
b. What is it used for?
c. What are the other methods used for it?
d. What is the disadvantage of transureteroureterostomy?

**Q18. Based on the figure, answer the following:**

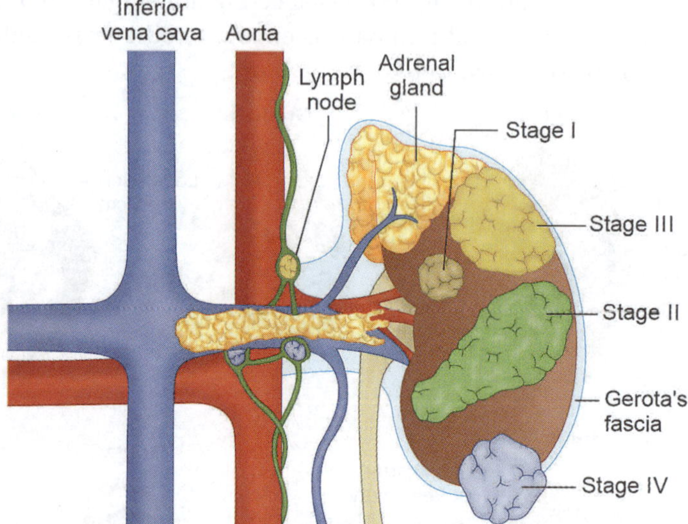


*Source:* Bailey and Love, 27th edition, page 1419.

a. Give the staging of RCC?
b. What are the risk factors?
c. Give a brief about management (inv and t/t).
d. What is the triad of RCC?
e. What are paraneoplastic syndrome a/w RCC?

**Q19. Based on the figure, answer the following:**

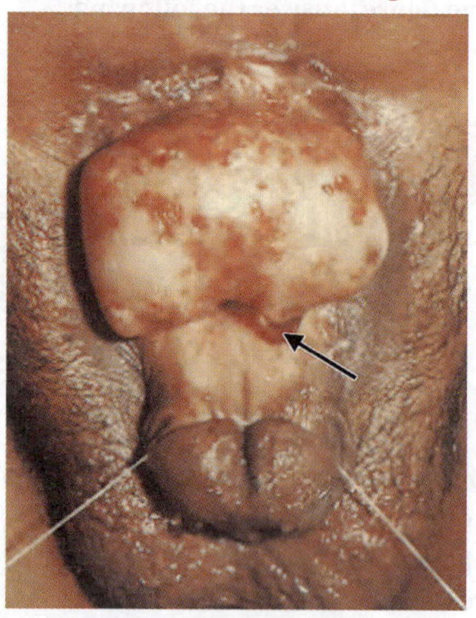

*Source:* Bailey and Love, 27th edition, page 1424.

a. What is the depicted condition?
b. What is etiopathogenesis?
c. What are associated anomalies?
d. What is the treatment?

**Q20. Based on the figure, answer the following:**

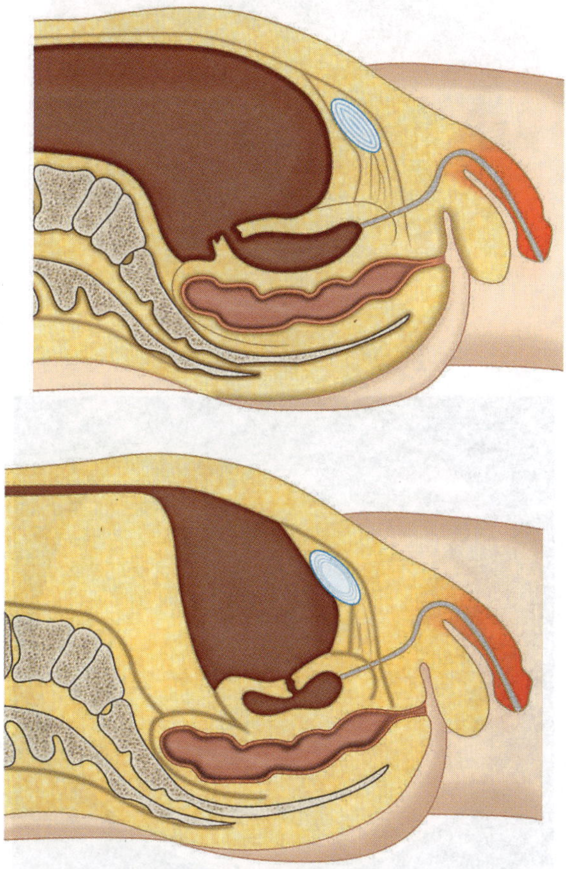

*Source:* Bailey and Love, 27th edition, pages 1419 and 1425.

a. Describe both the images?
b. What is the management?
c. If bladder is ruptured during operation (iatrogenic).
   i. In which operations bladder is often ruptured/injured?
   ii. What is the management?

**Q21. Answer the following:**

a. Elaborate the causes of acute retention of urine?
b. What are the clinical features of acute retention of urine?
c. What is the treatment option for this condition?

**Q22. Answer the following:**

a. From where does the secondary tumors of the bladder arise?

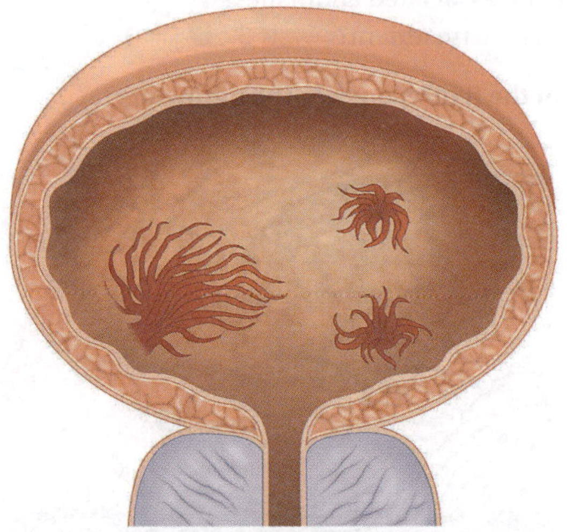

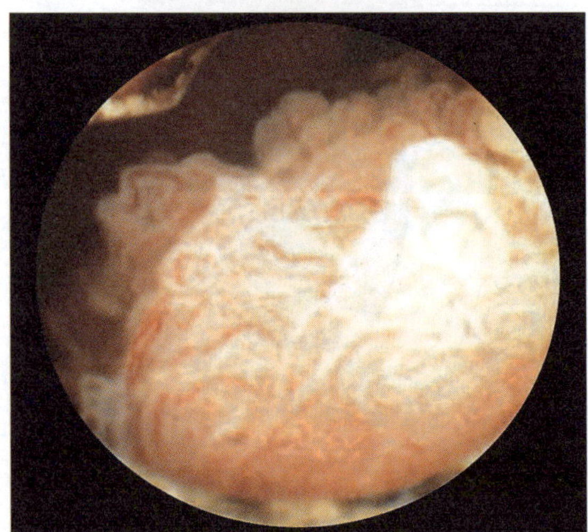

*Source:* Bailey and Love, 27th edition, pages 1445 and 1446.

b. What is depicted in these figures?

c. What are the types of bladder tumors?

**Q23. Answer the following:**

a. What are the risk factors for transitional cell cancer (TCC) of bladder?

b. What are the risk factors for squamous cell bladder (SCC)?

c. What are the occupational risk factors?

d. Elaborate the names of carcinogens of bladder cancer.

**Q24. Bladder cancer:**

a. What are its clinical features?
b. What is the investigation?
c. What is the staging?

**Q25. Bladder cancer:**

a. What are intravesical therapy agents used?
b. What is the treatment?

**Q26. Bladder cancer:**

Based on these figures, answers the following questions:

a. Describe in brief about radical cystectomy?

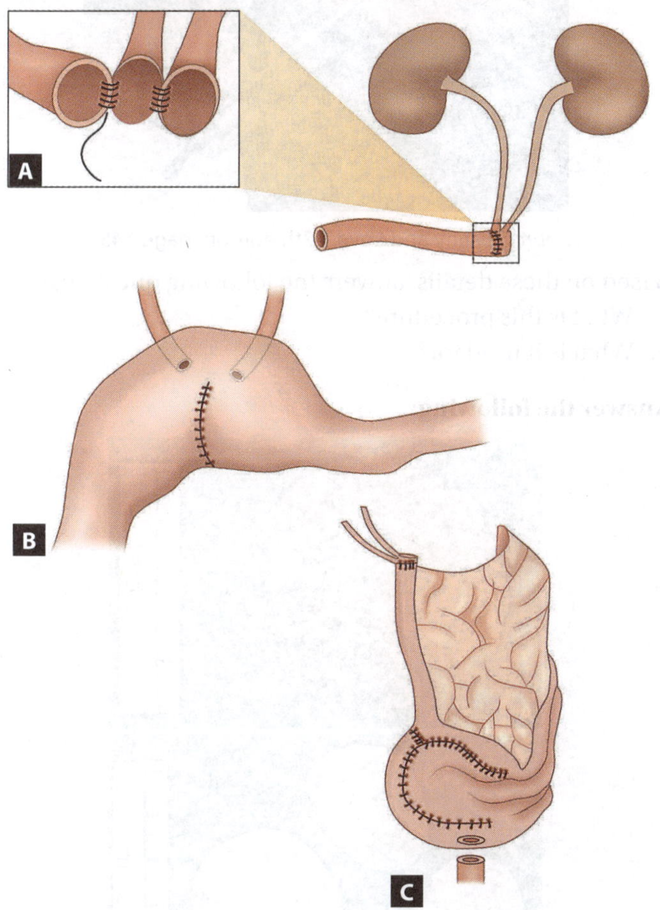


*Source:* Bailey and Love, 27th edition, page1453.

b. What are these methods?
c. What are these methods used for?
d. What are the complications of these methods?

**Q27. Patient with a pT3a cancer (ca) bladder who has previously undergone cystoprostatectomy and urethrectomy. A detubularized ileocecal reservoir has been made with the ureters and implanted in submucosal tunnels. The appendix has been implanted within the reservoir in a submucosal tunnel to provide the continence mechanism. The appendix has been brought to the umbilicus and is catheterized 4–6 hourly to empty the reservoir.**

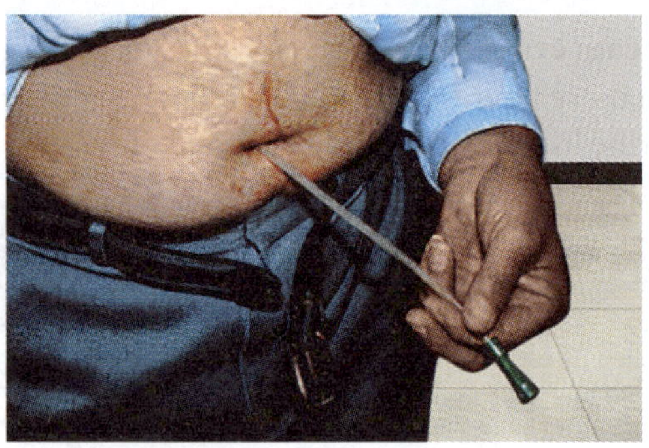

*Source:* Bailey and Love, 27th edition, page 1454.

Based on these details, anwers the following questions:

a. What is this procedure?
b. What is it used for?

**Q28. Answer the following:**

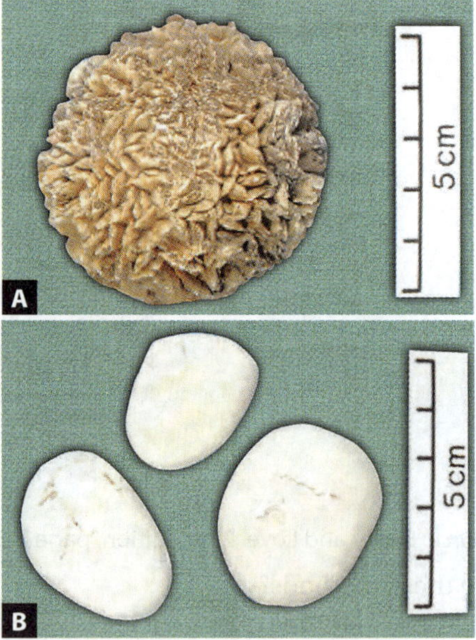


*Source:* Bailey and Love, 27th edition, page 1435.

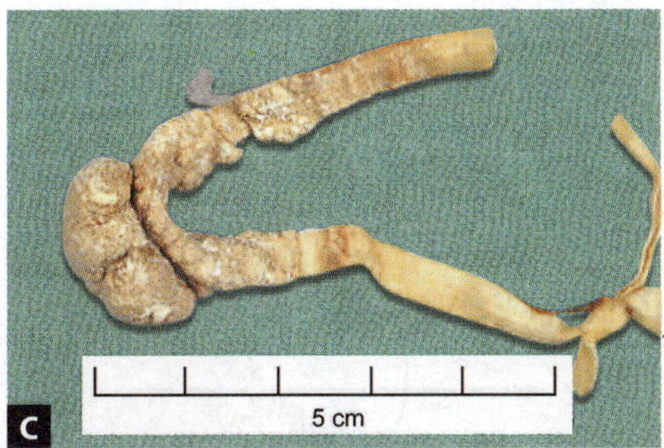


*Source:* Bailey and Love, 27th edition, page 1435.

Based on these images, answer the following questions:

a. What are these images depicted?
b. What are types of bladder stones and brief details?
c. What is the management?

**Q29. Answer the following:**

a. Give brief details about ESWL?
b. Give brief details about PCNL?

**Q30. Answer the following:**

a. What is skene's tubules?
b. Describe McNeal's surgical zones of prostate?
c. Elaborate the lobes of prostate.

**Q31. A 62-year-old male patient came with complains of frequency of urine and nocturia. He also gave history of unable to control urine flow and dribbling of urine. On uroflometry examination, peak urine flow rate was—<10 mL/sec and voiding pressure was—>80 cm $H_2O$. Serum PSA value was—6 ng/mL.**

Based on these findings, answer the following questions:

a. What is urine diagnosis?
b. What are the points in favor of urine diagnosis?

**Q32. Diagnosis of BPH**

Answer the following:

a. What are the symptoms of BOO (bladder outflow obstruction/ bladder outlet obstruction)?
b. What is the investigation for BPH?

**Q33. Treatment of BPH**

Answer the following:

a. What is the medical treatment?
b. What is the indication of surgery?

## Q34. Answer the following:

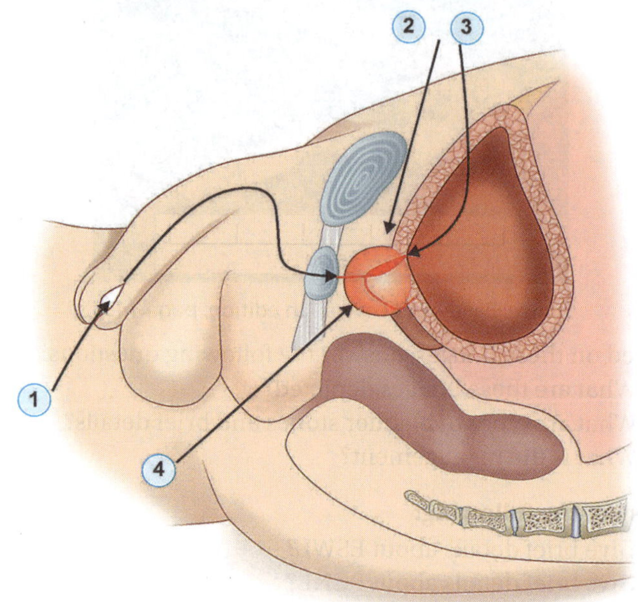


*Source:* Bailey and Love, 27th edition, page 1465.

a. What is 1, 2, 3, and 4?

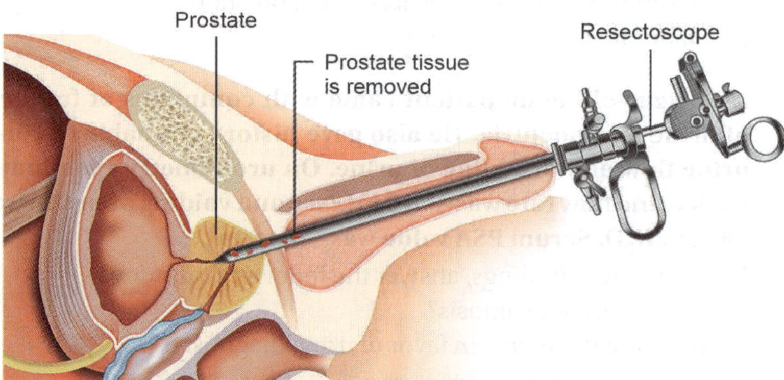


*Source:* Bailey and Love, 27th edition, page 1465.

b. Describe the procedure depicted here?
c. What are the complications of this procedure?

## Q35. Answer the following:

a. Describe the image depicted here?
b. What is it used for?

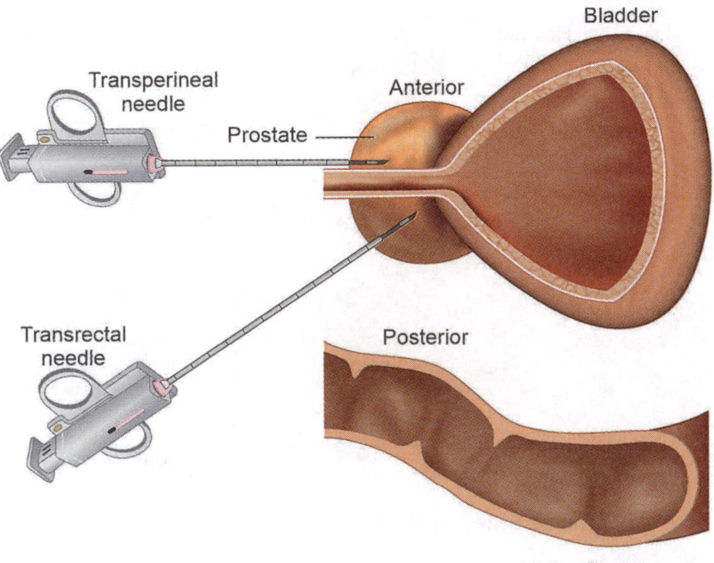


*Source:* Bailey and Love, 27th edition, page 1471.

**Q36. Answer the following:**

a. Describe different types of most common calculi in our body organs?
b. What is corpora amylacea?

**Q37. Cancer prostate**

a. What is the screening protocol?
b. Discuss in brief about prostate-specific antigen (PSA)?
c. What is the investigation?

**Q38. Cancer prostate**

a. What is the staging?
b. What is the management?
c. Elaborate Gleason score.

**Q39. Based on the figure, answer the following questions:**

a. What condition is depicted here?
b. What are its clinical features (c/f)?
c. What are its associated anomalies?
d. What are its types?
e. What is its management?

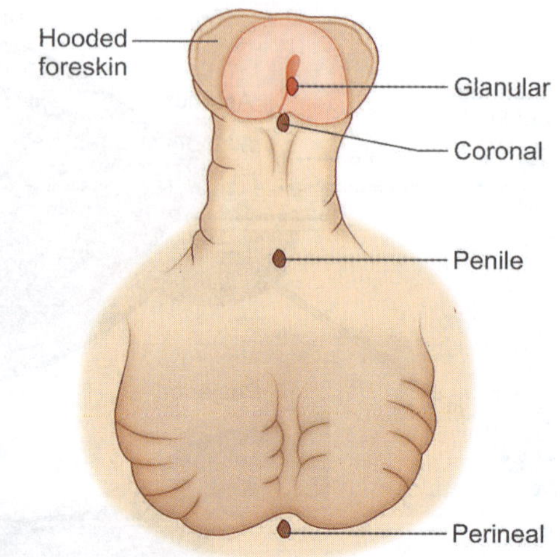


*Source:* Bailey and Love, 27th edition, page 1478.

**Q40. Answer the following:**

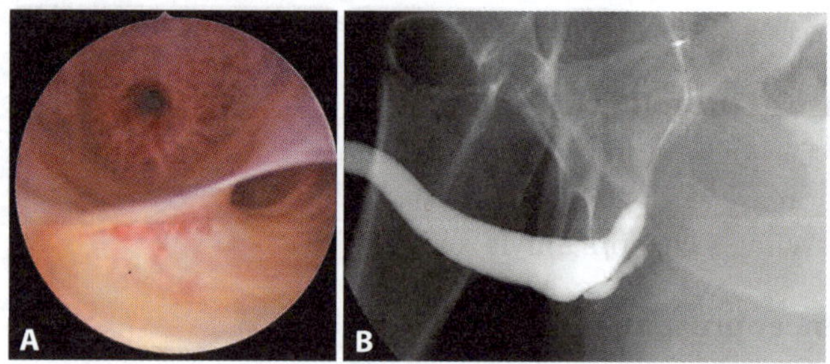


*Source:* Bailey and Love, 27th edition, page 1479.

a. What is this depicted condition?
b. Describe in brief about this condition?

**Q41. Answer the following:**

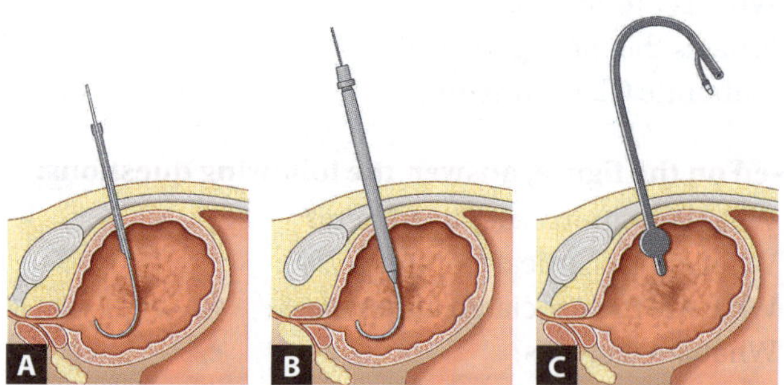


*Source:* Bailey and Love, 27th edition, page 1480.

a. What procedure is depicted in the image?
b. What are the indications of this procedure?

## Q42. Answer the following:

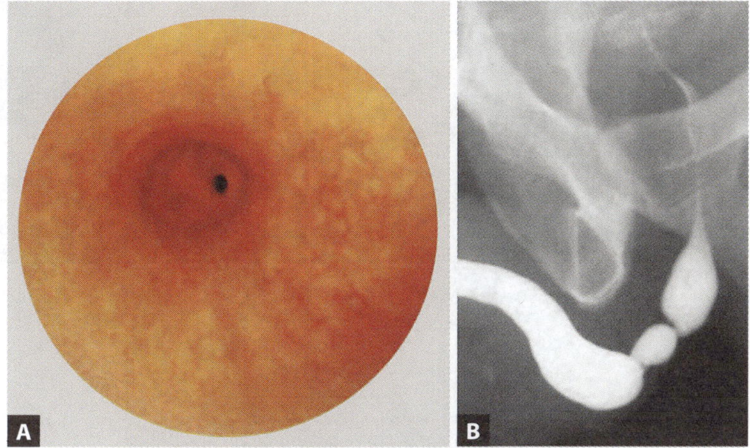


*Source:* Bailey and Love, 27th edition, page 1483.

a. What are the pictures depicted here?
b. Enumerate the causes of it.
c. What is their treatment?

## Q43. Answer the following:

a. What is the classification of urethra?
b. What are the clinical features (c/f) of urethral injury?
c. Enumerate the classification of urethral injuries.
d. How will you manage urethral injury?

## Q44. Answer the following:

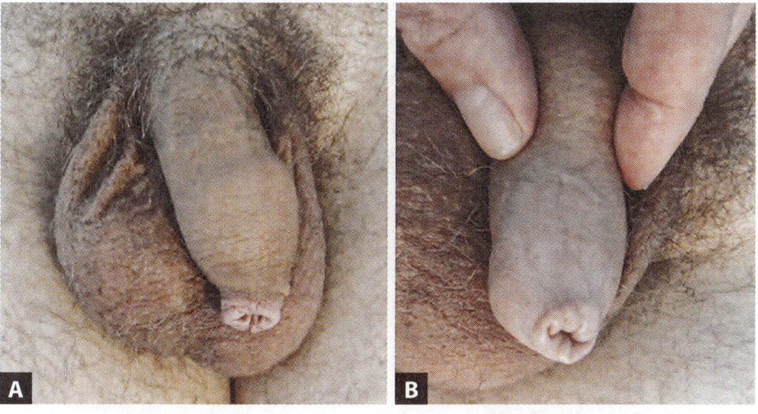


*Source:* Bailey and Love, 27th edition, page 1487.

a. What is depicted in the image?
b. What is the etiology?
c. What are its types?

**Q45. Answer the following:**

(a)

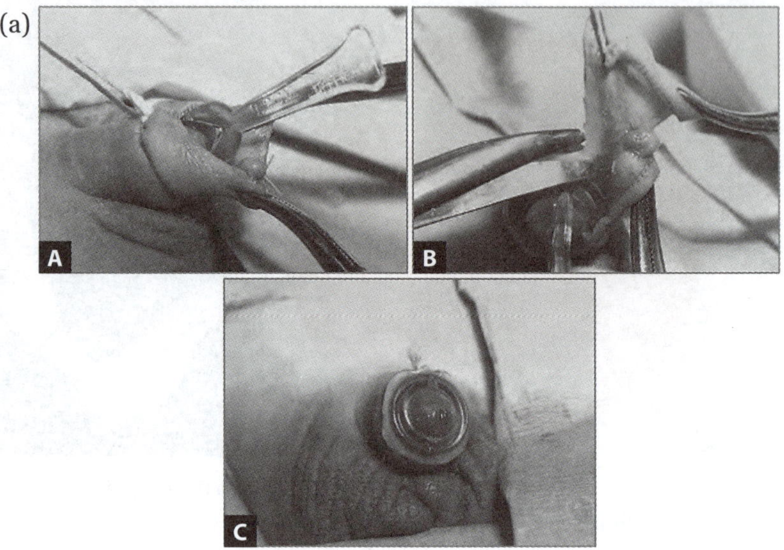


*Source:* Bailey and Love, 27th edition, page 1488.

(b)

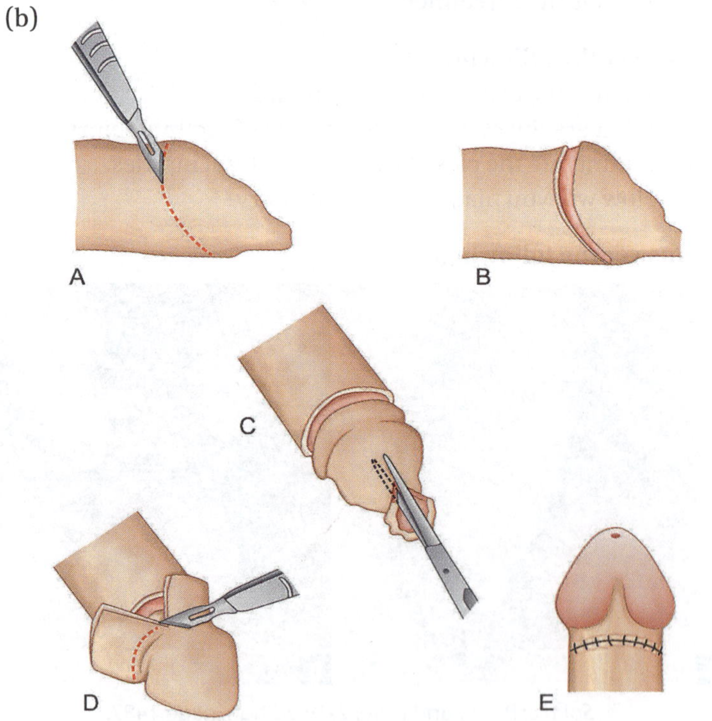


*Source:* Bailey and Love, 27th edition, page 1488.

a. What procedure is shown here?

b. What are its indication?

**Q46. Answer the following:**

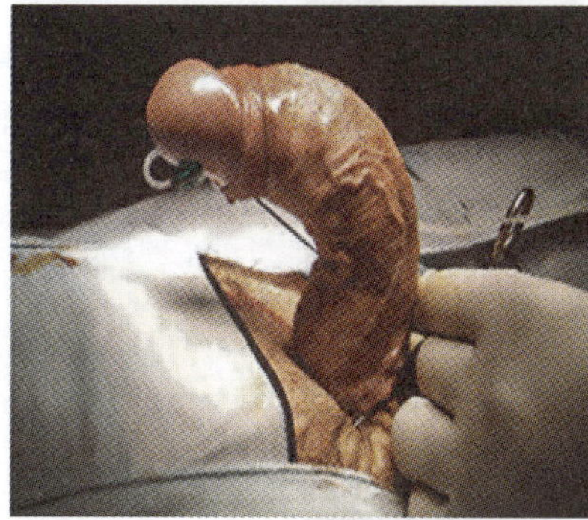

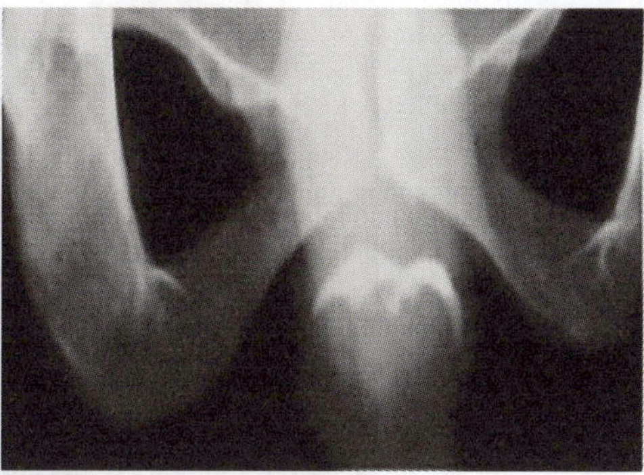

*Source:* Bailey and Love, 27th edition, page 1490.

a. What is the condition depicted here?
b. What is it associated with?
c. What are its clinical features (c/f)?
d. Name the surgery used for it.

**Q47. Answer the following:**

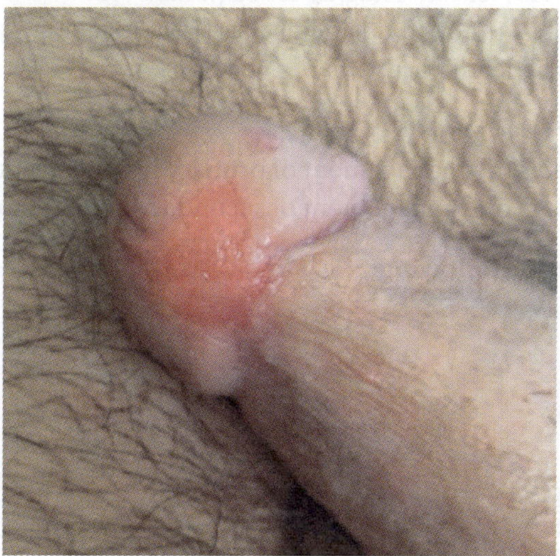

*Source:* Bailey and Love, 27th edition, page 1492.

a. What is the image depicted here?
b. Elaborate in brief.

**Q48. Answer the following:**

a. What is the picture depicted here?
b. What are its types?
c. What are the common sites?
d. What are its predisposing conditions?

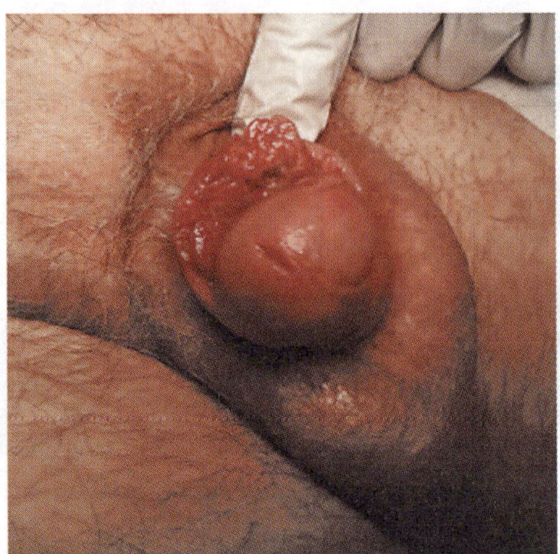

*Source:* Bailey and Love, 27th edition, page 1492.

**Q49. Cancer (Ca) penis**

a. What are its clinical features?
b. What is Jackson's staging for ca penis?
c. What is tumor, node, metastasis (TNM) staging?
d. Mcc of death in capenis?

**Q50. Cancer (Ca) penis**

a. What is the management of primary lesion in capensis?
b. What is the management of secondary nodal lesion?

**Q51. Answer the following:**

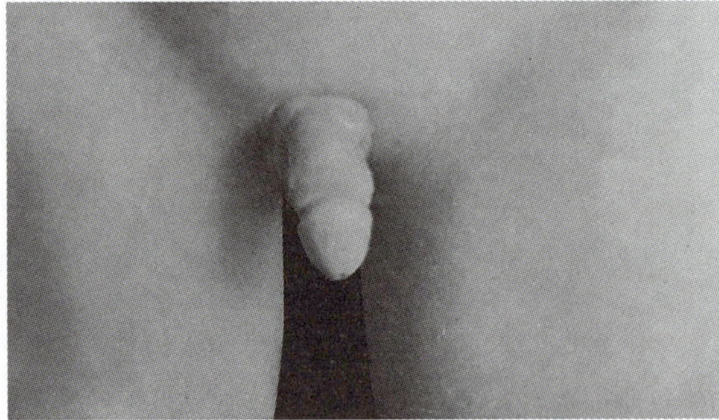

*Source:* Bailey and Love, 27th edition, page 1498.

a. What is this?
b. Describe the normal course of testes in fetal life to descend in scrotum from abdomen.
c. What is the difference between undescended testis (UDT) and ectopic testes?

**Q52. Answer the following:**

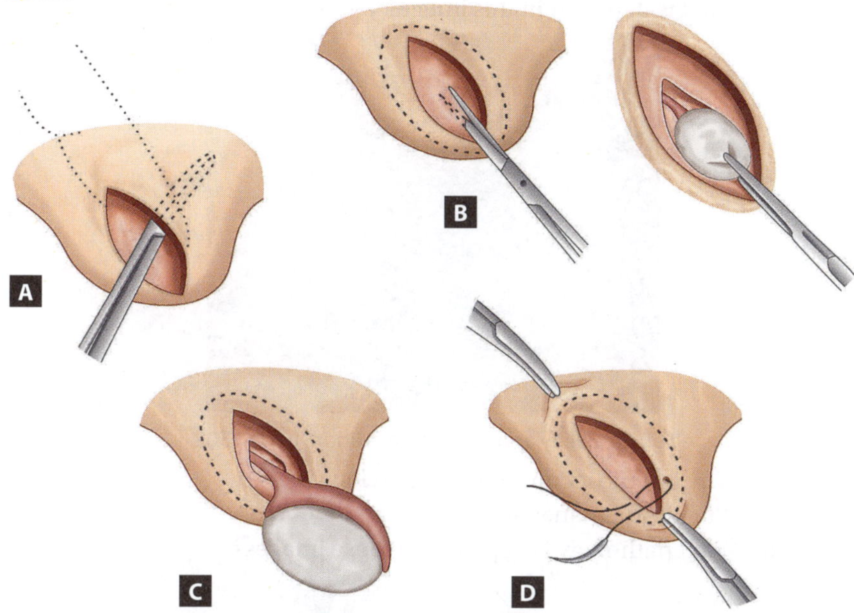


*Source:* Bailey and Love, 27th edition, page 1499.

a. What is the procedure shown here?
b. Describe the management of UDT?

**Q53. Answer the following:**

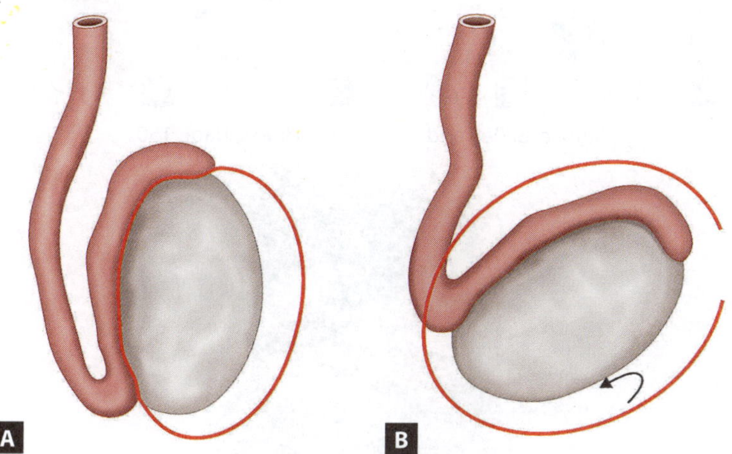


*Source:* Bailey and Love, 27th edition, page 1500.

a. What is the condition?
b. What is the etiopathogenesis?
c. What are the different signs?
d. What is its management?

**Q54. Answer the following:**

a. What is depicted in this image?

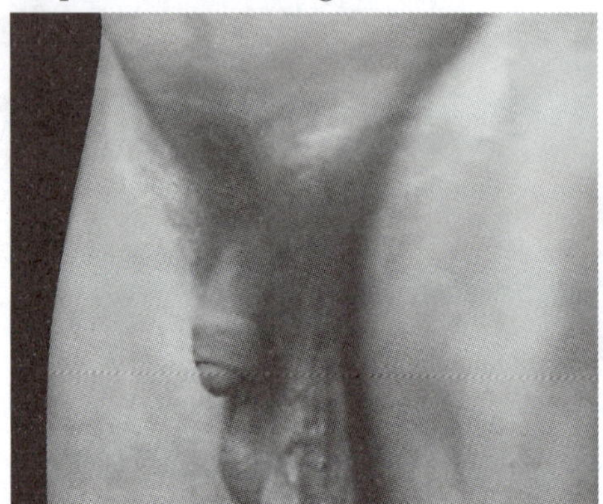

*Source:* Bailey and Love, 27th edition, page 1502.

b. Why is it most common (mc) on left side?

c. What is the management?

d. What pathology is depicted in these images?

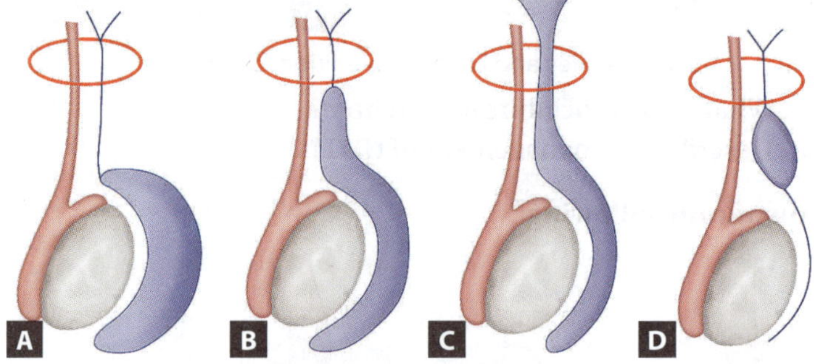


*Source:* Bailey and Love, 27th edition, page 1502.

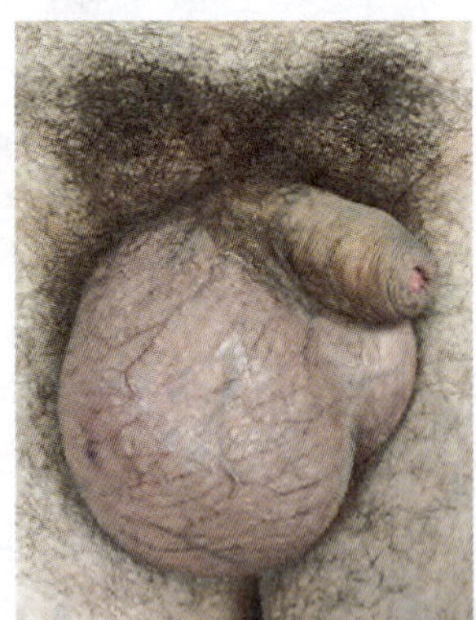

*Source:* Bailey and Love, 27th edition, page 1503.

e. What are its types?

f. What procedures are shown in these figures?

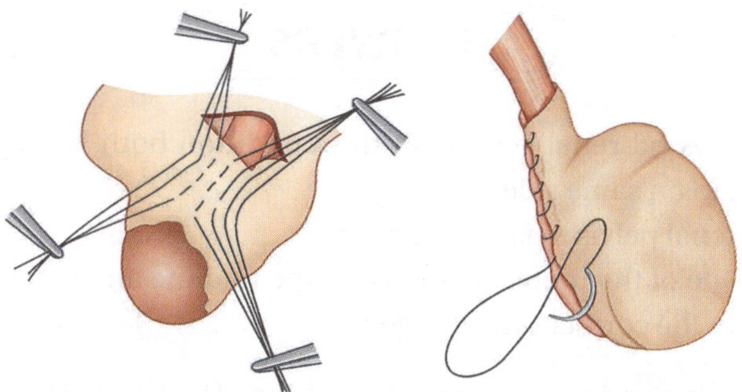

*Source:* Bailey and Love, 27th edition, pages 1503 and 1504.

**Q55. Answer the following:**

a. What pathology is shown in this image?

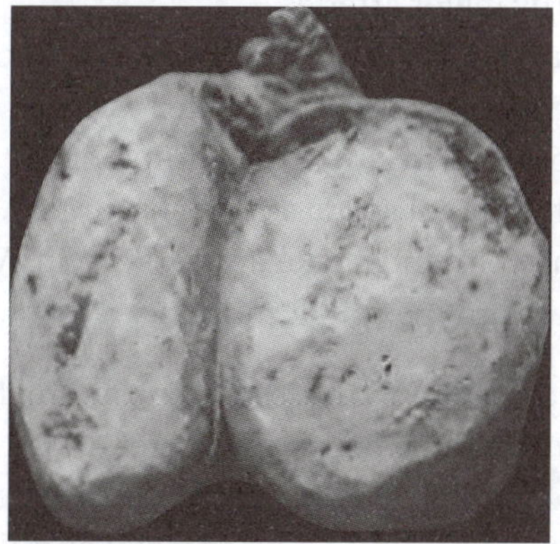

*Source:* Bailey and Love, 27th edition, page 1506.

b. What is the classification?
c. What are its predisposing factors?
d. What are its clinical features (c/f)?
e. What is the investigation?
f. What is the treatment?

**Q56. Describe the given images.**

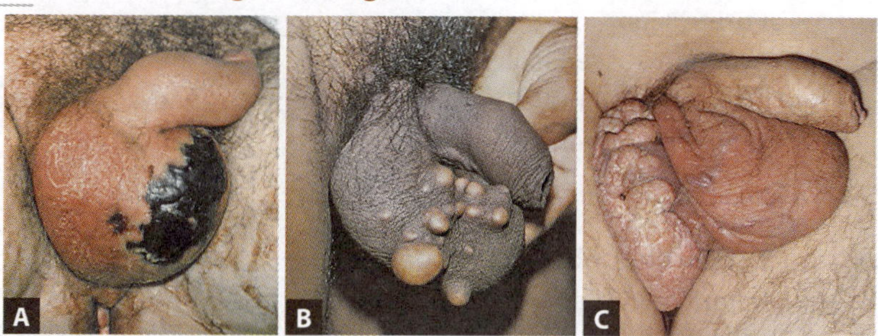


*Source:* Bailey and Love, 27th edition, pages 1510 and 1511.

## ANSWERS

**Ans. 1**
a. Crossed renal ectopia in this condition both kidneys are fused and on same side.
b. Renal pelvis to face anteriorly.
c. One of the ureter is crossed to the midline and enter the bladder on the correct side of trigone.

**Ans. 2**
a. This condition is horseshoe kidney (HSK). Incidence—1/1,000 people, most common (mc) in men. Most patients (pts) are asymptomatic. Pregnancy is not a contraindication for surgery but urinary infection is common for them. Blood supply of HSK is from nearby major arteries.
b. Ureters passing in front of the fused lower poles.
c. Prevented by the inferior mesenteric artery.
d. Reflux, obstruction, and stone formation.
e. Only in abdominal aortic aneurysm surgery.
f. Flower vase or hand shake appearance in IVP. Rarely, all calyces directed toward the spinal column.

**Ans. 3**
a. Duplication of ureter (most common anomaly of urinary system—duplication of renal pelvis and ureters).
b. Lower pole ureter is associated with vesicoureteral reflux (VUR), upper pole of ureter end ectopically and due to obstruction or dysplasia is often associated with (a/w) severe scarring of upper pole moiety.
c. Upper pole (ectopic) ureter's orifice inserts inferomedially to normal ureter.
d. Opening of ectopic ureter in boy—prostatic urethra girls—distal to external urethral sphincter or into the vagina. Hence, girls will have paradoxical urinary incontinence and continuous dribbling of urine seen.
e. Yoyo reflex—seen in ectopic ureter.
f. IVP is IOC and in IVP—drooping lily appearance is seen (ectopic ureter with ureterocele).

*This sign is also seen in neuroblastoma.*

**Ans. 4**
a. Ureterocele, Cobra head appearance.
b. Ureteric reimplant
c. Advance unilateral cases with hydronephrosis or pyonephrosis

**Ans. 5** a. Spider leg appearance found in autosomal dominant polycystic kidney disease (ADPKD) in IVP [IOC—computed tomography (CT)—kidneys, ureters, and bladder (KUB)].

b. Gene—*PKD1* and *PKD2* gene
Protein—polycystin-1 and polycystin-2, autosomal dominant pattern, bilateral condition (95%), no sex predilection (M = F) (but in end stage renal failure M>F).

c. On ultrasonography (USG) one kidney have three cysts or B/l kidney have two cysts each.

d. <40 years age—hypertension
>40 years age—kidney failure
Rarely, hematuria, renal stones

e. Uric acid stone/calcium oxalate stone or both

f. • Cysts seen in liver, spleen, pancreas, ovary [polycystic ovarian disease (PCOD)], arachnoid membrane, cyst not seen in lungs.
- Berry aneurysm—sudden headache
- Mitral valve prolapse—sudden cardiac failure
- Colonic diverticulosis—sudden abdominal pain
- Liver fibrosis

g. Rovsing operation (obsolete now)
Tolvaptan—vasopressin receptor antagonist, first approved drug for ADPKD. It increases urine excretion and increase sodium content in the body.
TOC—renal transplantation (until transplant they survive by dialysis)

**Ans. 6** a. *Escherichia coli* (also mc cause of prostatitis)

b. • Men >1,000,000 colony forming units (CFU/mL) (midstream urine).
- Female >1,000 CFU/mL (catheterized urine)

**Ans. 7** a. Golf hole ureter and blunting of calyx, found in genitourinary tuberculosis (TB)
Genitourinary TB—mc—kidney
Route of entry—hematogenous route

b. Earliest and mc features of renal TB—increased frequency (DD for increased frequency—[diabetes mellitus (DM), UTI, TB)].

*Diagnosis:*
- On examination of urine in renal TB—sterile pyuria [bacteria is absent but white blood cell (WBC) count is increased] (sterile pyuria is also found in *Neisseria gonorrhoeae* and mycoplasma genitalium infection)

- Early morning urine specimen for 3 days—Acid fast bacilli to diagnose TB.
- IOC to diagnose early TB
  - Earliest feature in TB kidney—blunting of calyx
  - CT pyelogram (IOC) for early TB.

c. • Cement or putty kidney
- Golf hole ureter
- Thimble small bladder

Treatment—resection and reconstruction (optimum after 6–12 weeks after ATT starts)

**Ans. 8** a. VUR (IOC is MCU)

b. Longitudinal bladder muscle deficiency

c. • Grade 1—reflux into the nondilated ureter
- Grade 2—reflux into the nondilated ureter and pelvis
- Grade 3—reflux is a/w mild-to-moderate dilatation on IVP (blunting of calyx seen)
- Grade 4—additional blunting of fornices with dilated ureter.
- Grade 5—absent papillary impressions.

d. • Grade 1 and 2—no surgery, only medical treatment (for UTI—antibiotics).
- Grade 3, 4, and 5—surgery (reimplantation of ureter).

**Ans. 9** a. Renal cyst

b. Bosniak classification of renal cyst

Category
- 1—simple cyst
- 2—benign cyst

1 and 2 do not require follow-up images.
2F—complex cyst (requires follow-up images)
3—indeterminate cyst
4—malignant cystic mass

c. 1 and 2—no risk of malignancy—no intervention required
2F—<5% risk of malignancy—no intervention required
3—biopsy is done
4—resection

**Ans. 10** a. 1

b. • A is calcium oxalate crystal—bipyramidal/envelope shaped, mc type of crystal in urine.
- B is calcium oxalate monohydrate crystal—dumbbell shaped or hour glass shaped crystals.
- C is uric acid crystal—multifaceted, irregular plates, rosettes like

- D cystine crystal—hexagonal, benzene ring like
- E struvite—coffin lid shaped
- F brushite—needle shaped

**Ans. 11** a.
- Idiopathic calcium urolithiasis;
- Hypercalcemic disorder;
- Renal tubular syndromes;
- Uric acid lithiasis;
- Enzyme disorders;
- Secondary urolithiasis; and
- Other factors

b. Calcium oxalate stone

c. <10 mm—no treatment needed, fluid intake >2.5 liter/day.
*Restrict:* Protein, salt, and oxalate diet
- Increase consumption—Calcium supplements
- Juice—Cranberry juice is used in management of renal stones

d. Drug causing renal stone (mnemonic—TIMES-CALL)
- T—Triamterene
- I—Indinavir
- M—Mg trisilicate (Antacids)
- E—Ephedrine
- S—Septran
- C—Ciprofloxacin
- A—Acetazolamide
- L—Loop diuretic
- L—Laxatives containing magnesium (Mg)

**Ans. 12** *Markings:*
1. Ureteropelvic junction
2. Crossing the iliac artery
3. Juxtaposition of vas deferens and broad ligament
4. Entering the bladder wall
5. Ureteric orifice

**Ans. 13** a.
- Ureteroscopy guided dormia basket ureteric stone retrieval.
- Basket introduced past stone.
- Opened
- Enclosing stone, ready for withdrawal.

b. Ureteric stone retrieval

c. Lithotripsy employing different energy source (ultrasound, electrohydraulic—rarely used these days, laser, and electrokinetic).

Stones can also be fragmented using mechanical disintegration using the LithoClast. Examples are extracorporeal shock wave lithotripsy (ESWL) and percutaneous nephrolithotomy or stone extraction (PCNL).

**Ans. 14** a. Image of ultrasound of a hydronephrotic kidney.
b. A: artery; C: calyces; P: pelvis.

**Ans. 15** a. Anderson–Hynes pyeloplasty
b. In congenital pelviureteric junction (puj) obstruction

**Ans. 16** a. Renal injury/renal trauma
Grading of renal injury—
- *Grade I:* Contusion or nonenlarging subcapsular perirenal hematoma, and no laceration.
- *Grade II:* Superficial laceration <1 cm without extension into the renal pelvis or collecting system (no evidence of urine extravasation). Nonexpanding perirenal hematoma confined to retroperitoneum.
- *Grade III:* Laceration >1 cm without extension into the renal pelvis or collecting system (no evidence of urine extravasation).
- *Grade IV:*
    - Laceration extends to renal pelvis or urinary extravasation.
    - *Vascular:* Injury to main renal artery or vein with contained hemorrhage.
    - Segmental infarctions without associated lacerations.
    - Expanding subcapsular hematomas compressing the kidney.
- *Grade V:*
    - Shattered kidney
    - *Avulsion of renal hilum:* Devascularization of a kidney hilar injury
    - Ureteropelvic avulsions
    - Complete laceration or thrombus of the main renal artery or vein.

b. Penetrating injuries
- Gross hematuria
- Shock in combination with microscopic hematuria
- *Children:* in whom the kidneys are much lower and less well protected

c. If this occurs, then an on-table intravenous urogram is required. If significant extravasation, nonfunction, poor opacification, or caliceal distortion is found then renal exploration is indicated. An expanding or pulsatile retroperitoneal hematoma should be explored but only after vascular control has been achieved.

**Ans. 17** a. Boari operation (In this surgery a strip of bladder wall is fashioned into a tube to bridge the gap between the cut ureter and the bladder.)

b. For repairing a damaged ureter

c. *Following are the methods for repairing a damaged ureter:*
- If there is no loss of length—Spatulation and end-to-end anastomosis without tension.
- If there is little loss of length—Mobilize kidney, Psoas hitch of bladder, and Boari operation.
- If there is marked loss of length—Transureteroureterostomy, interposition of isolated bowel loop, or mobilized appendix, nephrectomy.

d. The disadvantage of implanting the ureter in end-to-side into the contralateral ureter (a transureteroureterostomy) is that risk of converting a unilateral injury into a bilateral one

**Ans. 18** a. The staging RCC is based on size, position, and lymph node involvement:
- *Stage I:* Tumor 7 cm in the largest dimension, limited to the kidney.
- *Stage II:* Tumor >7 cm in the largest dimension, limited to the kidney.
- *Stage III:* Tumor in the major veins or adrenal gland with intact Gerota's fascia, or regional lymph nodes involved.
- *Stage IV:* Tumor beyond Gerota's fascia

b. Risk factors for RCC include:
- Age;
- Sex;
- Obesity;
- Hypertension; and
- Cigarette smoking

c. IOC—Contrast-enhanced computed tomography (CECT) whole abdomen

Treatment (T/T)—Radical nephrectomy partial nephrectomy (nephron sparing procedure)
- Structures removed
  - Kidney
  - Adrenal gland
  - Perinephric pad of fat
  - Regional nodes
  - Ureter
  - Gerota's fascia
- Indication of partial nephrectomy (nephron sparing procedure)
  - T1—<7 cm (even with normal opposite kidney)
  - Single functioning kidney

- VHL mutation—B/L RCC cases
- Renal failure (DM, HTN)

d. • Hematuria
- Pain
- Palpable loin mass

e. • Increased erythrocyte sedimentation rate (ESR) (M/C)
- Hypertension (Second m/c)
- Anemia (Third m/c)
- Hypercalcemia (5%)
- Polycythemia (3%)
- Stauffer's syndrome—nonmetastatic liver enzyme elevation
- Other features—Neuropathy, amyloidosis, pyrexia of unknown origin (PUO), and weight loss

**Ans. 19** a. Ectopia vesicae (bladder exstrophy) in a man. A drop of urine shown in arrow is seen at the left ureteric orifice, the corona gland is being retracted by threads.

b. The basic defect in exstrophy bladder is abnormal over development of the cloacal membrane and its rupture.

c. • Male
  - Umbilical hernia
  - Inguinal hernia
  - Epispadias
  - Undescended testis
- Female
  - Umbilical hernia
  - Epispadias
  - Split Clitoris
  - Wide open pelvis (duck like waddling gait)
  - Wide labia
  - Urinary incontinence

d. Plastic surgery reconstruction

**Ans. 20** a. Above image shows intraperitoneal rupture of bladder (20%) (intraperitoneal extravasation of urine) (mc due to direct blow in the dome of distended bladder)
- Cause uremic peritonitis
- Immediate surgery needed
- Below image shows extraperitoneal rupture of bladder/ extraperitoneal extravasation of urine (80%)
- Due to fracture of pelvis or blunt trauma injury or surgical damage.

- Superficial extravasation of urine seen with urine extravasated from nipple level to Holden's line level.
- Catheter inserted immediately.
- Wait and watch—gradually the injury heal.

b. IOC for bladder injury—Retrograde cystography
- Management of bladder trauma
- Extravesical injury—catheter drainage for 10 days.
- Intraperitoneal injury—laparotomy, repair and bladder drainage

c. i. The bladder may be injured in:
  - Inguinal or femoral herniotomy
  - Hysterectomy
  - Excision of the rectum

ii. If the injury is recognized, the bladder must be repaired and catheter drainage maintained for 7 days. If it is not recognized, the treatment is similar to that of rupture of the bladder.

**Ans. 21** a. The most common causes of acute retention
- Male
  - Bladder outlet obstruction (the most common cause)
  - Urethral stricture
  - Acute urethritis or prostatitis
  - Phimosis
- Female
  - Retroverted gravid uterus
  - Bladder neck obstruction (rare)
- Both
  - Blood clot
  - Urethral calculus
  - Rupture of the urethra
  - Neurogenic (injury or disease of the spinal cord)
  - Smooth muscle cell dysfunction associated with ageing
  - Fecal impaction
  - Anal pain (hemorrhoidectomy)
  - Intensive postoperative analgesic treatment
  - Some drugs
  - Spinal anesthesia

b.
- No urine is passed for several hours.
- Pain is present.
- The bladder is visible, palpable, tender, and dull to percussion.
- Potential neurological causes should be excluded by checking reflexes in the lower limbs and perianal sensation.

c. Treatment is to pass a fine urethral catheter (14F—French gauge is defined as the circumference in millimeter) and arrange urological management. Occasionally, in postoperative retention a warm bath can help.

**Ans. 22** a. Secondary tumors of the bladder are common and most frequently arise from the sigmoid and rectum, the prostate, the uterus or the ovaries, although bronchial neoplasms may also spread to the bladder.

b. Papillary tumor with daughter implantation ("kiss" cancer) endoscopic photograph of a pTa bladder tumor about to be resected.

c. *M/c type:* Transitional cell cancer (90%)
   - 2nd m/c—SCC
   - 3rd m/c—Adenocarcinoma (arises from urachal remnants)

**Ans. 23** a. M/C risk factor—smoking
   - Schistosomiasis
   - Occupational
     - β-naphthylamine (coal)
     - Diaminobiphenyl (aniline)
     - Aminobiphenyl
     - Nitrophenyl

b.
   - Stones
   - Schistosomiasis
   - Special diseases—diverticula diseases, long-term catheters

c.
   - Textile workers;
   - Dye workers;
   - Tyre rubber and cable workers;
   - Petrol workers;
   - Leather workers;
   - Shoe manufacturers and cleaners;
   - Painters;
   - Hairdressers;
   - Lorry drivers;
   - Drill press operators;
   - Chemical workers;
   - Rodent exterminators and sewage workers

d.
   - 2-naphthylamine;
   - 4-aminobiphenyl;
   - Benzidine
   - Chlornaphazine
   - 4-chloro-o-toluidine
   - o-Toluidine
   - 4,4′-methylene bis (2-choloroaniline);

- Methylenedianiline;
- Benzidine-derived azo dyes

**Ans. 24** a.
- M/c presentation—painless terminal hematuria
- M/c site—Dome and lateral wall of bladder
- Cancer from anterior wall producing spread to posterior wall is known as Kissing cancer.
- Balkan nephropathy is a/w an increased incidence of upper tract urothelial tumors.
- Adenocarcinoma of bladder arises in fundus part or area of glandular metaplasia.
- Mc site for superficial tumor are trigone and lateral wall of bladder.

b.
- *Urine examination:* Screening test for
  - Nuclear matrix protein (NMP)-2 protein
  - Mini-chromosome maintenance (MCM) protein
- IOC for staging—MRI > CECT abdomen/pelvis
- IOC for diagnosis—cystoscopic biopsy

c. Staging
- pTa—noninvasive papillary cancer
- p Tis—Cancer in situ
- p T1—Subepithelial connective tissue
- p T2—Muscularis propria
- p T3—Perivesical tissue
- p T4—Adjacent organs—Prostate, seminal vesicles, vagina, and abdominal wall.

  N0—no lymph node present

  N1—1-3 lymph node present

  MC lymph node involvement/sentinel node for both bladder and prostatic cancer—obturator node.

**Ans. 25** a.
- Mitomycin-C
- Doxorubicin
- Thiotepa
- BCG (best)

b. Paste RRM notes page 384 diagram

**Ans. 26** a. *Radical cystectomy:* Structures removed
- Bladder + fat
- Prostate + seminal vesicles
- Uterus + cervix + fallopian tube + anterior vaginal wall
- ± Urethrectomy
- Pelvic lymphadenectomy

b. • In ileal conduit; the ureters are spatulated and anastomosed to ileum end to side (insert);
- Ureterosigmoidostomy;
- Ileal neobladder with antireflux long afferent limb.

c. For diversion of urine

d. • Ileal conduit
    - M/c type
    - M/c complication ureteroilial stricture
- Colon conduit
    - Drained into sigmoid colon
    - M/c complication—infection
    - Risk of malignancy++
- Important prerequisite for this procedure—Patient must be able to hold 200 mL saline in rectum with continence.

Extra edge—
- Neobladder can also be created if urethra is not involved using ileum.
- Continent urinary diversion procedure—Kock's Ileostomy (Ileum made like a valve).
- Mitrofanoff procedure—Appendix can be used as a drainage of urine procedure from bladder.

*Conduit associated metabolic complications:*
- Ileal—Metabolic acidosis + hyperchloremia
- Jejunum—Metabolic acidosis + hypochloremia
- Colon—Metabolic acidosis + hyperchloremia
- Stomach—Metabolic alkalosis + hyperchloremia—stomach conduit is used in renal failure patients.

**Ans. 27** a. Mitrofanoff procedure

b. Used for continent diversion of urine

**Ans. 28** a. • *Image A:* Stone on a vaginal sling that had eroded into the bladder.
- *Image B:* Smooth uric acid-type stones.
- *Image C:* A rough bladder stone.

b. • Primary bladder stone
    - Dropped from above (from kidney)
    - Common type is calcium oxalate stone
- Secondary Bladder stone
- Secondary to some pathologies such as bladder outlet obstruction (BOO), Benign prostatic hyperplasia (BPH), and stenosis
- Formed in bladder itself

- This is the most common Bladder stone
- Ammonium urate is the MC secondary bladder stone.
- The calcium apoplexy (coating of calcium over the ammonium urate stone) results in radio opaque.

c. Extracorporeal shock wave lithotripsy (ESWL)
- Percutaneous nephrolithotomy (PCNL)
- Retrograde intrarenal surgery (RIRS) (via ureter the stone removed from kidney)
- Open nephrolithotomy—Opening the kidney along the Brodel's line and remove the Stone
- Open pyelolithotomy—Opening the renal pelvis and removing the stone

**Ans. 29** a. ESWL
- Passing Piezo electric waves and breaking the stones.
- *Indication:*
  - <1.5 cm size
  - Mainly done for stone in kidney, pelvis, upper ureter (cannot use it for lower ureteric stone [due to (d/t) pelvic brim bone hindrance])
- *Contraindications:*
  - Absolute—pregnancy, bleeding diathesis
  - *Relative:*
    - Obstruction/distally
    - Infection
    - Hematuria
    - Renal dysfunction
- *Complications:*
  - Hematuria
  - Incomplete clearance
  - If stone >1.5 cm a rare complication known as steinstrasse (stone street) happens. To prevent this problem happening, we must keep a 20 cm double J stent before ESWL.

b. PCNL
- Indication
  - Stone >2 cm
  - Infected
  - Obstructed
  - Cysteine
  - Failed ESWL
- Anatomical abnormality—Calyceal diverticulum containing stones obese patient.
- Lower calyceal stone (its less likely to pass after ESWL)

- Stone composition—struvite stone
- *Procedure:*
  - Transcostal approach
  - Subcostal approach
  - We insert a guidewire under fluoroscopic guidance—we dilate the tract and insert the nephroscope via the tract and remove the stone.
- *Complications:*
  - Bleeding
  - Sepsis
  - Perforation of bowel
  - Transcostal approach—Pleural injury and hydrothorax can happen.
  - Subcostal approach—Duodenal injury, colon injury, and liver and spleen injury.
  - Injury to renal artery/vein/inferior vena cava (IVC)
- *Staghorn stone:*
  - Sandwich technique—ESWL followed by PCNL
  - If this technique is not mentioned—go with PCNL

**Ans. 30** a. Skene's tubules open on either side of the female urethra, are the homologue of the prostate.

b. *Basic anatomy:* Mc Neal's three surgical zones
1. Transition zone
2. Central zone
3. Peripheral zone

In BPH—Transition zone is more involved
In cancer—Peripheral zone is more involved

c. *Five lobes in prostate:*
- Two lateral lobes
- One median lobe
- One posterior lobe
- One anterior lobe

BPH arises from median lobes.
Cancer arises from posterior lobe.
(Remember: Cancer—P-P: peripheral zone, posterior lobe)

**Ans. 31** a. Benign prostatic hyperplasia leads to bladder outlet obstruction (BOO).

b. • Old age (62)
- Symptoms of bladder outlet obstruction; frequency of urine and nocturia and dribbling of urine.
- Uroflowmetry value of BOO.
- PSA value >4 ng/mL

**Ans. 32** a.
- Mc in old age
- Symptoms of BPH is given by bladder outlet obstruction.
- Symptoms associated with bladder outlet obstruction irritative symptoms.
- Increased frequency (MC symptom)
  - Nocturia
  - Urgency
  - Hesitancy
  - Hematuria
- Obstructive symptoms
  - Dribbling
  - Thin stream urine
  - Retention

b. IOC to detect bladder outlet obstruction—uroflometry
- For a voiding volume of >200 mL a peak flow rate of >15 mL/sec is normal.
- Flow rate <10 mL/sec is low
- Voiding pressure at <60 cm $H_2O$ is normal
- Voiding pressure >80 cm $H_2O$ is high
- *USG abdomen:*
  - Prostate enlargement
  - Postvoid residual urine
  - Bilateral (B/l) hydroureteronephrosis

**Ans. 33** a. Medical treatment

α-1a blockers
- Tamsulosin
- Decreases smooth muscle tone
- Quick action

  Other drugs such as prazosin and terazosin will cause postural hypotension.

5 α reductase inhibitors
- Finasteride 5 mg
- Slow action—needs 6 months
- Decreases the volume (up to 40%)

  Remember finasteride is used in 1 mg dosage

b. Indication of surgery
- *Retention*
  - Acute
  - Chronic [Postvoid residual (PVR) >200 mL]
- *Complications*
  - Diverticula
  - B/L hydronephrosis (HUN)

- Bladder stone
- Hematuria
- Urinary tract infection (UTI)
- Uroflometry value
  - <10 mL/s
  - >80 cm $H_2O$

**Ans. 34** a. Transurethral resection of the prostate (TURP) (gold standard) (1)
Open
- Retropubic—Millin's operation (2)
- Transvesical—Freyer's operation (3)
- Perineal—Young operation (4)

b. TURP is done here
For transurethral resection of the prostate the resectoscope is inserted transurethrally. Electric current is passed through a diathermy loop at the end of the instrument. The surgeon moves this back and forth to create a cavity using diathermy to cauterize as they go. The resultant chips are washed out of the bladder intermittently throughout the procedure. A visual image of the operative field is transmitted through lenses running in the middle of the resectoscope. Around this lens, irrigating fluid is instilled and flows out, washing blood away from the operative field. The procedure is complete when an adequate channel has been created through the prostate.

c. *Immediate postoperative complications:*
- Hemorrhage—Usually arises from Floch arteries arising from inferior vesical arteries
- TUR syndrome—patient confused, irrelevant words, if we use distilled water there is high chance of dilutional hyponatremia and water intoxication.

*Delayed complication:*
- Bladder neck stenosis
- Retrograde ejaculation (m/c complication overall) due to IUS injury
- Incontinence due to EUS injury

**Ans. 35** a. The prostate is biopsied by two routes. The biopsy needle inserted through skin between the scrotum and anus (perineum) or the rectum. In both cases the passage of the needle is usually guided to the correct place with transrectal ultrasonography (USG). Transrectal USG is not good for sampling the anterior prostate, particularly when the prostate is large. Transperineal biopsy is gaining popularity as an alternative to conventional transrectal biopsy.

b. For prostate biopsy in a suspected case of prostate cancer.

**Ans. 36** a. *Most common type of stones:*
- *MC stone in prostate:* Calcium phosphate
- *MC stone in kidney:* Calcium oxalate
- *MC stone in bladder:* Ammonium urate
- *MC stone in salivary gland:* Calcium carbonate
- *MC stone in gall bladder:* Mixed stones

b. Corpora amylacea are tiny calcified lamellated bodies found in the glandular alveoli of the prostates of elderly men and apes, but not in the prostates of animals lower in the phylogenetic scale than anthropoids. Corpora amylacea are probably the forerunners of endogenous prostatic calculi.

**Ans. 37** a. *Screening protocol:* Digital rectal examination + PSA

b. Prostate specific antigen
- *Normal value:* <4 ng/L
- *Men 50–69 year:* >4 ng/L—Indication for biopsy
- *>10 ng/L:* Localized Cancer +
- *>35 ng/L:* Metastatic cancer prostate +

Other values:
- PSA velocity
- PSA density
- Old-acid phosphatase

c. *Biopsy methods:*
- Transrectal ultrasound (TRUS) guided biopsy
  - Traditional
  - Increased risk of infection, septicemia, bleeding, etc.
  - Prophylactic antibiotics required
  - Less areas of biopsy possible
- Transperitoneal template biopsy (TPTBP)
  - Detect lesion in anterior aspect of prostate
  - 36 biopsy possible
  - No infection risk is there
  - Helps to evaluate TRUS guided negative biopsy case
- IOC to stage prostatic cancer—multiparametric magnetic resonance imaging (mpMRI) > contrast-enhanced computed tomography (CECT) abdomen/pelvis.

  The mpMRI has a crucial role in the detection and localization of cancer in men with a persistently elevated PSA but negative previous TRUS biopsy.
- MRI
  - Is used to stage many urological cancers
  - Multiparametric MRI has a significant role in the assessment of men with suspected prostate cancer.

- mpMRI is increasingly used prior to prostate biopsy
- Prebiopsy MRI permits selection of biopsy technique (TRUS v. TPTBP)
- Prebiopsy MRI assists with targeting of biopsies
- *First node involved in cancer prostate:* Obturator nodes

**Ans. 38** a. T-staging

- *T1:*
  - T1a—<5% of TURP specimen shows cancer
  - T1b—>5% of TURP specimen shows cancer
  - T1c—PSA increase
- *T2:*
  - T2a—Involved one lobe
  - T2b—Involved both lobes
- *T3:* Seminal vesicle; involved beyond the capsule
- T4: Spread to rectum, bladder, pelvic bone
- *T1 and T2:* Early disease
- *T3 and T4:* Locally advanced

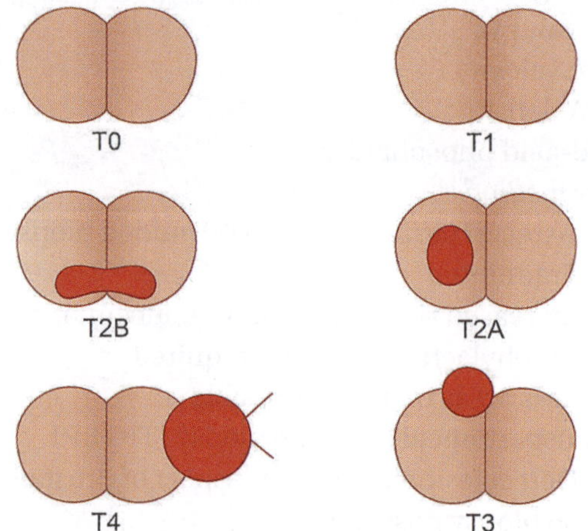


b.
- T1, T2—Radical prostatectomy
  - <70 years
  - Fit for surgery
- >70 years, unfit—T1/T2 prostatic cancer—wait and watch
- T3, T4, and M1—Androgen ablation (First step)
- *Androgen ablation methods:*
  - *Gold standard method for androgen ablation:* Subscapular orchidectomy or conventional orchidectomy + testicular prosthesis kept.
  - *If not willing for orchidectomy:* Medical castration methods—Luteinizing hormone-releasing hormone (LHRH) agonist such as flutamide; leuprolide, and goserelin

c. Gleason score—
   - Grade 1—Small uniform glands
   - Grade 2—More space between glands and increase in stroma
   - Grade 3—Distinct infiltration of cell margin
   - Grade 4—Irregular masses of neoplastic cells
   - Grade 5—Lack of glandular pattern
   - Old score—grade 1 (well differentiated)—grade 5 (poorly differentiated)
   - *New Gleason score:* Extends from grade 1 to grade 10
   - MC site of metastasis—Lumbar vertebra; More of osteoblastic secondaries

**Ans. 39** a. *Hypospadias:* Occurs in around 1 in 200–300 male live births and is the most common congenital abnormality of the urethra.

b. Three characteristic features. The external meatus opens on the underside of the penis anywhere from just short of the normal site as far back as the perineum, while the ventral aspect of the prepuce is poorly developed (the "hooded prepuce") and there is usually a ventral deformity of the erect penis (chordee).

c. • Associated cryptorchidism
   - Associated indirect inguinal hernia

d. Hypospadias is classified according to the position of the meatus **(Figure 79.2)**.
   - Glanular hypospadias (mc type). The ectopic meatus is placed on the glans penis, but proximal to the normal site of the external meatus, which is marked by a blind pit. Occasionally, the two are connected by a channel.
   - Coronal hypospadias. The meatus is placed at the junction of the underside of the glans and the body of the penis.
   - Penile and penoscrotal hypospadias. The meatus is on the underside of the penile shaft.
   - Perineal hypospadias. This is the rarest and most severe abnormality. The scrotum is bifid and the urethra opens between its two halves. In children with severe hypospadias, it is important to consider disorders of sexual development, which are usually associated with testicular maldescent and micropenis.

   The more severe varieties of hypospadias represent an absence of the urethra and corpus spongiosum distal to the ectopic opening. The absent structures are represented by a fibrous cord, which deforms the erect penis in a downward direction (chordee).

e. • Age group for surgery—6 months–1 year
- Circumcision is contraindicated
- Old method of surgery—Dennis brown 2 stage
- New and used procedure—Meatal advancement glanuloplasty incorporation (MAGPI)
- Order of reconstruction of MAGPI
    - Orthoplasty (Penile straightening)
    - Urethroplasty
    - Glanuloplasty
    - Meatoplasty
    - Scrotoplasty
    - Skin reconstruction and circumcision is done as last step

The most common procedure for distal hypospadias is the "tubularized incised plate" urethroplasty, while techniques that utilize the foreskin are commonly used for more proximal hypospadias.

**Ans. 40** a. Depicted condition urethral diverticulum.
- Cystoscopic appearance of a urethral diverticulum, normal urethra can be seen to extend superiorly to the urethral sphincter, while the blind ending diverticulum is seen inferiorly.
- Urethrogram showing a urethral diverticulum

b. Urethral diverticulum

This is usually congenital and represents a partial duplication of the urethra. Acquired cases are uncommon but are sometimes seen as a result of increased intraurethral pressure behind a stricture or due to stone or longstanding presence of foreign body.

**Ans. 41** a. Seldinger technique of supra pubic catheterization (SPC) in figure.

b. The percutaneous puncture of the bladder followed by passage of a guidewire into the bladder followed by dilatation of the track over the guidewire (b) allowing placement of a catheter into the bladder (c)
- Urethral injuries
- Urethral obstruction
- Bladder neck masses
- Prostate cancer

**Ans. 42** a. • Urethroscopic appearance of a urethral stricture.
- Ascending urethrogram showing urethral stricture of the bulbar urethra.

b. The common causes of urethral stricture are:
- Inflammatory
  - Secondary to urethritis
  - Secondary to balanitis xerotica obliterans (BXO)
- Traumatic
  - Bulbar urethral injury
  - Pelvic fracture urethral disruption injury
- Iatrogenic
  - Secondary to urethral instrumentation including catheterization and transurethral prostatectomy
  - Secondary to radical prostatectomy
  - Secondary to radiotherapy for prostate cancer
- Idiopathic

c.
- If stricture is short and single—we can use dilators
- If stricture is multiple and long—we plan stricturoplasty using Buccal mucosa

**Ans. 43** a. Four parts of urethra:
1. Most dilatable part—prostatic urethra
2. Least dilatable part—membranous urethra
3. Anterior urethra—penile and bulbar
4. Most narrow part of urethra—external urethral meatus

b. *Clinical feature of urethral injuries:*
- Blood at urethral meatus
- Retention of Bladder

c.
- Membranous urethral injury
- Mainly due to fracture pelvis
- *Per rectal examination:* Prostate—high lying and floating (Vermooten sign)
- The above examination is not advised in latest guidelines of ATLS
- Deep extravasation +++ of blood seen
- Bladder shape—Inverted tear drop
- Bulbar urethral injury
  - Mainly due to straddle injury
  - Typical presentation of urethral injury seen.

d. *Steps to be done in urethral injury*
- Never put Foley's catheter as it will cause more damage of the urethra
- Put suprapubic catheter (SPC)
- Via SPC we can do descending cystourethrogram/micturating cystourethrogram
- Other investigation—Retrograde urethrogram (via Foley's inserted only up to penile urethra and push contrast)

*Management:*
- Wait for 6–8 weeks after SPC insertion
- Gradually, the urethral injury goes for stricture
- If stricture is short and single—we can use dilators
- If stricture is multiple and long—we plan stricturoplasty using Buccal mucosa

**Ans. 44** a. Phimosis secondary to balanitis xerotica obliterans. (a) White and thickened appearance of the preputial skin, (b) with a constriction such that the foreskin cannot be retracted.

b. In true phimosis, there is scarring of the prepuce such that it will not retract without fissuring of the foreskin **(Figure 79.13)**.

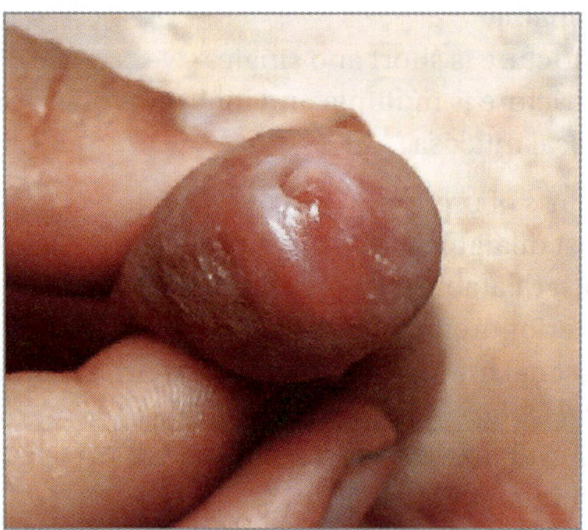

- Physiological phimosis
- Causes of acquired phimosis
    - Inflammation
    - Diabetes
    - BXO
    - Cancer
    - Trauma
    - Surgery is done for all acquired cases

c.
- Congenital phimosis
    - Physiological adhesions up to 6 years
    - No need to operate before 6 years
    - Wait up to 5–6 years
- Acquired phimosis
    - Inflammation
    - Diabetes
    - BXO

- Cancer
- Trauma
- Surgery is done for all acquired cases

**Ans. 45** a. The Plastibell (Hollister) device for circumcision in infants. (a) The foreskin is freed and retracted. (b) After the Plastibell device has been slipped into place over the glans penis, the foreskin is ligated over the groove of the bell and redundant foreskin is cut away. (c) This shows the completed operation.

- Less than 1 year child with severe ballooning of prepuce will need surgery as this is causing severe obstruction.
- Less than 1 year children can be operated by a Hollister/ Plastibell device—Sutureless method.

Figure showing (a–e) stages in circumcision

b. *Circumcision indications:*

- M/c performed for cultural reasons
- Is not indicated for failure of retraction caused by congenital adhesions between the glans penis and the prepuce
- Indicated when there is true phimosis
- Never use monopolar diathermy when performing circumcision

*Types of circumcision*

- Neonatal—at birth practiced by Jews, 100% protective of cancer penis.
- Infantile—<1 year practiced by Muslims, decreases incidence of cancer of penis.
- *Adults:* No relation with cancer.

**Ans. 46** a. Dorsal deformity of the erect penis that is typical of Peyronie's disease—Penile calcification in Peyronie's disease

b. Associated with Dupytrens, retroperitoneal fibrosis, Riedels

c. Clinical features

- Painful, persistent erection with deformity in a middle-aged man.
- Penis gets curved (dorsal curvature usually)

d. Nesbit procedure is done electively to straighten the penis.

**Ans. 47** a. Penile intraepithelial neoplasia affecting the glans penis.

b. PeIN typically seen as a red cutaneous patch on the penis. When it occurs on the glans penis, it is called as erythroplasia of Queyrat and when it occurs on the shaft of the penis it is called Bowen's disease.

**Ans. 48** a. A SC arising from the inner aspect of the prepuce.

b. M/c type: SCC
  - *Rare types:*
    - BCC
    - Adenocarcinoma (arises from Tyson glands)
    - Melanoma
    - Kaposi

c. • Common sites
    - Glans penis (50%)
    - Preputial skin (20%)
    - Other places—Shaft, corona glandis, etc.

d. • Predisposing condition
    - M/c—Smegma
  - *Other risk factors:*
    - Leukoplakia
    - BXO
    - Buschke Lowenstein tumor (caused by human papilloma virus)
  - Cancer in situ of Glans—Erythroplasia of Queyrat
  - Cancer in situ of shaft of penis—Bowen's disease

**Ans. 49** a. Clinical features
  - Fungating growth
  - Foul smelling odor [due to (d/t) secondary infection]
  - Sentinel node of cancer penis—Cabana node (superficial inguinal node)

b. Clinical staging (Jackson's staging)
  - I—Glans and perpuce involvement
  - II—Shaft involved
  - III—Node +
  - IV—Metastasis +

c. TNM Staging
  - T1—<2 cm growth
  - T2—2-5 cm
  - T3—>5 cm can invade corpus spongiosum, cavernosum, urethra (usually urethra not involved due to transitional epithelium inside)
  - T4—adjacent structure
  - N1: Single LN +
  - N2: Multiple LN (unilateral/bilateral)
  - N3: Deep inguinal/iliac node

d. One of the most common cause of death—Erosion of femoral artery by the nodes

**Ans. 50** a. Management of primary lesion;

- Nonsurgical
    - Radiotherapy
    - Interstitial brachytherapy
    - 5FU cream
    - Moh's micrographic
    - Laser excision
- Surgical treatment is best
    - 2 cm margin is given and after resection at least 2 cm of stump must be available for sexual activity and passing urine in standing position.
    - Usually partial amputation of penis is done for glans and distal growth.
    - *Indication of total amputation:*
        - <2 cm shaft
        - Urethral involvement++
    - Young operation—partial penectomy + bilateral ilioinguinal dissection
    - Piersey Gold operation—Total amputation + scrotum + testis (emasculation)—Not done

b. *Secondary nodal management:*

- *Node positive cases:* Lazy "S" incision done and Ilioinguinal block dissection done.
- *Node negative cases:*
    - Sentinel node biopsy of Cabana done in olden days
    - Superficial inguinal dissection of Dassler—all superficial nodes removed and sent for frozen section, If positive ilioinguinal block is done.
- Latest protocol for node negative cases
    - Modified ilioinguinal dissection of Catalona (superficial + deep nodes removal in a rectangular area) send for Frozen section—if nodes are positive ilioinguinal block is done.

Extra edge—

- *Verrucous cancer:*
    - A variety of SCC
    - Low malignant
    - Aggressive growth on RT

**Ans. 51** a. Figure showing undescended testes in male. B/l undescended testes with the underdeveloped scrotum. In cases of retractile testis, the scrotum is relatively well developed.

b. Testis is an organ of lumbar region.

*Course*
- 2nd month—lumbar region
- 3rd month—iliac fossa
- 7th month—deep ring.
- 7-8 month—travels in the canal
- 8th month—superficial ring
- 9th month—scrotum

c. Undescended testis (UDT)
- Arrest in normal path
- Underdeveloped
- Can cause
  - T—torsion
  - E—Epididymo-orchitis
  - S—Sterility
  - T—Trauma
  - I—Indirect inguinal hernia
  - S—Seminoma
- Scrotum not developed

Ectopic testis
- Deviation from normal path
- Normal development
- Can cause trauma as only complication
- Scrotum normal

Extra edge—
Retractile testis
- Cremasteric muscle overaction
- Testis will be retracted and lying in superficial ring and we can manually pull it back to scrotum which is impossible in ectopic testis.
- Scrotum normal

**Ans. 52** a. The testis is mobilized and retained in a pouch constructed between the dartos muscle and skin (subdartos pouch fixation) (orchidopexy)

b. *Clinical features:*
- M/c location—inguinal canal
- 70% of it resolve by 2 months
- M/c preterm babies
- Right side
- Leydig cell normal, Sertoli cell affected—so secondary sexual characters normal

*Investigation:*
- Gold standard—diagnostic laparoscopy
- Inguinal UDT—USG is enough (indirect inguinal hernia is also noted)
- *On diagnostic laparoscopy:*
    - Blind ending testicular vessels means the testis has gone for atrophy and no use of further exploration.
    - If vessels are seen entering deep ring—we will explore the inguinal canal

*Treatment:*
- Bilateral UDT—Measure β HCG level (may be hypertrophied clitoris looking like penis and the patient may be a female)
- Testosterone value
- Testis should be brought to scrotum back

*Uses*
- To prevent trauma
- To detect malignancy.
- Normal spermatogenesis returns if done early.
- Orchidopexy + fixation
    - Subdartus pouch (m/c)
    - Ombredanne procedure (kept in opposite side with normal tail)
    - Ladd and gross technique-2 sutures applied (testis and thigh)
    - Keetley Torek—temporarily keep it in thigh—after 3 months bring it back
- Testis unable to bring it to scrotum
    - Silbar—Disconnect the testicular artery, keep it in scrotum, and do microvascular anastomosis.
    - Fowler Stephen—Two stage procedure

**Ans. 53** a. *Testicular torsion:* (a) Normal attachment; (b) An abnormally high attachment of the tunica vaginalis predisposes to torsion—the "bell-clapper" deformity.

b. Torsion of the testis is uncommon because the normal testis is anchored and cannot rotate. *For torsion to occur one of several abnormalities must be present:*
- High investment of the tunica vaginalis causes the testis to hang within the tunica like a clapper in a bell. This is the M/C/C in adolescents and is typically a bilateral abnormality.
- Inversion of the testis. The testis is rotated so that it lies transversely or upside down.

- Separation of the epididymis from the body of the testis permits torsion of the testis on the pedicle that connects the testis with the epididymis.

c. • Prehn's sign
  - To differentiate between torsion and orchitis
  - On lifting the testis:
    - If pain increases—Suggestive of torsion
    - If pain decrease—Orchitis
  - Angel sign—Normal testis lying horizontally
  - Deming sign—Affected testis lying higher up

d. • Management of torsion testis:
  - 1st hour—manual detorsion
  - <4 hours—save testis (4 hours is golden period)
  - >4 hours—testis would be gangrenous
- IOC—Color Doppler scan
- Bilateral exposure is done for Torsion testis always:
  - Affected testis removed
  - Unaffected testis may have pathologies like Bell clapper deformity and hence do orchidopexy.

**Ans. 54** a. Large varicocele in a pendulous scrotum (bag of worm appearance). The left inguinal hernia.

b. Why varicocele is most common (mc) on left side?
- Left testicular vein drains at right angle.
- Left testicular vein is long.
- Left adrenal vein is near left testicular vein and hence can cause increased spasm.
- Sigmoid colon compresses left testicular vein.
- RCC can invade left renal vein and causes obstruction of left testicular vein.

Extra edge—The left varicocele not disappears on lying down—Left side RCC

c. Operation is not indicated for an asymptomatic varicocele. If the discomfort is significant, then percutaneous embolization of the gonadal veins is the first-line intervention. If this is not possible, or if it recurs (as it does in around 20% after embolization), then surgical ligation of the testicular veins is the appropriate treatment, although recurrence can occur even after such surgery.

Paloma operation—Retroperitoneal ligation of testicular veins
- Inguinal approach—Invanissevich procedure
- Transcortical approach
- After ligating vessels testis will drain through cremasteric vessel

d. (a) Vaginal hydrocoele (most common); (b) "Infantile" hydrocele; (c) Congenital hydrocele; (d) Hydrocele of the cord. A right-sided hydrocele.

e. *Types of vaginal hydrocele:*
- Primary hydrocele—testis not palpable
- Secondary hydrocele—Testis palpable separately
  - Primary—cause unknown
  - *Secondary:*
    - Infection—Filariasis, syphilis, etc.
    - Inflammation
    - Tumors
    - Trauma

*Types of hydrocele based on closure of tunica vaginalis:*
- Vaginal
  - Confined only to scrotum
  - Get above the swelling+
- Infantile hydrocele
  - Fluid collection seen up to superficial ring
  - Get above swelling not possible
- Congenital hydrocele
  - Communicating with the peritoneum
  - Reduced on lying down overnight
  - Inverted ink bottle effect is seen
- Encysted hydrocele cord
  - Decreased movement on traction

f. Lord's operation. A series of interrupted absorbable sutures is used to plicate the redundant tunica vaginalis. When these are tied, the tunica bunches at its attachment to the testis.
Jaboulay's procedure. The hydrocoele sac is everted and anchored with sutures.

**Ans. 55** a. Figure—seminoma of the testis

b.
- *Pathological types:*
  - Germ cell tumors
  - Seminomas
- *Nonseminomas:*
  - Choriocarcinoma
  - Yolk sac
  - Teratoma
  - Embryonal cell
- Sex cord tumors
  - Leydig cell tumors
  - Sertoli cell tumors

- Seminomas
  - 4th decade
  - Highly radiosensitive
  - LN metastasis > hematogenous metastasis
  - LDH increased
  - Good prognosis
- Nonseminomas
  - Seen in 30s
  - Radioresistant
  - Choriocarcinoma—Hematogenous metastasis+
  - LN metastasis also seen
  - Tumor markers—HCG, α-FP, LDH
  - Bad prognosis

c. • 3rd decade—nonseminomatous
- 4th decade—Seminomatous
- >5th decade—Lymphoma testis
- Predisposing factors
  - Undescended testis (seminoma)—Please remember even by doing orchidopexy the risk is not reduced; but helps in early diagnosis.
  - Klinefelter's
  - Testicular feminization syndrome
  - Maternal DES
  - Siblings history—history of (h/o) testicular cancer

d. *Clinical features:*
- Painless lump+
- Testicular sensation lost (syphilis and tumors have this clinical feature)
- Abdominal lump
  - Sentinel node on right side—Interaortocaval node
  - Sentinel node on left side—Preaortic node
- Hurricane tumor—Aggressive choriocarcinoma
- Sertoli cell tumors—Feminization and gynecomastia
- Leydig cell tumors—Precocious puberty

e. *Investigations for testicular tumors:*
USG must be done in every suspected case.
- IOC
  - To diagnose—Biopsy (inguinal method—Chevasu maneuver)
  - To stage—MRI
  - Tumor markers—HCG, AFP, LDH
- For biopsy testing—Chevasu maneuver biopsy

    - Don't do trans scrotal biopsy (violation of tumor principle will happen and you may disseminate the tumor via superficial inguinal nodes which is not its regular course).
    - Put an inguinal incision, pull the testis and examine the tumor, and take biopsy from tumor.
    - Do frozen section
    - If positive—High inguinal orchidectomy
    - If negative—Keep testis back in scrotum

f. Staging
- T1—Tumor confined to testis, no lymphovascular invasion.
- T2—Tumor confined to testis with lymphovascular invasion (+) and Tunica albuginea (+)
- T3—Tumor goes to spermatic cord
- T4—Tumor goes to scrotal wall
- N1—<2 cm nodal mass
- N2—2-5 cm nodal mass
- N3—>5 cm nodal mass
- M1—Metastasis

*Treatment*
- *After high inguinal orchidectomy:* Nodal secondaries must be managed.
- Seminoma is radiosensitive and hence RT given to nodes.
- Nonseminoma is not radiosensitive and hence we do retroperitoneal lymph node dissection (RPLND)
- *N1, N2 cases:*
    - Seminomatous—Radiotherapy to lymph nodes
    - Nonseminomatous—RPLND + Chemo
- N3 cases and M1
    - Seminoma—chemotherapy
    - Nonseminoma—chemotherapy
- *Radiotherapy in seminomatous tumors:*
    - Inverted "Y" field RT
- Chemotherapy
    - B—bleomycin
    - E—Etoposide
    - P-Cisplatin

**Ans. 56**
- *Image A:* Fournier's gangrene with an area of necrotic skin overlying an area of scrotal inflammation.
- *Image B:* Sebaceous cysts of the scrotum.
- *Image C:* Scrotal cancer or Chimney sweeps' cancer was the first reported occupational cancer. Rare cancer that has also been seen in other workers who come into contact with oil and coal products.

13

SECTION

# Transplantation

CHAPTER

# 53 Transplantation

## QUESTIONS

**Q1. Answer the following:**

a. When is world organ donation day?

b. Who did the first

- Kidney transplantation
- Liver transplantation
- Heart transplantation
- Pancreas transplantation

c. Define organ donation.

**Q2. Define the following:**

- Allograft
- Alloantigen
- Alloantibody
- Human leukocyte antigen (HLA)
- Xenograft
- Orthotopic graft
- Heterotopic graft

**Q3. Answer the following:**

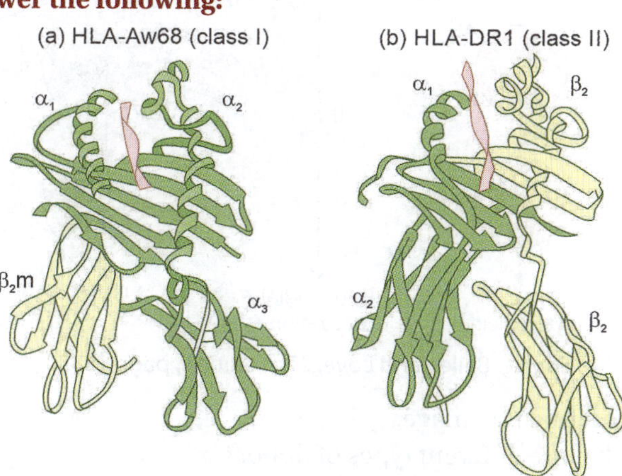


*Source:* Bailey and Love, 27th edition, page 1534.

a. Describe HLA.
b. Elaborate the class of HLAs.
c. HLA matching is not needed for and not possible for which organs?
d. Describe about orthotopic and heterotopic graft placement.

**Q4. Answer the following:**

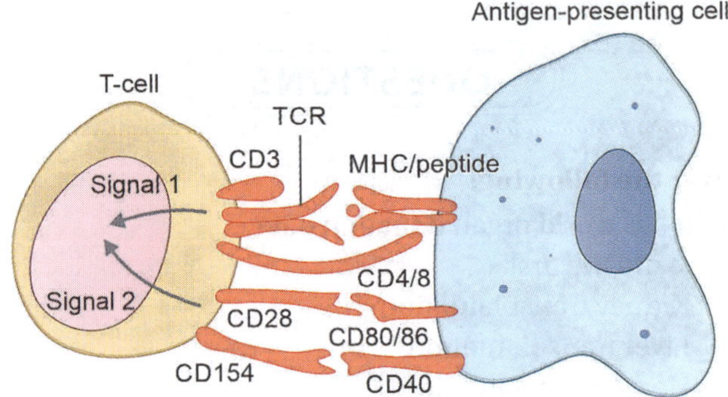


*Source:* Bailey and Love, 27th edition, page 1535.

a. Describe the image.
b. What are different types of allograft rejection?

**Q5. Answer the following:**

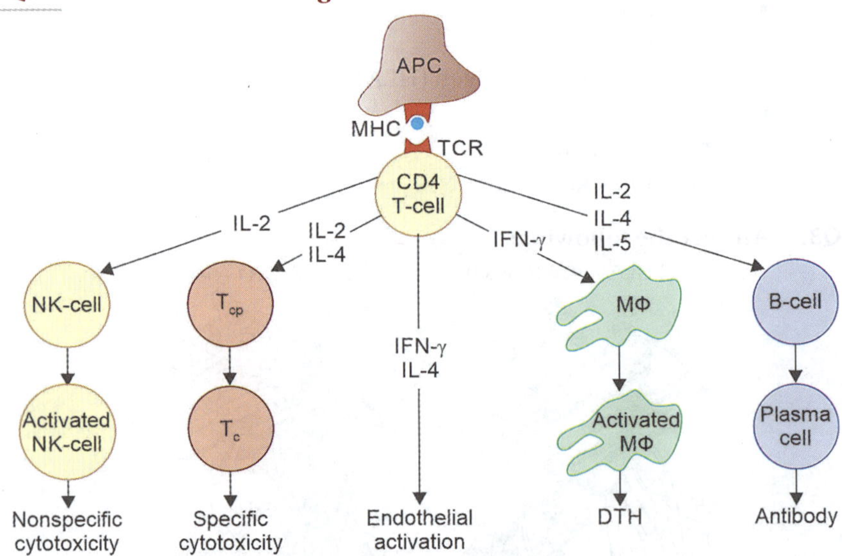


*Source:* Bailey and Love, 27th edition, page 1535.

a. Describe the image.
b. What are different types of donor?
c. What are the contraindication for organ transplant?

**Q6. Answer the following:**

a. Describe brain death donor?
b. Describe donation after cardiac death (DCD) donor: Maastricht classification.
c. Describe donor age group for different organs.

**Q7. Answer the following:**

a. What is extended donor criteria for liver and kidney transplant?
b. What is the process of organ extraction from donor?
c. What is Back Bench procedure?

**Q8. Answer the following:**

a. What is warm ischemic time?
b. What is cold ischemic time?
c. What is the cold ischemic solution?

**Q9. Answer the following:**

a. What are the risk factors for chronic rejection in kidney?
b. Describe immunosuppression in detail.
c. Describe post-transplant malignancy.

## LIVER TRANSPLANTATION

**Q10. Answer the following:**

a. What are the most common indications for liver transplant?

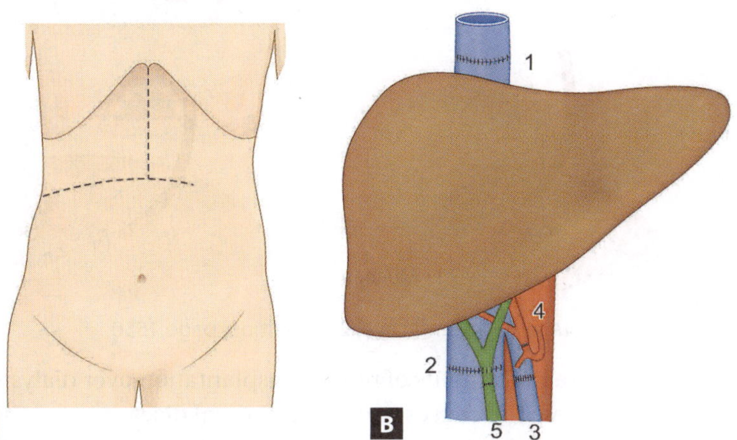


*Source:* Bailey and Love, 27th edition, page 1554.

b. What is the history of liver transplant?
c. What are Criteria for liver transplant?

**Q11. Types of liver transplant:**

a. What is auxiliary transplant?
b. What is domino liver transplant?
c. What is split liver transplant?
d. What is live donor?
e. What is reduced liver transplant?

**Q12. Answer the following:**

a. What are the steps in orthotopic liver transplant?
b. What is Piggyback transplant?
c. Describe rejection in liver transplantation.
d. What is Rotem device?

## KIDNEY TRANSPLANTATION

**Q13. Answer the following:**

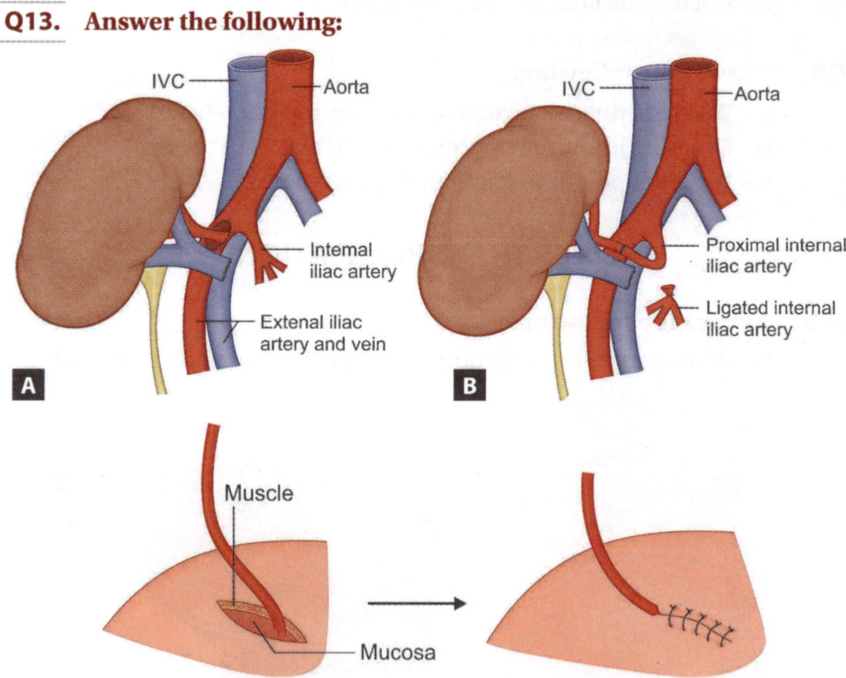


*Source:* Bailey and Love, 27th edition, page 1550.

a. What are the benefits of renal transplantation over dialysis?
b. Enumerate the causes of end-stage renal disease.
c. What is the most common (MC) indication/cause in children and adult?

**Q14. Answer the following:**

a. What are the types of renal graft?
b. What are the donor criteria for transplant?
c. What are the contraindications for donor in renal transplant?

**Q15. Answer the following:**

a. What are the steps in renal transplant (procedure)?
b. What are the complications of renal transplant?
c. What are the risk factors for chronic rejection in kidney transplant?

## PANCREAS TRANSPLANT

**Q16. Answer the following:**

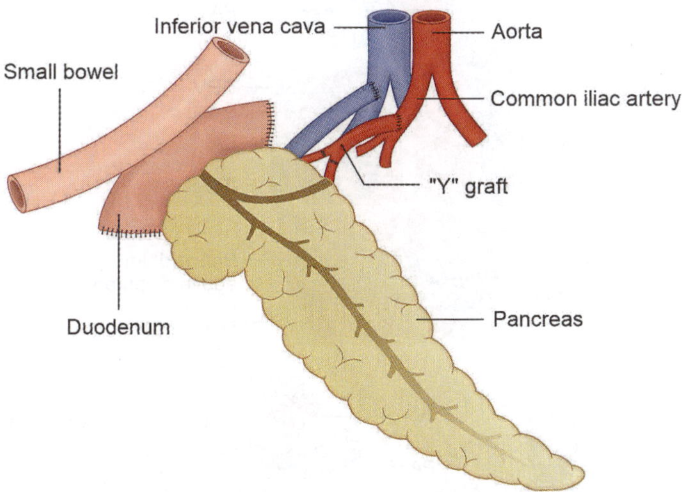


*Source:* Bailey and Love, 27th edition, page 1553.

a. Who does the first pancreas transplant?
b. What is Donerage?
c. What are types of pancreatic transplantation?
d. What are contraindications for donor?

**Q17. Answer the following:**

a. Describe procedure of pancreatic transplantation.
b. Describe two types of drainage procedure in pancreatic transplant.
c. What are the complications of pancreatic transplantation?
d. Describe islets cell transplant.

## INTESTINE TRANSPLANTATION

**Q18. Answer the following:**

a. What are the indications?
b. Who is the donor for small bowel transplant?
c. Describe cadaveric SI transplant.
d. What are the complications of small bowel transplant?

## HEART TRANSPLANTATION

**Q19. Answer the following:**

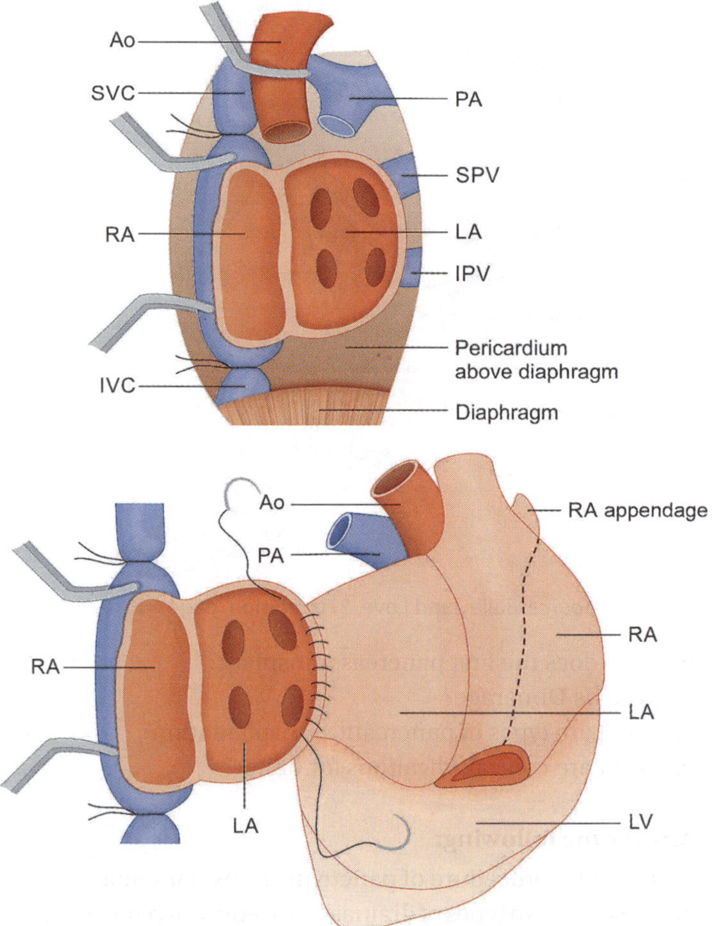


*Source:* Bailey and Love, 27th edition, page 1557.

a. What are the indication?
b. What are the procedures/steps of heart transplant?

## ANSWERS

**Ans. 1** a. August 13th—organ donation day every year

b. *The first:*
- Kidney transplantation is done by Murray in 1954.
- Liver transplantation is done by Starlz in 1963.
- Heart transplantation is done by Barnard.
- Pancreas transplantation is done by Kelly and Lillehei.

c. *Organ donation* is the process of surgical removal of organ or tissue (graft) from one person (donor) and placing it into another person (recipient) legally. It is performed by transplant surgeon.

**Ans. 2**
- *Allograft:* An organ or tissue transplanted from one individual to another.
- *Alloantigen:* Transplant antigen
- *Alloantibody:* Transplant antibodies
- *HLA:* Human leukocyte antigen, the main trigger to graft rejection.
- *Xenograft:* A graft performed between different species.
- *Orthotopic graft:* A graft placed in its normal anatomical site.
- *Heterotopic graft:* A graft placed in a site different from that where the organ is normally located.

**Ans. 3** a. *Human leukocyte antigen (HLA):*
- HLA are the most common cause of graft rejection.
- Their physiological function is to act as antigen recognition units.
- HLA are highly polymorphic (amino acid sequence differs widely between individuals).
- HLA-A, -B, -C (class I), and -DR, -DP and -DQ (class II) are most important in organ transplantation.

b. *There are two types of HLA molecule:* HLA class I and HLA class II. They are broadly similar in structure but have different cell expression profiles. HLA class I antigens are present on all nucleated cells, whereas HLA class II antigens have a more restricted distribution and are expressed most strongly on antigen-presenting cells, such as dendritic cells, macrophages, and B lymphocytes. T-cells recognize HLA molecules via their T-cell receptor, but full T-cell activation also requires the delivery of an additional or second signal by the interaction of costimulatory molecules on the surface of the antigen-presenting cell and T-cell.
Class I—HLA
HLA loci—HLA-A, -B, and -C

Structure—Heavy chain and β2-microglobulin
Distribution—All nucleated cells
Class II—HLA
HLA loci—-DR, -DP, and -DQ
Structure—α- and β-chain
Distribution—B-cells, dendritic cells, and macrophages

c. HLA matching is done for antigen recognition
   - HLA matching not needed for liver and cornea.
   - HLA matching is not possible for heart because cold ischemic time is 3 hours.

d. Based on placement of graft
   - *Orthotopic graft placement:* Graft is placed in same anatomical location, e.g., liver and heart.
   - *Heterotopic graft placement:* Graft is placed in a nonanatomical location, e.g., kidney and pancreas.

**Ans. 4** a. Molecular events involved in T-cell activation by an antigen-presenting cell. T-cell activation requires the delivery of two distinct signals to the T-cell. The first signal is delivered by ligation of the TCR/CD3 complex with the human leukocyte antigen (HLA)/peptide complex. The second signal is delivered after the interaction between pairs of co-stimulatory molecules such as CD28 with CD80/86 and CD154 with CD40.

b. *Types of graft rejection:*
   - Hyperacute rejection
     - Immediate graft destruction due to antibodies (ABO) or preformed antiHLA antibodies.
     - Characterized by intravascular thrombosis and interstitial hemorrhage.
   - Acute rejection
     - Usually occurs during first 6 months
     - T-cell dependent
     - May be cell mediated, antibody mediated, or both usually reversible.
   - Chronic rejection
     - Occurs after first 6 months.
     - Most common cause of graft failure.
     - Antibodies play an important role.
     - Nonimmune factors contribute to pathogenesis.
     - Characterized by myointimal proliferation in graft arteries leading to ischemia and fibrosis.

**Ans. 5** a. The central role of the CD4 T-cell in orchestrating the various effector mechanisms responsible for allograft rejection. (APC: antigen-presenting cell; DTH: delayed-type hypersensitivity; IFN-γ: interferon-gamma; IL: interleukin; MΦ: macrophage; MHC: major histocompatibility complex; NK: natural killer; Tc: T-cytotoxic cell; Tcp: T-cytotoxic precursor cell; TCR: T-cell receptor)

b. *Types of donor:*

*Liver donor:*

- Kidney
- Heart
- *Brain dead donor:* They are the donor's who have heart beat and circulation +
- *Donation after cardiac death (DCD):* They are the donor's who have no heart beat and cardiac arrest happened.
- *Xenograft donor:* Pigs are the ideal. Heart valves are used.

c. *Contraindication (CI) for organ donation:* The following persons should not donate organ:

- Human immunodeficiency virus (HIV) patient
- Creutzfeldt-Jakob (CJ) disease
- Malignancy within 5 years (exclude SCC, BCC, cancer in situ uterus, and brain tumors)
- Hepatitis B virus (HBV) patients
- Death due to sepsis

Extra edge—Donor matching of blood group:

- *O group can donate to:* O, A, B, AB
- *A group can donate to:* A, AB
- *B group can donate to:* B, AB
- *AB group can donate to:* AB
- O group is universal donor.
- AB group is universal recipient.
- Rh testing is not needed for organ transplantation. Only ABO and HLA matching is done.

**Ans. 6** a. *Brain dead donor:*

- Brain not working
- Heart is still beating

In UK two doctors should certify to declare as brain dead.

- One should be a consultant.
- None should be a transplant involved surgeon in the two doctors.

Two doctors should separately examine the following in two separate occasions: To condemn them as brain dead

- Cranial reflexes—CNS reflexes absent (pharyngeal, Gag reflexes, etc.)
- Motor response—No response
- No spontaneous breathing on raising $PaCO_2$ >60 mm Hg

b. *Donation after cardiac death (DCD) donor:*
Maastricht classification of DCD donor
- *Cat 1:* Dead on arrival at hospital
- *Cat 2:* Dead even after attempt of resuscitation
- *Cat 3:* Awaited cardiac arrest after withdrawal of supports (who is not brain dead)
- *Cat 4:* Cardiac arrest while brain dead
- *Cat 5:* Cardiac arrest in inpatient
- Cat 3 and 4 are good donors because they have circulation in organs until death they are controlled donors.
- *Cat 1, 2, and 5:* Uncontrolled donors

c. *Donor age group:*
- *Kidney:* 2 years—no upper limit
- *Liver:* No age limit
- *Heart:* 1–65 years
- *Lungs:* 5–65 years
- *Pancreas:* 10–60 years

**Ans. 7** a. The crisis in organ supply has required the use of extended donor criteria
*Extended donor criteria for kidney:*
- Age >60 years
- Age 50–59 years with history of two or more of the following:
  - Death due to cerebrovascular accident (CVA)
  - Impaired kidney function (serum creatinine >15 mg/dL)
  - History of (H/O) of hypertension (HTN)

*Extended donor criteria for liver:*
- Steatosis
- Age >65 years
- Hepatitis C virus (HCV) positive (+ve) patients
- HBV core Ag +ve patients

b. Process of organ extraction from donor
*On operating table procedure:*
- The brain dead patient is taken to the operation theater (OT)
- Anesthetist disconnects the supports
- The moment the heart beat stops
- All the organs needed are extracted by respective surgeons simultaneously

c. Back Bench procedure:
  - Immediately cold ischemic solution is infused into the organ.
  - The organ is kept in a ice bag and taken to the recipient.

**Ans. 8** a. Warm ischemic time is the time between the heart stops and infusion of ischemic cold solution into the organ. It should be as less as possible <30 minutes.

b. Cold ischemic time is the time of infusion of cold preservative solution to transplantation to the recipient is completed and there is reperfusion of recipient blood.

c. *Cold ischemic solution:* Most common (m/c) used is University of Wisconsin Solution. Eurocollin is another solution.

University of Wisconsin Solution components:
  - *Lactobionate:* Prevents cell swelling
  - *Adenosine:* Provides energy
  - *Allopurinol:* It is a free radical scavenger
  - *Glutathione:* Antioxidant

| *Organ* | *Optimum cold ischemic time* | *Maximum cold ischemic time* |
|---|---|---|
| Kidney | <18 hours | 36 hours |
| Liver | <12 hours | 18 hours |
| Heart | <3 hours | 6 hours |
| Lungs | <3 hours | 8 hours |
| Pancreas | <10 hours | 18 hours |
| Small intestine | <4 hours | 6 hours |

**Ans. 9** a. *Chronic rejection in:*
  - *Kidney:* Glomerular sclerosis
  - *Liver:* Vanishing bile duct syndrome
  - *Heart:* Accelerated coronary artery disease
  - *Pancreas:* Acinar loss
  - *Lungs:* Obliterative bronchiolitis

Risk factors for chronic rejection in kidney (NEET SS):
  - Previous episodes of acute rejection
  - Poor HLA matching
  - Prolonged cold ischemic time
  - Cytomegalovirus (CMV) infection
  - Increased blood lipids
  - Inadequate immunosuppression

b. *Immunosuppression is given to prevent graft getting rejection:*
  - *Induction phase:*
    - Is started immediately after surgery

- *Maintenance phase:*
  - Is continued for lifetime in many patient

Category of drugs for immune suppression drugs:
- *Calcineurin inhibitors:* Cyclosporine, tacrolimus
- *Antiproliferative agents:* Azathioprine, mercaptopurine, mycophenolate mofetil
- Steroids
- *mToR inhibitors (mammalian target of rapamycin inhibitor):* Sirolimus, everolimus

Monoclonal antibodies:
- Muromonab: Anti CD3 antibody
- Basiliximab: Anti CD25 antibody
- Rituximab: Anti CD20 antibody

M/C complication on immunosuppression—Infections:
- *Infections:* Recipient infection reactivation is most common.
- CMV reactivation in 6–12 weeks patient presents with CMV pneumonitis.

c. *Post-transplant malignancy:*
- M/C squamous cell carcinoma (SCC) > post-transplant lymphoproliferative disorder [PTLD M/C caused Epstein-Barr Virus (EBV)]
- *HHV 8 patients:* Kaposi's sarcoma
- HBV and HCV patients: HCC
- HPV: Cancer (Ca) cervix

Nonimmune mediated complications:

*Calcineurin inhibitors:*
- Chronic allograft nephropathy
- NoDAT: New onset diabetes mellitus (DM) after transplant happening in 30% <2 years

*Complications related to transplant:*
- M/C infection: CMV
- M/C parasitic infection: *Pneumocystis carinii*
- Polyoma BK virus: Ureteric stricture
- M/C malignancy is SCC

**Ans. 10** a.
- *M/C indication of liver transplant in adults:* Cirrhosis (HCV > HBV)
- *M/C indication of liver transplant in children:* Extra hepatic biliary atresia (EHBA)
- *M/C metabolic disorder:* α 1 antitrypsin deficiency
- *M/C indication for emergency transplantation:* Acute fulminant liver failure [paracetamol (PCM) toxicity]

b. *History:*
   - First liver transplant was done by Starzl—1963
   - First split liver transplant was done by Pichlmayr
   - First live donor liver transplant was done by Tanaka

c. *Modified child pugh score:* Child C > B
   - Bilirubin
   - Albumin
   - Ascites
   - PT
   - Encephalopathy

   Model for end liver disease (MELD)

   *Logarithmic score of:* C B I
   - Creatinine
   - Bilirubin
   - International normalized ratio (INR)
     - MELD score >35 priority
     - MELD score <15 put under waiting list

   *MELD exception:* In these patients we can do transplant in a lesser score also
   - HCC
   - Amyloidosis
   - Hepatopulmonary syndrome
   - Porto pulmonary hypertension (HTN)

   King's college criteria
   Liver transplant in acute fulminant liver failure

   *Paracetamol induced liver failure:*
   - pH <7.30 (irrespective of encephalopathy)
     or
   - PT >100 seconds + Serum creatinine >300 micro mol/L + grade 3 or 4 encephalopathy

   *Nonparacetamol induced liver failure:*
   - PT >100 seconds
     or
   - *Any three of the below:*
     1. Age <10 >40 Years
     2. *Etiology:* Non A/non B liver damage may be due to halothane or idiosyncratic drugs
     3. 7 days of jaundice before encephalopathy developed
     4. Serum bilirubin >300 micro mol/L
     5. PT >50 seconds

*Milan criteria:*
- Followed for hepatocellular carcinoma (HCC) patients with cirrhotic liver
- Single tumor <5 cm
- <3 lesions (all 1–3 cm diameter)
- No extra hepatic spread

**Ans. 11** a. *Auxiliary transplant:*
- Indicated for acute fulminant liver failure,
- Stop immunosuppressant drugs when the original liver recovers or can remove the transplanted liver,
- Auxiliary partial orthotopic liver transplant: Part of diseased liver is removed and part of new liver is placed in the same position.
- Auxiliary heterotopic liver transplant: New liver is placed just beneath the original liver.

b. *Domino liver transplant:*
- Amyloidotic liver is removed and given to someone in need of liver and new liver is given to amyloidotic patient.
- Patients are saved with 1 liver

c. *Split liver transplant:*
- Segments 5, 6, 7, 8 will be given to adult and segment 2, 3 alone is enough for children.

d. *Live donor (can donate only to relatives):*
- Segment 5, 6, 7, 8 is taken if donating to adult;
- Segment 2, 3 is taken if donation is for the pediatric patient.

e. *Reduced liver transplant:*
- The retrieved liver is trimmed to suit for the body weight of the recipient (mostly to children).

**Ans. 12** a. *Steps in orthotopic liver transplant:*
- Remove cadaveric liver along with supra hepatic inferior vena cava (IVC) and portal triad (portal vein, bile duct, and hepatic artery)
- *Recipient operation:* Remove liver along with hepatic vein and part of IVC and small amount of portal vein.
  Place the cadaveric liver in the donor and anastomose the structures in the following order:
- *First:* IVC (supra hepatic followed by infra hepatic)
- *Second:* Portal vein anastomosis (may develop reperfusion syndrome: Hypotension and bradycardia)
- *Third:* Hepatic artery

- *Fourth:* Bile duct (end to end anastomosis)
  Bile duct anastomosis is C/I in primary sclerosing cholangitis and extra hepatic biliary atresia for the above two conditions do a Roux en Y jejuna anastomosis.

b. *Piggy back transplant:*
- If liver alone is removed in recipient and donor liver is removed along with IVC do piggy back anastomosis. Advantage is blood flows throughout the process of surgery.

c. *Hyper acute rejection:* Rare or not happens in liver transplant
- *Acute rejection*—Manifests as hepatic artery thrombosis: Immediately need retransplant portal vein thrombosis no retransplant advised.
- *Chronic rejection*—Manifests as vanishing bile duct (rare).

d. *ROTEM:* Rotational thromboelastometry used to measure prothrombin (PT)/INR dynamically while transplantation is going on.

**Ans. 13** a. Renal transplantation is the preferred treatment for many patients with end-stage renal disease because it provides a better quality of life for them than dialysis. Transplantation releases patients from the dietary and fluid restrictions of dialysis and the physical constraints imposed by the need to dialyze. Transplantation is also more cost-effective than dialysis and improves patient survival.

b. The causes of end-stage renal disease are numerous and include the following:
- Glomerulonephritis;
- Diabetic nephropathy;
- Hypertensive nephrosclerosis;
- Renal vascular disease;
- Polycystic kidney disease;
- Pyelonephritis;
- Obstructive uropathy;
- Systemic lupus erythematosus;
- Analgesic nephropathy; and
- Metabolic disease (oxalosis, amyloid).

c.
- *M/C cause in adults:* Renal failure due to diabetic nephropathy.
- *M/C cause in children:* Chronic glomerulonephritis
- It is always a heterotopic graft [right (Rt) iliac fossa > left (Lt) iliac fossa]

**Ans. 14** a. *Types of graft:*
- Cadaveric
- *Live donor:* Kidney preferred is Lt kidney b/c Lt renal vein is longer

b. *Donor criteria:*
- Age 18–70 years
- Body mass index (BMI) <35
- BMI >40
- Diabetes mellitus (DM)
- No caner
- No active sepsis
- Kidney has normal function.
- ABO compatibility/human leukocyte antigen (HLA) matching

c. *C/I for donor:*
- BMI >40
- DM
- Malignancy
- HIV +ve, sepsis
- Hypertension (HTN)
- Glomerular filtration rate (GFR) < 70, albuminuria
- Horse shoe kidney
- Kidney stones

**Ans. 15** a. *Procedure:*
- In cadaveric kidney along with the renal artery small portion of the aorta is also removed known as Carrel patch.

*Ureter is anastomosed to the bladder by:*
- Short tunnel technique @ LichGregoir technique (M/C done).
- Long tunnel technique @ Lead Better Politano technique. Renal vein anastomosed to common iliac vein.

*Renal artery anastomosis:*
- *In cadaveric donor carrel patch is taken:* Do end to side wide anastomosis of carrel patch with external iliac artery
- *In live donor carrel patch is not possible:* Do end to end anastomosis of renal artery with internal iliac artery. Renal artery stenosis is M/C with live donor kidney transplant.

b. Complications of kidney transplant

*Complications to live donor:*
- M/C complication is urinary retention and paralytic ileus

*Complications to recipient:*
- Hemorrhage
- Renal vein thrombosis (1–5%)

- Renal artery thrombosis (1%)
- Renal artery stenosis (1–23%)
- Viral infections
- Bacterial infections'
- Lymphocele
- Polyoma BK virus produce multiple ureteric strictures

Extra edge—

*Allograft dysfunction of transplanted kidney:*

- Banff classification

c. *Risk factors for chronic rejection:*
- HLA mismatch
- History of (H/O) acute rejection
- Long cold ischemic time
- CMV infection
- Increased blood lipids
- Poor compliance to immune suppression

**Ans. 16** a. First done by Kelly and Lillehei

b. Donor age 10–45 years (only cadaveric transplant is possible)

c. Types of pancreas transplant

Simultaneous pancreas-kidney (SPK) (80%) simultaneous pancreas and kidney transplant.

- Has 85% 1 year graft survival rate (highest among the three types)
- Done in type I (IDDM) with severe C peptide deficiency
- Type II with C peptide levels <2 ng/mL
    - *PTA (15%):* Pancreas transplant alone
    - *PAK (5%):* Pancreas after kidney transplant

d. *Contraindication for donor:*
- Type I DM
- Pancreatic surgery
- Chronic pancreatic disorders
- Intraductal papillary mucinous neoplasm (IPMN)

**Ans. 17** a. *Procedure:*
- Pancreas is retrieved including C shaped duodenum, 1 vein superior mesenteric vein and two arteries superior mesenteric artery (SMA) and splenic artery (SA).
- Y shaped graft is also taken from the cadaver (common ileac artery with internal and external iliac arteries) anastomose the IIA with SA and environmental impact assessment (EIA) to superior mesenteric artery (SMA).

b. *Anastomosis of the graft can be done in two ways:*
- Enteric drainage
- Bladder drainage
  *Enteric drainage:* M/C performed
- *Advantages:*
  - It is physiological drainage.
  - No increased infection
  - No UTI
- *Disadvantage:* Leak is M/C
  Bladder drainage:
  *Advantage:* Graft failure can be identificd by looking at urinary amylase early rejection which can be diagnosed. Leak rate is less.
  *Disadvantage:* Urethritis, urinary tract infection (UTI), and metabolic acidosis.
  Extra edge—
- M/C complication following pancreas transplant is graft thrombosis.
- M/C cause of graft failure is graft thrombus [superior mesenteric vein (SMV) > artery]; Pancreas is to be removed.
- *M/C cause of death post-transplant:* Cardiovascular (CVS) cause.

c. *Complication:*
- Rejection
  - *Leak:* Debridement and reanastomosis
  - Bleeding (Rx octreotide)
  - Infection
  - Necrosis
  - Abscess

d. *Islets cell transplant:*
- 8,000—10,000 islets/kg body weight is needed to make him insulin free, to get this we need four donor pancreas
- These islets are injected into the portal vein.
- They live in the liver.
- *Complication:* Bleeding and portal vein (PV) thrombosis.
- Edmonton Protocol (NEET SS)
  - Steroids not to be used
  - Interleukin (IL) 2 antibodies (Abs) are used.

**Ans. 18** a.
- *M/C indication in adult/children:* Short bowel syndrome
- *M/C cause of short bowel syndrome in adults:* Acute superior mesenteric artery ischemia

- *M/C cause of short bowel syndrome in children:* Gastroschisis > Midgut volvulus
  Short bowel syndrome patients will be on *total parenteral nutrition* (TPN). Indications of SI transplant:
- TPN failure is the most common (m/c) indication of small intestine transplant
- Patient on TPN develops liver failure
- Patient on TPN develops central vein thrombosis
- Patient on TPN develops >2 episodes of infection
- Patient on TPN develops frequent dehydration.
- Single time fungal infection in central line.

b. *Small bowel can be taken from: Cadaveric donor*
   - Isolated SB graft
   - Combined SB and liver transplant
   - *Multivisceral transplant:* SB + Stomach ± Colon
   - *Modified multivisceral transplant:* Liver is not included
     *Live donor:* Last 150–200 cm of ileum is taken; it is based on ileocolic artery or ileocolic vein
     Xenograft—From figure
     Extra edge—
   - Body weight of donor should be 50–75% of the recipient.
   - Avoid prolonged cold ischemic time.

c. *Cadaveric SBT:*
   - Small bowel is anastomosed with duodenum and ileum is kept as ileostomy only.
   - Superior mesenteric vein is anastomosed with portal vein of the recipient.
   - Superior mesenteric artery is anastomosed to the infrarenal aorta.

d. *Complications of SB transplant:*
   *Rejection:*
   - Highest chance of rejection: 70–80%
   - Clinical features (C/F): Fever, abdomen pain, and increased stool.
   - Do ileoscopy and biopsy to look for rejection.
   - Graft versus host disease is M/C in SB transplant of all: 0–14%
   - *New markers for rejection:* Stool calprotectin and stool citrulline.
   - PTLD also M/C 10–20%.
   - M/C complication overall is bacterial infection 70–90%.
     Extra edge—

- Combined liver + SB transplant has better prognosis than isolated SB transplantation alone.
- M/C cause of death is infection (sepsis).
- M/C cause of graft loss is sepsis > graft rejection.

**Ans. 19** a. M/C cause for transplant is ischemic dilated cardiomyopathy.

b. Do sternotomy and remove the heart. Preserve the Lt atrial cuff, aorta, superior vena cava (SVC), inferior vena cava (IVC), and pulmonary arteries. Insert the donor heart and anastomose in the following order:
   - Left atrial cuff (1st)
   - SVC and IVC (2nd)
   - Aorta
   - Pulmonary artery

14

SECTION

# Miscellaneous

CHAPTER 54

# Biostatistics

## QUESTIONS

**Q1. What are the types of research studies?**

**Q2. What is:**

a. Case control study
b. Odds ratio

**Q3. What is:**

a. Cohort study
b. Relative risk
c. Attributable risk
d. Advantages and disadvantages cohort

**Q4. What is:**

a. Randomized control trial (RCT)
b. Randomization
c. Classification of RCTs
d. Advantages and disadvantages of RCT

**Q5. What is:**

a. Concept of blinding in RCT and classification.
b. Meta-analysis

**Q6. Answer the following:**

a. What is bias in clinical research?
b. What are the types of bias?
c. What are various methods to eliminate bias in RCT?

**Q7. What are the measures of central tendency, explain them (NEET SS 2023)?**

**Q8. Answer the following:**

a. What are the measures of dispersion of data?
b. What is *p* value?

**Q9. What are the types of error in statistics, explain them?**

**Q10. What is the concept of power of a study?**

**Q11. What are the statistical tests? And how will you choose them.**

**Q12. Answer the following:**

a. What is the concept of univariate and multivariate analysis?
b. What is the correlation?

**Q13. Explain the following:**

a. Regression
b. Incidence
c. Prevalence

**Q14. Explain screening test, types, uses, and characteristics.**

**Q15. Describe the evaluation of an investigative test.**

**Q16. Answer the following:**

a. What are Kaplan-Meier plots?
b. What are Forest plots?

**Q17. Answer the following:**

a. What is receiver operating characteristic curve?
b. What is evidence based medicine?

**Q18. Answer the following:**

a. What is Cochrane collaboration?
b. Explain ethics in research.

**Q19. What are levels of evidence?**

**Q20. What is informed consent?**

**Q21. Describe the Clavien-Dindo classification of surgical complications.**

**Q22. What are the types of data in statistics?**

**Q23. Answer the following:**

a. Identify the statistical diagram shown in the figure.

| | | | | | | | | | | | | |
|---|---|---|---|---|---|---|---|---|---|---|---|---|
| 52 | 0 | | | | | | | | | | | |
| 53 | 2 | 4 | | | | | | | | | | |
| 54 | 0 | 2 | 8 | | | | | | | | | |
| 55 | 0 | 0 | 4 | 4 | 5 | 5 | 5 | 6 | 6 | 7 | 9 | |
| 56 | 0 | 0 | 0 | 0 | 0 | 2 | 4 | 5 | 6 | 8 | 9 | 9 |
| 57 | 0 | 0 | 0 | 7 | 8 | 9 | | | | | | |
| 58 | 0 | 0 | 0 | 0 | 4 | 7 | | | | | | |
| 59 | 0 | 0 | 0 | 0 | | | | | | | | |
| 60 | 0 | 0 | 0 | 0 | 3 | 3 | 7 | 8 | | | | |
| 61 | 0 | 5 | | | | | | | | | | |

b. Identify the statistical diagram shown in photograph.

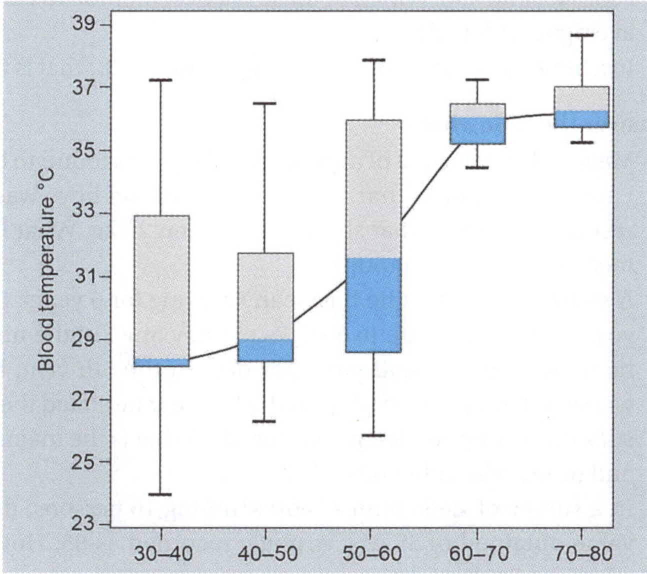


**Q24. Answer the following:**

a. An investigator into the life expectancy of intravenous (IV) drug abusers divides a sample of patients into human immunodeficiency virus (HIV)-positive and HIV-negative groups. What type of data does this division constitute?

b. In statistical literature data are broadly classified as interval scale data, ordinal scale data, and categorical data. For what, blood groups will be an example.
c. In a study following interpretation are obtained: Satisfied, very satisfied, and dissatisfied. Which type of scale is this?
d. A doctor is taking history from a diabetes patient and decides to make a chart to assess joint involvement. Which chart should he make?

**Q25. Answer the following:**

a. Out of 11 births in a hospital, 5 babies weighed over 2.5 kg and 5 weighed less than 2.5 kg. What value do 2.5 represent?
b. The number of malaria cases reported during the last 10 years in a town is given as, 250, 320, 190, 300, 5,000, 100, 260, 350, 320, and 160. The epidemiologist wants to find out the average number of malaria cases reported in that town during the last 10 years. What is the most appropriate measure of average for this data?
c. The incidence of malaria in an area is 20, 20, 50, 56, 60, 5,000, 678, 898, 345, and 456. Which of these is a best method to calculate the average incidence?
d. In a bimodal series, if mean is 2 and median is 3, what is the mode?

**Q26. Answer the following:**

a. Mean value of weight of a group of 10 boys was found to be 18.2 kg. Later, it was found that weight of one of the boys was wrongly recorded as 2.0 kg that should have been 20 kg. What is the true mean weight of the group?
b. A smoker states that he has been smoking for 6 years. In the first year he was taking up to 5 sticks per day only. In the next 3 years he increased it to half pack per day. In the 5th year, his habits worsened to 1 pack per day. In the last year he stated that his daily sticks consumption is 2 packs per day. What is the mean, median, and mode of number of sticks?
c. In a survey of sleep apnea scores among 10 persons, the highest value obtained of 58 was wrongly recorded as 85. How will this affect the final results?
d. What will be the median of the following data will be: 10, 9, 8, 8, and 7?

**Q27. Answer the following:**

a. What is calculated when the values are arranged in ascending and descending order?
b. What does "Centile" divides data into?

c. A bacterium can divide every 20 minutes. Beginning with a single individual, how many bacteria will be there in the population if there is exponential growth for 3 hours?

d. A measure of location that divides the distribution in the ratio of 3:1 is

**Q28. Answer the following:**

a. Blood pressure data of 200 persons were collected. The first quartile blood pressure (BP) of data was 94 mm Hg and 3rd quartile was 110 mm Hg. How many patients lie between the 3rd and 4th quartile?

b. A physician recorded diastolic BP in 125 women aged 18–60 years and found the mean to be 70 mm Hg with SD of 10 mm Hg. What will be the 5th percentile value? Z = – 1.645.

c. Median weight of 100 children was 12 kg. The standard deviation was 3. Calculate the percent coefficient of variance.

d. While calculating the incubation period for measles in a group of 25 kids, standard deviation is 2 and the mean incubation period is 8 days, calculate standard error.

**Q29. Answer the following:**

a. If the birth weight of each of the 10 babies born in a hospital in a day is found to be 2.8 kg, what will be the standard deviation of this sample?

b. Among a 100 women with average hemoglobin (Hb) of 10 g%, the standard deviation was 1, what is the standard error?

c. If each value of a given group of observations is multiplied by 10, what is standard deviation of the resulting observations?

d. The Hb level in healthy women has mean 13.5 g/dL and standard deviation 1.5 g/dL, what is the Z score for a woman with Hb level 15.0 g/dL?

**Q30. Answer the following:**

a. In a sample of 100 pregnant females, mean hemoglobin level estimated was 10 g% with a standard deviation of 1 g%. What is the standard error?

b. In a population of 100 prevalence of *Candida glabrata* was found to be 80%. If the investigator has to repeat the prevalence with 95% confidence, what will the prevalence be?

c. There is a population of 20,000 people with mean hemoglobin being 13.5 g% having a normal distribution. What proportion of population constitutes proportion >13.5 g%?

d. Correct relation between S = standard deviation and V = variance is

**Q31. Answer the following:**

a. The fasting blood levels of glucose for a group of diabetics is found to be normally distributed with a mean of 105 mg per 100 mL of blood and a standard deviation of 10 mg per 100 mL of blood. From this data is can be inferred that approximately 95% of diabetics will have their fasting blood glucose levels within the limits of:

b. A chest physician observed that the distribution of forced expiratory volume (FEV) in 300 smokers had a median value of 2.5 liters with the first and third quartiles being 1.5 and 4.5 liters, respectively. Based on this data, how many persons in the sample are expected to have a FEV between 1.5 and 4.5 liters?

c. 50% population having disease with estimated prevalence to be 45–55% with 95% of probability of identifying them minimum sample size required is:

d. What is detected by using Q-test?

**Q32. Answer the following:**

a. In a study, variation in cholesterol was seen before and after giving a drug. Which test would give its significance?

b. A cardiologist wants to study the effect of an atorvastatin drug. He notes down the initial cholesterol levels of 50 patients and then administers the drug on them. After a month's treatment, he measures the cholesterol level again. Which of the following is the most appropriate to test the statistical significance of the change in blood cholesterol?

c. In a particular trial, the association of lung cancer with smoking is found to be 40% in one sample and 60% in another. What is the best test to compare the results?

d. Height of group of 20 boys aged 10 years was 140 + 13 cm and 20 girl of same age was 135 cm ± 7cm to test the statistical significance of difference in height. What is the applicable test?

**Q33. Answer the following:**

a. The mean BP of a group of persons was determined and after an interventional trial, the mean BP was estimated again. Which is the best test to be applied to determine the significance of intervention?

b. An investigator wants to study the association between maternal intake of iron supplements (yes or no) and incidence of low birth weight (<2,500 or >2,500 g). He collects relevant data from 100 pregnant women as to the status of usage of iron supplements and the status of low birth weight in their newborns. Which is the appropriate statistical test of hypothesis advised in this situation?

c. A cardiologist wants to study the effect of an antihypertensive drug. He notes down the initial systolic blood pressure (mm Hg) of 50 patients and then administers the drug on them. After a week's treatment, which is the most appropriate statistical test of significance that he measures to test the statistical significance of the change in blood pressure?

d. A study was undertaken to assess the effect of a drug in lowering serum cholesterol levels. 15 obese women and 10 nonobese women formed the two limbs of the study. Which test would be useful to correlate the results obtained?

**Q34. Answer the following:**

a. In a particular trial, the association of lung cancer with smoking is found to be 40% in one sample and 60% in another. What is the best test to compare the results?

b. What test is used for testing the statistical significance of the difference in heights of school children?

c. Mean bone density among two groups of 50 people each is compared, which would be the best test?

d. An antihypertensive drug is studied before and after using it for treatment of a patient, what is this study?

**Q35. Answer the following:**

a. An investigator finds out that five independent factors influence the occurrence of a disease. By what we can assess comparison of multiple factors that are responsible for the disease?

b. Mean blood alcohol levels are measured in patients before and after using an interventional drug. Which statistical test of significance is to be applied?

c. In a study, two groups of newborns are checked for their weights based on whether mothers received food supplements or not. What is the appropriate statistical test that can be used?

d. A study which planned to find out the effect of iron supplementation during pregnancy on the birth weight of new born children. Two groups, one with iron supplementation and the other without iron supplementation during pregnancy were compared. Birth weight of newborns were recorded as means + SD. Which significant test (statistical) is appropriate for comparison of birth weights between the two groups?

**Q36. Answer the following:**

a. The correlation between variables A and B in a study was found to be 1.1. What does this indicate?
b. A lecturer states that the correlation coefficient between prefrontal blood flow under cognitive load and the severity of psychotic symptoms in schizophrenic patients is – 1.24. What can you conclude?
c. An investigator wants to study the association between maternal intake of iron supplements (Yes/No) and birth weights (in g) of newborn babies. He collects relevant data from 100 pregnant women and their newborns. What statistical test of hypothesis would you advise for the investigator in this situation?
d. A randomized trial comparing the efficacy of two drugs showed a difference between the two with a $p$ value of <0.005. In reality, however, the two drugs do not differ. What example is shown here?

## ANSWERS

**Ans. 1** *Types of research studies*

- Descriptive studies
- Analytical studies
  1. Ecological studies
  2. Case control studies
  3. Cohort studies
  4. Cross sectional studies
- Experimental studies
  1. Randomized control trial
  2. Uncontrolled trial
- Integrative studies
  1. Systematic review
  2. Meta-analysis

**Ans. 2** a.

- *Definition:* It is a type of observational study comparing characteristics of individuals with the disease of interest with a suitable control group of individuals without the disease.
- Since, it is an observational study no intervention is attempted or no attempt is made to alter the course of disease.
- Case control studies are commonly retrospective in nature.
- It is also known as effect to cause study (backward looking study), disease to risk factor study, and outcome to exposure study.
- It provides odds ratio, which is an estimate of relative risk (RR).

b. It is a measure of the strength of association between the risk factor and outcome.

| | Case | Control |
|---|---|---|
| Exposed | a | b |
| Nonexposed | c | d |
| | | |

- Odds ratio (OR) = ad/bc
- *Interpretation:*
    - *OR = 1:* Exposure to risk factor is identical in both case and control group.
    - *OR < 1:* Exposure to risk factor is lower in cases than in control.
    - *OR > 1:* Exposure to risk factor is greater in cases than in control.

**Ans. 3** a
- Cohort study—Type of analytical study which is undertaken to obtain evidence to support or refute existence of association between suspected cause and disease.
- *Also known as:* Prospective study, forward-looking study, incidence study, cause-effect study, longitudinal study, and exposure to outcome study.
- Since, it is an observational study no intervention is attempted or no attempt is made to alter the course of disease.
- Analysis may be both retrospective and prospective.
- *Definition of cohort:* Defined as a group of people who share a common characteristic or experience within a defined time period.
- *Example:* All those born in 2019 form birth cohort of 2019.
- *Types of cohort studies:*
    - Prospective cohort studies
    - Retrospective cohort studies
    - Combination of retrospective and prospective studies
    - Prospective study is also known as current cohort study and retrospective cohort study is also known as historical cohort study.
- Analysis

| Exposure | Deceased | Nondiseased |
|---|---|---|
| Yes | a | b |
| No | c | d |

- Incidence in exposed: a/a + b
- Incidence in nonexposed: c/c + d

*Interpretation:*

- If incidence in exposed is more than incidence in nonexposed: Risk is present
- If incidence in exposed is equal to incidence in nonexposed: There is no risk
- If the incidence in exposed is less than that in nonexposed: The exposure is protective

b. *Relative risk:*

- Is the ratio of incidence of disease among exposed to incidence of disease among nonexposed.
- Relative risk is direct measure of strength of association between suspected cause and effect.
- *Interpretation of relative risk:*
    - *If RR >1:* Risk is present.
    - *If RR = 1:* There is no risk.
    - *If RR <1:* Exposure is protective.
    - Larger the RR greater the strength of association between suspected factor and disease.
    - *Example:* Relative risk of 2 indicates that the incidence rate of disease is two times higher in exposed subjects as compared to nonexposed ones.

c. Attributable risk (AR)

- Defined as the difference in incidence rate of disease in exposed group and unexposed group
- Expressed as percentage

$$AR = \frac{\text{Incidence in exposed} - \text{Incidence in unexposed} \times 100}{\text{Incidence in exposed}}$$

- *Uses:* It indicates the extent to which the disease under study can be attributed to the exposure.

  Population attributable risk =

$$\frac{\text{Incidence rate in total sample} - \text{Incidence in exposed} \times 100}{\text{Incidence rate in total sample}}$$

    - *Use:* It gives an estimate of the amount by which the disease could be reduced in that population if the suspected factor was eliminated or modified.

d. • *Advantages of cohort study:*

- In case of prospective study, data is of better quality.
- It yields incidence rate, relative risk, and attributable risk.
- Multiple diseases resulting from an etiological factor under study can be simultaneously looked at several possible outcomes related to exposure can be studied simultaneously.
- No recall bias as in case control study.

- *Disadvantages:*
    - Long duration of study.
    - Unsuitable for study of rare diseases.
    - Attrition is a problem.
    - It is expensive.
    - It can be difficult to find a suitable cohort group.
    - Administrative and ethical problems.
    - *Hawthrone effect:* Change in behavior of study subjects.
    - If retrospective, there will be problem with data quality.

**Ans. 4** a. *Randomized control trial:*

- It is a type of experimental study design which aims to reduce bias when testing a new treatment/intervention.
- *Basic steps:*
    - Drawing up a protocol:
        - One of the essential features of RCT is that this study is conducted under a strict protocol.
        - The protocol specifies the aims and objectives of the study, questions to be answered, inclusion and exclusion criteria for selection of study and control group subjects, sample size, treatment, or intervention to be performed.
    - Selecting a reference and experimental population:
        - *Reference population:* It is the population to which the findings of the trial if found successful will be applicable
        - *Study/experimental population:*
            - Derived from reference population
            - Should be randomly chosen
            - Should be representative of reference population
            - Should be eligible for the trial and should give consent for the same
            - Is also called as experimental population

b. *Randomization*

- It is the heart of randomized control trial.
- *Definition:* Randomization is a statistical procedure by which the participants are allocated into either study or control groups, to receive or not receive the intervention under study.
- Randomization is done in an attempt to eliminate bias and allow for comparability between the study and control group.
- It ensures that the investigator has no control over the allocation process and this helps eliminate selection bias.
- It means that every individual study subject has an equal chance of being allocated to either study or control group.
- It is best done by using a table of random numbers.

*Intervention/manipulation:* Deliberate application of treatment/intervention to be tested or withdrawal/reduction of suspected causal factors.

*Follow-up:* Examination of the experimental and control group subjects at defined interval of time to look for desired study outcome.

- *Attrition:* It is loss to follow-up which may happen due to either death, migration, loss of interest, or withdrawal of consent. Every effort should be made to minimize this. Losses are inevitable.

  Assessment of data to derive results

c. Classification of RCTs:
- *On basis of hypothesis:*
  - Superiority trial
  - Noninferiority trial
  - Equivalence trial
- *On basis of outcome of interest:*
  - Explanatory
  - Pragmatic
- *Study designs in randomized control trial:*
  - Concurrent parallel study design
  - Crossover type study design
- *Types of RCT:*
  - Animal experiment
  - Human clinical trial
  - Preventive trial
  - Risk factor trial
  - Cessation experiment

d. *Advantages of RCT:*
- Considered most reliable form of scientific evidence (level 1 evidence)
- Used to find cause and effect relationship
- No selection bias
- Multiple outcome variables can be measured in a single study

*Disadvantages of RCT:*
- Expensive
- Longer study duration
- Ethical restrictions and administrative issues
- Participant and observer bias
- Noncompliance of controls threatens the validity of study

**Ans. 5** a. *Concept of blinding in RCT*:
- It refers to the concealment of group allocation from one or more individuals involved in the research study

- It is also called as "masking".
- *Classification:*
    - *Single blind:* Participant is not aware whether he belongs to study or control group.
    - *Double blind:* Neither the participant nor the investigator is aware of the group allocation and treatment or manipulation received.
    - *Triple blind:* Participant, investigator as well as the person analyzing the data are unaware of the group allocation and treatment or manipulation received.
- *Purpose:*
    - Randomization minimizes the differences between the treatment and control groups.
        - Reduces bias in a study
    - Since the participant is unaware about which treatment group they are in, their beliefs about the treatment are less likely to influence the outcome.
    - Also, since the researcher is unaware of which subjects are receiving the tested treatment, they are less likely to influence the outcomes.

b. Meta-analysis
- First done by Karl Pearson in 1904, term coined by Gene V Glass in 1940.
- Meta-analysis is a statistical analysis that systematically combines the results of several studies which address a specific research question.

**Ans. 6** a. It is a systematic error which is defined as disproportionate weight in favor of or against one thing, person or group compared with another. It is in a way considered to be unfair.

b. *Types of bias:*

*Selection bias*
- It is also called as Berksonian bias.
- It involves individuals being more likely to be selected for study than others.

*Funding bias:* It refers to bias which has been introduced to derive outcomes which favor the study's financial sponsor.

*Reporting bias:* It refers to bias which is introduced when reporting observations; such that observations of a certain kind are more likely to be reported than others.

*Analytical bias:* It refers to bias which is introduced while analyzing the study results.

*Exclusion bias:* It refers to bias which is introduced due to systematic exclusion of certain individuals from the study to alter study results.

*Attrition bias:* It refers to bias which is introduced due to loss of participants/attrition; Example: death or loss to follow-up.

*Recall bias:* It refers to bias which arises as a result of inability of the participant to recollect past events accurately.

*Observer bias:* It refers to bias which is introduced by the researcher/observer. It is the subconscious cognitive bias of judgment by the researcher.

*Confounding bias:*

- It refers to a situation in which association between exposure and outcome is distorted by presence of a confounding factor/variable
- Confounding variable (exposure/outcome)
- *Types:*
    - *Positive confounding:* Observed association is biased away from null.
    - *Negative confounding:* Observed association is biased toward null.

c. Various methods to eliminate bias in RCT
- Randomization
- Blinding
- Allocation concealment

**Ans. 7** *Measures of central tendency:*

- Mean
- Median
- Mode

*Mean*

It is derived by adding all the individual observations and then dividing it by the total number of observations.

*Example:*

- If individual observations are a, b, c, and d; the mean = a + b + c + d/4

*Advantages:*

- Easy to calculate.
- Easy to understand.
- All values in the distribution are included in its calculation.
- It is most commonly used statistical measure of central tendency.

*Disadvantage:*

- It is affected by the extreme values which may result in skewed results.
- The value at times may look ridiculous.

*Median*

It is derived by first arranging the data in ascending or descending order; the value of the observation in the middle of the set is the median.

It is a better indicator of central tendency as compared to mean, when the lowest and highest observation are wide apart or when they are unevenly distributed.

*Advantage:*

- It is easy to calculate.
- Easy to understand.
- Not affected by sampling variations.

*Disadvantage:*

- It does not consider all values in the distribution.

*Example:*

- If individual observations are 1, 2, 3, 4, and 5, then the median is 3.
- If individual observations are 1, 2, 3, 4, then the median is 2 + 3/2 = 2.5.

**Ans. 8** a. • *Measures of dispersion of data:*

- Also called as variability of data.
- Measures of dispersion or variability of a data give an idea of the extent to which the values are clustered or spread out.
- Gives an idea of homogeneity and heterogeneity of data.
- Two sets of data can have similar measures of central tendency but different measures of dispersion.
- Therefore, measures of central tendency should be reported along with measures of dispersion.

*The measures of dispersion include:*

I. *Range:*
   - Simplest measure of dispersion.
   - It can be represented as the difference between maximum and minimum value or simply as maximum and minimum value.
   - Range is given with median.

II. *Mean deviation:* It is the average of deviation from arithmetic mean

III. *Standard deviation:*
   - Always given with mean.
   - It denotes the extent of variation of values from the mean.
   - *Example:* If the standard deviation is 10, then the values tend to be about 10 units above and below the mean.

- Higher values of standard deviation represent higher variability in the data and vice versa.
- Zero represents no variability.

b. *p* value = Probability value
   - *Definition:*
     - It is the probability of occurrence of an event by chance.
     - It is the probability of null hypothesis being true (null hypothesis assumes that there is no significant difference between specified populations).
     - It is the probability of type 1 error.
     - Lesser the *p* value, lesser is the probability of the event occurring by chance.
     - As the confidence interval increases, previously significant value becomes nonsignificant.
   - *Interpretation of p value:*
     - $p = 0.5$ means probability of occurrence of an event by chance is 50 in 100 or 50%.
     - $p = 0.05$ means the probability of occurrence of an event by chance is 5 in 100 or 5%.
     - $p = 0.01$ means the probability of the occurrence of an event by chance is 1 in 100 or 1%.
     - $p = 0.001$ means the probability of occurrence of an event by chance is 1 in 1,000 cases.
     - *p* value for null hypothesis is usually kept at $<0.05$, it means that null hypothesis is true in <5% cases. So, if $p < 0.05$, the null hypothesis is rejected, that is alternative hypothesis is accepted and the difference is statistically significant.
   - *Significance:*
     - $p < 0.05$ is considered statistically significant.
     - Lesser the *p* value, lesser is the probability of occurrence of the event by chance.
     - Higher the *p* value lesser the significance.
     - As the confidence interval increases, previously significant values will become insignificant.

**Ans. 9** Types of error in statistics

- There are four possible outcomes at the end of statistical analysis in a research study.
  1. True positive
  2. True negative
  3. False positive
  4. False negative

- Error in research results when false positive or false negative outcomes are accepted.
- *Type I error:* To reject the null hypothesis when it is true or
    - False positive error, or
    - $\alpha$ error
    - *Example:* Type I error would mean that the effects of two drugs studied were found to be different by statistical analysis, when in fact there was no difference between them.
- *Type II error:* To accept the null hypothesis when it is false or
    - False negative error or
    - $\beta$ error
    - *Example:* Type II error would mean that the effects of two drugs studied were not found different by statistical analysis, when in fact there was a difference.
- One has to increase sample size to reduce error.

**Ans. 10**
- The power of a statistical hypothesis test measures the test's ability to reject the null hypothesis when it is actually false—that is, to make the correct decision.
- Statistical power = Rejection of null hypothesis when alternate hypothesis is true.
  = Making a correct decision
  = 1-$\beta$ (type II error)
- The maximum power a test can have is 1 and the minimum is 0.
- Ideally, we want a test to have high power, close to 1.
- Increasing the sample size is the best way to increase the power of a statistical test.

**Ans. 11** Statistical tests

*Nonparametric tests:* Statistical test used in the case of nonparametric data.
- Chi square test
- Mann-Whitney U test
- Fisher exact test
- Wilcoxon test

*Parametric tests:* Statistical test used in the case of parametric data.
- *Large sample size:* Z test
- *Small sample size:*
- Paired T test
- Unpaired T test
- One-way analysis of variance (ANOVA)
- Two-way ANOVA

Choosing a statistical test:

- Once data has been collected and tabulated into the spreadsheet, we need to decide what statistical test needs to be performed for different variables tabulated into the spreadsheet.
- *Choice of different tests depends on the following factors:*
  - Whether the variable is categorical or continuous?
  - Whether the data in that variable is normally distributed (parametric) or not normally distributed (nonparametric)?
  - Whether the data is paired or unpaired?

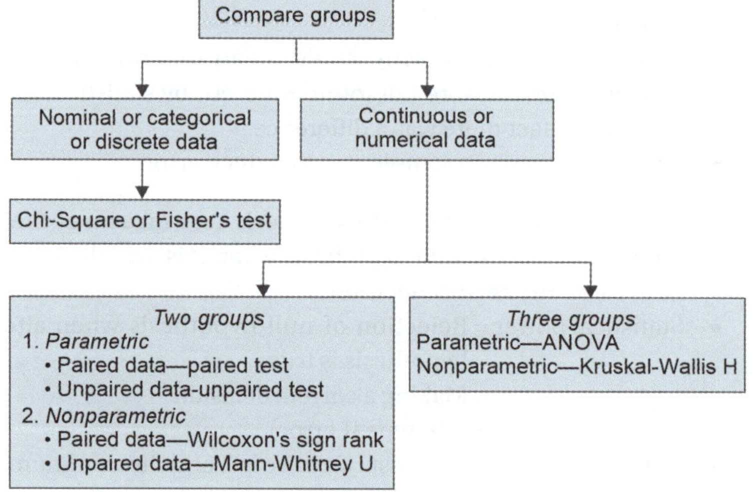


**Ans. 12** a.
- *Univariate analysis:* It analyzes whether one variable is associated with another or not.
  - That is only one variable which is analyzed at a time.
  - Such association does not necessarily mean causation.
- *Multivariate analysis:* It simultaneously tests effect of multiple factors on an outcome.
- That is more than two variables is analyzed at a time.
- It helps in inferring the independent factors that are associated with the outcome.

b. Correlation
- Correlation is relationship between the two sets of continuous data
  - *Example:* Relationship between height and body weight; relationship between fasting blood sugar and body weight.
- Correlation statistics is used to determine the extent to which two independent variables are related and yields a number called coefficient of correlation.

- Correlation coefficient may be positive or negative and may vary from -1 to +1.
- Positive correlation means that values of two different variables increase and decrease together (direct relationship).
    - For example, speed of running and pulse rate correlates positively.
- Negative correlation means that if value of one variable decreases then value of the other variable increases (inverse relationship).
    - For example, age and number of scalp hair may correlate negatively.
- The strength of a correlation is determined by absolute value of correlation coefficient
- Closer is the value to 1, stronger is the correlation.
- Correlation between two variables is shown by scatter plot.
- *p* value in a correlation statistics indicates whether the correlation (or no correlation) observed is real or by chance.
- Correlation analysis is important because it can be used to predict values of one variable on the basis of value of other variable.
- A correlation does not mean causation but it also does not mean absence of causation, that is, if two variables exhibit strong correlation then one of the variables may cause the other.
- Correlation data is therefore not sufficient evidence for causation.
- Pearson correlation is applied for parametric data while Spearman correlation is applied for nonparametric data.
- Combined effect of a group of variable upon a variable not included in the group is called as multiple correlation.

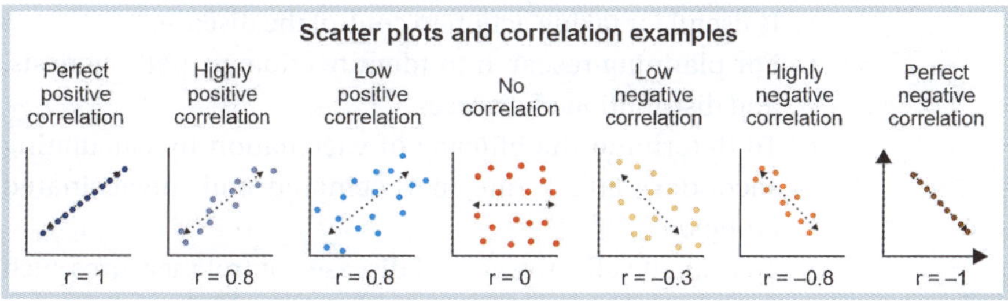


**Ans. 13** a. *Regression*

- Regression analysis is used to predict the values of a quantitative dependent variable based on the values of one or more independent variables.

- In simple regression analysis, there is one quantitative-dependent variable and one independent variable.
- In multiple regression analysis, there is one quantitative-dependent variable and two or more independent variables.
  - For example, one may derive a formula to predict liver span (dependent variable) from the height of a person (independent variable).
- Linear regression statistics finds the best-fit line (line of regression) that predicts dependent variable from independent variable.
- Linear regression statistics is applied to data where independent variable is continuous.
- If the independent variable is categorical (e.g., present vs. absent) then logistic regression is used.

b. *Incidence:*

- Incidence rate is defined as the number of new cases occurring in a defined population during a specified period of time.

$$\text{IR} = \frac{\text{Number of new cases of specific disease diagnosed during a given time period}}{\text{Population at risk during this time period}} \times 1{,}000$$

- Thus, incidence rates refer to:
  - Only new cases
  - Diagnosed during a given time period
  - In a specified/at risk population
- Uses
  - It measures the rate at which new cases are occurring in the population.
  - Helps describe the magnitude of the illness.
  - It acts as a health status indicator.
  - Is useful for taking action to control the disease.
  - For planning research to identify etiology, pathogenesis, and distribution of disease.
  - To determine the efficacy of vaccination by calculating secondary attack rate in vaccinated and unvaccinated groups.
  - To evaluate effectiveness of disease control measures such as isolation, immunization, and disinfection.
- Special incidence rates
  - Attack rate
  - Secondary attack rate
  - Hospital admission rate

c. *Prevalence*

- *Definition:* It is the total number of all individuals who have the disease at particular time period divided by the population at risk of having the disease in this time period.
- Prevalence is a ratio.
- The term refers to all current cases (new and old existing cases) at a given time period in a given population.
- *There are two types:*
  1. Point prevalence
  2. Period prevalence
- *Relationship between incidence and prevalence*
  - Prevalence depends on incidence and duration of illness.
  - If population is stable and the incidence and duration of illness is unchanging.
  - Prevalence = Incidence × duration of illness

**Ans. 14** ▪ *Screening test*

- It is defined as the search for unrecognized disease or conditions by means of rapidly applied tests, examinations or other procedures in an apparently healthy individual.

| ***Screening test*** | ***Diagnostic test*** |
|---|---|
| • Applied on healthy individuals<br>• Applied to groups of individuals<br>• Based on a cutoff point<br>• Less accurate<br>• Less expensive<br>• Not basis of initiation of treatment; it is basis for further evaluation with diagnostic tests<br>• *Example:* Newborn screening, screening of anemia in pregnant women | • Applied to a diseased individual<br>• Applied on a specific individual and not on a group<br>• Based on evaluation of number of symptoms, signs, and test findings<br>• It is more accurate<br>• More expensive<br>• Used as a basis for initiation of treatment<br>• *Example:* HbA1c in diabetics |

▪ *Uses of screening tests*

*Case detection:* Also known as prescriptive screening

- Peoples are screened primarily for their own benefits.
- *Example:* Neonatal screening

*Control of diseases:* Also known as prospective screening

- People are screened for the benefit of others.
- *Example:* Screening of immigrants for detection of infectious diseases; example: yellow fever.

*Research purpose:* Screening may sometimes be performed for research purposes; example in chronic diseases whose natural history is not fully known.

▪ Educational purposes

*Types of screening*

- *Mass screening:* Screening of whole population or sizable subgroup of population.
- *High risk screening:* Screening of a particular subgroup of population which is deemed to be at high risk for the particular disease. It is more productive.
- *Multiphasic screening:* Application of two or more screening test.

*Characteristics of screening test*

- *Acceptability:* It should be acceptable to the individuals in whom it has to be done.
- *Repeatability*
  - The test must give consistent results when repeated more than once on the same individual under the same conditions
  - Factors which *affect repeatability of the test*
    - *Observer variation:* It may be either intraobserver variation (one observer finding different values in the same patient) or interobserver variation (two different observers finding different value in same patient).
    - *Biological variation*
- *Validity:* Also known as accuracy.
  - It is defined as the ability of the test to separate or distinguish those who have the disease from those who do not.
  - *It has two components:* Sensitivity and specificity.
  - Both are expressed as a percentage.

**Ans. 15** *Evaluation of an investigative test:*

- Sensitivity
- Specificity
- Positive predictive value
- Negative predictive value

| *Screening test results* | *Diseased* | *Nondiseased* | *Total* |
|---|---|---|---|
| Positive | a<br>True positive | b<br>False positive | a + b |
| Negative | c<br>False negative | d<br>True negative | c + d |
| *Total* | a + c | b + d | a + b + c + d |

*Sensitivity*

- Defined as the ability of a test to correctly identify all those who have the disease that is true positive.
- Sensitivity = (a/a + c) × 100

*Specificity*

- Defined as the ability of the test to correctly identify those who do not have the disease that is true negative.
- *Specificity* = (d/b + d) × 100

*Positive predictive value:* Proportion of individuals with a positive test result who have the disease.

- *Positive predictive value* = (a/a + b) × 100

*Negative predictive value:* Proportion of individuals with a negative test who do not have the disease.

- *Negative predictive value* = (c/a + c) × 100

Predictive value reflects diagnostic power of the test.

*Diagnostic accuracy (DA):* Accuracy is the proportion of all test results (positive and negative) that are correct.

- Diagnostic accuracy = a + d/a + b + c + d
- An ideal screening test should be 100% sensitive and 100% specific.
- However, when sensitivity increases specificity of the test decreases; that is sensitivity is inversely proportional to specificity and vice versa.
- *In general:*
  - Screening test should have high sensitivity
  - Diagnostic test should have high specificity.

**Ans. 16** a. Kaplan-Meier plots

- It is a nonparametric statistical analysis used to estimate survival function form lifetime data.
- In medical research, it is often used to measure the fraction of patients living for a certain amount of time after treatment, that is survival.
- They are named after Edward L Kaplan and Pual Meier.
- *Basic concepts:*
  - Kaplan Meier plots is a series of declining horizontal steps, which, with a large enough sample size approaches the true survival function for that specific population.
  - In order to generate Kaplan-Meier (KM) plots at least two pieces of data are required for each patient.
    1. The status of the last observation.
    2. Time to event (or time to censoring).
- Length of horizontal lines along the x-axis represent survival duration for that interval.
- Vertical axis represents estimated probability of survival.
- *Example:* Kaplan-Meier survival analysis.

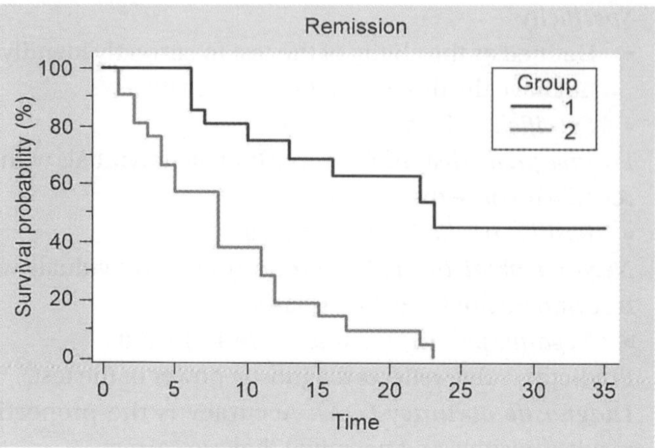


The survival of patients in surgery plus adjuvant chemotherapy group (group 1) is better than patients in surgery only group (group 2).

*Advantage:*

- The advantage of KM plots is the possibility of inclusion of censored data which means that the information about patients who are lost at any point of time, for any reason, can be used for the analysis.
- With the use of these plots professionals have an improved understanding of the disease processes.
- Kaplan-Meier plots can be used in clinical practice for counseling while dealing with patients with different types of diseases.

b. *Forest plots*

- Forest plot is graphical manner of presenting means and confidence interval of studies, so that they can be easily reviewed and compared.
- It is convenient and easily understandable manner of presenting study results in a systematic review/meta-analysis.
- It is used mainly to present results of individual study in a systematic review/meta-analysis as well as the systematic review/meta-analysis itself.
- It shows effect size of all studies and results of meta-analysis.
- Example of a forest plot.

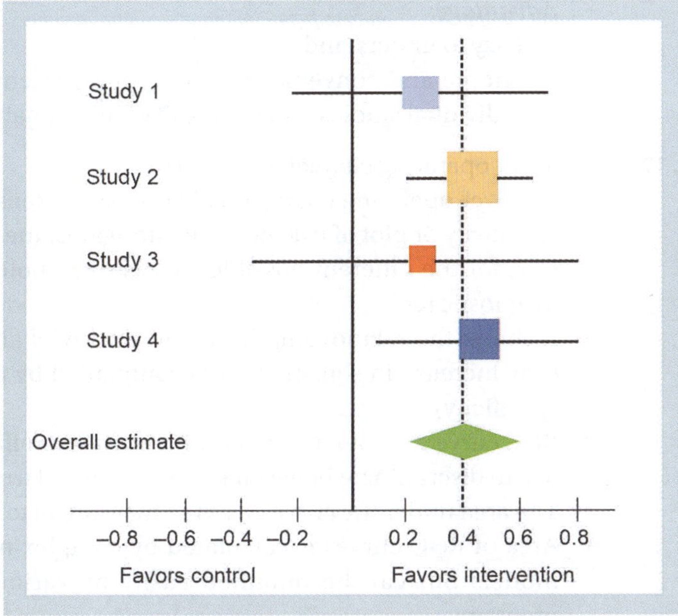


*Example of a forest plot:* The squares represent the effect estimate of the individual studies and the horizontal lines indicate the confidence interval; the dimension of the square reflects the weight of each study.

The diamond represent the summary point, estimate is usually represented with a diamond at the bottom of the graph with the horizontal extremities indicating the confidence interval.

- *Parts of a forest plot:*
  - *Left side:* It enumerates the names of various studies which have been included in the meta-analysis in a chronological order.
  - *Right side:* It represents the measure of effect of the studies included.
  - The square in diagram is a measure of effect of the study (*example:* Mean, odds ratio, and relative risk) and the horizontal line represents the 95% confidence interval of the study.
  - Size of each square or the area of a square is proportional to the weight of the study in the meta-analysis.
  - The diamond in the plot represents the overall measure of effect of the meta-analysis.
  - The vertical line represents the line of no effect/null hypothesis.

*Advantage:*
- Easy to understand.
- Simple and convenient method of representing result of individual studies and net result of meta-analysis.

**Ans. 17** a. Receiver operating characteristic curve
- Receiver operating characteristic is a plot of sensitivity versus specificity or plot of true positive rate against the false positive rate, for the different possible cutoffs (threshold values) of a diagnostic test.
- It shows the relationship between sensitivity and specificity (any increase in sensitivity is accompanied by a decrease in specificity).
- ROC curve gives an idea of accuracy of a test (efficiency of the test to discriminate between true positive and true negative).
- The area under the curve gives the measure of test accuracy.
- Area of ROC curves is calculated by complex mathematical models but can be obtained easily by various computer programs.

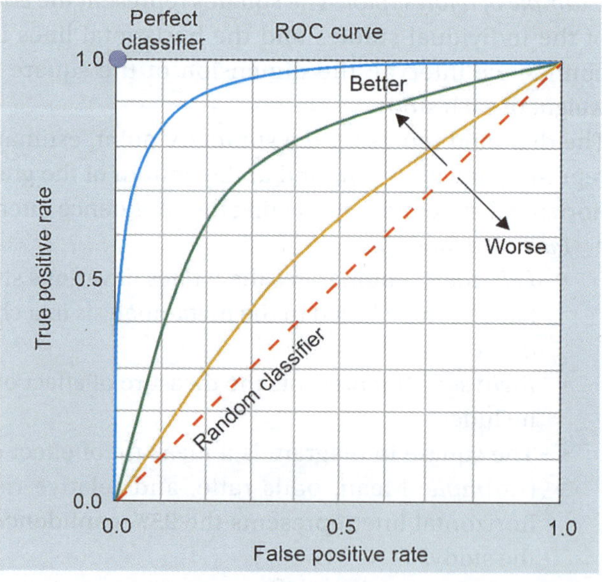


b. Evidence-based medicine
- It is defined as the process of turning clinical problems into questions, then answering them by systematically locating, appraising, and using research findings to finally help with clinical decision making.
- It is also known as evidence-based clinical practice.
  Components of evidence-based medicine

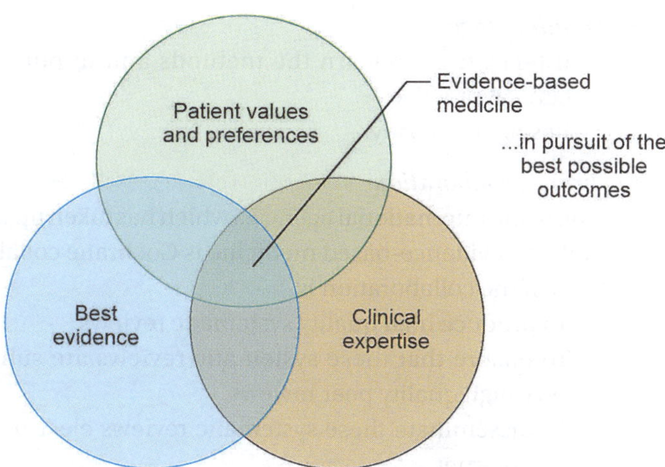


- Steps in evidence-based medicine
  - *Evaluate your patient in form of:* History, clinical examination, and laboratory investigations.
  - Ask appropriate clinical questions.

The question should include all components of PICO, that is:

- *P:* Description of patient population
- *I:* Intervention
- *C:* Comparison group
- *O:* Outcome
- Acquire the best evidence in the form of research available.
- Appraise the evidence.
- Apply the evidence to patient care.
- Self-evaluation
- Rules of evidence-based medicine:
  - Not all evidence is equivalent.
  - Evidence alone cannot help make clinical decisions.
- *Advantages:*
  - It helps upgrade the knowledge base of the clinician.
  - It helps improve the understanding of the clinician in aspects of research and its methods.
  - It improves the confidence of the clinician in managing clinical situations.
  - It improves the computer literacy and data searching skills.
  - It allows group problem solving and teaching.
  - It improves our reading habits.
  - Wasteful practices can be abandoned.
  - It helps with more effective use of resources.
  - Helps keep the clinician up-to-date.
  - Helps in decision making process.

- *Disadvantages:*
    - It takes time to learn the methods and to put them into clinical practice.
    - Research is costly.

**Ans. 18** a. *Cochrane collaboration:*

- One of the international agencies which has taken up the task of building evidence-based medicine is Cochrane collaboration.
- Goal of the collaboration is
    - To produce high quality systematic reviews.
    - To ensure that these systematic reviews are subjected to very high quality peer reviews.
    - To disseminate these systematic reviews electronically via the internet.

b. *Ethics in research:*

- It is defined as the philosophy of morality.
- *Principles of ethics:*
    - Respect for autonomy
    - Beneficence
    - Nonmaleficence
    - Justice
- *Respect for autonomy:*
    - It is obligation to respect the decision-making capacity of the individual.
    - You need to consult research participants and obtain their agreement before you start your work.
    - Informed consent is obligatory.
    - This principle gives the individual subject, the right to gather as much information as possible so that they can make their informed choice whether to go forward with the intervention or not.
    - Patient need not give any reason for withdrawal.
- Beneficence (means: to do good) and nonmaleficence (means: first do no harm).
    - This principle confers the responsibility of protecting the physical, mental, and social well-being of the research participant during a research to the researcher.
    - The researcher must consider the principles of beneficence and nonmaleficence together and aim at producing net benefit over harm.
- *Justice:* Justice precludes exposing one group of individuals to risks of research for benefit of another group.

**Ans. 19** Level type of evidence:

- *1A:* Systematic review (with homogeneity) of randomized controlled trials (RCTs).
- *1B:* Individual RCT (with narrow confidence intervals)
- *1C:* All or none study.
- *2A:* Systematic review (with homogeneity) of cohort studies.
- *2B:* Individual cohort study (including low quality RCT, e.g., <80% follow-up)
- *2C:* "Outcomes" research; Ecological studies.
- *3A:* Systematic review (with homogeneity) of case-control studies.
- *3B:* Individual case-control study.
- *4:* Case series and poor quality cohort and case-control study.
- *5:* Expert opinion without explicit critical appraisal or based on physiology bench research or "first principles."

| ***Grades of recommendation*** | |
|---|---|
| A | Based on level 1 studies |
| B | Based on level 2 or 3 studies or extrapolations from level 1 studies |
| C | Based on level 4 studies or extrapolations from level 2 or 3 studies |
| D | Based on level 5 evidence or troublingly inconsistent or inconclusive studies of any level |

"Extrapolations" are where data is used in a situation that has potentially clinically important differences than the original study situation.

**Ans. 20**

- It is defined as consent given by a competent individual who has received the necessary information in the language he best understands, has adequately understood the information, and after considering the information has arrived at the decision without having been subjected to coercion, undue influence, inducement, or intimidation.
- If an individual is willing to participate in a research, the investigator should take the participants' informed consent.
- In case of minor or other vulnerable participant, parents/guardians are legally authorized representative who can give consent on their behalf.
    - *Vulnerable participants:* Any individual who lacks the ability to fully consent to participate in a study; example: minor, illiterate person.
    - However, in case of minors above 7 years of age, their consent (also known as assent) should be obtained to the extent of the child's capabilities.

  - For children below 7 years of age, consent has to be obtained from parents/guardians alone.
- *Elements of informed consent:*
  - Volunteerism
  - Information disclosure
  - Decision-making capacity
  - Investigator should give information about following to the participant before taking consent
  - Purpose of the study
  - Expectation from the participant
  - Responsibilities of the investigator
  - Risk and benefits of the intervention under study
  - Alternatives available
  - Option to withdraw from the study
  - In case of complication, whom to contact

**Ans. 21** *Clavien–Dindo classification of postoperative complications*

*Grade I*

- Any deviation from the normal postoperative course without the need for pharmacological treatment or surgical, endoscopic, or radiological intervention.
- Acceptable therapeutic regimens are—drugs as antiemetics, antipyretics, analgesics, diuretics and electrolytes, and physiotherapy. This grade also includes wound infections opened at the bedside.

*Grade II:* Requiring pharmacological treatment with drugs other than such allowed for grade I complications. Blood transfusions and total parenteral nutrition are also included.

*Grade III:* Requiring surgical, endoscopic, or radiological intervention.

- *IIIa:* Intervention not under general anesthesia
- *IIIb:* Intervention under general anesthesia

*Grade IV:* Life-threatening complication (including central nervous system (CNS) complications, e.g., brain hemorrhage, but excluding transient ischemic attack (TIAs) requiring intensive care unit (ICU) management.

- *IVa:* Single-organ dysfunction (including dialysis)
- *IVb:* Multiorgan dysfunction

*Grade V:* Death of a patient

**Ans. 22** Data refers to observed values of a variable.

*Types of data:* Qualitative or categorical or nonparametric data: It refers to data which can be separated into different categories.

*Ordinal data*

- It refers to data which can be arranged in an ascending or descending order.
- *Example:* Stages of cancer (1, 2, 3, and 4)

*Nominal data*

- It refers to data which cannot be arranged in ascending or descending order.
- *Example:* Sex, eye color.
- Quantitative or numerical or parametric data: It refers to data which can be measured.

*Interval data*

- It refers to data which is measured along a scale in which each data point is equidistant from one another.
- *Example:* Level of pain rated from 1 to 10 on scale.

*Ratio*

- It refers to data which can be measured as multiples of one another.
- That is data which can be multiplied or divided.

**Ans. 23** a. Stem and leaf plot
- *Description:* A special table where each data value is split into a "stem" (the first digit or digits) and a "leaf" (usually the last digit).
  - *Stem:* Vertical column of numbers listed downward.
  - *Leaves:* Each horizontal row of numbers.
- *Utility:* Detailed quantitative data presentation, a method for showing the frequency with which certain classes of values occur.

b. Box and whisker plot
- *Description:* A convenient way of graphically depicting groups of numerical data through their quartiles.
- *Line in box:* 2nd quartile (median)
- *Whiskers end:* 1st quartile and 3rd quartile

**Ans. 24** a. *Nominal:* In the given question, an investigator into the life expectancy of IV drug abusers divides a sample of patients into HIV-positive and HIV-negative groups; Since, there is no order of characteristic and it cannot be measured directly, it cannot be an ordinal data or metric data, respectively. Thus, it is nominal data (based only on names, i.e., HIV-positive and HIV-negative groups).

b. Categorical data

c. Ordinal
d. Tree diagram
  - A tree diagram is simply a way of representing a sequence of events along with their probabilities.
  - Tree diagrams are particularly useful in probability since they record all possible outcomes in a clear and uncomplicated manner.
  - In the given question, branches can indicate different joints involvement in the case of diabetes; Further, branches can indicate if test conducted was positive or not.
  - It can further help in decision making for treatment joint wise and overall.

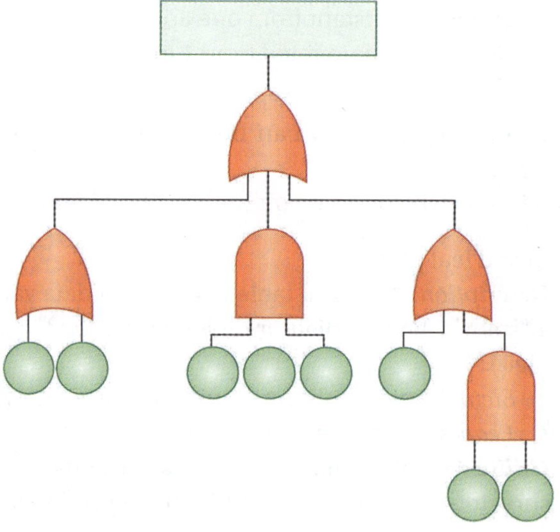

**Ans. 25** a. Median
b. Median
c. Median
d. 5

In a bimodal series Mode = 3, Median—2 mean. In the given question, mean is 2 and median is 3 in a bimodal series. Thus, Mode = 3(3) – 2(2) = 9 – 4 = 5.

**Ans. 26** a. 20 kg

*Mean [averag(e)]:* Is obtained as sum of all values divided by the no. of values. Mean = Sex/n; in the given question, = 18.2 kg and n = 10. Thus, sex = 182. Also, weight of one of the boys was wrongly recorded as 2.0 kg that should have been 20 kg. True sex = 182 + (20 – 2.0) = 200. So, true mean = sex (true)/n = 200/10 = 20.0 kg.

b. 16, 10, and 10.

c. Increased mean, no change in median

In the given question, sleep apnea scores of 10 students is recorded. If the highest value (obtained 58) is wrongly recorded as 85 then,

- *Mean will increase:* As total sum in numerator will increase while denominator (number of persons 10) remain same
- *Median will not change:* As only the highest value changes, middle value in the distribution (ascending order) remains same.
- *Mode:* Is unlikely to change (unless 58 was the mode, it may change)?

d. 8

**Ans. 27** a. Median

b. 100 equal parts

*Centile (percentile):*

- Divides a distribution into 100 equal parts, after arranging in an ascending order, such that each part/segment has equal number (n/100) of subjects.
- Requires 99 intercepts (cutoff points) for division into 100 parts.
- *Total percentiles:* 99.
- *The nth percentile implies:* When all values are arranged in ascending order, n% are below this value.
- *Methods for location of percentiles:*
    - *Graphical method:* Cumulative frequency diagram
    - *Arithmetic method:* Cumulative frequency table
- *Applications and uses of percentiles:*
    - Location of a percentile
    - Preparation of a standard percentile (Q2, median) for particular age, sex, etc.
    - Comparison of a percentile value of a variable (between samples or populations)—To study growth in children (using growth charts).
    - As a measure of dispersion (interquartile/semi-interquartile range).

c. 512

$p$ = C (1 + r) n where, $p$ = Final value, C = Initial value, r = Fraction increase, n = no. of times increase. In the given question, a bacterium can divide every 20 minutes and exponential growth is for 3 hours, Thus, C = 1, and r = 1 (it doubles every time) n = 3 hours/20 minutes = 9 times. Thus, $p$ = C (1 + r) n = 1 (1 + 1) 9 = 29 = 512.

*One other simple way of doing it:*

- *Given information:* A bacterium can divide every 20 minutes (3/hour).
- Thus, in 3 hours, it will total divide 3/hours × 3 hours = 9 times
- Thus, 9 times multiplication will successively yield 2, 4, 8, 16, 32, 64, 128, 256, and 512 bacteria.
- So, at end of 9 hours, there will be 512 bacteria.

d. Third quartile

- *Quartile:* Divides a distribution into four equal parts, so the number of intercepts required will be 3, i.e., Q1, Q2, and Q3.
    - So, zero – Q1 covers 25% values.
    - Similarly, Q2 – Q1, Q3 – Q2, and 100 – Q3 all cover 25% values each.
    - Thus, Q2 – zero, 100 – Q2, and Q3 – Q1 all cover 50% values each.
    - Q1 divides a distribution in a ratio of 25:75 or 1:3.
    - Q2 divides a distribution in a ratio of 50:50 or 1:1, thus, second quartile is equivalent to median.
    - Q3 divides a distribution in a ratio of 75:25 or 3:1.

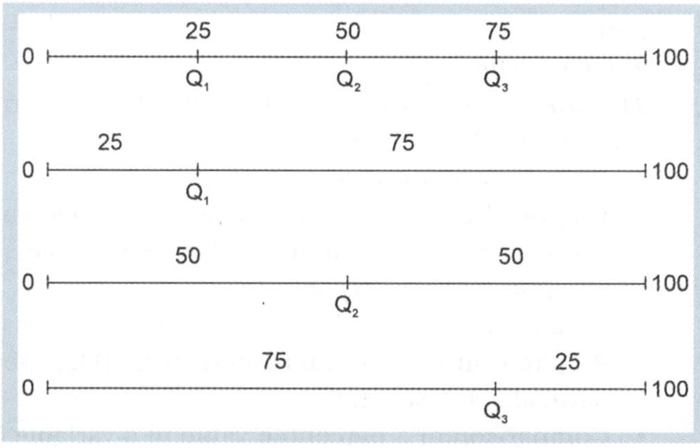


**Ans. 28** a. 50

- Among 200 persons, Q1, Q2, and Q3 would be located at 50th, 100th, and 150th person, respectively.
- This would divide data of 200 persons into four equal parts of 50 each.
- Also, Q3 (3rd quartile) divides a distribution in a ratio of 3:1, i.e., 150:50.
- So, last quarter would include 50 persons.

b. 53.6

*Percentile calculation*

- Standard normal distribution is also be useful for computing percentiles:
  - *Median:* 50th percentile
  - *First quartile:* 25th percentile
  - *Third quartile:* 75th percentile
- *Percentile formula:* $X = \mu + Z\sigma$ (where $\mu$ is mean, $\sigma$ is standard deviation (SD) and Z is value from normal distribution for desired percentile)
- *Z values for commonly used percentiles:* In the given question, mean = 70 mm Hg, SD = 10 mm Hg, Z = – 1.645, and X = 5th percentile value. So, X5 = 70 + (– 1.645) 10 = 53.6 mm Hg.

c. 25%

*Coefficient of variation:*

- Is a measure used to compare relative variability
- Is a unit-free measure to compare dispersion of one variable with another
- Is SD expressed as percentage of mean

$$CV = \frac{SD}{Mean} \times 100 = \frac{\sigma}{\mu} \times 100$$

In the given question, median weight (m) = 12 kg, n = 100, standard deviation (s) = 3. Thus, coefficient of variance = s/m × 100 = 3/12 × 100 = 25%.

d. 0.4

Standard error of mean (SEMEAN)

- SEMEAN is the measure of difference between sample and population values: Whatever be the sampling procedure or the care taken while selecting sample, the sample estimates (statistics) will differ from population values (parameters).
- SE is a "measure of chance variation", and it does not mean an error or mistake.

$$SE_{mean} = \frac{\text{Standard deviation (SD)}}{\text{Sample size}} = \frac{\sigma}{\sqrt{n}}$$

In the given question, $n$ = 25 kids, standard deviation (s) = 2, mean incubation period ($\mu$) = 8 days. Thus, standard error = 0.4.

- Greater the standard deviation (s), greater will be the standard error (SE), especially in small samples.
- SE can be minimized by reducing SD: By taking a large sample.
- SE is a measure of variability of sample summaries: SEMEAN is the SD of sample means.
- Uses of standard error of mean (SEMEAN) in large samples:

- To work out limits of desired confidence within which population mean would lie
- To determine if sample is drawn from a known population or not.
- To find SE of difference between 2 means (to know if difference is real and statistically significant)
- To calculate sample size (within desired confidence limits).

- Standard error of difference between 2 means:

$$SE_{\text{diff bet mean}} = \sqrt{(\sigma_1^2/n_1 + \sigma_2^2/n_2)}$$

**Ans. 29** a. 0

In the given question, the birth weight of each of the 10 babies born in a hospital in a day is found to be 2.8 kg, thus, SD = Zero. So, the standard deviation of this sample will be:

$$SD\ (\sigma) = \sqrt{(\text{Variance})} = \sqrt{\frac{\Sigma(x-\bar{x})^2}{n}} = \text{Zero.}$$

b. 0.1

In the given question, n = 100 women, mean hemoglobin (m) = 10 g%, standard deviation (s) = 1.

Thus, standard error:

$$(SE) = \frac{(SD)}{\sqrt{\text{Sample size}}} = \frac{\sigma}{\sqrt{n}} = \frac{1}{\sqrt{100}} = 0.1$$

c. Original standard deviation × 10

$$SD\ (\sigma)\ \text{new} = 10\sqrt{\Sigma(x-\bar{x})^2/n} = 10 \times \text{Original SD.}$$

d. 1.0

Z score (standard score):

- Is also known as "normal deviate."
- Is difference of a value from group mean, in terms of how many times of SD (s).

$$Z\ \text{score} = \frac{\text{Individual level} - \text{Mean}}{(SD)} = \frac{(x-\mu)}{\sigma}$$

- The standard score indicates how many standard deviations an observation is above or below the mean.
- Z scores are frequently used in assessing how far a child is in his relative growth to a standard
  - *Z score = 2:* Any measurement of at least 2SD away is considered too far away to be normal.

*In the given question,*

x = 15.0 g/dL, m = 13.5 g/dL, s = 1.5 g/dL

Thus, Z score = (x – m)/s = (15.0 – 13.5)/1.5 = 1

**Ans. 30** a. 0.1 g%

b. 72–88%

Confidence intervals for population proportions (for 95% confidence)

$$CI = P + 2\ SEP = P + 2\sqrt{pq/n}$$

In the given question, P = 0.80 (80%); p = 0.80; q = 1-p = 1–0.80 = 0.20; $n$ = 100 CI = 0.80 + 2 $\sqrt{0.8*0.2/100}$ = 0.80 + 0.08 = 0.72, 0.88 (72%, 88%)

c. 0.50

In a normal distribution, 50% of values lie above mean (or median or mode).

d. S = square root of V

**Ans. 31** a. In the given question, the fasting blood levels of glucose for a group of diabetics is found to be normally distributed with a mean of 105 mg per 100 mL of blood and a standard deviation of 10 mg per 100 mL of blood. Thus, mean (μ) = 105 mg/dL and SD (s) = 10 mg/dL.

95% of diabetics will have their fasting blood glucose levels within the limits of mean ± 2SD (μ ± 2s), i.e., within 105 + 2(10).

b. 150

*Quartile:* Divides a distribution into four equal parts, so the number of intercepts required will be 3, i.e., Q1, Q2, and Q3.

- So, zero – Q1 covers 25% values
- Similarly, Q2 – Q1, Q3 – Q2, and 100 – Q3 all cover 25% values each.
- Thus, Q2 – zero, 100 – Q2, and Q3 – Q1 all cover 50% values each.
- Q1 divides a distribution in a ratio of 25:75 or 1:3.
- Q2 divides a distribution in a ratio of 50:50 or 1:1. Thus, second quartile is equivalent to median.
- Q3 divides a distribution in a ratio of 75:25 or 3:1.

In the given question, n = 300, Q3 = 4.5 liters and Q1 = 1.5 liters. Thus, Q3 – Q1 will cover 50% values, i.e., 50% of 300 = 150 values.

c. 400

Minimum sample size for prevalence calculation in cross-sectional studies (field surveys):

Sample size = $4\ pq/L^2$

Where, p = prevalence; q = 1-p; l = error in estimation of prevalence.

In the given question,

p = 50% (50/100); q = 1-p = 1-0.50 = 0.50 (50/100);

L = 5% (5/100 as range permissible is 45–50%, i.e., + 5%)

So, sample size = $(4*50/100*50/100)/(5/100)^2$ = 400

d. Outliers

Dixon's Q test

- *Use:* To find out and eliminate outlier from a distribution.
- *Method:* Measure the difference between a suspect value and next closest value, and then compare it with total range of observations.
- *Alternative method to detect outliers:* Grubb's T procedure.

**Ans. 32** a. Paired T-test

In the given question, variation in cholesterol was seen before and after giving a drug. Thus, comparison of mean (cholesterol levels) is done in paired data for which Paired student's T-test is done.

b. Paired T-test

In the given question, a cardiologist wants to study the effect of an atorvastatin drug; he notes down the initial cholesterol levels of 50 patients and then administers the drug on them and after a month's treatment, he measures the cholesterol level again.

- Since, mean cholesterol levels are being measured in the same group of individuals before and after an intervention, this is paired data.
- Thus, the most appropriate to test the statistical significance of the change in blood cholesterol will be student's [paire(d)] T-test.

c. Chi-square test

In the given question, in a particular trial, the association of lung cancer with smoking is found to be 40% in one sample and 60% in another, since, two proportions are to be compared best test will be Chi-square test.

d. In the given question, mean ± SD of 20 boys (140 ± 13 cm) and 20 girls (135 cm ± 7 cm) of the same age are compared.

Thus, most appropriate statistical test of significance would be unpaired student's T-test.

**Ans. 33** a. Paired "T" test

In the given question, the mean BP of a group of persons was determined and after an interventional trial, the mean BP was estimated again. The best test to be applied to determine the significance of intervention would be paired student's T-test.

b. Chi-Square test

In the given question, an investigator wants to study the association between maternal intake of iron supplements (yes or no) and incidence of low birth weight (<2,500 or >2,500 g).

Thus, association is to be studied between two qualitative variables, i.e., status of usage of iron supplements and status of low birth weight in their newborns.

So, most appropriate test would be Chi-square test.

c. Paired T-test

In the given question, a cardiologist wants to study the effect of an antihypertensive drug. So, he will compare mean BP of 50 patients before and after administering the drug. Thus, paired T-test will be most appropriate test of significance.

d. Student's T-test

In the given question, the study to assess the effect of a drug in lowering serum cholesterol levels was undertaken in 15 obese women and 10 nonobese women (two limbs of the study).

Thus, mean lowering of serum cholesterol would be obtained in the two samples, thereby making "two-sampled student's T-test" as the test of choice.

**Ans. 34** a. Chi-square test

In the given question, association of lung cancer with smoking is found to be 40% in one sample and 60% in another. So, the best test to compare the results will be Chi-square test.

b. One way analysis of variance (one way ANOVA)

In the given question, we have to test the statistical significance of the difference in heights of school children; thus, mean heights of schools children in different classes/standards/schools will be done Thus, ANOVA test (F—test/F—ratio) is most suitable.

c. Student T-test

- In the given question, mean bone density among two groups of 50 people each is compared,
- Thus, means are to be compared in two different groups,
- So, unpaired student's T-test is most appropriate to test significance of association.

(Remember McNemar's Chi-square test is a nonparametric test used to test significance of association between two sampled paired data or for paired nominal data in sample.)

d. Paired "T" test

**Ans. 35** a. Multiple logistic regression

- *ANOVA:* Analysis of variance is a parametric test used for polytomous independent variable.
- *Chi-square test:* It is nonparametric test used for testing association between two or more qualitative variables.

- *Multiple linear regression:* It is used if the target variables are dimensional having multiple possible values (e.g., blood pressure, serum cholesterol, and body temperature).
- *Multiple logistic regression:* It is used if the target variables are binary having only two possible values (e.g., hypertension, smoking, and geriatric age group).

In the given question, the investigator finds out that five independent factors influence the occurrence of a disease. So, to compare these five factors (each factor being dichotomous) one should use multiple logistic regression.

b. Paired student's T-test

c. Chi-square test

In the given question, significance has to be tested between receipt of maternal food supplements (yes/no) and subsequent weights of newborns (values or categories), hence, Chi-square test would be more appropriate.

d. Unpaired "T" test

**Ans. 36** a. *Computational mistake in calculating correlation*

*Correlation:*

- Is the relationship between two quantitative or continuous variables.
- *Correlation coefficient (r):* Measures the degree or strength of relationship in a correlation - Correlation coefficient (r) lies between: –1 to +1 ($-1 < r < +1$)
- *Correlation is represented by* "Scatter diagram"—In a scatter diagram, two imaginary lines are drawn along the distribution of dots/scatter.

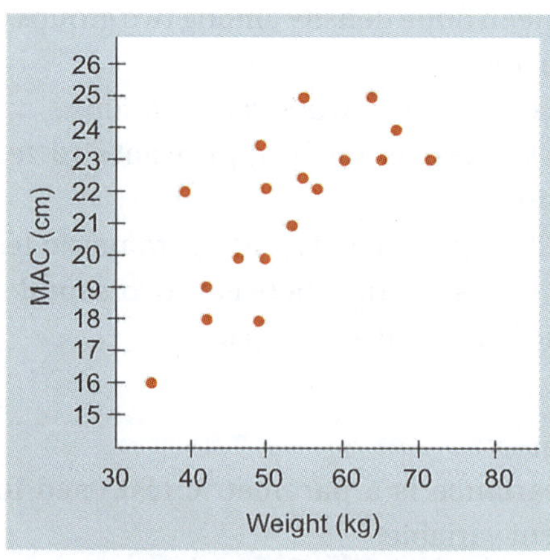


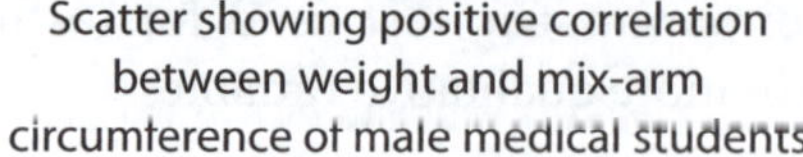
Scatter showing positive correlation between weight and mix-arm circumference of male medical students

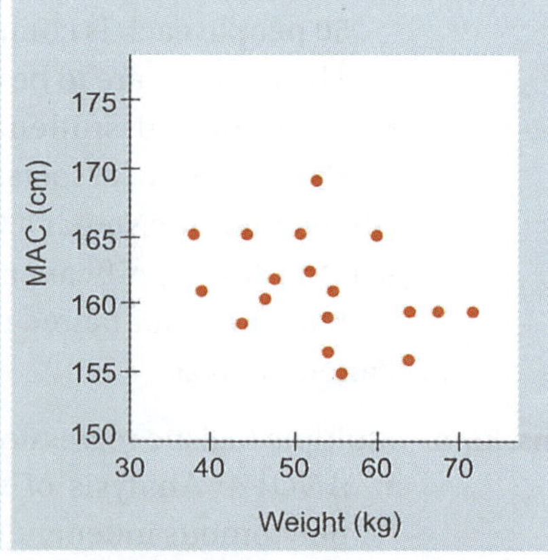


Scatter diagram showing negative correlation between weight and weight and height of male medical students

*Correlation coefficients:*

- *Pearson's correlation coefficient:*
    - It is used in ungrouped series.
    - It is used when associated variables are normally distributed.
    - Symbol is "r"
- *Spearman's rank correlation coefficient*:
    - It is used in a grouped series
    - It is used when associated variables are not normally distributed
    - Symbol is "rho (r)"

*Point to remember*

- *Multiple correlation coefficient:* It is used for calculation of correlation between one variable (dependent) and the combination of two or more variables (independents).
- *Coefficient of determination:*
    - It is the percentage of variation in a variable that is explained by one or more of the others.
    - It is generally obtained in a regression setup.
    - Coefficient of determination = (Correlation coefficient)$^2$ = $r^2$
- *Coefficient of variation:*
    - It is a measure used to compare relative variability.
    - It is a unit-free measure to compare dispersion of one variable with another

$$CV = SD/mean \times 100 = s/m \times 100.$$

b. The lecturer has reported the correlation coefficient incorrectly:

*Correlation coefficient (R):*

- Measures the degree or strength of relationship in a correlation (relationship between two quantitative or continuous variables).
- Correlation coefficient (r) lies between: –1 to +1 ($-1 < r < +1$)
- *Strength of correlation:*
    - *Weak positive correlation:* $0 < r < 0.3$
    - *Moderate positive correlation:* $0.4 < r < 0.6$
    - *Strong positive correlation:* $r > 0.7$
- *Correlation is represented by:* "Scatter diagram" in the given question, a lecturer states that the correlation coefficient between prefrontal blood flow under cognitive load and the severity of psychotic symptoms in schizophrenic patients is - 1.24.

  Since, correlation coefficient (r) lies between –1 to +1 only, a value of r = - 1.24 is not possible. There is some computational mistake in calculation.

c. Chi-square test

In the given question, association is to be studied between maternal intake of iron (yes/no) and birth weights of newborns (to see the proportion of low birth weight), i.e., between two qualitative characteristics, thus Chi-square test is most suitable.

d. Type I error ($\alpha$ error)

*A test with a high specificity has a low type I error rate:*

- False positive rate (a) = 1 - specificity
- False negative rate (b) = 1 - sensitivity

# CHAPTER 55

# Previous Year Recalls

## QUESTIONS

**Q1. A 30-year-old female had undergone hysterosalpingography 48 hours ago. Few hours later, she had abdominal pain which was relieved by some pain killers. This morning, she had mild abdominal pain for which abdominal X-ray was done and attached.**

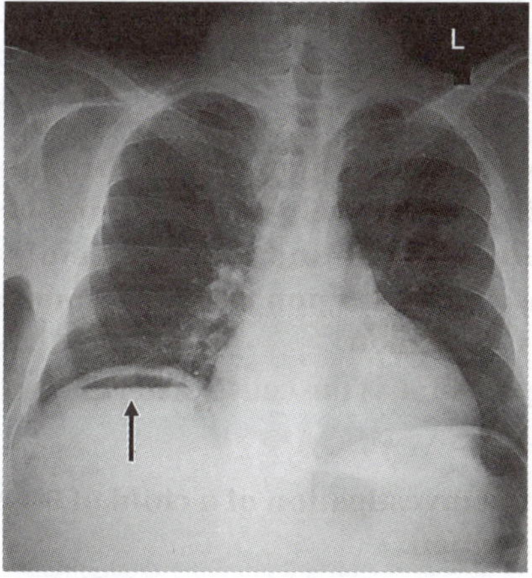


a. What is the most likely diagnosis?

b. What is the next step?

Resuscitation and patient to be posted for surgery.

c. What treatment is suggested to her?

**Q2. A 25-year-old male is brought to the emergency with history of motor vehicle accident. He is unconscious on arrival with a Glasgow Coma Scale (GCS) of 9/15. On examination, he is found to be pale with a thready pulse and cold extremities. The BP is 80 systolic.**

a. Outline the initial management of this patient.

b. Which is the ideal intravenous (IV) fluid for this patient?

c. Interpret these findings.

d. What is your next step in the management of this patient?

**Q3. A 35-year-old while driving cycle and was brought to A and E with altered sensorium and severe pain abdomen. On evaluation, she was found to have stable vitals, GCS of 13/15. X-ray chest done is attached.**

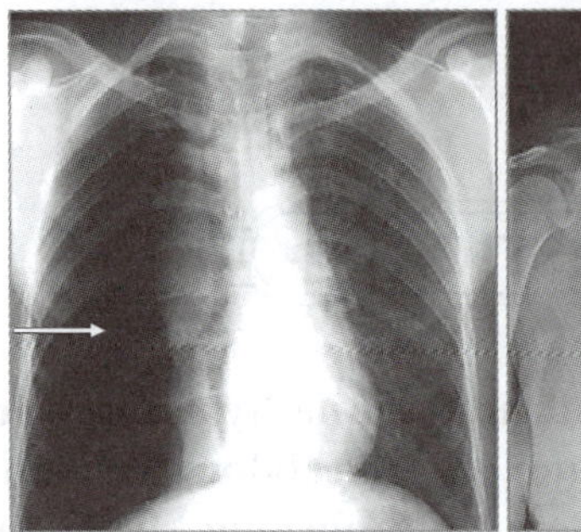

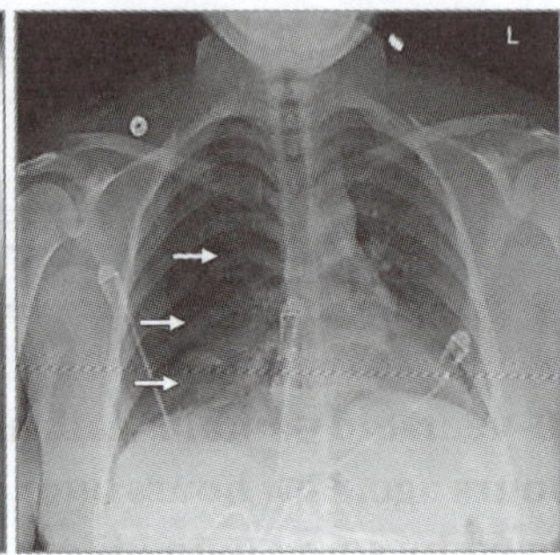


a. What is the clinical diagnosis?
b. What is the next step in management priority wise?
c. She is also found COVID positive. What steps are recommended by you?

**Q4. A 50-year-old female pillion rider is brought to the emergency after a fall in a motor vehicle collision. She had a momentary dizziness after the fall and an episode of vomiting. However, she lost consciousness upon reaching home an hour later and is unconscious since then.**

a. What do you think is the cause of her clinical condition?
b. What is the next step?

**Q5. Attached is the investigation of a child of 6-year-old complaining of pain in abdomen.**

a. Name the investigation shown in the film.

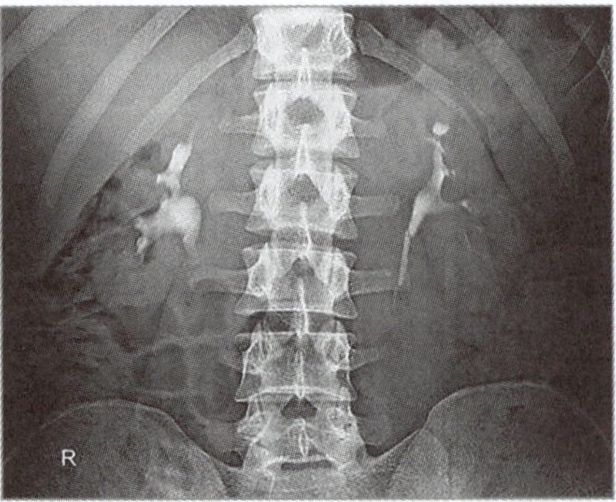


b. Enumerate positive radiological findings.
c. What is the cause of such findings?
d. What investigation is suggested next?

**Q6.**

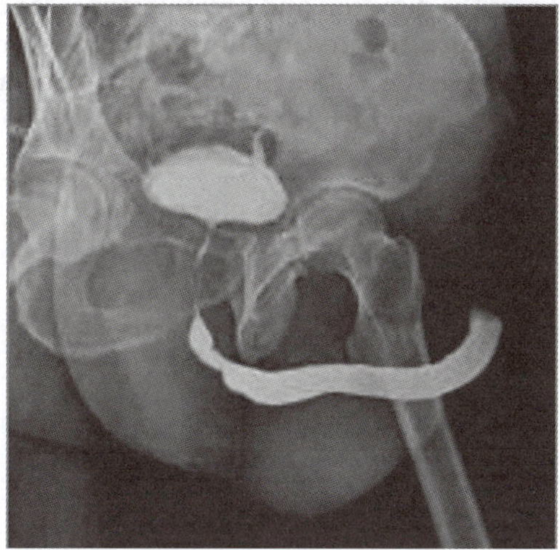

a. Name the investigation.
b. Enumerate the radiological findings seen.
c. What is the most common cause of this condition?
d. What treatment is suggested?

**Q7A.** **A 35-year-old woman, homemaker, complains of a lump in her left breast since last 2 years. The lump is painless. It is progressively increasing in size. Enumerate four important points that you will like to elicit in the history in this patient.**

**Q7B.**

- No past history of breast lump excision.
- History of breast cancer in her elder sister diagnosed at 40 years of age.
- Menarche at 12, still menstruating, regular.
- 2 children, first child at 20 years of age, both breast fed.
- No history of hormone use.

What important signs will you look for in the local examination in this patient?

**Q7C.**

- 3 × 3 cm lump in outer upper quadrant of left breast.
- Smooth, firm; well defined margins; freely movable.
- Overlying skin is unremarkable; Nipple areola complex normal; Axilla is clear.

How will you confirm the diagnosis?

**Q8. A 32-year-old female comes with history of h/o altered bowel habit of 2 months duration and breathlessness for the last 1 month. Abdominal exam reveled moderate distension and evidence of fluid in the peritoneal cavity. She consulted a physician who advised chest X-ray which is enclosed.**

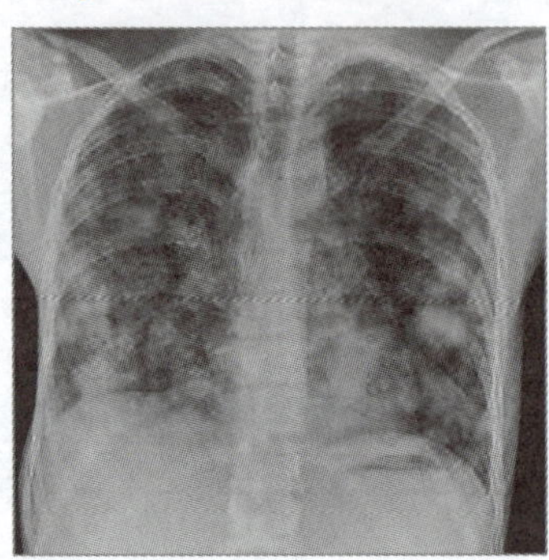

a. What is the provisional clinical diagnosis?
b. What is the next investigation suggested?
c. What is the line of management?
d. How will you explain the prognosis of this patient to her attendants?

**Q9. A 50-year-old rickshaw puller complains of dragging sensation in the left side of abdomen since last 6 months. It is associated with abdominal distension and difficulty in breathing. He is an alcoholic since last 20 years.**

a. What are the likely causes of these symptoms?
b. What additional information would you elicit in the present history?

**Q10.**

- There is no history of previous prolonged illness
- No history of jaundice
- No history of bleeding
- No history of altered sensorium

What would you look for in general physical examination (GPE)?

**Q11. A 53-year-old gentleman presented in OPD with clinical features of pallor and mild icterus. Examination findings are pulse 70/min, BP 110/70 mm Hg, abdomen uniformly distended, umbilicus is everted, splenomegaly present crossing the midline and fluid thrills present.**

a. What is your diagnosis?
b. Name one investigation to confirm the diagnosis.

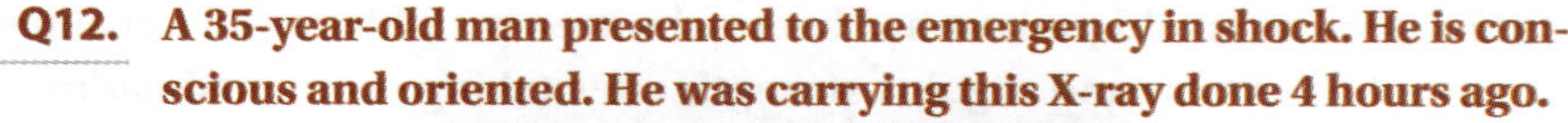

**Q12. A 35-year-old man presented to the emergency in shock. He is conscious and oriented. He was carrying this X-ray done 4 hours ago.**

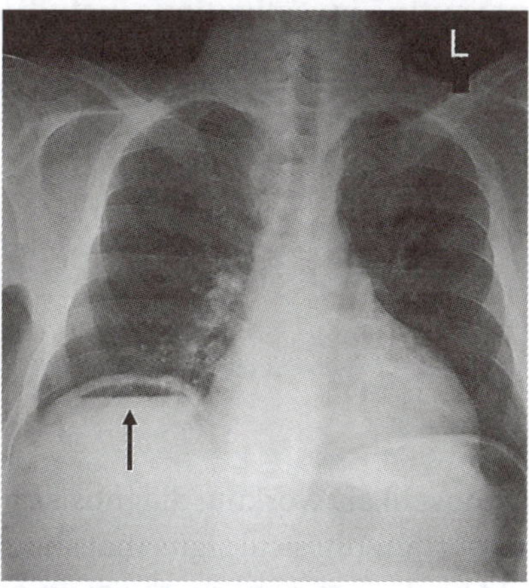


a. What is the finding on this X-ray?
b. What is your diagnosis?
c. What important history will you like to elicit with regards to the diagnosis?
d. What is the Initial management of this patient? Enumerate two of the most important points.
e. What is the definitive management of this patient?

**Q13. A 35-year-old female patient presents with history of a swelling in the front of neck since 7 years. The swelling has started increasing in size since 6 months.**

a. Enumerate two relevant points in history that you will ask this patient.
b. Point out four important signs that you will look for in the GPE.
c. Enumerate four important signs on clinical examination.

**Q14. A 30-year-old lady with recent preference for cold weather. Increased appetite. Noticed recent weight loss since 3–4 months. No significant family history, lives in Jaipur. No change in voice; slowly increased in size, painless. Pulse—100/min, regular, skin moist; sitting comfortably on the chair; face unremarkable; no eye signs; no hand tremors, 2 × 3 cm nodular enlargement of right lobe of the thyroid; left lobe not palpable; firm, nontender; trachea central; and no neck nodes. Carotids in normal position.**

a. What is your diagnosis?
b. Name two important investigations to further manage the patient.

**Q15. A 66-year-old patient has been admitted with history of episodes of weakness and regains strength after taking some medications. He underwent routine investigations including attached X-ray.**

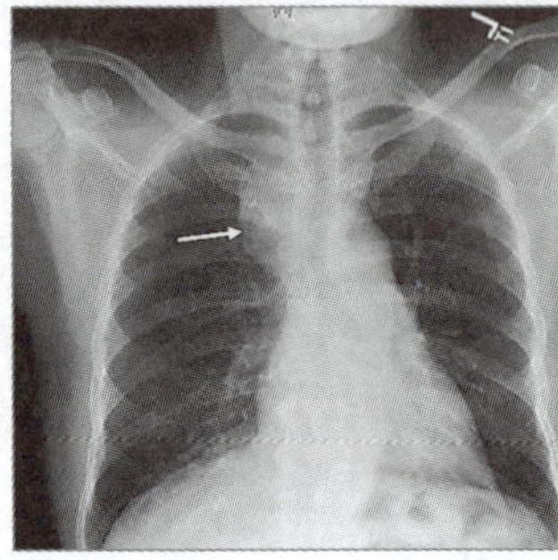

a. What is the most likely working diagnosis?
b. What are important physical signs that should be elicited?
c. What should be done to confirm the diagnosis?
d. What treatment is planned?

**Q16. A 55-year-old man presents with multiple swellings on right side of neck for 3 months.**

a. What are the likely causes of this presentation?
b. What additional information would you elicit in the history?

**Q17. A 72-year-old gentleman with history of dry cough since 2–3 months. Occasional hemoptysis, history of smoking bidis for 50 years. Occasional alcohol intake, no history of fever.**

a. What signs would you look for in the local examination?
b. Name two important investigations for making a diagnosis in this case.

**Q18. A 24-year-old male presented with complaints of pain in the right lower abdomen since 1 day, he underwent a surgical procedure in emergency and the specimen is as shown in the image.**

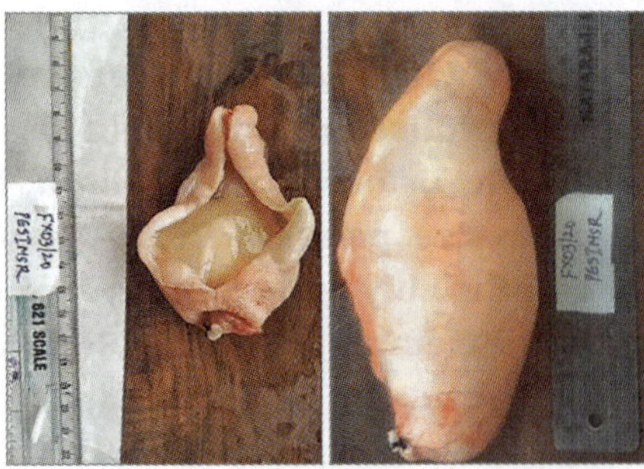

a. Identify the specimen shown in the picture.
b. What is the likely diagnosis?

c. Name the other organ where this pathology is found.
d. Name single most dreaded complication of this condition.

**Q19. A 20-year-old male presents to outpatient department (OPD) with a painless swelling in right side of scrotum for 2 years. The swelling is slowly increasing.**

a. Enumerate two important points that you would like to ask in the history.
b. What is your provisional diagnosis?
c. Name the important signs that you will elicit in examination to confirm the diagnosis.

**Q20. On examination fluctuation is present. Testes is not palpable separate from the swelling.**

a. What is your diagnosis?
b. How would you investigate and treat this case?

**Q21. A 55-year-old male presented with pain right upper abdomen and fever for 5 days, he is febrile with pulse rate 110/min. On examination, he was found to be having tender hepatomegaly 5 cm below costal margin. His CECT film is shown in the image.**

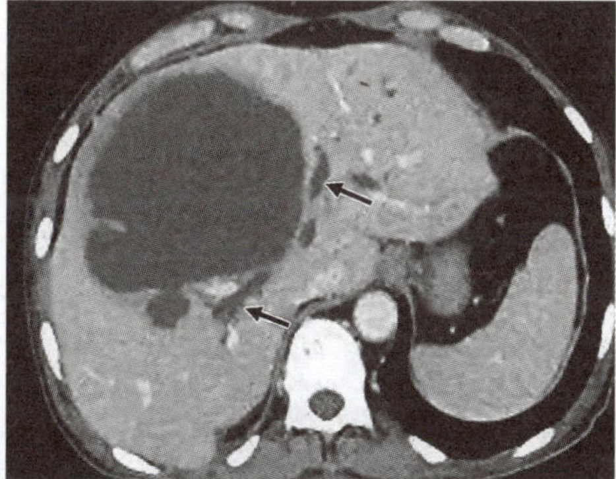

a. What is the most likely diagnosis?
b. Name the etiology of this condition.
c. Write four serious complications of this disease.
d. Name two main modalities to treat this disease.

**Q22. A preterm male baby of 1 month of age is brought with absence of both testes in the scrotum, as a surgical resident on duty, you are called to examine and advise the parents.**

a. What would you advice the anxious parents of the boy and why?
b. What is the most common location of testes in such a patient?
c. Which is the earliest postnatal histologic abnormality in the testes of such a patient?

d. What are the various anomalies associated with this condition? (Name any three).
e. What are the complications associated with this condition? (Name any four).

**Q23.**

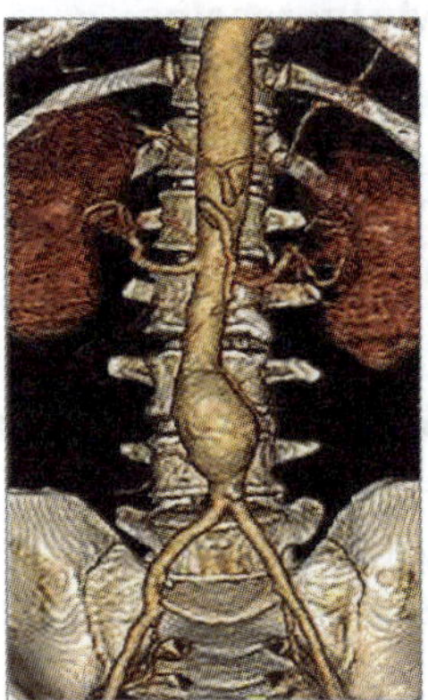

a. Mention the diagnosis seen in the image.
b. Mention any two etiological factors of this condition.
c. Mention any four complications of this condition.
d. Mention two methods of definitive treatment of this condition and one complication of each method.

**Q24.**

a. Write any four information to be disclosed during the discussion for "informed consent".
b. Who cannot provide an informed consent? (Any two).

**Q25.**

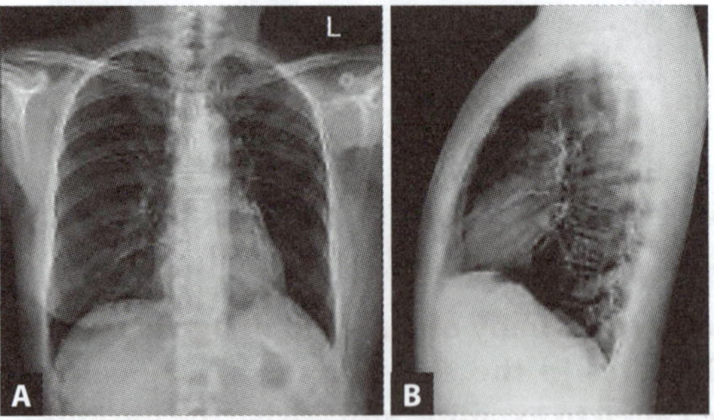


a. Identify the X-rays marked A and B and mention the finding seen.
b. Name the procedure that has been performed on this patient.
c. Name two indications for this procedure.
d. Name two complications of this procedure.

**Q26. A 75-year-old female underwent difficult laparoscopic cholecystectomy for symptomatic gallstone disease 5 weeks ago. She sustained iatrogenic CBD injury during the surgery. The injury was repaired laparoscopically and a T-tube was placed. However, the patient had persistent bile leak through the epigastric port for which she was investigated (see film).**

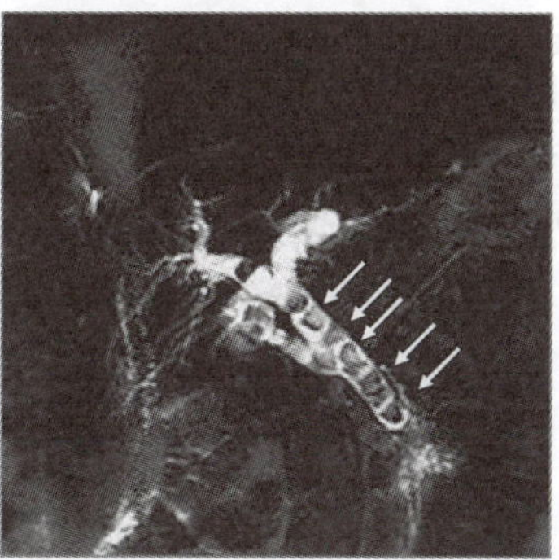

a. Name the investigation in full and enumerate the salient findings seen.
b. What are the endoscopic options for management of this case?
c. What is the best option if endoscopy fails/is not available?

**Q27. A 32-year-old male rickshaw puller comes to the OPD complaining of severe pain in his right lower limb for 2 months and blackening of little toe for 3 weeks. He has been smoking at least two bundles of bidis for last 20 years. He has a history of increasing pain in the calf for last 2 years, now he is unable to walk even to the toilet because of pain. He either hangs his legs or holds it in his palms to get some relief. On examination, the affected foot is cooler. There is a clear line of demarcation between the blackened area and the normal area, all peripheral pulses are present though dorsalis pedis and posterior tibial are weak in the affected limb.**

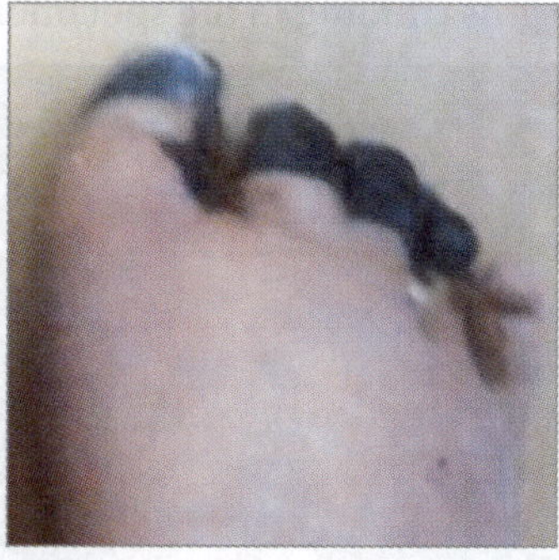

a. What is the clinical diagnosis?
b. What are the points in favor of your diagnosis?

c. Why does the patient get relief on hanging his leg or holding his foot in his palm?
d. How will you confirm your diagnosis?

## MARCH 2021

**Q28. A 40-year-old female presented to the OPD with history of swelling in the front of the ear since last 3 years. The swelling is slowly increasing in size and is painless.**

**Additional information: The patient was taken up for an educational procedure.**

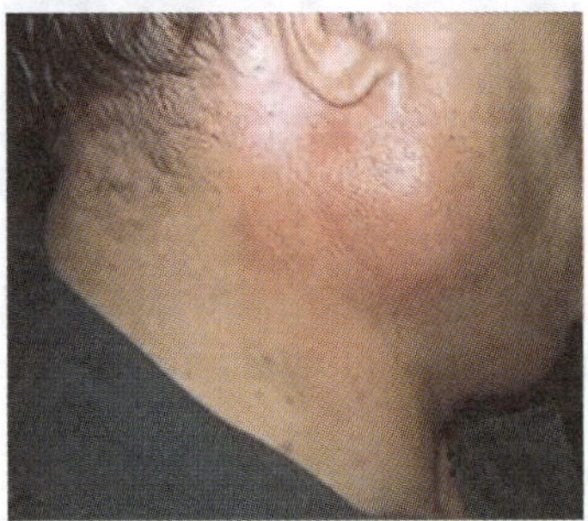

a. Name three important structures that the surgeon should be aware of while performing this surgery.
b. Name two essential anatomical landmarks that the surgeon should be aware of while performing this procedure.
c. Name two important postoperative complications of this procedure.

**Q29. A 45-year-old male presented in emergent with features of perforation peritonitis for which he underwent a surgical procedure. The surgical specimen was opened and is as shown in the picture.**

a. Describe the gross finding in the specimen.

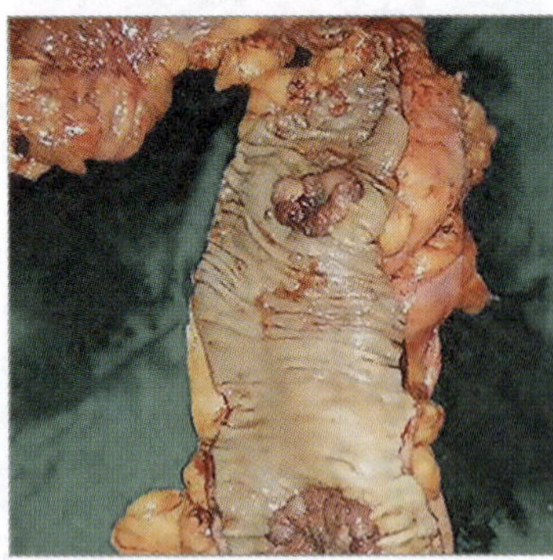

b. What is the likely diagnosis?

c. What are the two characteristic findings on histopathological examination of this condition?
d. What is the definitive treatment of this condition?

**Q30. A 50-year-old female presented with neck swelling for >15 years, initially small in size that increased rapidly to the present size in last 1 month with change in voice for last 20 days.**

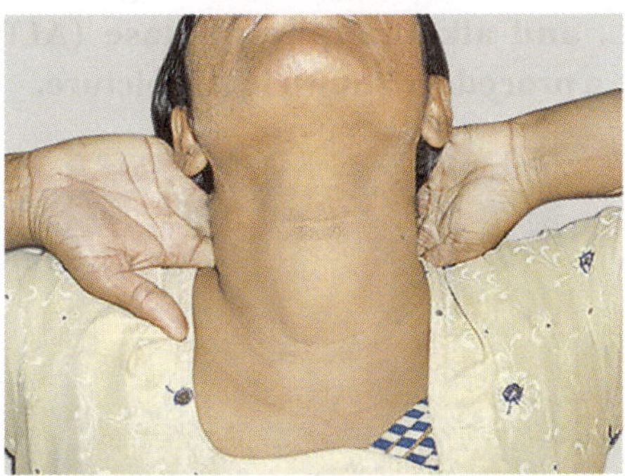

a. What is the name of the maneuver shown in the picture? Why is it done?
b. If carotids are not palpable, what is its implication?
c. What is likely pathological diagnosis of the condition shown in the picture?
d. What is the operative treatment of this condition?
e. Name two specific complications of the operative procedure.

**Q31. A 30-year-old male presented to emergency with penetrating injury to anterior abdomen 2 hours ago. On examination, his vitals are—pulse 100/min and BP—82 mm Hg systolic with findings as depicted in the picture.**

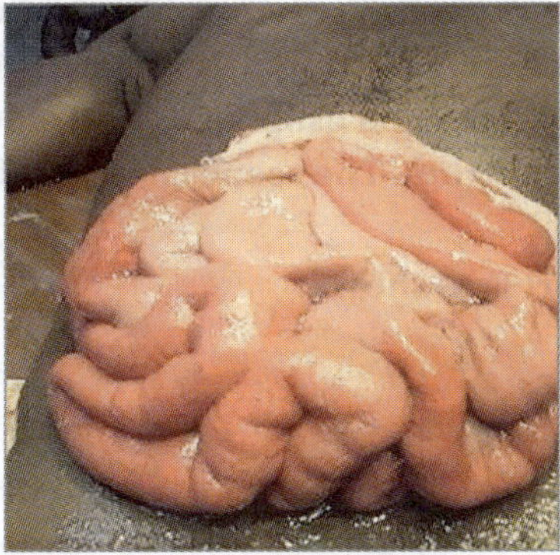

a. What is the definitive management of this patient?
b. Would you consider CECT abdomen in this patient at this stage and why?

c. If a single stab perforation is seen on antimesenteric border of small gut, what will be your approach?
d. If on exploration there is zone II retroperitoneal hematoma, what is your approach?

**Q32. A 35-year-old female presented with right hypochondrium pain, fever with serum bilirubin—10.0 mg/dL, direct component 7.0 mg/dL, and alkaline phosphatase (ALP)—560 U/L. She underwent a procedure shown in the picture.**

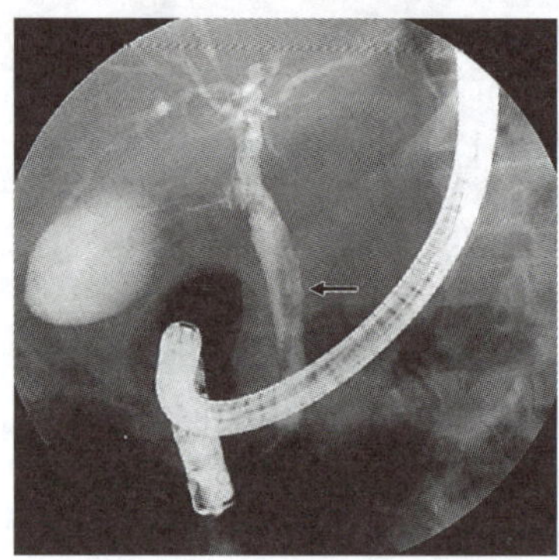

a. Name the investigation in full.
b. Name two findings seen in the picture.
c. What is the indication of this procedure in this case?
d. After on day of the procedure, the patient developed severe epigastric pain with abdominal distention.
e. What are the likely causes for this?

**Q33. A 21-year-old girl is bought to casualty with history of corrosive ingestion 10 days back. She is not able to take solids or liquids and is having repeated vomiting. Upper gastrointestinal (GI) endoscopy revealed a normal esophagus and a deformed, edematous, and narrowed antrum. The scope could not be negotiated beyond the antrum.**

**Her ABG report is as shown:**

| | |
|---|---|
| *pH* | 7.48 |
| *$HCO_3^-$* | 30 mEq/L |
| *$pO_2$* | 98 mm Hg |
| *$pCO_2$* | 46 mm Hg |
| *Na* | 127 mmol/L |
| *K* | 2.9 mmol/L |

a. Interpret the ABG report.
b. Mention two modes of maintaining nutrition in this patient.
c. What are the definitive surgical options? (Any two).

**Q34.**

a. What is a double blind study? What is its advantage?
b. What is impact factor of a journal?
c. What is h-index?

**Q35.**

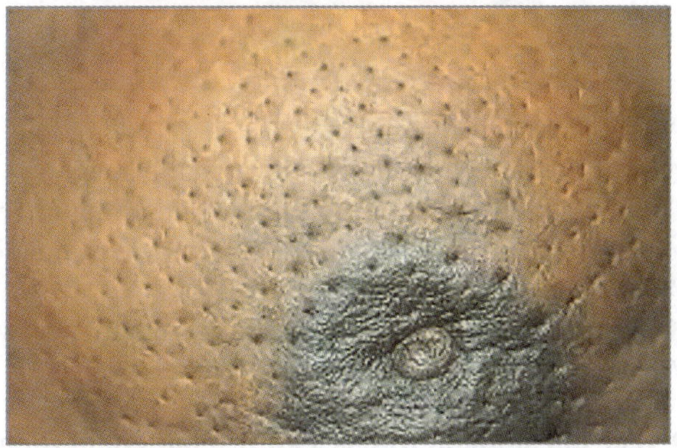

*In palpation of breast lump:*

a. What physical sign is shown in figure?
b. What is the anatomical basis of this physical sign?

**Q36. What will be the N stage of carcinoma breast if lymph node marked at number 5 is involved?**

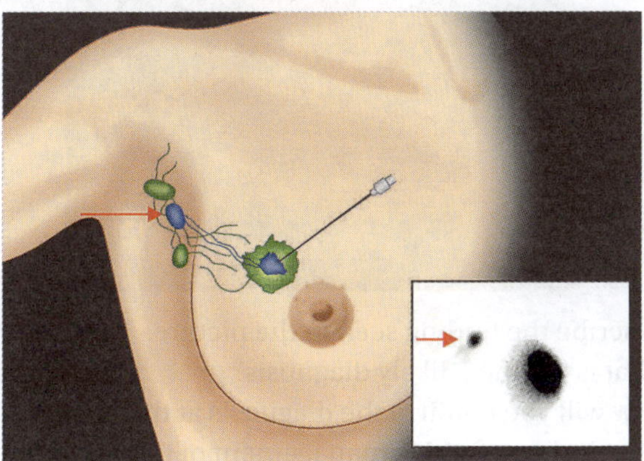

**Q37. A 37-year-old male sustained polytrauma in a road traffic accident. At presentation, his BP was 90 mm Hg systolic and HR 130/mL. His oxygen saturation at admission was 75 with absent breath sounds on the right side. 2 liters of warm saline is started.**

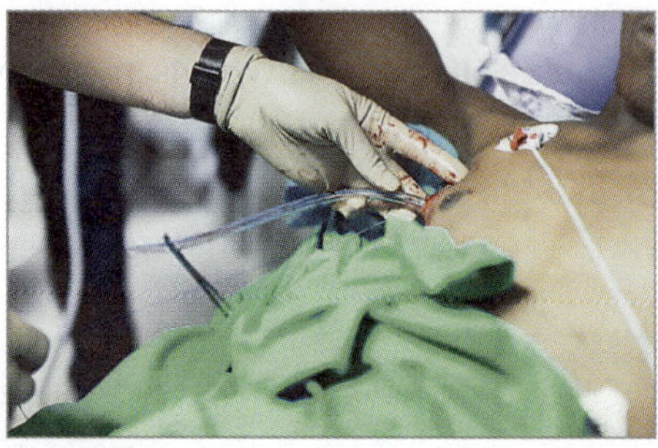

a. What is the likely diagnosis?
b. What is the procedure being shown in the image?
   The saturation continues to dip in spite of the intervention and he has to be incubated. Saturation improves dramatically.
c. What is the possible cause?
   Nurse reports fall in saturation with prominent neck veins.
d. What has happened now?

**Q38. A 40-year-old smoker, who is a known patient of rheumatic heart disease, presented in the emergency with acute pain in left lower limb for the last 3 hours. The left leg was cold and pulsations of the left popliteal artery, posterior tibial artery, and dorsalis pedis artery were absent.**

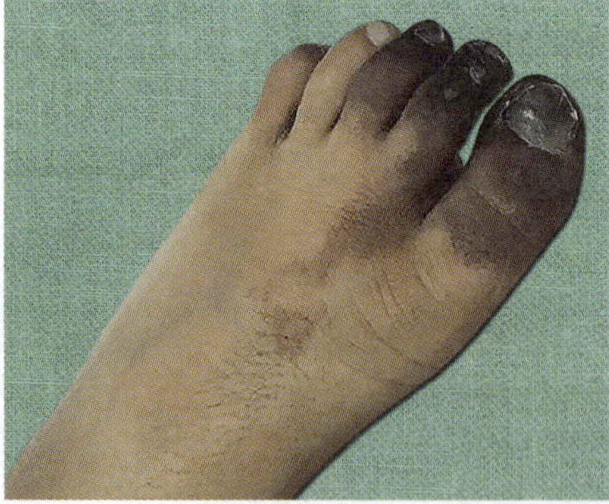

a. Describe the finding seen in the picture.
b. What is the most likely diagnosis?
c. How will you confirm the diagnosis at this stage?
d. What is the definitive management of this condition?

**Q39. A mother has bought her 11-month-old child with complaint of abnormality in his accepting.**

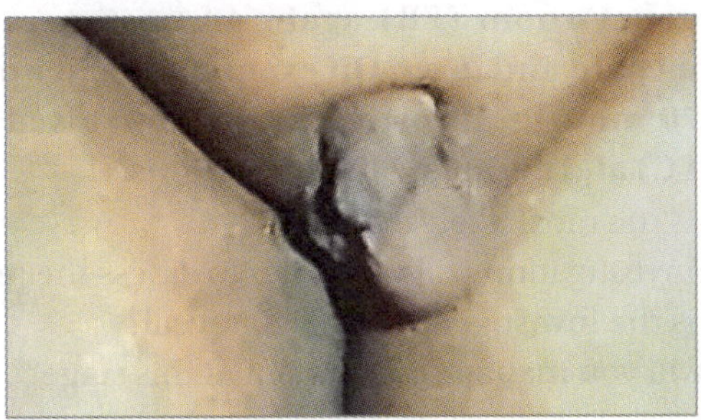

a. What are the findings seen in scrotum?
b. What is the diagnosis?
c. Name one investigation that is mandatory in this case.
d. What is the most dreaded complication of this condition?
e. What advice will you give to the mother?

**Q40. A 54-year-old male presents to the A & E with a 4-day history of central colicky abdominal pain followed by abdominal distention, vomiting, and constipation. He has past history of right-hemicolectomy 2 years ago for colonic carcinoma.**

**Examination revealed normal blood pressure and temperature. Pulse was 100/min. He has abdominal distention. Rectum is empty on digital examination. The bowel sounds are exaggerated. Abdominal X-ray of this patient is displayed here.**

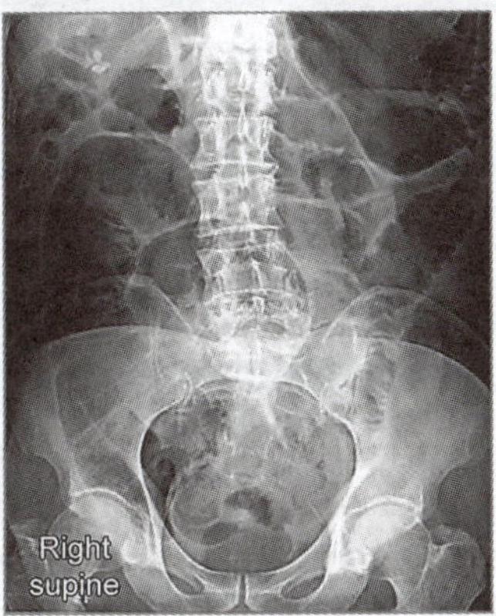


a. What is the clinical diagnosis?
b. What features on the X-ray point toward this diagnosis?
c. What are the two probable causes of this condition?
d. When would you consider this case for surgical exploration? (Any two).

**Q41. A 30-year-old lady underwent laparoscopic cholecystectomy. She was discharged after 24 hours of surgery. She has presented in emergency room (ER) again on postoperative day 3 with abdominal pain and fever. On examination her pulse is 100/min, BP 110/70 mm Hg. Investigations show raised total leukocyte count (TLC) and deranged liver functions.**

a. What is the most likely diagnosis?
b. What investigation will you order to assess the problem?
c. What is the investigation likely to reveal?
d. How will you manage this patient at this stage?

**Q42. A 30-year-old male was admitted with complaints of abdominal pain, episodic headache, and palpitations. Echocardiography revealed cardiomyopathy. This patient was managed surgically by complete removal of the organ shown in the picture.**

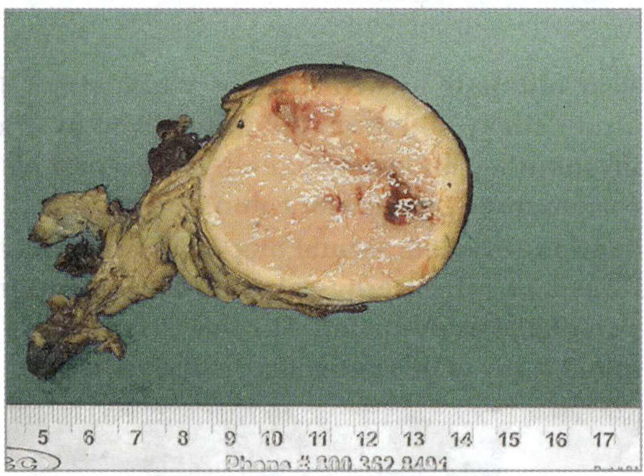


a. Identify the organ and its pathology.
b. What are the two specific diagnostic investigations for this condition?
c. Name two important preoperative preparations control of blood pressure.

**Q43. A 46-year-old female presented to the surgical OPD with complaints of off-and-on pain in right upper abdomen since 2 months. The physical examination is unremarkable. The ultrasonography (USG) shows features of chronic calculous cholecystitis. A laparoscopic cholecystectomy was performed which took 4 hours due to difficulty dissection. Gauze inserted during dissection is stained yellow when retrieved.**

a. What is the likely cause?
b. What is the management?

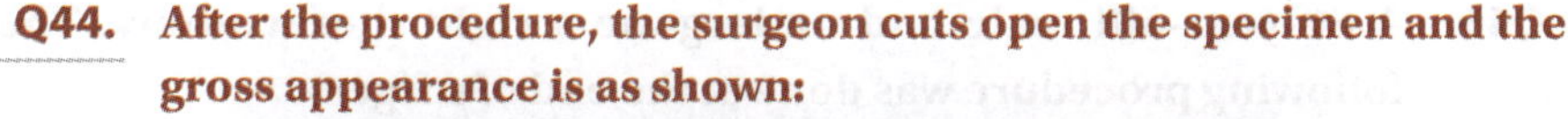

**Q44. After the procedure, the surgeon cuts open the specimen and the gross appearance is as shown:**

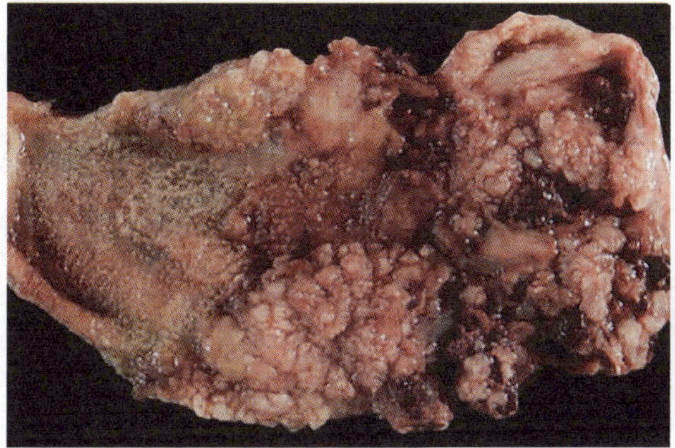

a. Describe the microscopic findings. What is your impression?
b. With this picture of the gross specimen, what additional information do you want?

**Q45. A 50-year-old rickshaw puller presented to surgery OPD with nonhealing ulcer on the inner aspect of cheek. On examination, an ulcer of size 1.5 × 1.5 cm is seen which is 2 cm away from gingivobuccal fold. Its margins are indurated.**

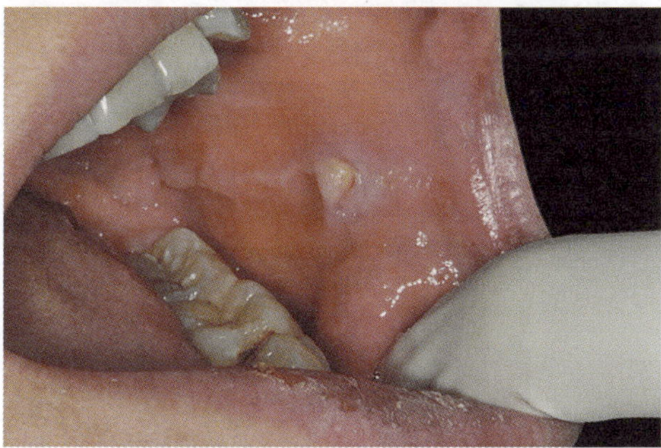

a. What are the risk factors associated with this condition? Name any two.
b. Name two important physical signs that will help in deciding the management of this patient.
c. How will you confirm the diagnosis?
d. Name one investigation that is mandatory in this case.
e. How will you manage this patient?

**Q46. A 60-year-old male had undergone a right thoracotomy. The following procedure was done at the end of surgery.**

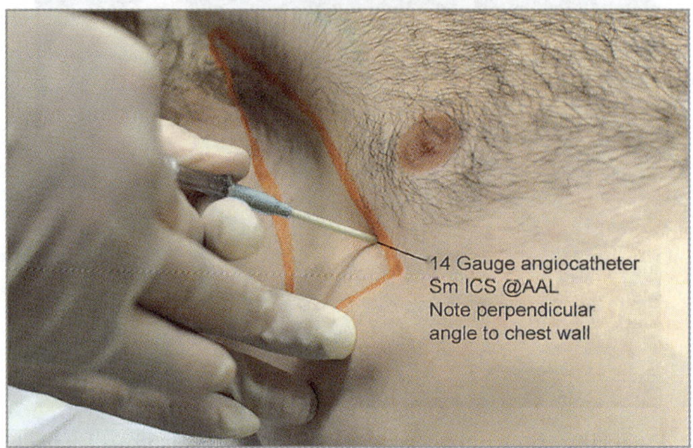


a. What is the procedure being performed?
b. What are the physiological benefits after this procedure?
c. Name two complications of this procedure.

**Q47. This 35-year-old woman has presented with dysphagia for liquids for the last 1 year. The image of the radiological investigation performed is shown.**

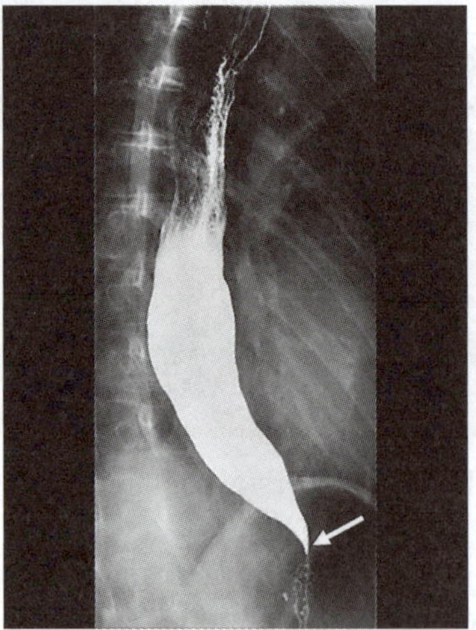

a. Identify the radiological abnormality.
b. Name the most likely diagnosis.

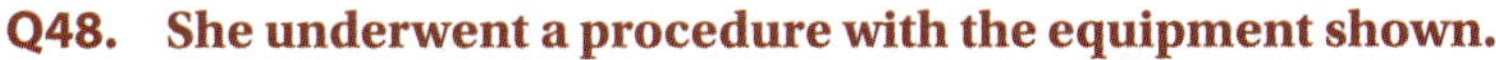

**Q48. She underwent a procedure with the equipment shown.**

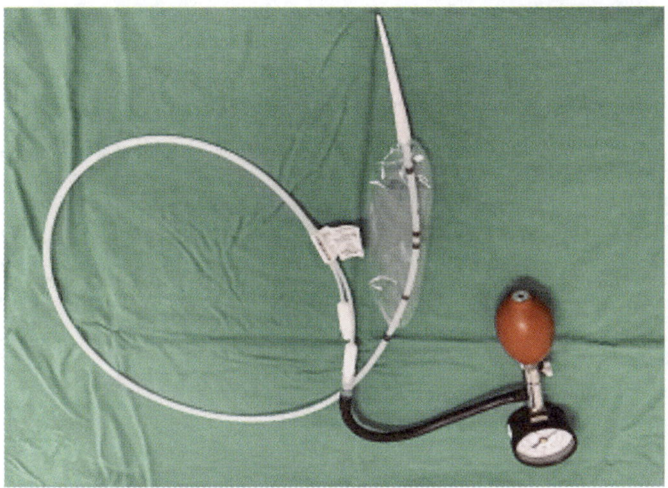

Name the procedure performed.

**Q49. 2 hours after the procedure, patient developed severe retro-sternal chest pain and respiratory distress image of the emergency contrast study is shown.**

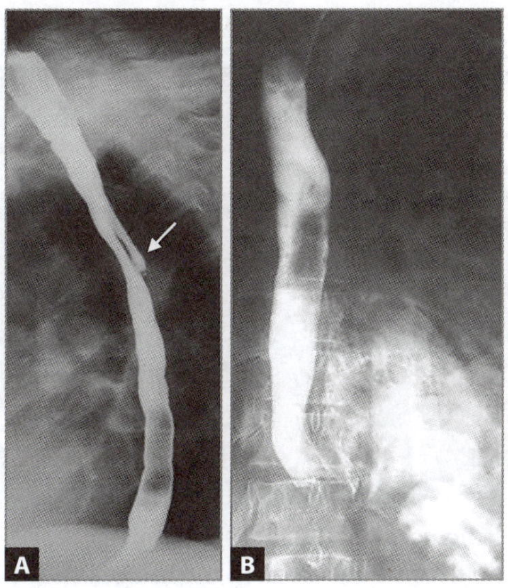


a. Identify the abdominal finding.
b. Name the complication.

**Q50.**

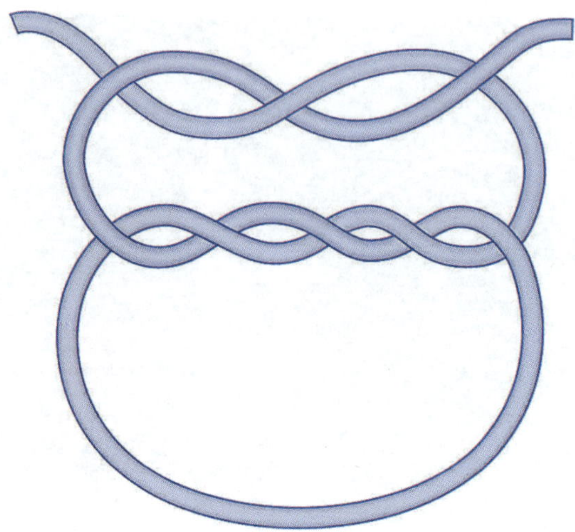

a. Identify the knot shown in the image.
b. Name two indications of use of this knot.

## MARCH 2022

**Q51. A 12-year-old boy complains of left upper abdominal pain. An investigation was performed and some images are as shown.**

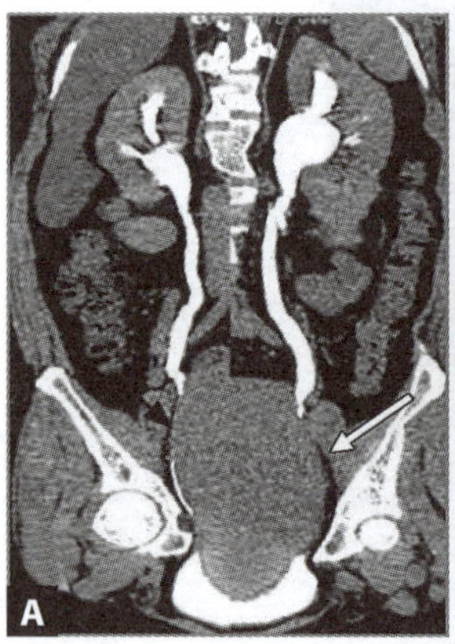


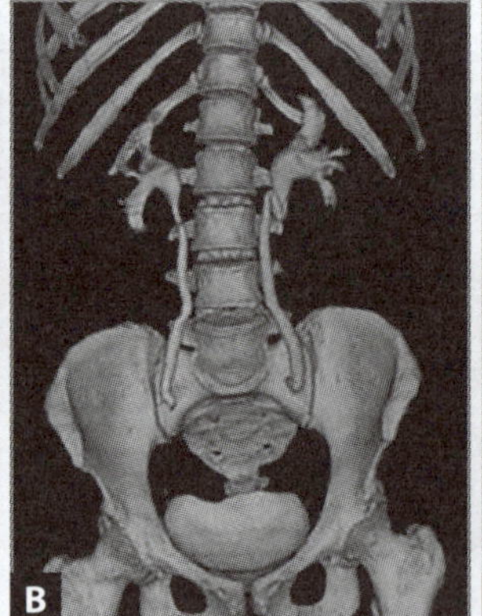


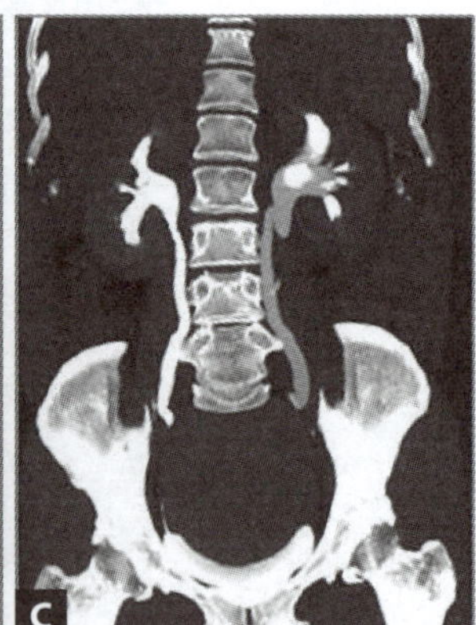


a. What is the name of the investigation?
b. What are the findings seen in the images shown?
c. Name one confirmatory investigation that you would like to do to decide the treatment in this patient.
d. What is the appropriate treatment for this condition?

**Q52. A 40-year-old lady underwent exploratory laparotomy and the operative photograph is shown below:**

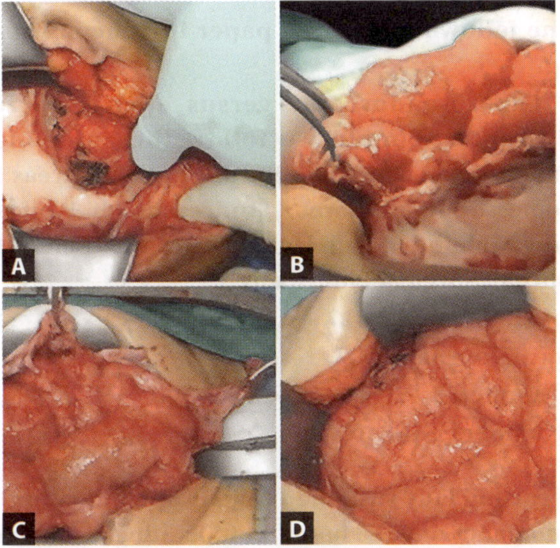


a. Describe the lesions seen in the photograph.
b. What is the most likely diagnosis?
c. What would have been the clinical presentation of this case?
d. Name the segment of small bowel commonly affected by this condition.
e. What will be your specific advice to this patient while discharging after surgery?

**Q53. A 60-year-old bedridden lady presented to casualty with abdominal pain distension and nonpassage of feces and flatus. Her X-ray abdomen was carried out as shown here.**

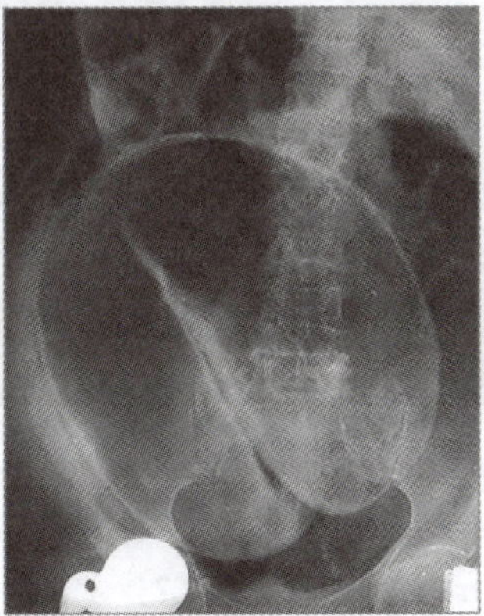

a. What is the most likely radiological diagnosis?
b. What are the risk factors of this condition?

c. Name the classical radiological signs of this condition.
d. What are the treatment options?

**Q54. Cite the following research paper in Vancouver style of referencing.**

**Title: Laparo-endoscopic versus open recurrent inguinal hernia repair: Should we follow the guidelines? Authors: Ferdinand Kockerling, Reinhard Bittner, Andreas Kuthe, Bernd Stechemesser, Ralph Lorenz, Andreas Koch, Wolfgang Reinpold, Henning Niebuhr, Martin Hukauf, Christine Schug-Pass. Name of the Journal: Surgical Endoscopy.**

**Year of Publication: 2017**

**Volume of Journal: 31**

**Issue Number: 8**

**Page Numbers: 3168 to 3185**

**Q55. A 30-year-old lady sustained road traffic injury and is brought to the emergency after 36 hours, complaining of abdominal pain and vomiting. Her pulse is 100/min, BP is 110/70 mm Hg. Respiratory rate is 20/min. An investigation was performed and is shown here.**

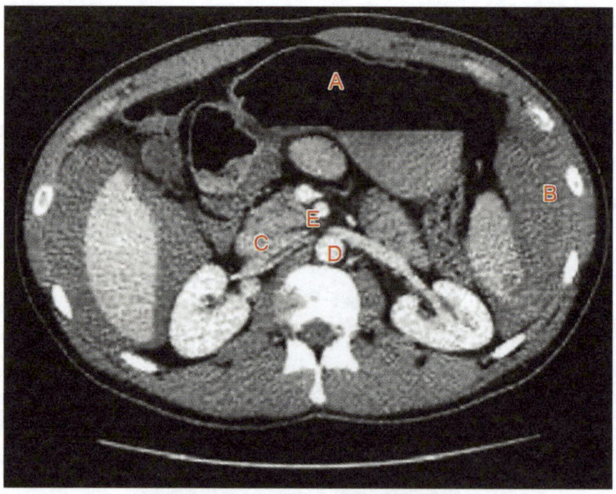


a. Which structure is labeled as A?
b. Which structure is labeled as B?
c. Which structure is labeled as C?
d. Which structure is labeled as D?
e. Which structure is labeled as E?

**Q56. A 36-year-old woman is undergoing laparoscopic IPOM repair of lower abdominal incisional hernia. A special mesh is used for the repair.**

a. What is special about the mesh used for IPOM?
b. Enumerate five complications of IPOM repair.
c. What is the difference in plane of mesh placement in laparoscopic IPOM repair and eTEP repair of incisional hernia?

**Q57. In the photograph shown:**

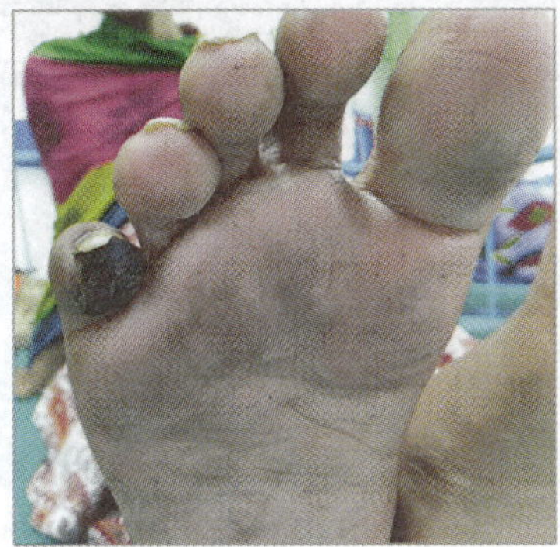

a. What is the diagnosis?
b. What are the findings seen?
c. What is the diagnosis if the patient is a 32-year-old male with history of chronic smoking?
d. What is the appropriate management of this condition?

**Q58.**

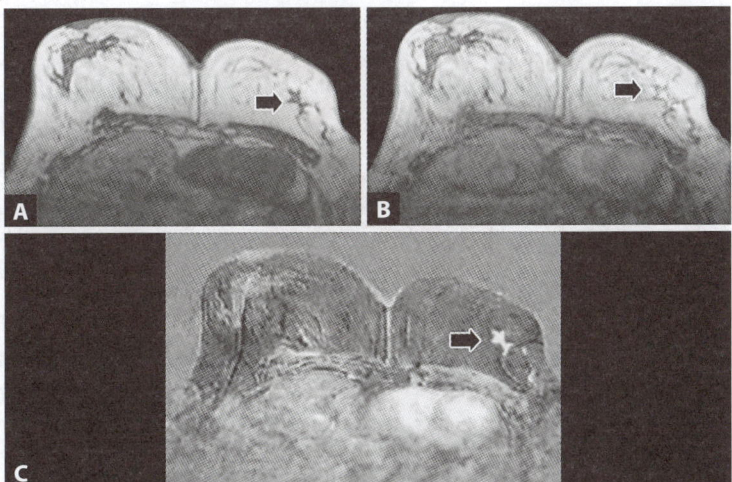


a. Name the investigation shown.
b. What is depicted in figure A?

c. What is depicted in figure B?
d. What is depicted in figure C?
e. What is the diagnosis based on figures A, B, and C?

**Q59. A 28-year-old male suffering from atrial fibrillation presented with acute severe pain in his left leg of 4 hours duration. On examination, the left leg was found to be cold with absent peripheral pulses. The device shown in the photograph was used for his treatment.**

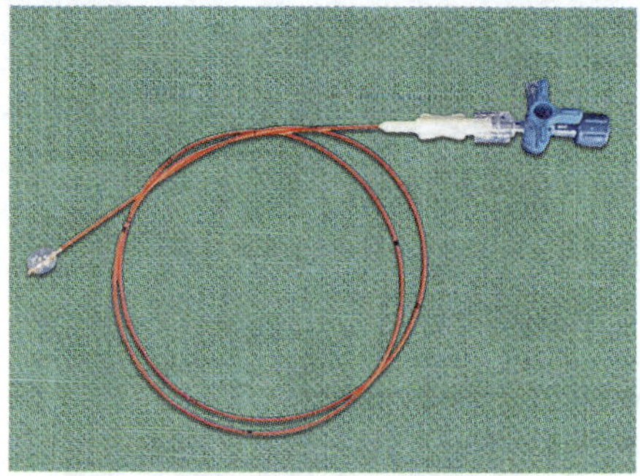

a. Name the device shown in the photograph.
b. Write three uses of this device.
c. Write three complications associated with use of this device.
d. What systemic complication can occur if the device is used late in the course of the disease?
e. What treatment will be offered to the above described patient after this procedure?

**Q60.**

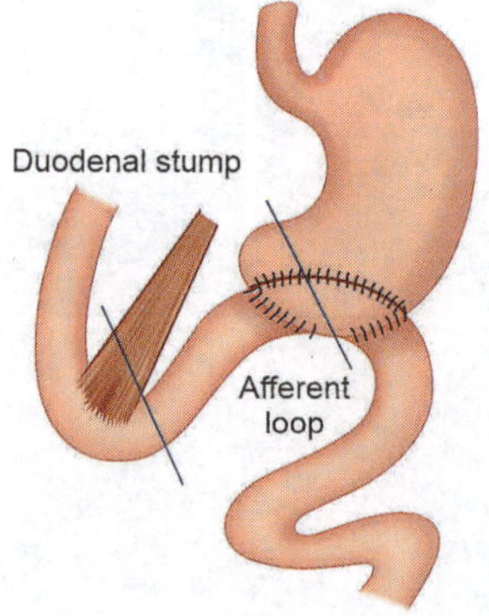


a. Name the procedure shown in the diagram.
b. What is the most common indication of this procedure?
c. How is the duodenal stump managed?
d. What is the most common cause of morbidity after this procedure?

**Q61.**

a. What is the radiological diagnosis in the CT film shown?
b. What is the origin of this pathology?
c. What is the most common clinical presentation of this condition?
d. What is the primary modality of treatment of this condition?
e. What is the adjuvant treatment for this condition?

**Q62.**

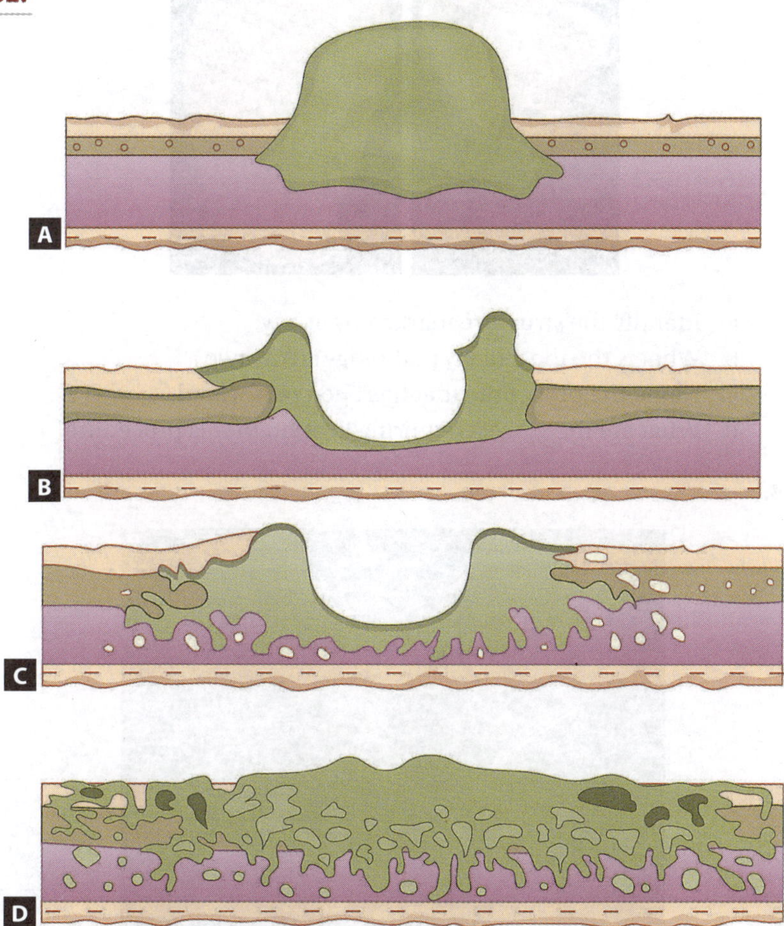


a. Name this classification.
b. What is this classification used for?
c. What does A depict?
d. What does B depict?
e. What does C depict?
f. What does D depict?
g. Name one more classification used for the same condition.

## Q63.

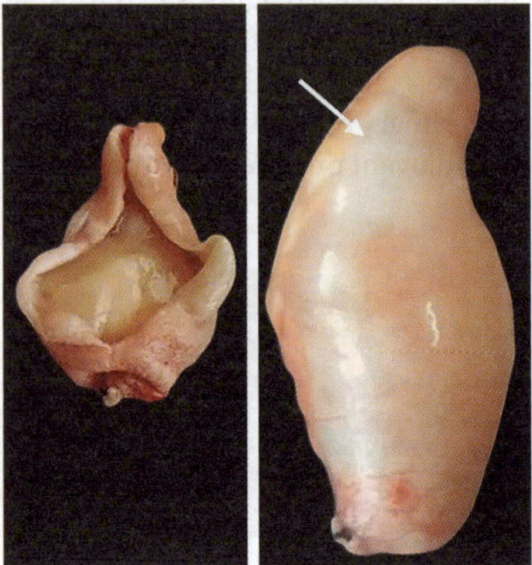

a. Identify the structure marked by arrow.
b. What is the most likely pathology? (Any two).
c. Name the procedure that has been performed.
d. What are the vessels requiring ligation in this procedure.

## Q64.

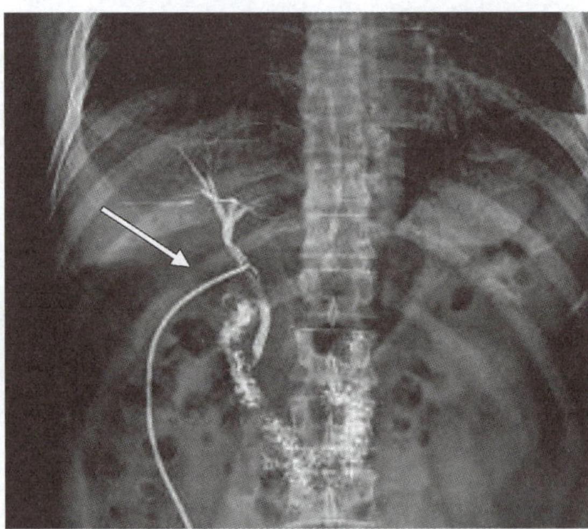

a. Name the investigation shown.
b. Name the procedure performed in this patient.
c. What does this arrow show?
d. Name one indication of this procedure.

**Q65.**

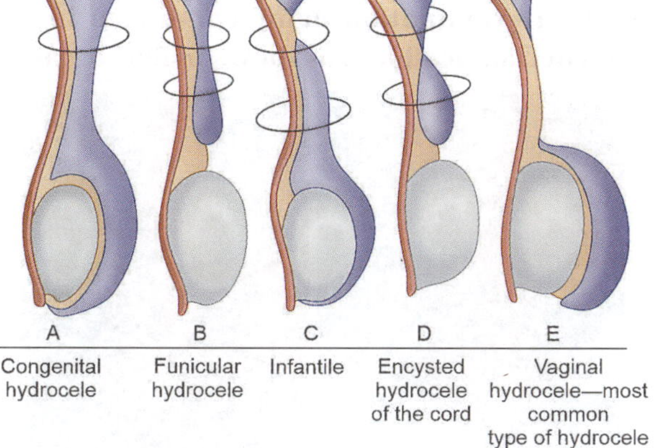


a. What does (A) depict?
b. What does (B) depict?
c. What does (C) depict?
d. What does (D) depict?
e. What does (E) depict?

What is the treatment of (A) shown in the diagram?

**Q66.**

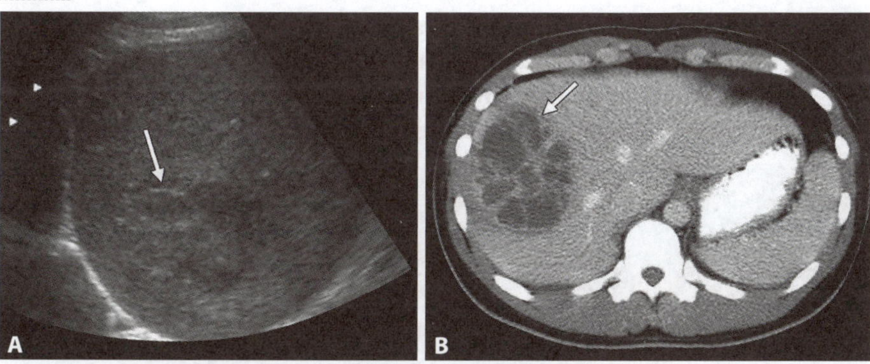


a. What are the findings seen in the CT film shown here?
b. What is the most likely etiology of the condition?
c. What treatment is suggested for the conditions A and B?

**Q67. A 45-year-old female patient with history of neck swelling for last 10 years, now presents with a pulsatile forehead swelling of 3 months duration.**

a. What is the most probable diagnosis?
b. What is the appropriate treatment of this condition?
c. What is the suggested plan of management for this patient?

## JAN 2024

**Q68. Image of an examination being conducted in a patient with intermittent claudication is as shown in figure A and B.**

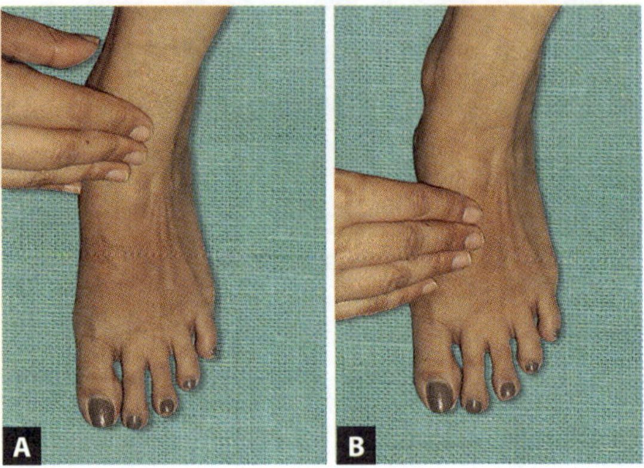


*Source:* S Das.

a. Which structure is being palpated in figure A?
b. Which structure is being palpated in figure B?
c. What are the landmarks of palpation of femoral artery? What is the structure against which it is palpated?
d. Which cervical vertebrae has carotid tubercle?

**Q69. A 20-year-old gentleman presents with scrotal swelling in right hemiscrotum for 6 months. On examination, there is no evidence of fluctuation or transillumination. The patient underwent an operative procedure and images are shown.**

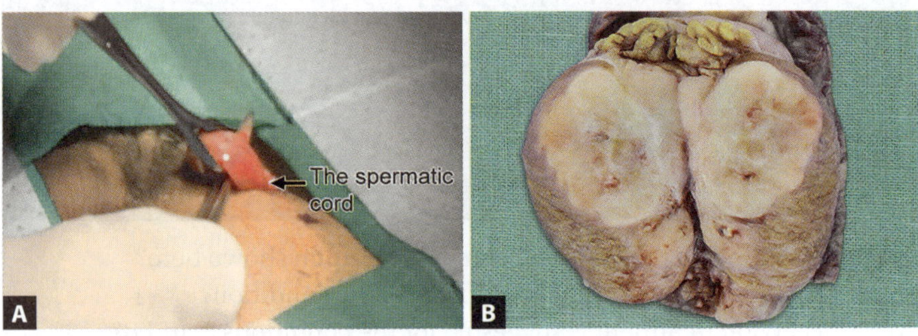


a. Name the structure looped in image A.
b. Name the procedure performed.
c. What is the likely pathology?
d. What is the role of preoperative fine or core needle biopsy in confirming the diagnosis?
e. Which investigation done preoperatively to confirm the diagnosis will help in follow-up?

**Q70. A 58-year-old woman presented with redness and scaling on and around nipple.**

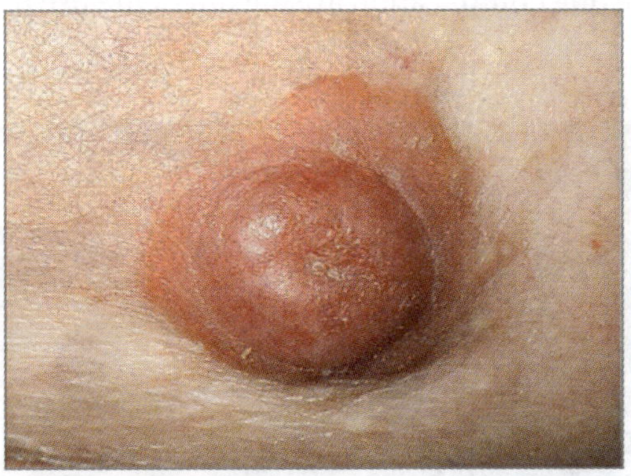

a. Identify the lesion. What is it associated with?
b. How will you confirm the diagnosis?
c. What is the characteristic histopathologic criteria?
d. What is the treatment?

**Q71. A 50-year-old woman presented to the emergency department with complaints of abdominal distension, vomiting, and absolute constipation of 1 day duration. On examination, the patient has central abdominal distension with high pitched exaggerated bowel sounds. The patient has previous history of on and off episodes of right upper abdominal pain, lasting few hours to days. A plain X-ray of the abdomen was performed as shown.**

a. What is the clinical diagnosis after examination and X-ray?
b. Name two important findings on X-ray that are essential to make the diagnosis.
c. What is the definitive management of this patient?

**Q72.**

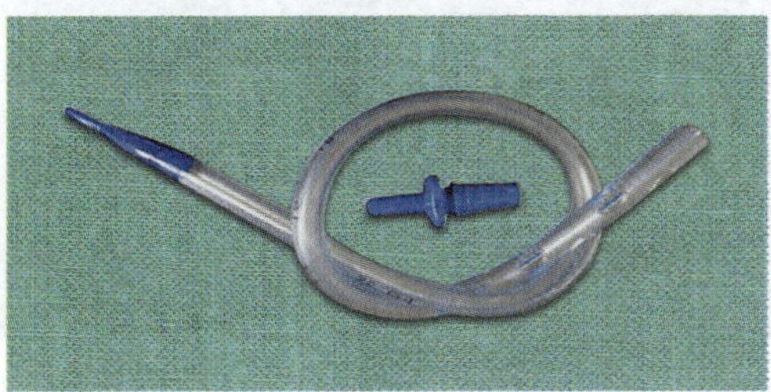

a. Identify the tube.
b. Name the material that is made of.
c. What is the purpose of green line marked with an arrow?

d. Name two technical considerations to keep in mind while introducing the tube.
e. Name one complication arising out of the use of this tube.

**Q73.**

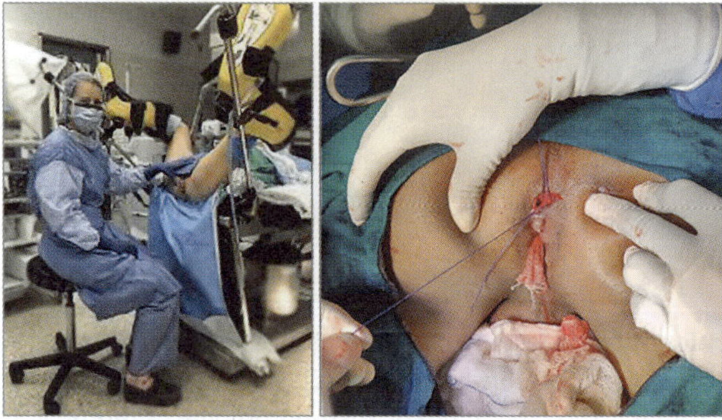

a. Name the likely clinical diagnosis shown in the photograph.
b. Name the operative position of the patient.
c. Name the three operative procedures for management of this condition.

**Q74. A 35-year-old male, motorcycle rider is brought to the emergency department with the history of being hit by truck. On examination, PR: 110/min, BP: 100 mm Hg, systolic RR: 18/min, and $SpO_2$: 94%. There is bruising and tenderness in the lower abdomen and the emergency department resident doctor was unable to introduce a urethral catheter. The surgeon on call has ordered a radiograph and the findings are as shown.**

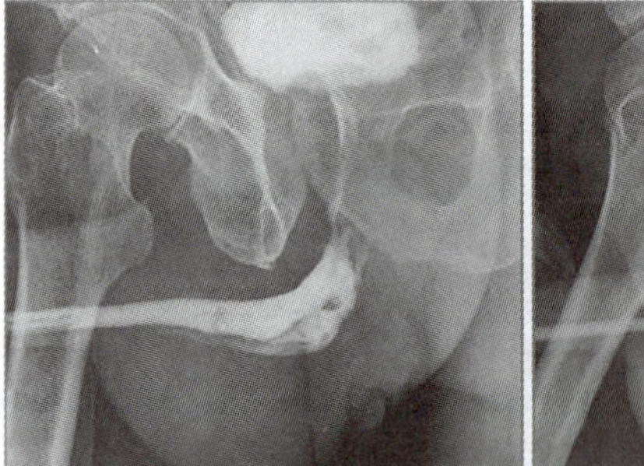

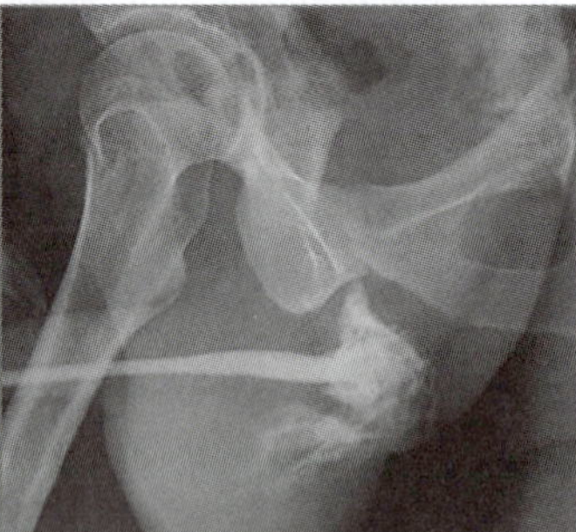

a. Name the investigation.
b. Name two significant findings seen on this image.
c. Enumerate four important principles/steps in the management of this patient.

**Q75. A 60-year-old gentleman presents with abdominal swelling and cachectic appearance. There is a history alcohol intake for last 20 years. On examination, a large mass was felt in right upper abdomen. CT scan revealed a large space occupying region in the right lobe of liver.**

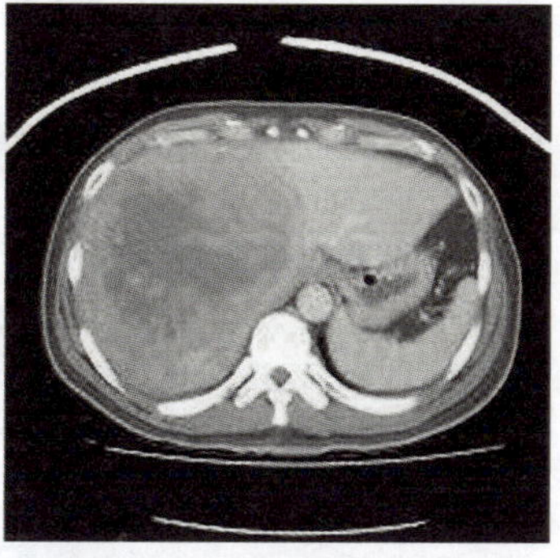

a. Give the complete clinical diagnosis.
b. What further blood investigations are needed to manage this patient? (Any four).
c. What is the criteria to decide the suitability of such patients for liver transplantation?
d. Which clinical test can you perform to decide the etiology of dilation of abdominal wall veins.

**Q76. A 45-year-old gentleman presents to the surgery OPD with a history of recurrent episodes of left flank pain for last 1.5 years. The pain radiates to the back and is severe enough to need IV analgesics. The physical examination is essentially normal apart from slight tenderness in the left flank. A radiological investigation was performed and is as shown.**

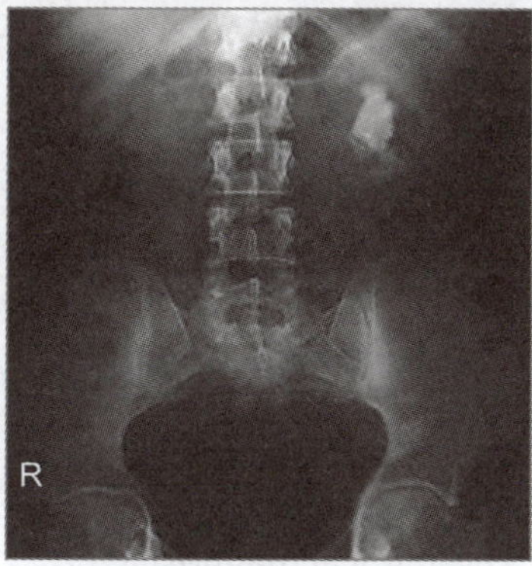


a. Name the investigation in full.
b. Name the findings seen on this radiograph.

c. Name one important investigation needed for deciding the management of this patient.
d. What is the definitive management of this patient?

**Q77.**

a. Based on the gross appearance and cross section shown in the figure, name the type of suture material A, B, C, and D.

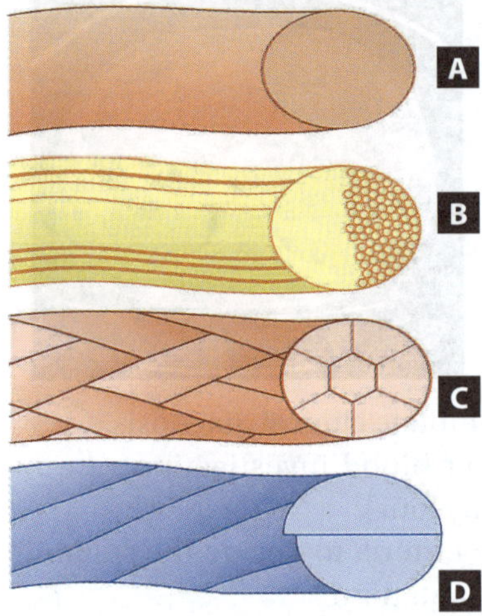


b. Which of these suture materials will you ideally use for suturing a skin incision?

**Q78. A 20-year-old gentleman presents with a discharging sinus in the right supraclavicular area with an underlying palpable lump. Patient has completed 6 months of antitubercular treatment. The specimen obtained from the surgical procedure performed is shown in image.**

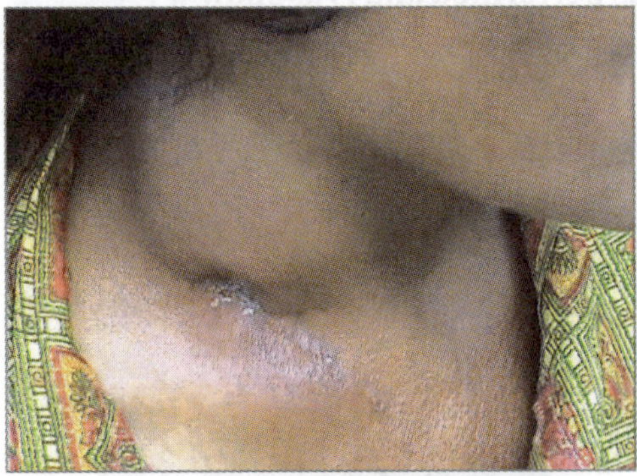

a. What is the likely clinical diagnosis?
b. Name the operative procedure performed, specimen obtained is as shown in image

c. What investigation must be performed on the tissue removed to confirm the diagnosis and manage the condition?

**Q79.**

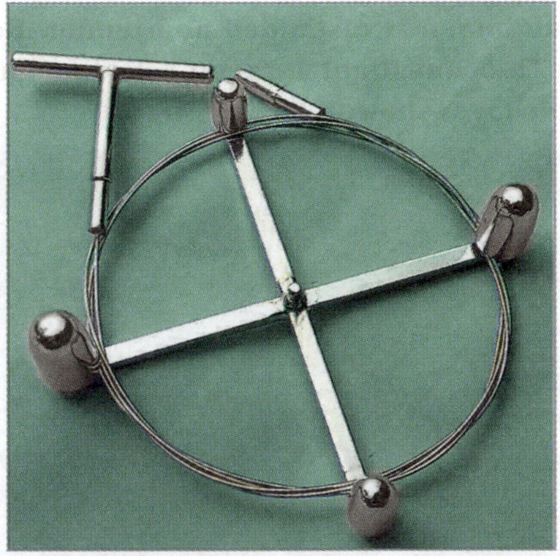

a. Identify the instrument shown.
b. Name the surgery where this instrument is used.
c. What is the absolute contraindication for this surgery?
d. What are the alternative methods of treatment for the clinical condition treated by this surgical procedure? (Any two) endovascular laser therapy (EVLT).

**Q80. A 30-year-old gentleman presents in surgical emergency with acute onset of pain in perianal area and tender palpable swelling as shown in the image.**

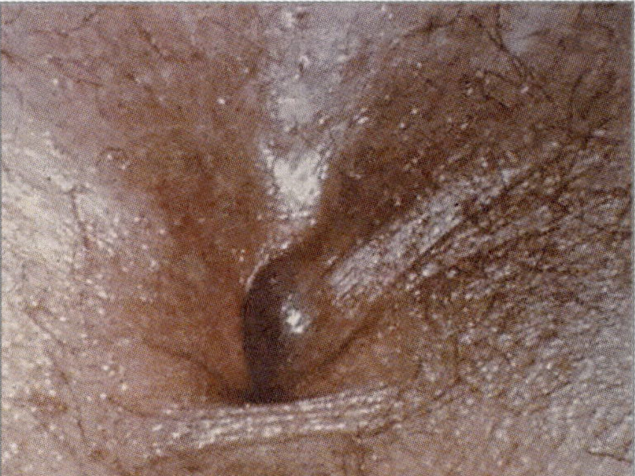

a. Name the likely clinical diagnosis.
b. What are the options of management of this condition?
c. Name two complications of the condition.

**Q81. A 25-year-old lady underwent an uneventful surgical procedure for gall stones 2 days back and was discharged the next morning. She presents to the emergency on POD 3 complaining of abdominal pain and uneasiness. On examination, her PR is 120/min and the abdomen is distended and tender. Bowel sounds are sluggish. The consultant surgeon asked for an urgent investigation which is as shown.**

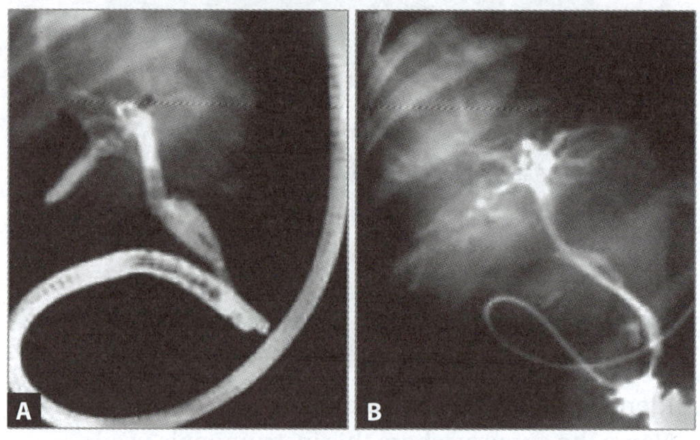


a. Name the investigation shown in full.
b. Name two significant findings seen on this image.

**Q82.**

a.

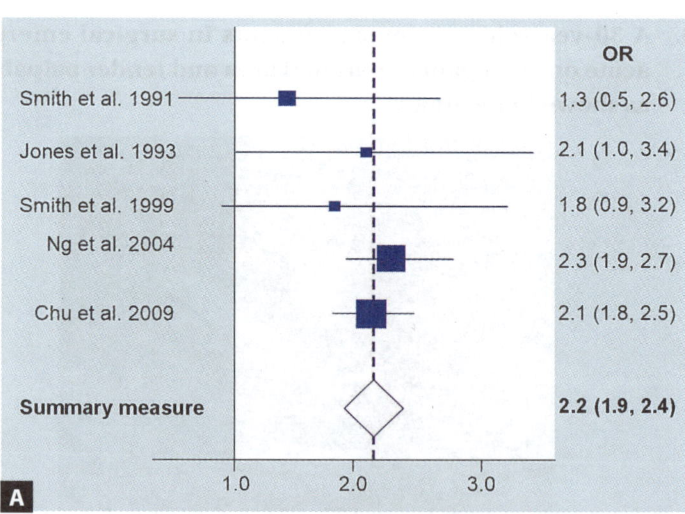


i. Identify the type of graph in figure A.
ii. Which statistical method is it used for?

b.

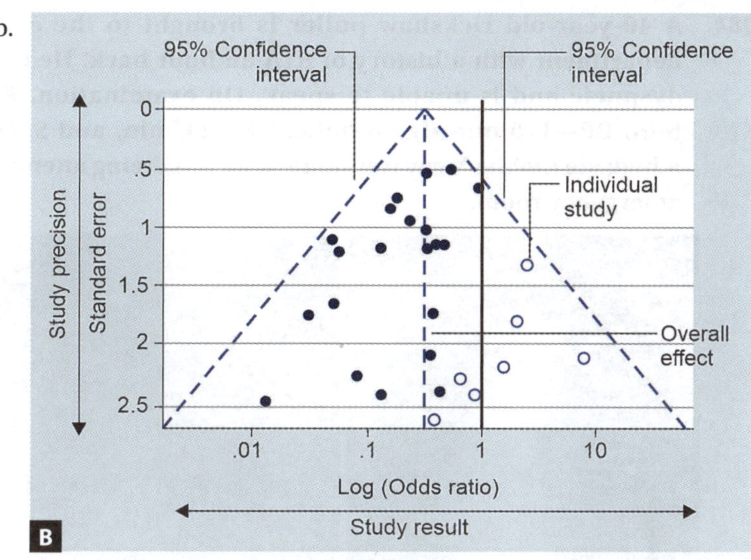


i. Identify the type of graph in figure B.

ii. Which statistical method is it used for?

c. Name one strength of each of these graphs.

## Q83.

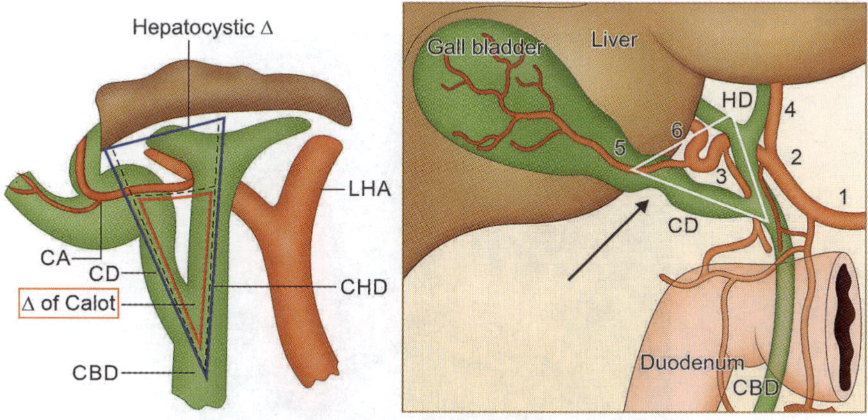


a. Identify the triangle shown marked in blue.

b. What are the boundaries of this triangle?

c. What are the contents of this triangle?

d. What is the anomaly marked with the arrow called?

**Q84. A 40-year-old rickshaw puller is brought to the emergency department with a history of RTA an hour back. He is severely dyspneic and is unable to speak. On examination, PR—120/min, BP—110 mm Hg, systolic, RR—24/min, and $SpO_2$—88%. A bedside mobile X-ray was done as he was, being attended to this emergency room.**

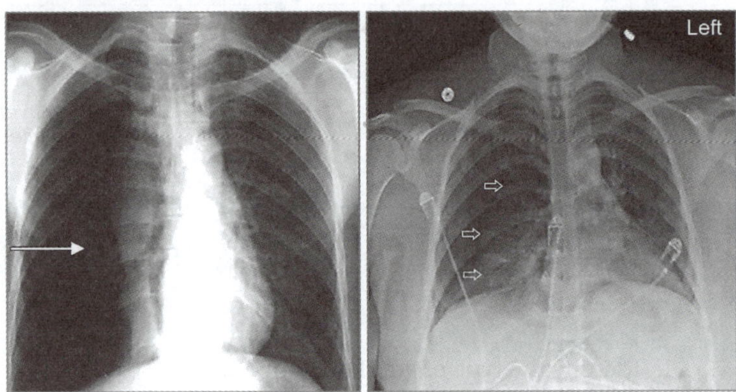


a. Name two important findings seen on this radiograph.
b. What is the diagnosis?
c. Enumerate the sequential management of this condition as per ATLS protocol.

**Q85.**

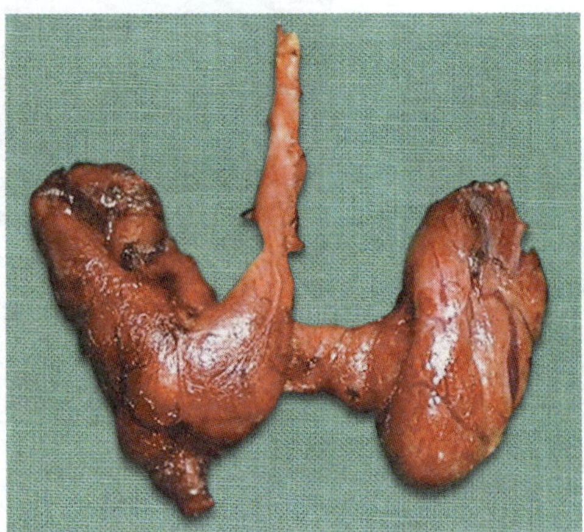

a. Identify the organ and the procedure performed.
b. Write the name of the cytopathological grading used for this organ.
c. Write a metabolic complication specific to this procedure and two clinical tests to confirm it.

## ANSWERS

**Ans. 1** a. Gas under the diaphragm suggestive of uterine perforation.
b. Resuscitation and patient to be posted for surgery.
c. Exploratory laparotomy and repair of the perforation.

**Ans. 2** a. ABCDE
b. SO is 85%; PR is 100/min; arterial blood gas (ABG): pH—7.21; PO—70; PCO—32; HCO—18. Crystalloids as a bridge till blood is available.
c. There is bruising over left lower chest; bony crepitus over the area; decreased air entry in left basal zone; abdomen is distended and tense. Left-sided pneumothorax along with? splenic injury (hemoperitoneum). Left-sided tube thoracostomy for decompressing.
d. Serial monitoring of hemoglobin along with contrast-enhanced computed tomography (CECT). Patient to be taken in the operation theater (OT), if hemodynamically unstable.

**Ans. 3** a. Right-sided pneumothorax with right lung collapsed.
b. F Angiocatheter in 5th intercostal space in mid axillary line f/b tube thoracostomy
c. ICU management along with high flow oxygen and starting the patient with IV antibiotics.

**Ans. 4** a. Head injury due to RTA.
*On further examination: Airway was patent; Pulse 60/min; Respiratory rate: RR 25/min; BP—160/100 mm Hg.*
b. Check for the pupils and get a noncontrast computed tomography (CT) brain (NCCT) head immediately.
*On examination:* There is a bruise and swelling over left temporoparietal area
i. She opens eyes to pain.
ii. Verbal response is only incomprehensible sounds.
iii. She produces withdrawal to pain.
iv. Interpret the GCS of this patient.

**Ans. 5** a. Intravenous pyelography
b. B/L urolithiasis, B/L ureteric strictures, B/L ureterocele
c. Noncontrast computerized tomography kidneys, ureters, and bladder (NCCT KUB)
d. Bilateral pelvicalyceal dilatation

**Ans. 6** a. Retrograde urethrogram
b. Proximal bulbar urethral strictures
c. Pelvic fracture
d. Progressive perineal urethroplasty (PPU)

**Ans. 7A** 1. Onset of lump
2. Duration of lump
3. Progression of lump
4. Family history

**Ans. 7B** Tethering, puckering, peau d'orange, fixity to breast, fixity to skin, fixity to muscle, and axillary lymphadenopathy.

**Ans. 7C** Core cut biopsy of the lump.

**Ans. 8** a. Carcinoma of colon with malignant ascites with lung metastasis.
b. Positron emission tomography computed tomography (PET CT)
c. Colonoscopy with biopsy along with palliative management.
d. Poor prognosis, hospice treatment

**Ans. 9** a. Splenic vein thrombosis with splenomegaly.
b. Complete blood count to look for pancytopenia history of (h/o) hematemesis h/o Melena

**Ans. 10** Icterus, pallor, and generalized edema.

**Ans. 11** a. Alcoholic liver disease with portal hypertension with splenomegaly with gross ascites.
b. CECT (A+P)

**Ans. 12** a. Gas under the diaphragm
b. Perforation peritonitis
c. History of (h/o) nonsteroidal anti-inflammatory drugs (NSAIDs), h/o peptic ulcer disease, h/o alcohol consumption
d. Resuscitation with fluids and output monitoring, central venous pressure, urine output, and arterial blood gas analysis.
e. Exploratory laparotomy with primary repair of the perforation.

**Ans. 13** a.
- Rapid loss of weight and appetite.
- Compressive symptoms such as dysphagia and dysphonia.

b.
- Eye signs
- Tachycardia
- Neck swellings
- Hand tremors

c.
- Swelling movement with protrusion of the tongue
- Swelling movement with deglutition
- Compressible/reducible swelling
- Consistency of the swelling

**Ans. 14** a. Thyroid swelling with hyperthyroid state
b. Serum thyroid-stimulating hormone (TSH) value, USG neck

**Ans. 15** a. Thyroid swelling with retrosternal extension
b. Pemberton sign
c. USG-guided fine-needle aspiration (FNA) and CT thorax
d. Total thyroidectomy with median sternotomy (If retrosternal extension present)

**Ans. 16** a.
- Tubercular lymphadenopathy
- Viral adenopathy
- Lymphomas

b.
- History of Koch/Koch contact
- History of loss of weight/appetite
- History of evening rise of temperature
- History of night sweats

**Ans. 17** a.
- Examination of lymph nodes—usually occur as cervical and supraclavicular nodes.
- Initially affected nodes are discrete, mobile, nontender, but later become matted.
- Look for other stigmatas of TB-lupus vulgaris, scrofuloderma, phlyctenulosis, tinea versicolor, and erythema nodosum.

b.
- Excisional biopsy of lymph node
- Tissue for AFB staining and culture.
- Chest X-ray

**Ans. 18** a. Appendix
b. Acute appendicitis (mucocele)
c. Gallbladder
d. Perforation of appendix causing peritonitis

**Ans. 19** a.
- Reducible on lying down
- History of (h/o) trauma
- H/o pain

b. Right-sided hydrocele
c. Transillumination, fluctuation, getting above the swelling, cough impulse, and palpation of testes.

**Ans. 20** a. Right-sided hydrocele
b.
- Hydrocele is a clinical diagnosis, however, to rule out testicular malignancy, we shall do an ultrasonography of the scrotum.
- Treatment is surgical, however, the technique depends of the size of the hydrocele.
- Small hydrocele—lords plication

- Moderate hydrocele—Jabouley's repair
- Gross hydrocele—Excision of the sac and repair

**Ans. 21** a. Liver abscess

b. Amebic liver abscess/pyogenic liver abscess

c. 
- Rupture and peritonitis
- Rupture into lung
- Bronchopleural fistula
- Subphrenic abscess

d. 
- Medical management—antibiotics and antipyretics
- Percutaneous drainage
- Surgical drainage

**Ans. 22** a. About 3% of full term and 30% of premature infants are born with one or both undescended testes. About two-thirds of these reach the scrotum during the first 3 months of life, but full descent after that is uncommon. The incidence of maldescent at the age of 1 year is 1%.

b. High scrotal (60%) (*Source:* Bailey, 28th edition/superficial inguinal pouch (*Source:* Campbell)

c. Impaired transformation of gonocytes to spermatogonia is reported.
Number of spermatogonia per tubule is reduced.

d. 
- Classic prune belly (triad or eagle barret) syndrome
- Spigelian hernia
- Cerebral palsy
- Myelomeningocele
- Omphalocele

e. T: Torsion
E: Epididymo-orchitis
S: Sterility
T: Trauma
I: Indirect inguinal hernia
S: Seminoma

**Ans. 23** a. Abdominal aortic aneurysm

b. Major risk factors involving smoking and hypertension.
Rare but important causes include syphilis and connective tissues disease such as Ehlers Danlos type 1 and Marfan's syndrome.

c. 
- Rupture (most common)
- Peripheral embolization
- Aortic thrombosis
- Fistula formation

d. 
- Open repair and endovascular repair (EVAR)

- *Open repair Cx:* Cardiac ischemia, renal insufficiency, colonic insufficiency, pulmonary complications, and graft limb thrombosis.
- EVAR repair Cx:
  - *Early:* Endoleak, hematoma, psuedoaneurysm, local wound complication
  - *Late:* Rupture, endoleak, sac enlargement, and migration of stent.

**Ans. 24** a. A comprehensive informed consent consists of four basic elements: (1) description of the clinical problem, the proposed treatment, and alternatives including no treatment; (2) discussion of the risks and benefits of the proposed treatment with comparisons to the risks and benefits of alternatives, and discussion of medical/clinical uncertainties regarding the proposed treatment; (3) assessment of the patient's understanding of the information provided by the medical provider; and (4) solicitation of the patient's preference and consent for treatment.

b. i. Temporary incapacity to give consent:
  - Illness
  - Intoxication
  - Anesthesia

ii. *Consent in child:* Parents will give on their behalf. Child should be explained about the surgery and deal with child's response.

**Ans. 25** a. X-ray anteroposterior (AP) view chest, X-ray lateral view chest

b. Barium swallow

c. • High/low dysphagia
  - Gastroesophageal reflux disease (GERD)
  - Assessment of hiatus hernia
  - Assessment of fistula
  - Inability to pass upper gastrointestinal (UGI) scope

d. • Contrast allergy
  - Massive pulmonary edema (high osmolarity water soluble contrast agent)

**Ans. 26** a. Magnetic resonance cholangiopancreatography (MRCP)

b. Endoscopic retrograde cholangiopancreatography (ERCP)-guided stone removal, stenting, and sphincterotomy for clearance.

c. Common bile duct (CBD) exploration (LAP/Open)

**Ans. 27** a. Peripheral vascular disease (Berger's disease)
b. Smoker, blackening of toe, claudication symptoms, and relief of hanging foot.
c. On hanging the limb—arterial claudication decreases and venous claudication increases.
d. Investigation of choice would be computed tomography (CT) angiography
However, to support my diagnosis I can go ahead with—duplex Doppler USG and general hematological investigation.

## MARCH 2021

**Ans. 28** a. • Branches of facial nerve
• Greater auricular nerve
• Intraparotid lymph nodes
• Auriculotemporal nerve
• Retromandibular vein
b. Tragal pointer
Tympanomastoid suture line
Digastric tendon insertion
Stylomastoid foramen
c. • Temporary facial nerve palsy
• Sialocele
• Hematoma
• Frey's syndrome

**Ans. 29** a. Ulcerative proliferative growth present in small bowel
b. Right-sided small bowel malignancy (adenocarcinoma)
c. • Glandular pattern
• Clear cells
• Granular cells solid pattern
d. Right hemicolectomy

**Ans. 30** a. Pizillo's maneuver, thyroid gland can be made more prominent.
b. Large goiters may result in deviation of the trachea causing prominence of the ipsilateral sternocleidomastoid muscle (Trails sign). They may also cause obliteration of the carotid pulsations due to displacement of the vessels (Berry's sign).
c. Thyroid malignancy
d. Total thyroidectomy
e. • Vocal cord palsy
• Hemorrhage
• Injury to surrounding vessels

**Ans. 31** a. Immediate exploratory laparotomy
b. Transfer the patient to OR immediately, clinical diagnosis.
c. Primary repair of the perforation if small since mesenteric vessels are not damaged. If large, perforation may require resection and anastomosis.
d. Since, it is a penetrating injury, expose ipsilateral renal vessels at base of transverse mesocolon. Obtain proximal control of renal vessels.

**Ans. 32** a. Endoscopic retrograde pancreatocholangiography
b. • Multiple filling defects present
• Dilated CBD
c. Diagnostic and therapeutic procedure
d. Post-ERCP pancreatitis
e. Mechanical injury to the pancreas due to prolonged manipulation of the ducts or surrounding organs.

**Ans. 33** a. Metabolic alkalosis
b. Enteral feeding and parenteral feeding
c. Subtotal gastrectomy with HSV with drainage procedure (pyloroplasty) antrectomy with drainage procedure.

**Ans. 34** a. A type of clinical trial in which neither the participants nor the researcher knows which treatment or intervention participants are receiving until the clinical trial is over.
b. Impact factors are used to measure the importance of a journal by calculating the number of times selected articles are cited within the last few years. The higher the impact factor, the more highly ranked the journal. It is one tool you can use to compare journals in a subject category.
c. The h-index is a metric for evaluating the cumulative impact of an author's scholarly output and performance; measures quantity with quality by comparing publications to citations. The h index corrects for the disproportionate weight of highly cited publications or publications that have not yet been cited.

**Ans. 35** a. Peau d'orange
b. A phenomenon in which hair follicles become buried in edema, giving the skin an orange peel appearance. Peau d'orange can be caused by cutaneous lymphatic edema, which causes swelling. Parts of the edematous skin are tethered by hair follicles and sweat glands such that pinpoint pitting occurs within areas of swelling, leading to the characteristic appearance.

**Ans. 36** Clinical staging N2

**Ans. 37**
a. Tension pneumothorax
b. Intercostal drain tube insertion
c. Mediastinal injury
d. Air embolism

**Ans. 38**
a. Blackening of toes, mummification
b. Peripheral vascular disease
c. CT angiography
d. Autoamputation of the toes and considering revascularization of limb

**Ans. 39**
a. Absence of right hemiscrotum
b. Undescended testes
c. Ultrasonography of the scrotum and testes
d. Seminoma (testicular malignancy)
e. The incidence of testicular maldescent at the age of 1 year is around 1%

**Ans. 40**
a. Acute colonic obstruction
b. Dilated bowel loops, loss of haustration, caliber of large bowel is 5–8 cm.
c. 
   - Stricture formation
   - Recurrent growth
d. Acute intestinal obstruction, perforation peritonitis, and recurrent malignant growth.

**Ans. 41**
a. Biliary peritonitis
b. CECT (A + P)
c. Cystic duct blow out causing biliary leak
d. Loculated collection—external drainage by USG guidance pigtailing followed by ERCP with stent placement for internal drainage.

**Ans. 42**
a. Adrenal, pheochromocytoma
b. Plasma and urinary metanephrines or catecholamine measurement
c. Alpha blockade is used to block the effects of catecholamine excess and its consequences during surgery. Additional β blockade if tachycardia or arrhythmias develop.

**Ans. 43**
a. Gallbladder perforation
b. Adequate wash and put an abdominal drain

**Ans. 44**
a. Glandular adenocarcinoma with perineural invasion, extending into gallbladder belt and invading gallbladder carcinoma

b. • Cauliflower like proliferative growth CA 19-9, CEA (tumor markers)
   • Spread of the tumor and liver invasion.

**Ans. 45** a. • Smoking
   • Alcohol
   • Betel quid human papillomavirus (HPV)

b. Size of the lesion, invasion into surrounding structure, and depth of invasion

c. Edge biopsy of the lesion

d. Multidetector CT (MDCT) face and magnetic resonance imaging (MRI)

e. Surgical management—the gold standard of oral cavity squamous cell carcinoma (OCSCC) is resection with 1 cm clinical margin circumferentially, vital structures permitting.

**Ans. 46** a. Wide bore needle insertion in triangle of safety

b. Release of tension pneumothorax and getting back the hemodynamics quickie. Act as a bridging procedure.

c. Hemothorax, pulmonary/diaphragmatic laceration, and intercostal neuralgia

**Ans. 47** a. Bird beak appearance in barium swallow

b. Achalasia cardia

**Ans. 48** Pneumatic balloon dilator

**Ans. 49** a. Esophageal perforation

b. Bleeding and perforation

**Ans. 50** a. Surgeons knot

b. Approximation of wound edges, ligation of large critical vessels.

## MARCH 2022

**Ans. 51** a. CT intravenous pyelogram (IVP) or intravenous urography (IVU) with reconstruction.

b. The findings are likely related to the urinary system. Common findings might include hydronephrosis, ureteral obstruction, or kidney stones.

c. A confirmatory investigation could be a CT scan of the abdomen and pelvis with contrast to provide more detailed images of the urinary tract and any associated pathology.

d. The treatment depends on the specific findings:
   • For kidney stones, treatment options could include pain management, hydration, lithotripsy, or surgical removal.

- For an obstruction, treatment might include placing a stent or performing surgery to remove the obstruction.
- For infections, antibiotics would be appropriate.

**Ans. 52** a. Multiple tubercles noted with cocoon abdomen.
b. Abdominal tuberculosis.
c. Small bowel obstruction
d. Ileocecal junction, ileum, cecum
e. Postoperative AKT, dietary advice

**Ans. 53** a. Sigmoid volvulus
b. • High fiber diet
• Chronic constipation
• Neuropsychiatric disorder
c. • Coffee bean sign
• Frimann-Dahl sign
d. • Flatus tube insertion and decompression
• Sigmoidopexy
• Resection and anastomosis with proximal anastomosis
• Hartmann's procedure

**Ans. 54** Kockerling F, Bittner R, Kuthe A, Stechemesser B, Loranze R, Koch A, et al. Laparo-endoscopic versus open recurrent inguinal hernia repair: should we follow the guidelines. Surg Endosc. 2017;31(8): 3168-85.

**Ans. 55** a. Stomach
b. Spleen
c. Pancreas
d. Aorta
e. Superior mesenteric artery

**Ans. 56** a. • Composite mesh
• Peritoneal side—Polytetrafluoroethylene (PTFE) material
• Abdominal wall side—Polypropylene material
b. • Mesh migration
• Adhesion
• Bowel perforation
• Shrinkage
• Pain
c. Intraperitoneal onlay mesh (IPOM) mesh is placed intraperitoneally whereas extended totally extraperitoneal (eTEP) repair mesh is placed preperitoneally without breaching peritoneum.

**Ans. 57** *In the photograph shown:*
a. Dry gangrene of left little toe
b. Blackish discoloration of small toe with line of demarcation noted.

c. Beurger's disease

d. • Investigation—Duplex USG and hematological profile
   • Treatment
     - General mx—Abstinence from smoking and dietary modification
     - Medical mx—antiplatelets, cilostazole, phosphodiesterase type (PDE 5) inhibitors
     - Nonsurgical mx—stenting
     - Surgical mx-amputation of toe—if line of demarcation present
     - Bypass grafts and revascularization

**Ans. 58** a. Magnetic resonance imaging showing carcinoma of the left breast

b. Precontrast

c. Postgadolinium contrast

d. Subtraction image

e. Carcinoma of the left breast

**Ans. 59** a. Fogarty catheter

b. 1. Embolectomy
   2. Retrieval of common bile duct stones
   3. In pediatric cases placement of occlusive balloon (Fogarty catheter through a rigid bronchoscope into the tracheoesophageal fistula may be useful)

c. 1. Intimal tears and dissections
   2. Vascular perforation
   3. Catheter track infections

d. • Pulmonary embolism
   • Septicemia

e. Because of the ensuing stasis, a thrombus can extend distally and proximally to the embolus. The immediate administration of 5,000 U of heparin IV can reduce the extension and maintain patency of the surrounding (particularly the distal) vessels until the embolus is treated. The relief of pain is essential because it is severe and constant. Embolectomy and thrombolysis are the treatment available for patients with limb emboli.

**Ans. 60** a. Billroth 2 gastrectomy

b. Gastric ulcer

c. Conservative management with external drainage

d. • Dumping syndrome
   • Afferent loop syndrome

**Ans. 61** a. Single well-circumscribed lesion? Carcinoma of gallbladder.
b. Gallbladder
c. Obstructive jaundice
d. Radical cholecystectomy
e. Chemotherapy—taxanes and gemcitabine.

**Ans. 62** a. Bormann's classification
b. Staging of early gastric cancer
c. Polypoidal
d. Fungating
e. Ulcerative
f. Diffuse gastric cancer
g. Laurens classification

**Ans. 63** a. Appendix
b. • Mucocele
 • Appendicular carcinoid
c. Right hemicolectomy
d. • Ileocolic artery
 • Right colic artery
 • Middle colic artery

**Ans. 64** a. T tube cholangiogram
b. Therapeutic removal of stones (Burhenne technique)
c. T tube
d. Removal of retained/residual stones

**Ans. 65** a. Congenital hydrocele
b. Funicular hydrocele
c. Infantile hydrocele
d. Hydrocele of cord
e. Vaginal hydrocele
Herniotomy

**Ans. 66** a. Infective space occupying lesion in liver.
b. Pyogenic liver abscess.
c. Medical treatment with pigtailing for external drainage of pus.

**Ans. 67** a. Follicular carcinoma
b. Radiotherapy
c. Radiotherapy followed by neoadjuvant chemotherapy/I131 and total thyroidectomy.

## JAN 2024

**Ans. 68** a. The posterior tibial artery felt just behind the medial malleolus midway between it and tendo-Achilles.

b. The dorsalis pedis artery is felt just lateral to the tendon of extensor hallucis longus (EHL).
c. Landmarks of femoral artery—It is felt at the groin just below the inguinal ligament midway between the anterior superior iliac spine and symphysis pubis.
d. Sixth cervical vertebrae against carotid tubercle (also known as Chassaignac tubercle).

**Ans. 69** a. Spermatic cord and cord structures
b. High inguinal orchidectomy
c. Carcinoma testes (most likely seminoma)
d. Testicular biopsy performed for the investigation of infertility. Contralateral testis biopsy in patient with giant cell tumors (GCT) or within the affected testis in patient undergoing testis sparing surgery.
e. Serum tumor markers [alpha-fetoprotein (AFP), lactate dehydrogenase (LDH), beta human chorionic gonadotropin [β-hCG].

**Ans. 70** a. Paget's disease of breast. 95% associated with an underlying breast carcinoma.
b. In patients without underlying mass diagnosis is obtained by skin biopsy.
c. Large periodic acid-Schiff (PAS) positive Paget's cell invading the epidermis are seen on histology.
d. Management can usually be done by wide local excision of central sector with axillary staging and RT in Paget's disease without an underlying mass followed by 3D skin tattooing.

**Ans. 71** a. Large bowel obstruction (SBO)
b.
  i. Small bowel lies centrally in the abdomen unlike large bowel which lies peripherally.
  ii. The valvulae conniventes (folds) of the small bowel traverse the entire width of lumen while the haustra of large bowel do not.
  iii. The caliber of small bowel is typically less than the large, even when obstructed (typical measurement in obstruction (small bowel: 3.5–5 cm; large bowel: 5–8 cm).

c. Depending on the cause of small bowel, management is decided. Surgical treatment is necessary for most cases of intestinal obstruction but should be delayed until resuscitation is complete, provided there is no sign of strangulation or evidence of closed bowel obstruction.

**Ans. 72** a. Intercostal drainage tube
b. It is made up of polyvinyl chloride (PVC), soft silicone, polyethylene, and Portex.

c. It usually has a radiopaque stripe running through the most proximal hole (allowing for it location to be visualized on chest X-ray) and markings to indicate distance in centimeter from the most proximal hole.
d. The implantable cardioverter-defibrillator (ICD) is placed above the upper surface of the rib to avoid damage to the neurovascular bundle on the inferior surface. An oblique tract, so that skin incision and the hole in the parietal pleura do not overlie each other and the drain is in a short tunnel, which reduces the chances of entraining air. A drain for pneumothorax and hemothorax should aim toward the apex of the lung. A drain for pleural effusion or empyema should be nearer the base. The retaining stitch should be secure but should not obliterate the drain.
e. Hemorrhage damage to intercostal vessels and nerves lung and mediastinal injury infection.

**Ans. 73** a. Fistula in ano
b. Patient is placed in lithotomy position
c. Simple short fistula—lay open fistulotomy
- Fistulectomy: Newer techniques:
  - Plugging tract
  - LIFT: Ligation of intersphincteric fistula tract
  - VAFT: Video-assisted fistula tract excision

**Ans. 74** a. Retrograde urethrogram (RGU)
b. • Injury to the bulbar urethra
- Extravasation of dye

c. i. According to the latest edition of Bailey, if the tear is partial a gentle attempt of Foley's catheterization can be done.
ii. If failed, suprapubic catheterization
iii. Through suprapubic catheterization (SPC), we can do descending cystourethrogram/micturating cystourethrogram.
iv. Other investigation—RGU (via Foley's inserted up to penile urethra and push contrast).
v. Emergency laparotomy is required for bladder rupture and bladder neck injuries.
vi. A diverting colostomy is performed in associated rectal injuries.

**Ans. 75** a. Hepatocellular carcinoma
b. AFP, LDH, SGOT, SGPT, bilirubin, prothrombin (PT)/international normalized ratio (INR)
c. Child Pugh criteria

d. *Harvey's test:* Test for assessment of venous insufficiency. Empty a segment of vein with two fingers and the distal fingers released. The movement of the blood flow is seen, filling from above downward is superior vena cava (SVC) obstruction and vice versa for inferior vena cava (IVC) obstruction.

**Ans. 76** a. X-ray kidney, ureter, and bladder (KUB)
b. Left-sided staghorn calculi
c. Noncontrast computed tomography (NCCT) KUB, diethylene-triamine pentaacetic acid (DTPA) scan (functionality of the kidney)
d. Endourology—percutaneous nephrolithotomy (PCNL), open—pyelolithotomy, and laparascopic pyelolithotomy

**Ans. 77** a.
- Polypropylene/polyamide
- Silk
- Polyglycolic acid
- Polyester

b. Polyamide (nylon)

**Ans. 78** a. Cervical tuberculosis
b. Excision of the lymph node
c. Tissue for AFB, ZN staining, and tissue culture

**Ans. 79** a. Cambia vein stripper
b. Trendelenburg vein stripping surgery
c. Deep vein thrombosis
d. Radiofrequency ablation (RFT), mechanoablation, sclerotherapy, and venaseal

**Ans. 80** a. Thrombosed hemorrhoids
b. Emergency evacuation of the clot, excision of the hemorrhoids (open method—Milligan Morgan, closed method—Fergusson)
c.
- Immediate—Hemorrhage, pain, sphincter injury
- Late—Anal stenosis

**Ans. 81** a. ERCP
b. Cystic duct blowout with extravasation of dye

**Ans. 82** a. i. Forest plot
ii. Used to describe the distribution of effect sizes.
b. i. Funnel plot
ii. They are simple scatter plots of the treatment effects estimated from individual studies (horizontal axis) against a measure of sample size (vertical axis). It is used to look for publication bias.

c. A forest plot is the most effective tool for showcasing the heterogeneity and the pooled results. However, it cannot display potential bias to readers. A funnel plot can do that instead.

**Ans. 83** a. Hepatocystic triangle

b. Superiorly by inferior surface of liver, laterally by cystic duct and the medial border of the gallbladder, and medially by common hepatic duct.

c. Important landmark as the cystic artery usually can be found within its boundaries. The cystic lymph node often lies superficial to the cystic artery and acts as a landmark to locate this artery in difficult cases.

d. Caterpillar turn/Moynihan hump

**Ans. 84** a. Radiolucent shadow on right side, hyperinflated lung 2nd and 3rd right sided rib fracture, left-sided tracheal shift.

b. Right-sided pneumothorax

c. 14F angiocatheter in 5th intercostal space in mid axillary line (it causes sudden expansion) followed by tube thoracotomy in 5th intercostal space in mid axillary line.

**Ans. 85** a. Thyroid, total thyroidectomy

b.
- The Bethesda system of reporting thyroid cytology
- Royal College of Pathologists (RCP). One of the classification fine needle aspiration cytology (FNAC) grading

c.
- Hypocalcemia
- Serum calcium, serum parathyroid hormone (PTH)

15

SECTION

# Revision Spotter

# 56 CHAPTER Clinical Images

## CLINICAL IMAGES SPOTTERS AND REVISION POINTS

**1.**

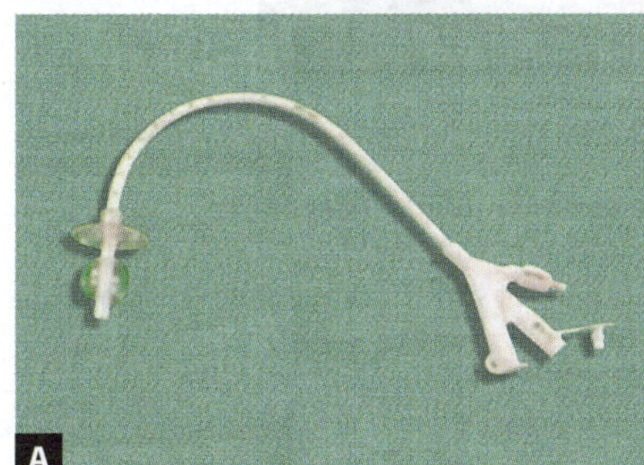

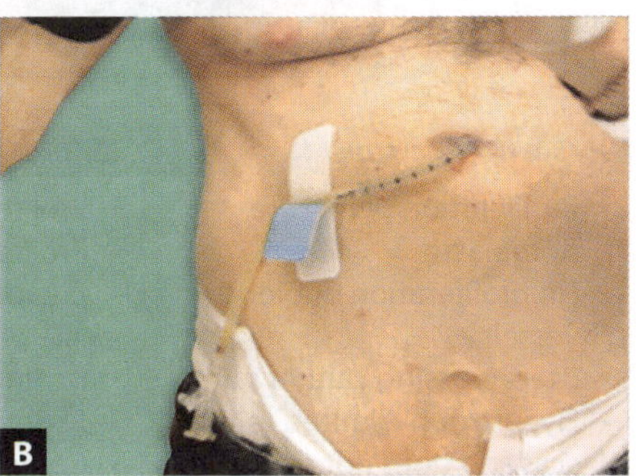

(A) Percutaneous endoscopic gastrostomy (PEG) tube; (B) inserted PEG tube.

Associated revision points:

- Indications for total parenteral nutrition (TPN)

| *As primary therapy* | *As supportive therapy* |
|---|---|
| • Gastrointestinal (GI) fistulas<br>• Renal failure (acute tubular necrosis)<br>• Short gut syndrome<br>• Severe burns<br>• Hepatic failure<br>• Crohn's disease<br>• Anorexia nervosa | • Radiation enteritis<br>• Acute chemotoxicity<br>• Prolonged ileus<br>• Weight loss preliminary to surgery |

- Complications of enteral nutrition:

| *Tube-related gastrointestinal* | *Gastrointestinal* |
|---|---|
| • Malposition<br>• Displacement<br>• Blockage<br>• Breakage/leakage<br>• Local complications (erosion of skin and mucosa) | • Diarrhea<br>• Bloating<br>• Vomiting<br>• Abdominal cramps<br>• Aspiration<br>• Fecal impaction (constipation) |

## 2. Keloid

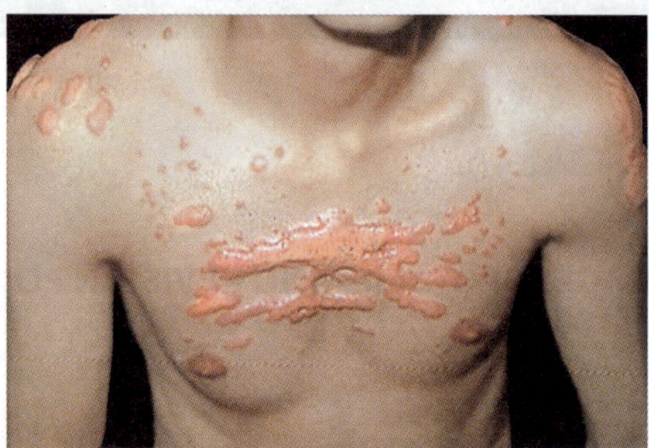

| *Hypertrophic scar* | *Keloid* |
|---|---|
| • Proliferation of mature fibroblasts<br>• No proliferation of blood vessels<br>• Scars crossing Langer's lines<br>• Hypertrophy limited to the scar and does not encroach adjacent tissue<br>• No claw-like process<br>• No itching<br>• Equal in male and female<br>• Common in children<br>• Gradually regress after 6 months<br>• Does not recur after excision | • Proliferation of immature fibroblasts<br>• Proliferation of immature blood vessels<br>• Encroachment of surrounding tissues by claw-like process<br>• Itching and blanching<br>• Slightly warm and slightly tender<br>• Commonly seen in black negroes, has genetic association<br>• Females > males<br>• Common age: 10–30 years<br>• Occasionally malignant change (Marjolin's ulcer)<br>• Recurrence after excision common<br>• Intrakeloidal—steroid, hyaluronidase, vitamin A, and methotrexate to prevent recurrence |
| *Common site:* Flexor surfaces | *Common site:* Sternum |

## 3. Burst abdomen

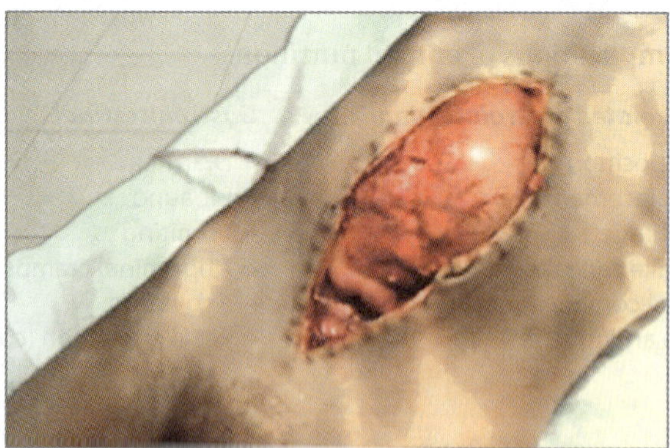

- *First sign of burst abdomen*: Serous/serosanguinous drainage
- Most commonly observed between 5th and 8th postoperative day (POD)
- *Wound dehiscence*: Partial or total disruption of operative wound with Evisceration after rupture extrusion of bowel.
- *Management*: Elective closure at the earliest
- Thorough saline wash is given and abdomen resutured—tension sutures are made.

**4.** Kocher's technique

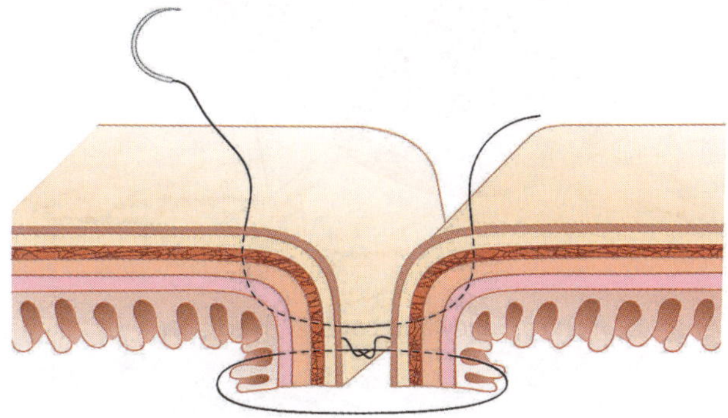

*Source:* Bailey and Love, 27th edition.

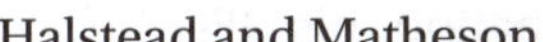

Halstead and Matheson

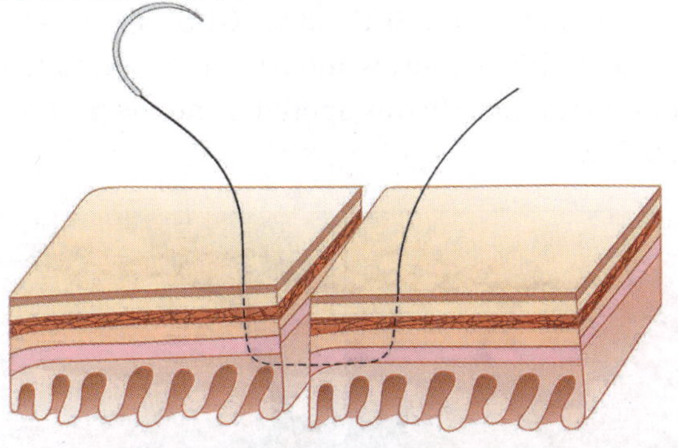

*Source:* Bailey and Love, 27th edition.

- Kocher's technique of bowel anastomosis—two-layer closure of bowel anastomosis
- Halstead and Matheson method—single layer extramucosal intermittent anastomosis (submucosa included)
- Most stable of the layers used for anastomosis—submucosa because it contains high amount of collagen.
- Current preferred method for anastomosis is Halstead and Matheson extramucosal method.

**5.** Cheatle cut.

- Cheatle cut is made in the small diameter bowel during end to end anastomosis.
- It is made on antimesenteric border.

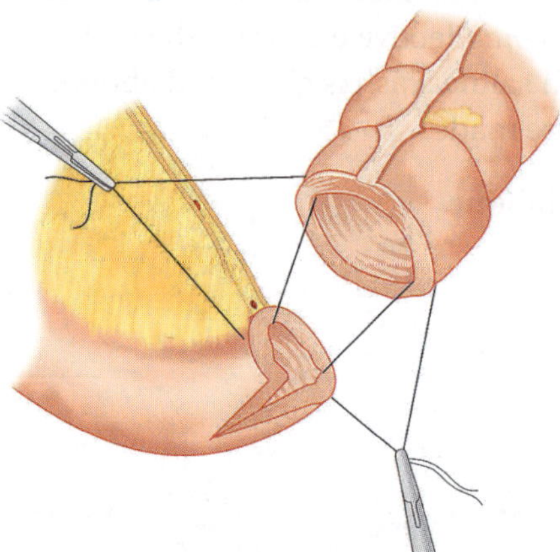

*Source:* Bailey and Love, 27th edition.

**6.**

A 26-year-old young male met with a road traffic accident and came to the emergency room. On examination, his BP—90/56 mm Hg, pulse—140 beats/min, $SpO_2$ 86%, GCS—8. On examination, the patient had multiple injuries and FAST ultrasound screening positive in all four quadrants. He was operated and the postoperative pictures shown below.

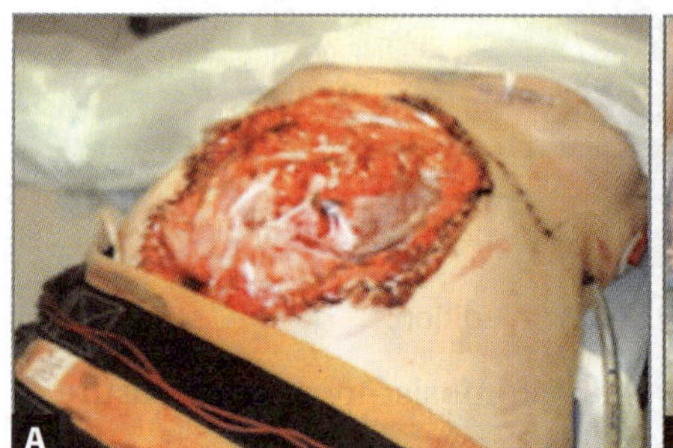


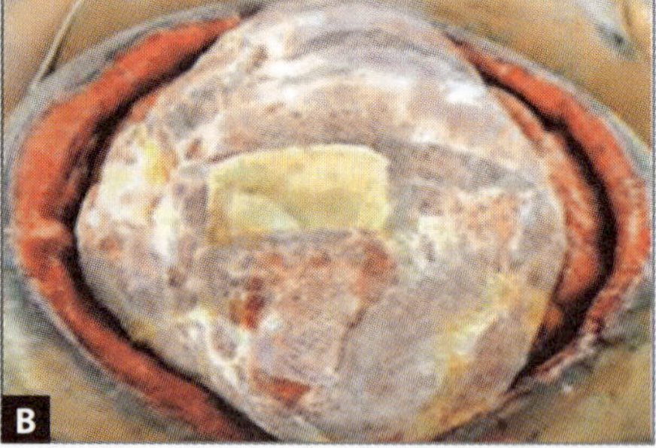


- Damage control surgery (DCS) is also known as abbreviated laparotomy.
- The initial focus is hemorrhage control, followed by control and limitation of contamination, achieved using a range of abbreviated techniques including simple ligation of bleeding

vessels, shunting of major arteries and veins, drainage, temporary stapling off of bowel, and therapeutic packing.

*Stages of DCS are:*
- Stage I patient selection
- Stage II control of hemorrhage and control of contamination
- Stage III resuscitation continued in the intensive care unit
- Stage IV definitive surgery
- Stage V abdominal closure

As per stage II, after hemorrhage control the abdomen is closed in a temporary fashion using a sheet of plastic (e.g., Opsite) over the bowel, an intermediate pack to allow suction, and a further sheet of adherent plastic drape to the skin to form a watertight and airtight seal abdominal fluid. This technique is known as the "Vacpac" or "Opsite sandwich". The first image is showing the closure of abdomen using a plastic bag known as "Bogota bag".

**7.** Triangle of safety.

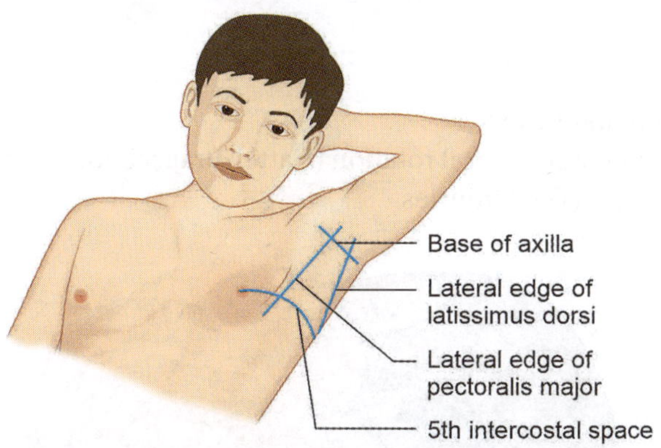


*Tube thoracostomy:*
- Skin incision made at the level of nipple
- Triangle of safety—anteriorly by lateral border of pectoralis major, posteriorly by mid axillary line and inferiorly by an imaginary horizontal line drawn at level of nipple to meet mid axillary line
- Subcutaneous tunnel created in superior direction and chest entered bluntly in an interspace above the skin incision
- Underwater drainage device providing 20 cm water suction

**8.** Mattox maneuver:

Left medial visceral rotation (Mattox maneuver)—needed for supracolic injuries [aorta, celiac axis, proximal superior mesenteric artery (SMA), and left renal arteries]

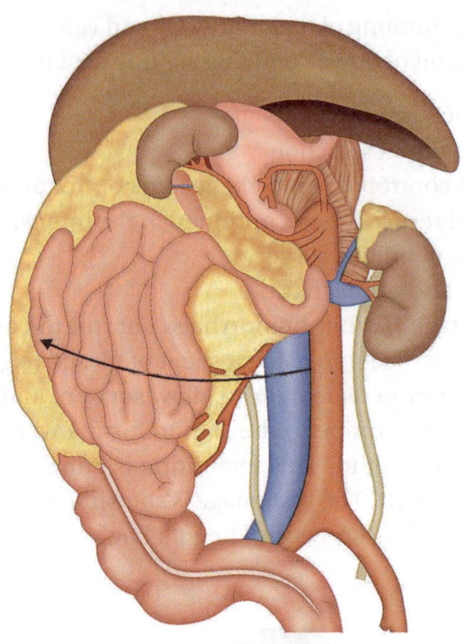

Cattell maneuver
Right medial visceral rotation (Cattel-Braasch maneuver) for inferior vena cava (IVC) injuries

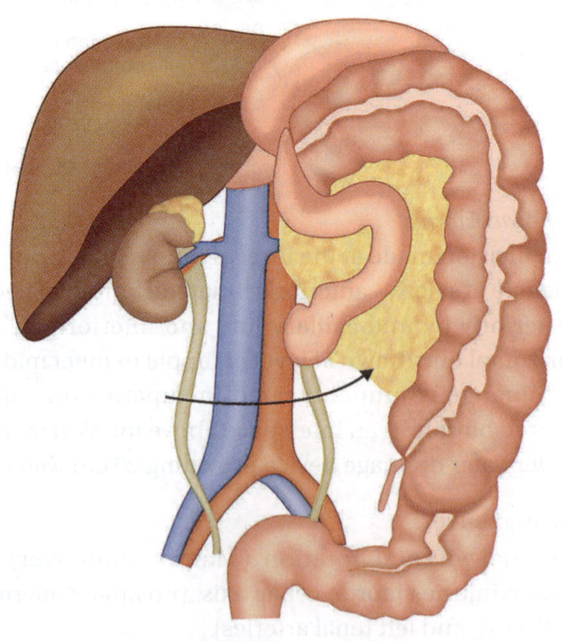

**9.** Clam shell thoracotomy

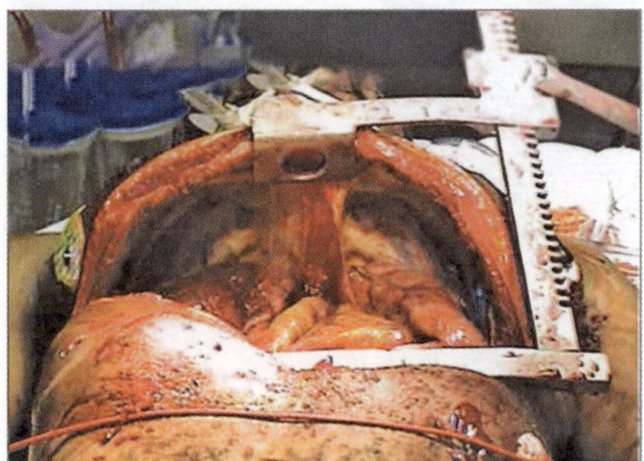

In emergency, the chest cage is opened fully at diaphragm level to look for major vessel injury and repair—this is known as clam shell thoracotomy.

**10.** Fasciotomy

- Done when pressure >30 mm Hg.
- Two incisions running deep is needed to decompress all the compartments.
- Myoglobinuria and renal failure can occur in late cases.

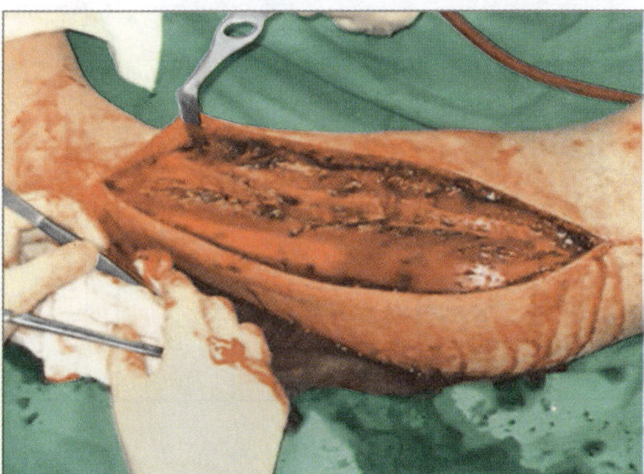

**11.** Diagnostic peritoneal lavage (DPL):

- DPL is said to be positive if >10 mL is aspirated as frank blood.
- DPL showing blood may need surgery, but if patient is stable, do contrast-enhanced CT (CECT) abdomen and we proceed based on the findings.

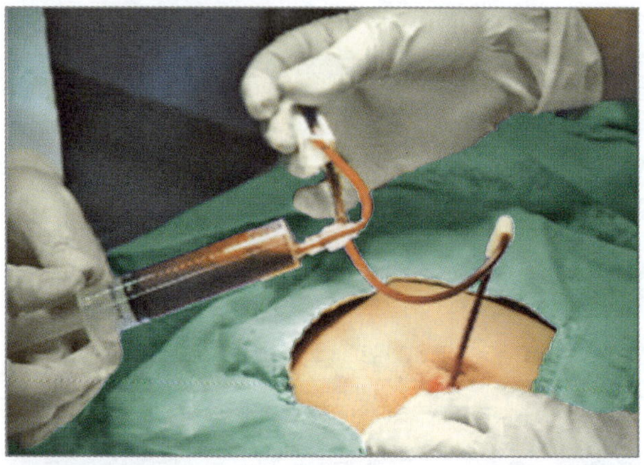

**12.** Retroperitoneal hemorrhage

- Hematoma behind the portal vein is known as zone 4. Otherwise there are only 3 zones.
- Zone 1, is marked as B, needs immediate exploration.
- Zone 2 is C and D
- Zone 3 is pelvic at E
- Zone 2 and 3 can be observed.
- Zone 4 is occasionally referred to collection of hemorrhage in the retroportal vein area.

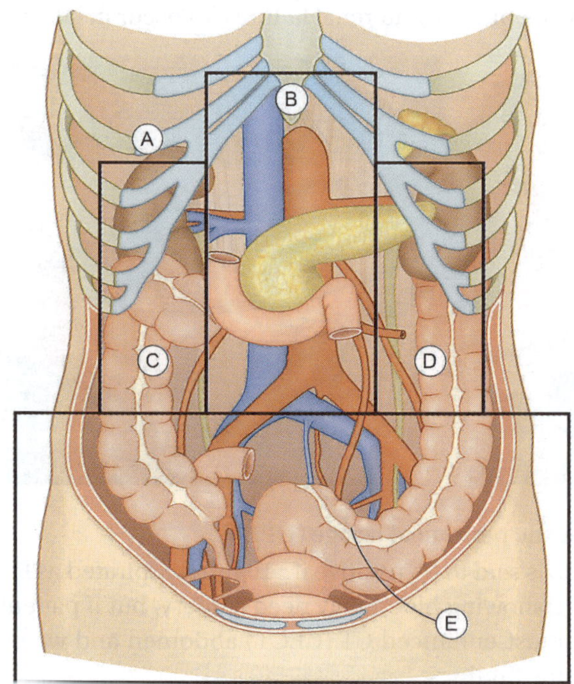

**13.** Log roll for spine examination

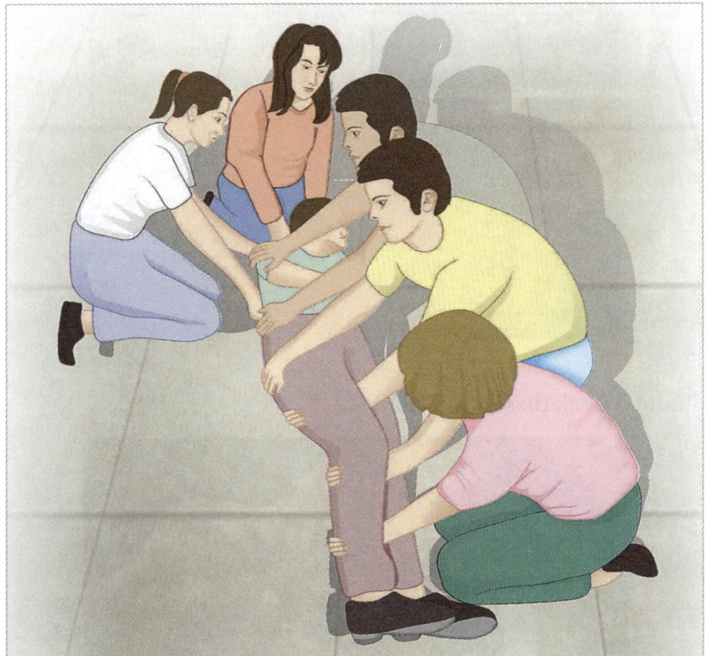

**14.**

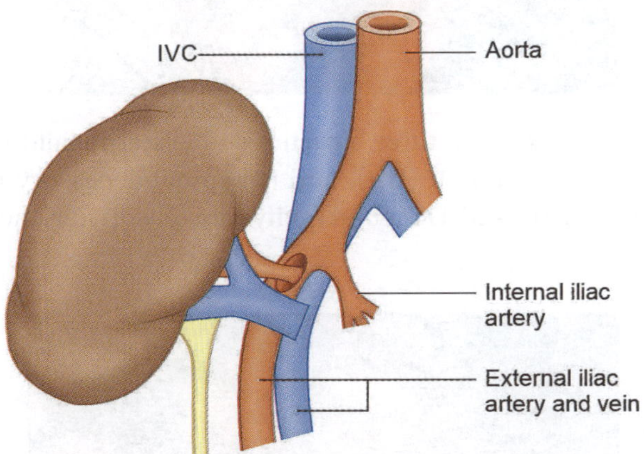


*Cadaveric donor:*

- This is the kidney from cadaveric donor because there is carrel patch seen in the image.
- Carrel patch containing cadaveric donor renal artery anastomosed to external iliac artery.

**15.** Johansen step ladder flap

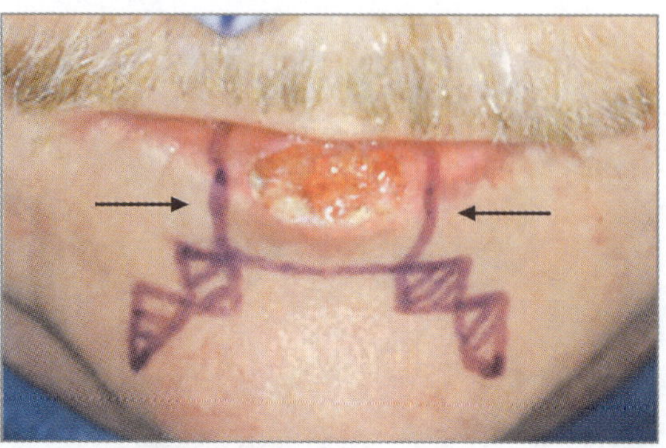

**16.** Radical neck dissection (RND)

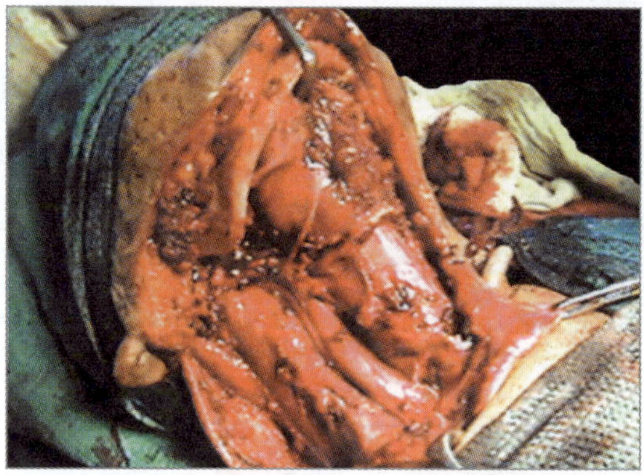

We can observe the three structures—(1) sternocleidomastoid, (2) internal jugular vein (IJV), and (3) spinal accessory nerve being removed. This is RND for oral cavity cancer with neck nodes.

**17.**

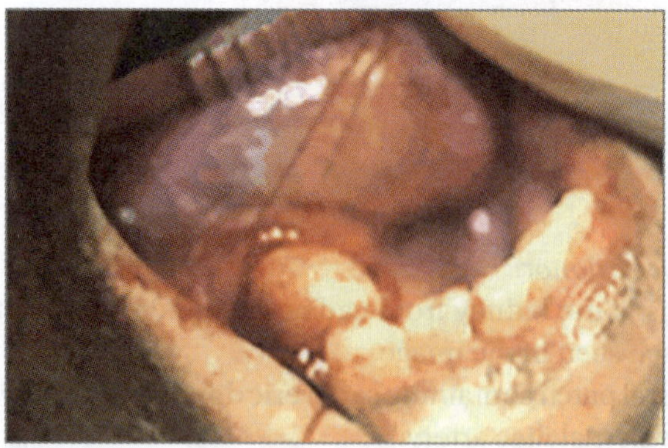

- This is a case of submandibular duct stone distal to the lingual nerve.
- The treatment is by lay opening of the duct and stone removal.
- No need to remove the gland

**18.** A 20-year-old female presents with a cystic swelling in the neck—it moves up with protrusion of tongue.

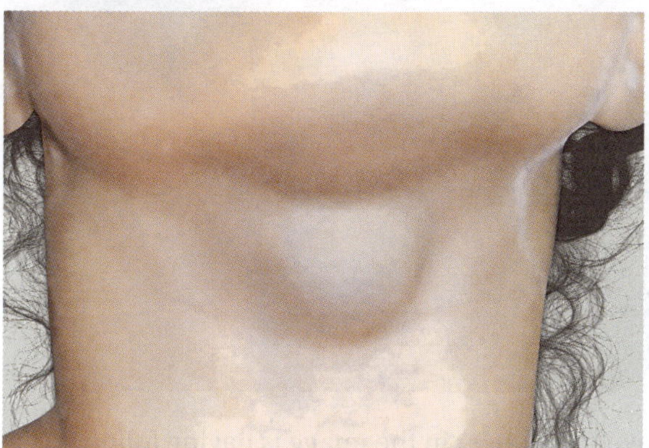

*Source:* Bailey and Love, 27th edition.

- Thyroglossal cyst moves with protrusion of tongue
- Other swellings which move only with deglutition are—subhyoid bursitis, midline dermoid cyst, and thyroid swelling.

**19.** Adson's test

Test done here for thoracic outlet syndrome.

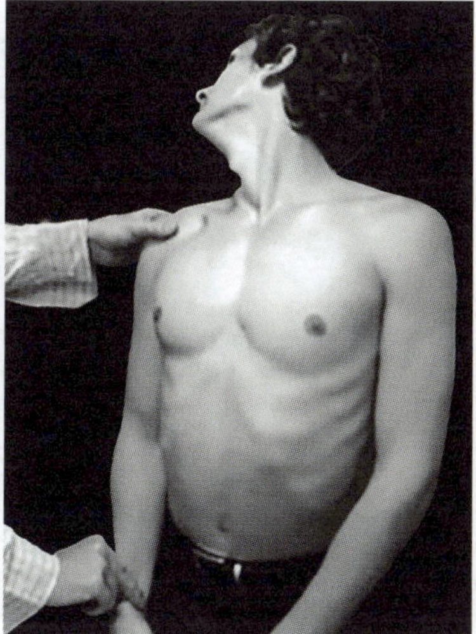

*Source:* Bailey and Love, 27th edition.

Feel for radial pulse becoming thin on taking deep breath and extending the backward.

**20.** Branchial cyst

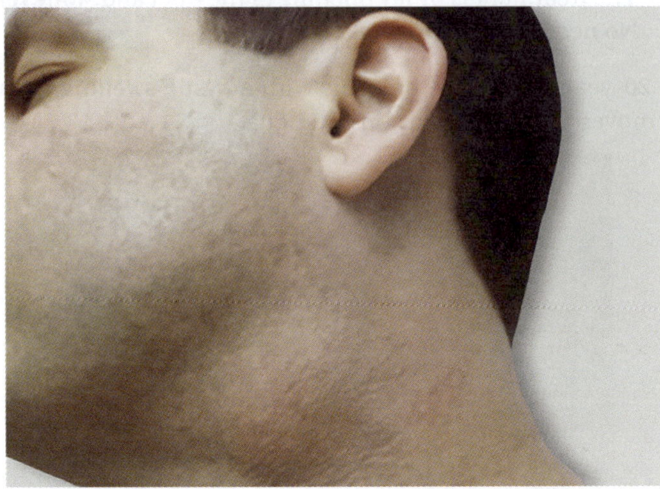

The swelling shown in the image is having following features:
- Anterior triangle swelling (so pharyngeal pouch ruled out)
- Not in midline (hence dermoid cyst and pretracheal bursa ruled out)
- Only swelling which suits the location at upper one-third level of sternocleidomastoid muscle is branchial cyst.

**21.** Cystic hygroma

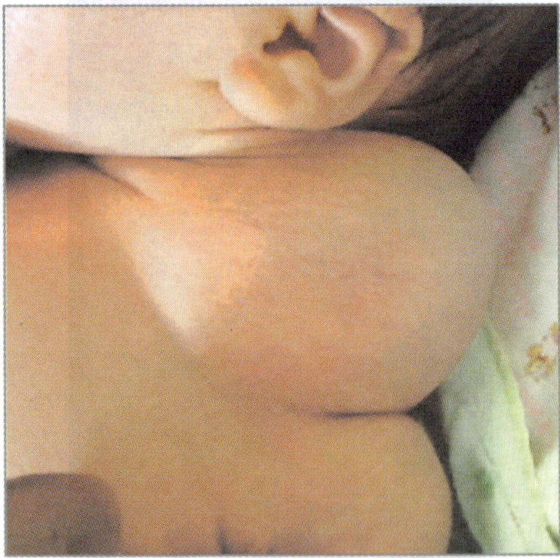

*Source:* Bailey and Love, 27th edition.

- This is due to congenital sequestration of lymphatics.
- Brilliant trans illumination+

**22.** Identify the disease in this young girl. On palpation, there is a hard swelling seen in the base of posterior triangle.

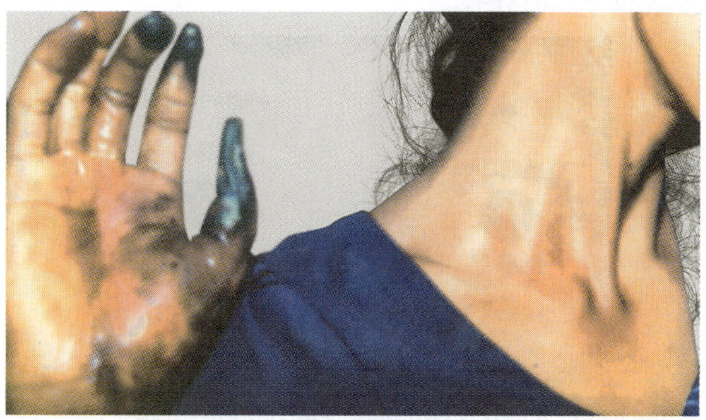

*Cervical rib with thoracic outlet syndrome (TOS):*

- This is a typical case of cervical rib with clinical features of thoracic outlet syndrome.
- Patient has developed gangrene due to the compression of subclavian artery.

**23.**

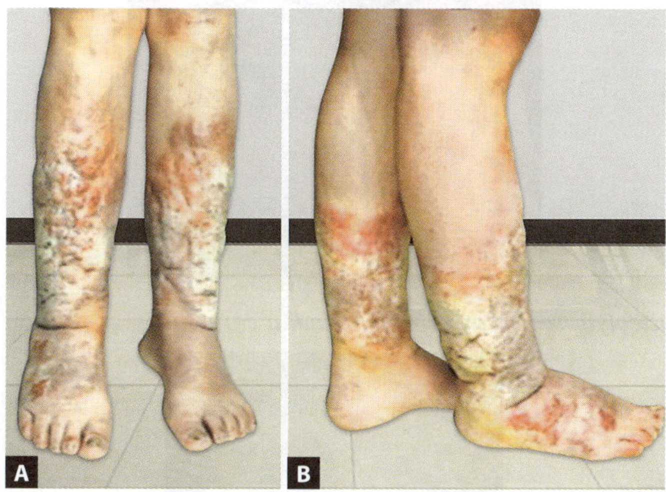

- Dermatopathy seen in hyperthyroidism known as pretibial myxedema
- Glycosaminoglycans deposition in the pretibial region
- Pretibial myxedema name is a misnomer as it is seen in thyrotoxicosis and not in myxedema.

**24.** The patient having visible upper sclera on examination. This sign in thyrotoxicosis is known as *Visible upper sclera is known as Dalrymple's sign.* (INI SS 2023):

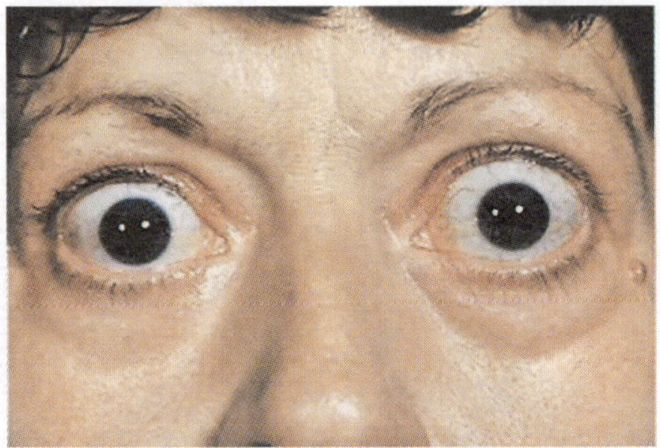

*Visible upper sclera is known as Dalrymple's sign.*

**25.** Patients operated for thyroid cancer has now presented after 5 months with a pulsatile swelling in scalp. What may be the pathological diagnosis she would have had before?

Follicular carcinoma produces pulsatile skull secondaries: Osteolytic in nature.

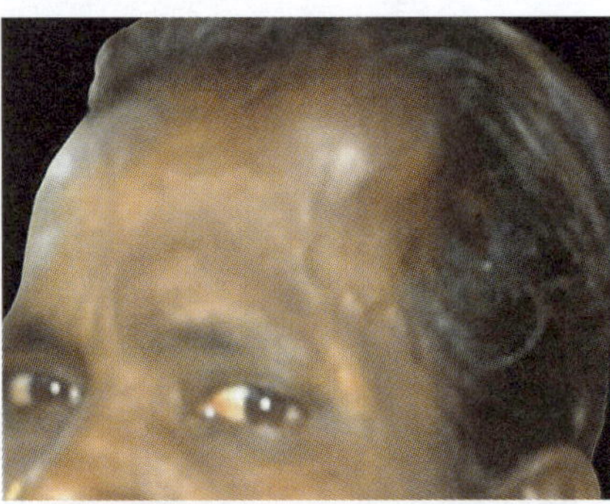

*Osteolytic secondaries from follicular cancer*

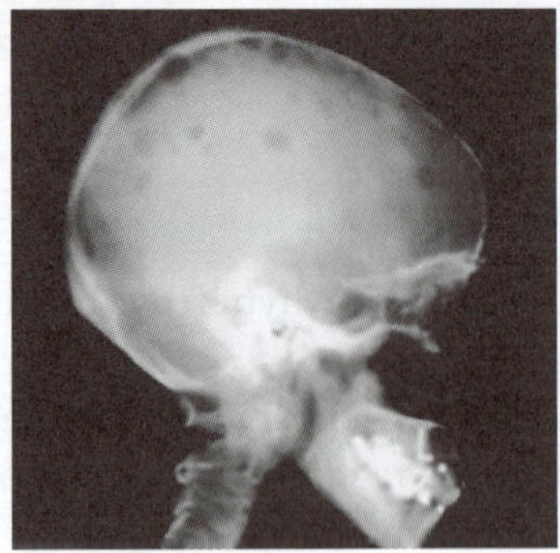

**26.** This young girl presented with a swelling in the neck which moves on deglutition. She complains of dyspnea and venous engorgement in face. She is examined with the following test. The name of this sign is:

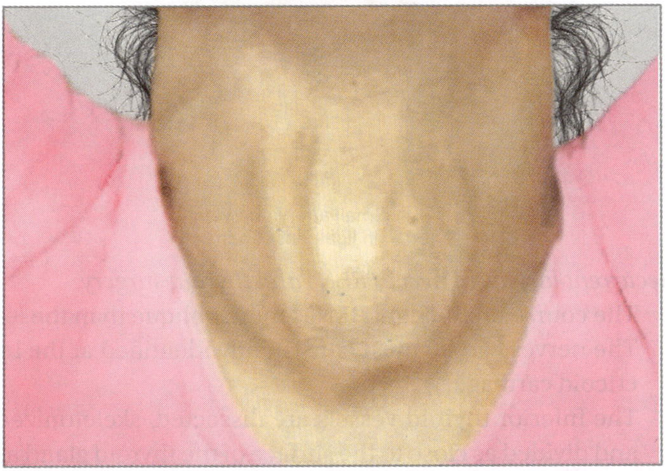

*After arm raising significant dilatation of neck veins (positive Pemberton's sign):*

- Pemberton sign is done in cases where lower border of the thyroid swelling is not visible.
- This test is to confirm that retrosternal goiter is causing compression.

**27.** On 5th, POD on a ward rounds—the post-total thyroidectomy patient shows the following finding spot diagnosis:

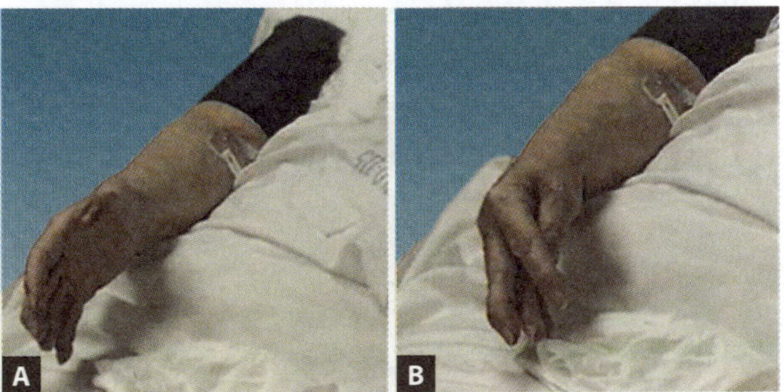


*Source:* Bailey and Love, 27th edition.

*Hypocalcemia:*

- *Trousseau sign:* Seen in hypoparathyroidism
- Carpal spasm happens on raising the BP.

**28.**

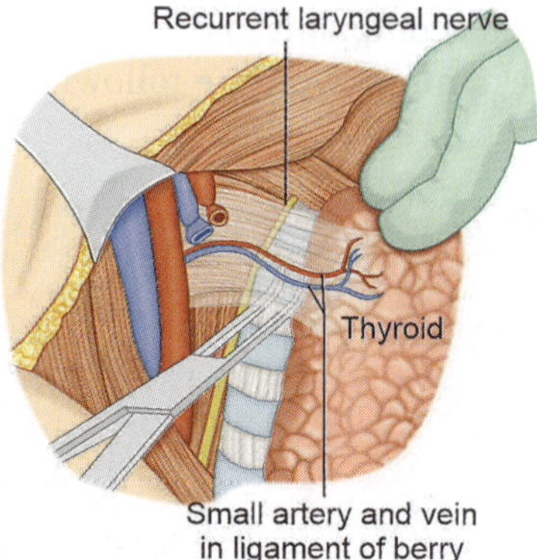


*Recurrent laryngeal nerve (RLN) and thyroid surgery:*

- The course on the right RLN is more oblique than the left RLN.
- The nerves can be most consistently identified at the level of the cricoid cartilage.
- The inferior thyroid vessels are dissected, skeletonized, ligated, and divided as close to the surface of the thyroid gland as possible to minimize devascularization of the parathyroids (extracapsular dissection) or injury to the RLN.
- The RLN is most vulnerable to injury in the vicinity of the ligament of Berry.
- The nerve often passes through this structure along with small crossing of arterial and venous branches (Fig.).
- Any bleeding in this area should be controlled with gentle pressure before carefully identifying the vessel and ligating it.
- Use of the electrocautery should be avoided in proximity to the RLN.

**29.** Gamma Camera looking for high radioactivity.

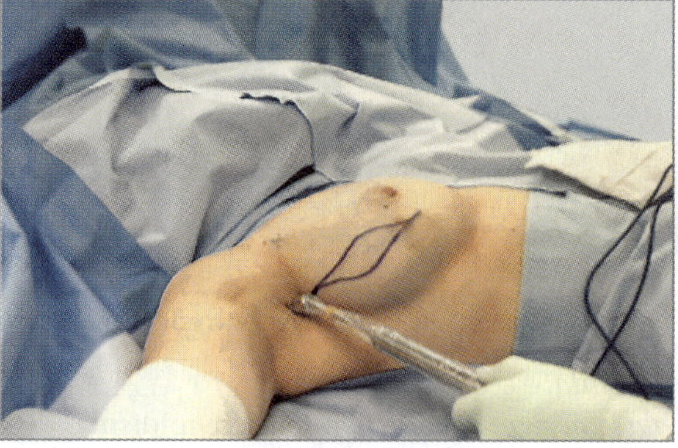

*Source:* Bailey and Love, 27th edition.

- Day before surgery or on the same day of surgery inject technetium 99m, Sulfur colloid in the breast parenchyma or around the tumor, this activity can be measured using Gamma probe during surgery. The node with high activity is sentinel node.
- At the same time, we also inject isosulfan-blue in the operating table. The node which appears blue is the sentinel node.
- With a small incision, we take the node and send it for *Frozen section* biopsy. If node is negative, no more dissection needed. If node is positive, do complete axillary dissection.

**30.** Identify the disease shown here, where the entire nipple is completely getting eroded:

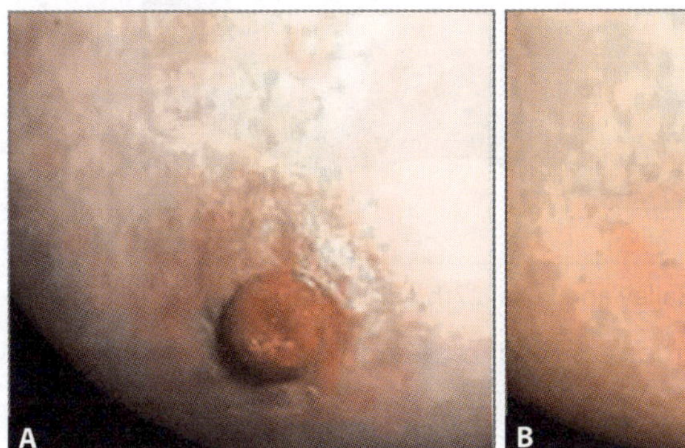


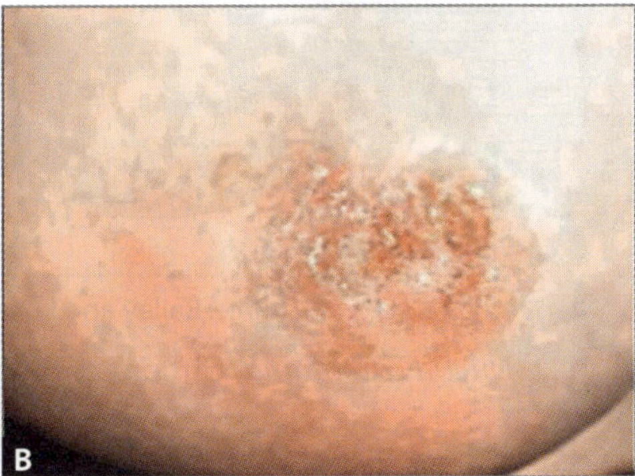


*Paget's disease:*
- Paget's disease is a superficial manifestation of an underlying cancer breast.
- *Treatment:* Modified radical mastectomy

**31.** Identify the disease in this patient having cord-like appearance in breast.

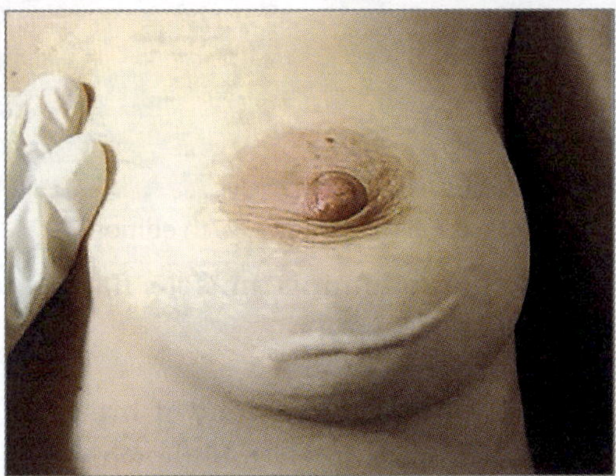

*Source:* Bailey and Love, 27th edition.

*Mondor disease:*

- It is a superficial vein thrombophlebitis seen over the breast.
- Treated conservatively

**32.** This patient shows circumferential nipple retraction, your diagnosis:

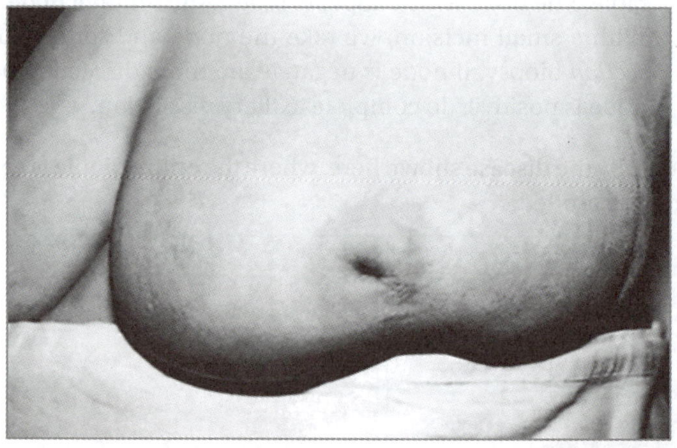

*Source:* Bailey and Love, 27th edition.

*Ductal carcinoma:* Circumferential retraction is seen in carcinoma.

**33.** Name the flap used here for surgical reconstruction.

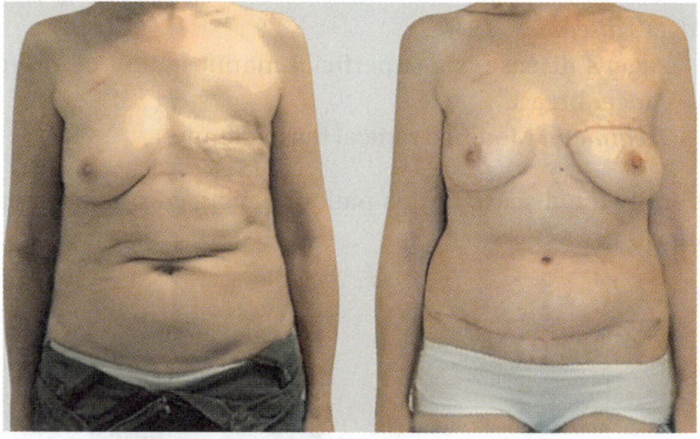

*Source:* Bailey and Love, 27th edition.

Transverse rectus abdominis muscle flap is used for breast construction.

**34.** Identify the cause for enlargement of breast in this lady aged 40 years. The swelling is freely mobile with no attachment with muscles. No axillary nodes are seen. USG showed cystic spaces.

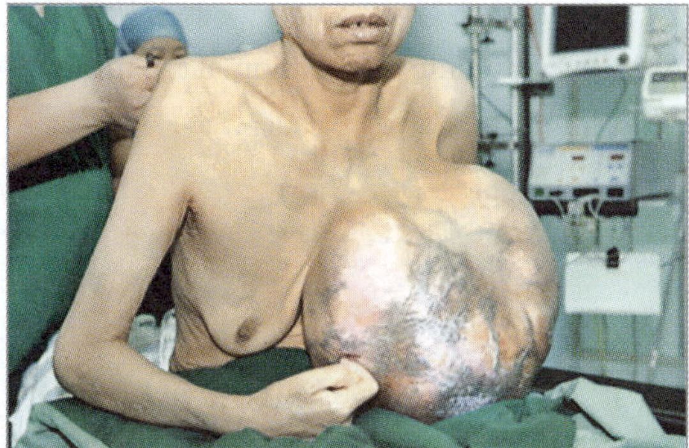

Phyllodes tumor has no nodal mets and shows cystic spaces.

**35.** Identify the T staging of this cancer breast.

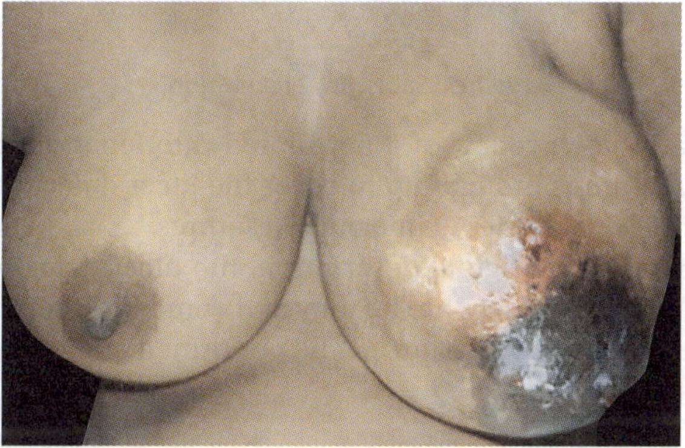

*T4b:*

- T4b stands for skin involvement.
- This patient has skin ulceration.

**36.** Identify the T-staging in this cancer breast.

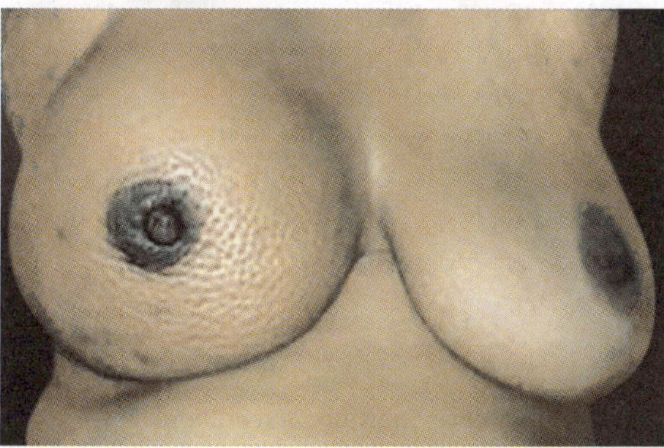

*Source:* Bailey and Love, 27th edition.

*T4:*
*Peau d'orange:* Lymphatic permeation of the tumor (T4b)

**37.**

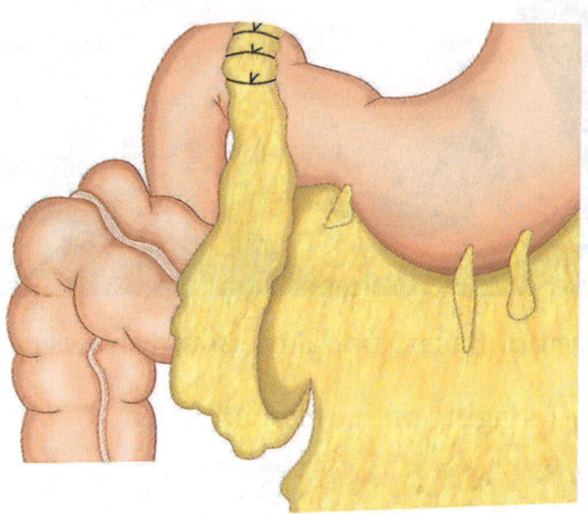

*Source:* Sabiston, 21st edition.

Graham patch repair of a perforated duodenal ulcer. A "tongue" of omentum is brought up to cover the ulcer defect and secured in position with a series of interrupted sutures.

In Graham's original description, the ulcer defect is not closed, but if the tissue edges are healthy and come together without undue tension, a primary closure can be performed and reinforced with an omental patch.

**38.**

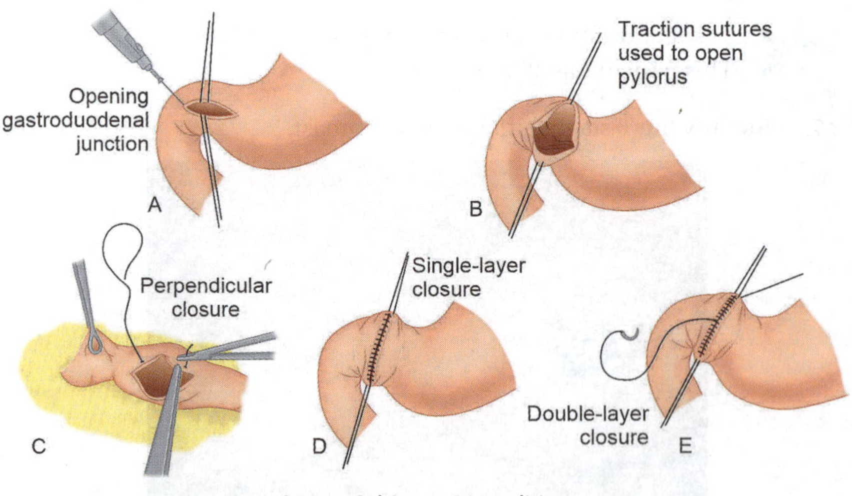


*Source:* Sabiston, 21st edition.

A to E Heineke-Mikulicz pyloroplasty

**39.**

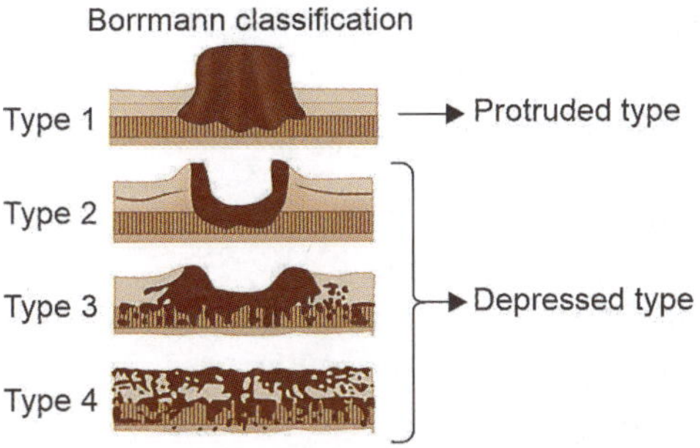


*Source:* Sabiston, 21st edition.

Borrmann pathologic classification of gastric cancer based on gross appearance.

*Lauren classification system for gastric cancer:*

| ***Intestinal*** | ***Diffuse*** |
|---|---|
| Environmental | Familial |
| Gastric atrophy, intestinal metaplasia | Blood type A |
| Men > women | Women > men |
| Increasing incidence with age | Younger age group |
| Gland formation | Poorly differentiated, signet ring cells |
| Hematogenous spread | Transmural, lymphatic spread |
| Microsatellite instability | Decreased E-cadherin |
| *APC* gene mutations | |
| p53, p16 inactivation | p53, p16 inactivation |

**40.**

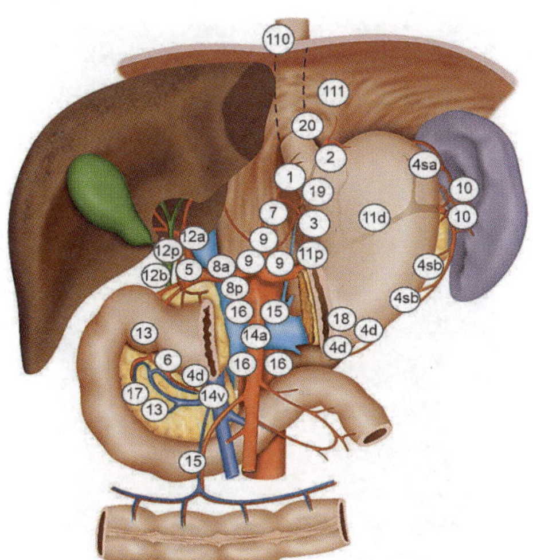


*Source:* Sabiston, 21st edition.

Lymph node station numbers as defined by the Japanese Gastric Cancer Association.

| | |
|---|---|
| 1 | Right paracardial |
| 2 | Left paracardial |
| 3 | Lesser curvature |
| 4sa | Short gastric |
| 4sb | Left gastroepiploic |
| 4d | Right gastroepiploic |
| 5 | Suprapyloric |
| 6 | Infrapyloric |
| 7 | Left gastric artery |
| 8a | Anterior common hepatic |
| 8p | Posterior common hepatic |
| 9 | Celiac artery |
| 10 | Splenic hilum |
| 11p | Proximal splenic |
| 11d | Distal splenic |
| 12a | Left hepatoduodenal |
| 12b, p | Posterior hepatoduodenal |
| 13 | Retropancreatic |
| 14v | Superior mesenteric vein |
| 14a | Superior mesenteric artery |
| 15 | Middle colic |
| 16aI | Aortic hiatus |
| 16a2, b1 | Para-aortic, middle |
| 16b2 | Para-aortic, caudal |

**41.**

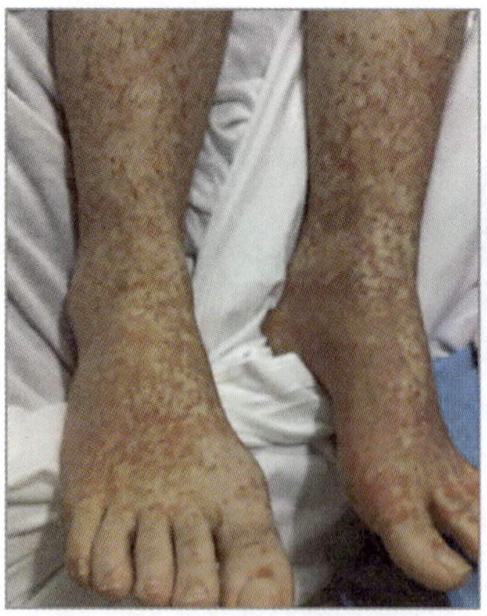

*Source:* Sabiston, 21st edition.

Crohn disease patient with erythema nodosum. The most common extraintestinal presentations of Crohn disease are skin lesions, which include erythema nodosum and pyoderma gangrenosum.

*Montreal classification of Crohn disease (INISS 2023 NEET SS 2023, 2022):*

- *Age at diagnosis (years)*:
  - *A1:* ≤16
  - *A2:* 17–40
  - *A3:* >40
- *Behavior:*
  - *B1:* Nonstricturing/nonpenetrating
  - *B2:* Stricturing
  - *B3:* Penetrating
  - *P:* Perianal disease modifier (can add to B1-3)
- *Location*:
  - *L1:* Ileal
  - *L2:* Colonic
  - *L3:* Ileocolonic
  - *L4:* Isolated upper GI tract (can add to L1-3)

**42.** Multiple recurrent enterocutaneous fistula patient with scarred skin and abdominal wall. CT scan shows a bowel obstruction and separation of the rectus muscles of 6 cm. The patient had already undergone an anterior components release.

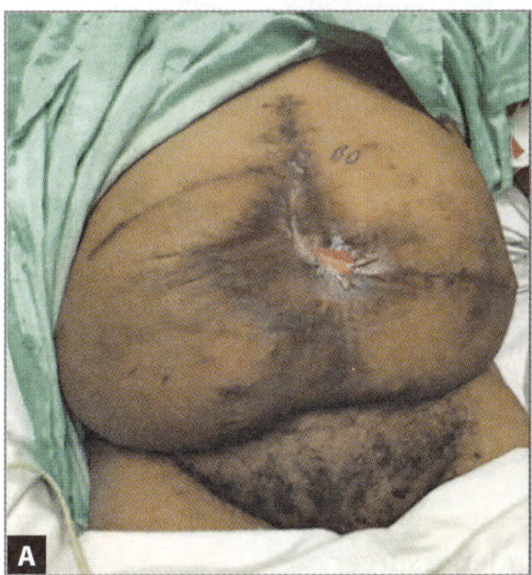


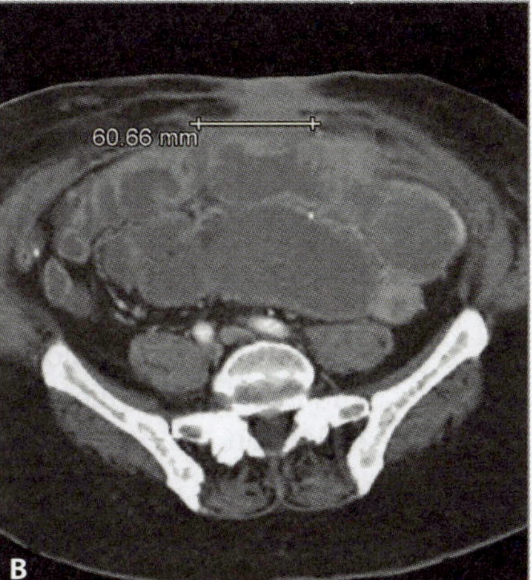


*Source:* Sabiston, 21st edition.

Factors predictive of nonoperative fistula closure:

| Favorable | Unfavorable |
|---|---|
| • Surgical etiology<br>• Appendicitis or diverticulitis<br>• Transferrin >200 mg/dL<br>• No evidence of bowel obstruction, discontinuity, infection, and inflammation<br>• Length >2 cm, end fistula<br>• Output <200 mL/24 hours<br>• No sepsis, balanced electrolytes<br>• Initial referral to tertiary care center and subspecialty care | • Ileal, jejunal, and nonsurgical etiology<br>• Inflammatory bowel disease, cancer, and radiation<br>• Transferrin <200 mg/dL<br>• Distal small bowel obstruction, bowel is in discontinuity, adjacent infection, and adjacent inflammation<br>• Length <2 cm, lateral, or multiple fistulas<br>• Output >500 mL/24 hours<br>• Sepsis, electrolyte disturbances<br>• Delay getting to tertiary care center and subspecialty care |

Treatment strategy in patients with an enterocutaneous fistula.

*Sepsis control:*
- Radiologic drainage of abscess
- Relaparotomy on demand, minimally invasive if possible
- Consider other infectious foci: intravenous line, urinary tract infection, and pulmonary

*Optimization of nutritional status:*
- Rehydration and electrolyte supplementation
- Enteral nutrition is preferred.
- Parenteral nutrition to meet calorie requirements, small bowel ECF
- Allow 500 mL/day clear liquids orally.

*Wound care:*
- Gauzes for low-output ECF
- Collect ECF fluids with bag (wound manager, fistula bag), paste to protect the skin
- Drainage of excessive ECF fluid with sump suction
- Proton pump inhibitors

*Anatomy of ECF:*
- Macroscopic
- Biochemical analysis of ECF fluid (bilirubin/amylase)
- Methylene blue
- *Preoperatively*: Fistulography or contrast CT; length of intestine and localization of origin of ECF, stenosis, obstruction, and fluid collection

*Timing of surgery:*
- Clinically stable (above)
- Psychologically willing to undergo surgery
- Albumin >25 g/L period of convalescence >6 weeks

*Surgical strategy:*
- One-stage procedure
- Careful adhesiolysis
- Wedge excision of intestinal resection
- Limit number of anastomoses to minimum
- Cover sutures with healthy, viable tissue
- Keep away from compromised area

**43.**

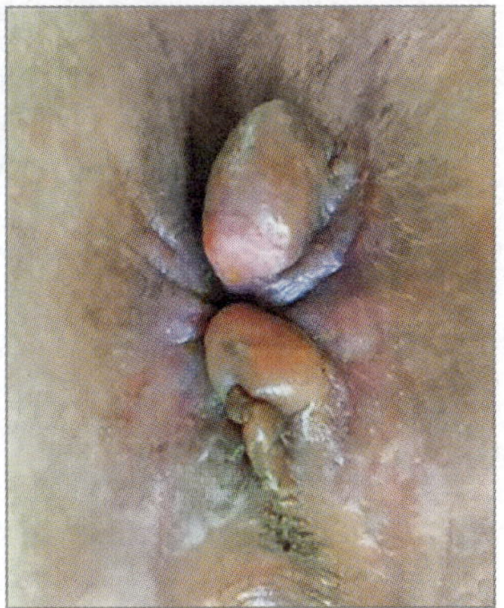

*Source:* Sabiston, 21st edition.

Large anal Crohn tags. Note the bluish coloring and waxy appearance of the perianal skin

**44.**

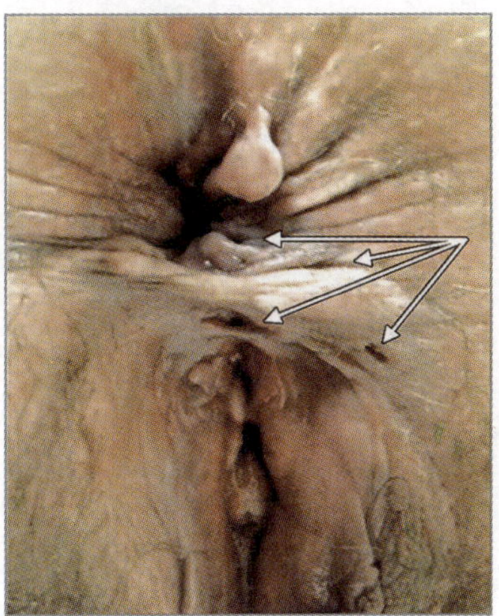

*Source:* Sabiston, 21st edition.

A woman with significant fistulizing perianal Crohn disease. Note the multiple external fistula openings shown by the white arrows. These all had a common internal opening in the anterior midline, which was also associated with a rectovaginal fistula. This patient ultimately elected to undergo ileostomy diversion.

**45.**

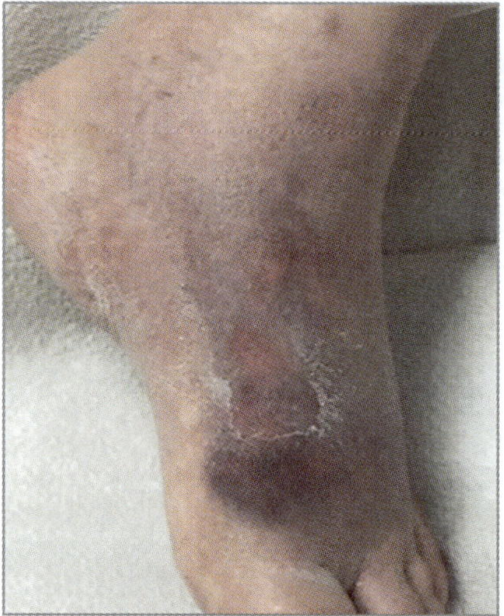

A patient with a Crohn disease flare and active erythema nodosum. Note the red purplish nodule on the dorsum of the foot.

**46.**

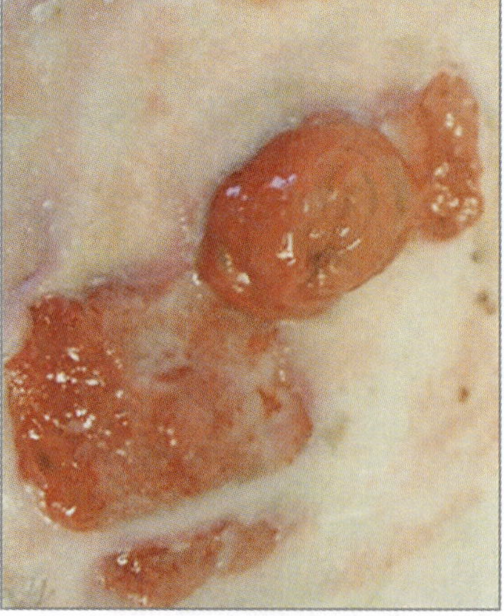

*Source:* Sabiston, 21st Edition

Pyoderma gangrenosum adjacent to an end ileostomy in a patient with Crohn disease. Here, the lesions have started to heal with granulation tissue.

**47.** Choledochal cyst classification

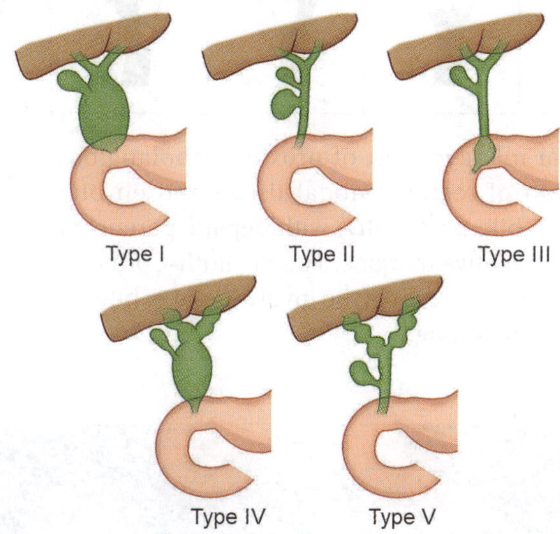


*Source:* Bailey and Love, 27th edition.

**48.**

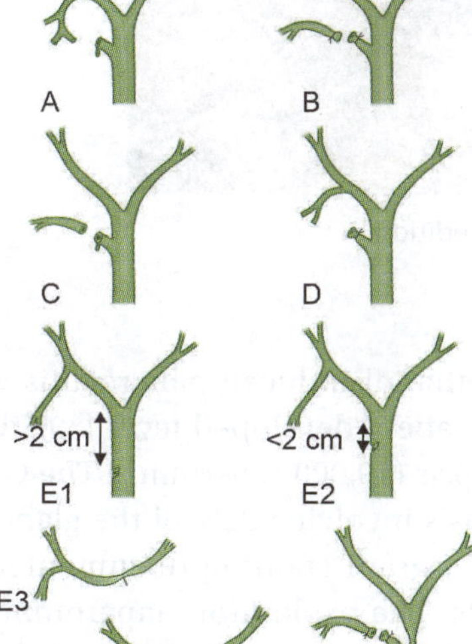


Strasberg classification of postoperative bile duct strictures.

(A) Injury to small ducts in continuity with the biliary system with a leak in the duct of Luschka or the cystic duct. (B) Injury to a sectoral duct, causing obstruction of portion of the biliary system. (C) Injury to a sectoral duct with bile leak; leak from a duct not continuous with the biliary system. (D) Lateral injury to the extrahepatic biliary ducts. (E1) Bismuth type 1: Injury more than 2 cm from the confluence. (E2) Bismuth type 2: Injury less than 2 cm from the confluence. (E3) Bismuth type 3: Injury at the confluence; confluence intact. (E4) Bismuth type 4: Destruction of the biliary confluence. (E5) Complete occlusion of all bile ducts, including sectoral ducts.

*Source:* Bailey and Love, 27th edition.

**49.** Bismuth-Corlette classification of tumor involvement.

| Type I | Type II | Type IIIa | Type IIIb | Type IV |
|---|---|---|---|---|
| | | | | |

Surgical management of proximal cholangiocarcinoma involves resection of regional nodal tissue and en bloc resection of the common bile duct (CBD) with hepatic parenchyma as necessary to achieve negative margins. The Bismuth-Corlette classification of the tumor by assessment of the involvement of biliary radicals helps with operative planning.

**50.**

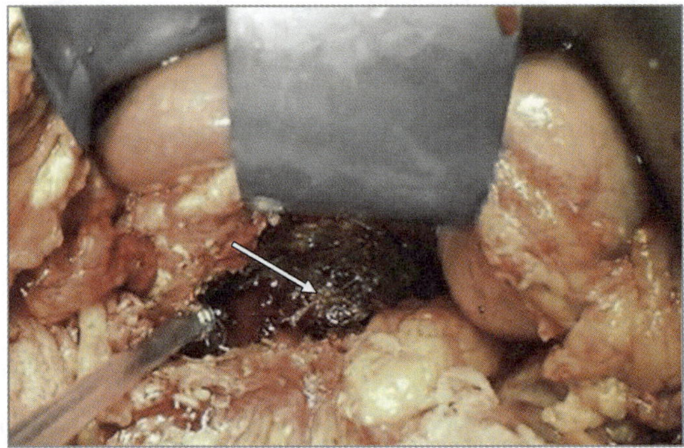

*Source:* Sabiston, 21st edition.

*Infected pancreatic necrosis:*
This 45-year-old man had severe ethanol-induced pancreatitis. 4 weeks after the initial episode, the patient developed fever [39.5°C (103°F)], hypotension, and leukocytosis (19,000 cells/mm$^3$). The CT scan documented pancreatic necrosis involving 35% of the gland. After fine-needle aspiration (FNA), gram staining documented the presence of gram-negative rods. The exploratory laparotomy indicated pancreatic necrosis involving mainly the body of the gland (arrow). The patient was treated with necrosectomy, closed drainage, and intravenous meropenem. Final culture documented

the presence of *Escherichia coli*. The patient was discharged home 56 days after the initial episode.

**51.**

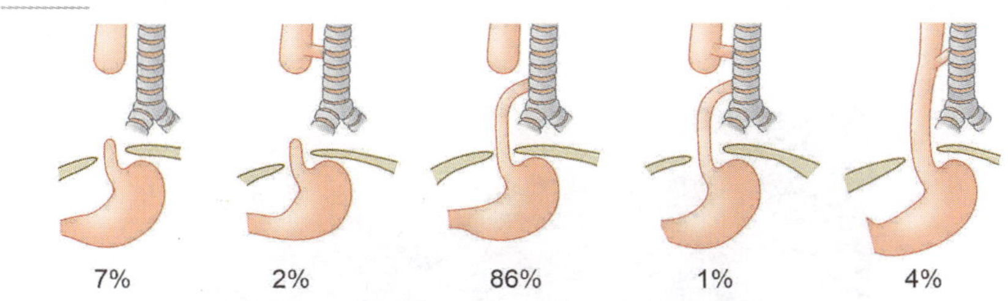


*Source:* Sabiston, 21st edition.

Anatomic variants and incidence of esophageal atresia with tracheoesophageal fistula.

**52.**

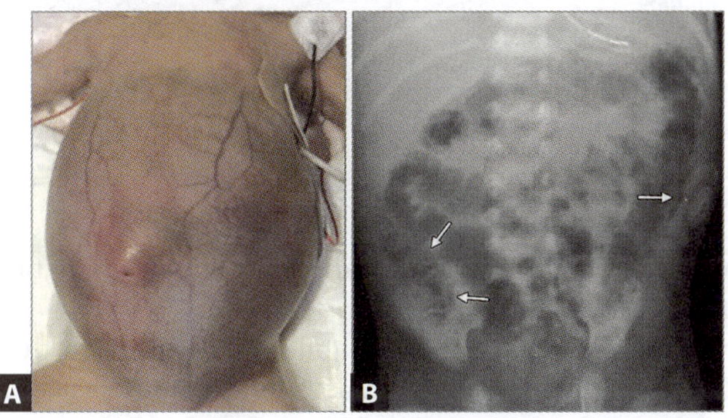


*Source:* Sabiston, 21st edition.

(A) Premature infant with necrotizing enterocolitis. Abdominal distention with marked cellulitis and dusky abdominal indicates intraabdominal catastrophe. (B) Pneumatosis intestinalis (arrows), a pathognomonic radiographic sign for necrotizing enterocolitis.

**53.**

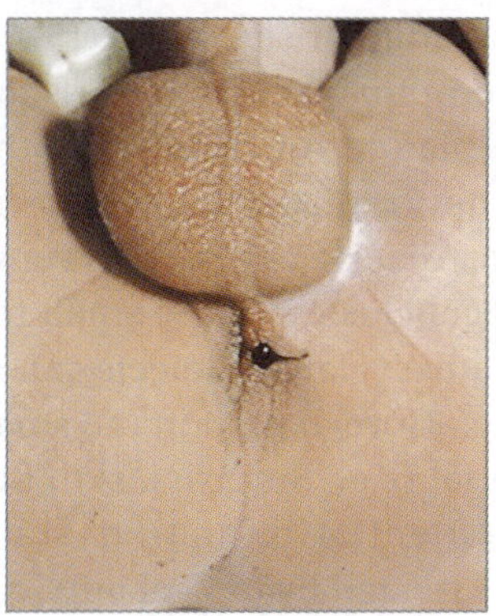

*Source:* Sabiston, 21st edition.

Imperforate anus with perineal fistula opening demonstrating meconium. Gluteal and scrotal anatomy appear relatively normal, consistent with characteristic findings in blind rectal pouch close to perineal skin amenable to anorectoplasty without an ostomy.

**54.**

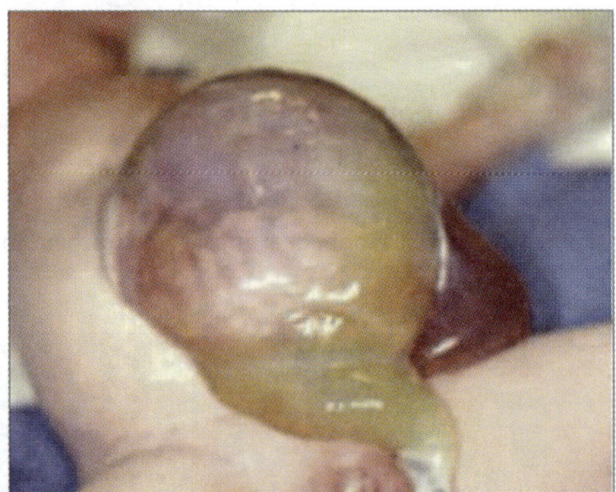

*Source:* Sabiston, 21st edition.

Omphalocele with intact sac and centrally located abdominal wall defect.

An omphalocele is a central abdominal wall defect that is generally >4 cm in diameter, with an intact membranous sac composed of an outer layer of amnion and an inner layer of peritoneum.

Defects <4 cm in diameter are arbitrarily designated as umbilical cord hernias. Infants with an omphalocele have a high incidence (~50%) of associated anomalies, such as Beckwith-Wiedemann syndrome: A combination of gigantism, macroglossia, and an umbilical defect, either hernia or omphalocele. Chromosomal abnormalities, including trisomies 13, 15, 18, and 21, have also been associated with omphalocele. Other associated anomalies include exstrophy of the bladder or cloaca and the pentalogy of Cantrell: Omphalocele, anterior diaphragmatic hernia, sternal cleft, ectopia cordis, and intracardiac defect, such as ventricular septal defect.

Primary surgical closure of the small to medium-sized defect is preferred. Alternatively, larger defects can be closed with prosthetic patch closure (e.g., Gore-Tex), porcine small intestinal submucosa-derived biomaterial (e.g., Surgisis), skin flap closure, or placement of a silo for sequential reduction and staged closure. Giant omphaloceles are treated by topical application of escharotic agents such as povidone-iodine (betadine) ointment or silver nitrate, which allows the sac to thicken and epithelialize. The overall survival for infants with an omphalocele largely depends on their lung maturity and severity of associated anomalies.

**55.**

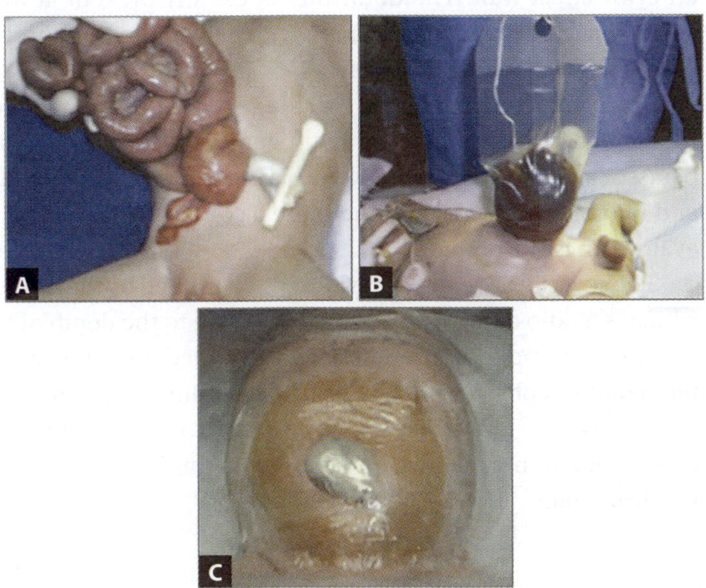

*Source:* Sabiston, 21st edition.

(A) Gastroschisis with eviscerated bowel. Note the abdominal wall defect is to the right side of an intact umbilical cord. (B) Silastic bag with ringed edge can be placed at bedside and bowel loops are gradually reduced into abdominal cavity. (C) Sutureless closure of gastroschisis. After reducing eviscerated bowel loops into the abdominal cavity, the umbilical cord is folded over the defect and a clear watertight dressing is placed.

**56.**

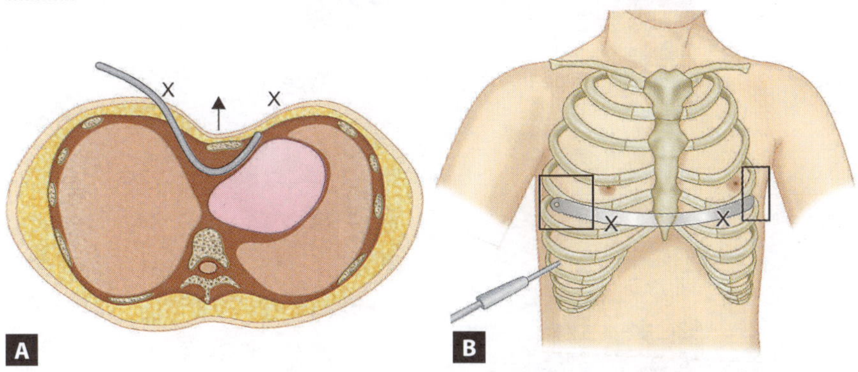


*Source:* Sabiston, 21st edition.

(A) Pectus excavatum. A tunneler is used to dissect the retrosternal place under thoracoscopic guidance. (B) A Nuss bar is placed beneath the sternum and secured onto the chest wall with stabilizers.

Pectus excavatum, a chest wall structural deformity where the anterior chest wall is caved-in or sunken, is five times more common than pectus carinatum, an abnormal outward protrusion of the anterior chest wall. The deformity is usually present at birth and steadily becomes more prominent with age until past puberty with a male-to-female ratio of 3 to 4:1.

Abnormalities in costal cartilage development have been implicated in the underlying pathogenesis. Pectus excavatum can be associated with mitral valve prolapse, Ehlers-Danlos syndrome, and Marfan syndrome, and therefore a comprehensive preoperative evaluation is warranted.

The severity of pectus excavatum is quantified by the Haller index, which is a ratio of the width of the chest wall to the depth of between the sternum and the vertebral body on limited chest CT or two-view plain radiographs. A Haller index of >3.2, pulmonary function testing indicating restrictive disease, mitral valve prolapse, murmurs, or conduction abnormalities on echocardiography are indications for surgical repair.

**57.**

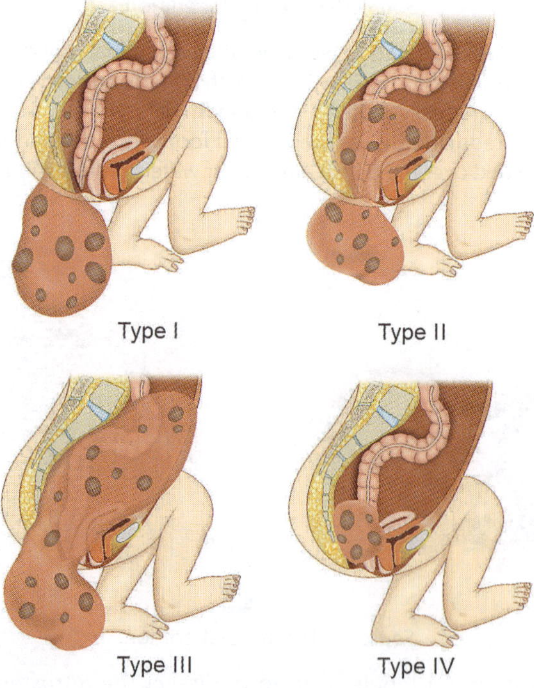


*Source:* Sabiston, 21st edition.

*Sacrococcygeal teratoma Altman classification types I to IV:* Type I is resected entirely from perineal approach. Types II and III require combination of perineal and abdominopelvic approach. Type IV is resected entirely via abdominal approach.

*Sacrococcygeal teratoma:*

- Teratoma occurs frequently in neonatal period and MC site is sacrococcyx.
- They arise from primitive streaks.
- Most common in females
- Most of them appear as external mass.
- Most neonatal teratomas are benign.
- Development of hydrops and placentomegaly during intrauterine screening is bad prognosis.
- Complete surgical excision is to be done.

**58.** A patient with advanced carcinoma stomach is presenting with a nodule in umbilicus. Your diagnosis.

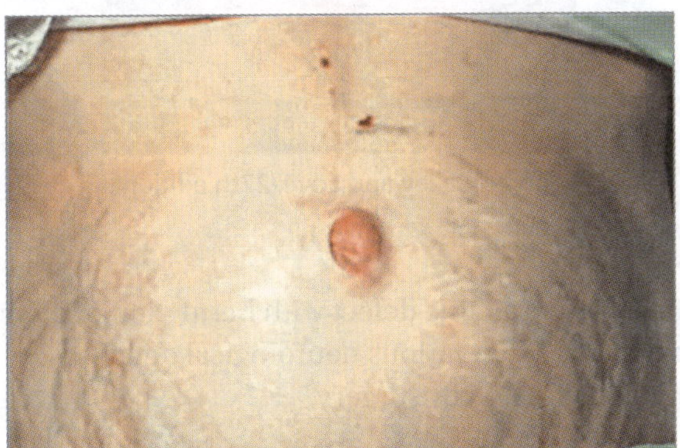

Transcoelomic spread of metastasis to umbilicus is sister joseph nodule.

**59.** Raynaud disease

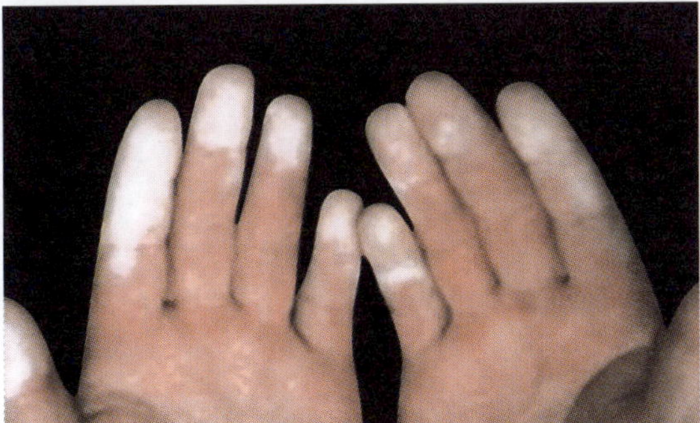

*Source:* Bailey and Love, 27th edition.

*Stages:*
1. Local syncope—white
2. Local asphyxia—blue
3. Recovery—crimson red

**60.** Identify the disease shown below.

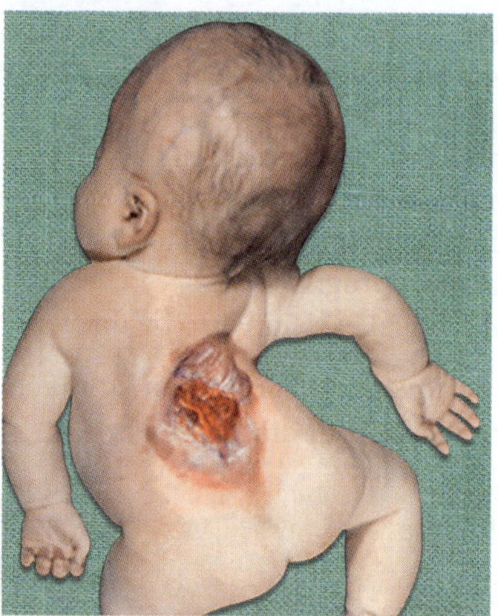

*Source:* Bailey and Love, 27th edition.

*Meningocele:*
- A type of neural tube defect with herniation of meninges.
- Characterized by various neurological deficits.
- Should be treated by surgery.

# CHAPTER 57 Endoscopic View

## ENDOSCOPIC IMAGES SPOTTERS AND REVISION POINTS

**1.**

Herpes simplex esophagitis

Common in immunocompromised patients.

Characterized by small raised herpetic vesicles few days before on the lips.

Endoscopy reveals vesicles and small ulcers with raised margins (punched out) usually in upper half of esophagus.

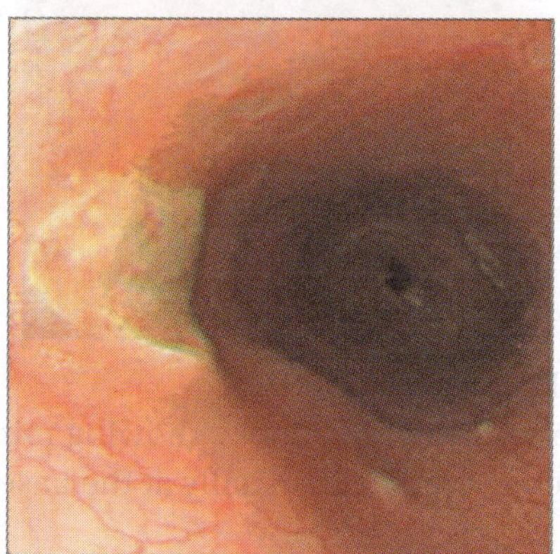

**2.** CMV esophagitis

- Seen in graft versus-host disease following bone marrow (BM) transplantation.
- Endoscopy shows characteristic— geographical or serpentine border.
- Serpentine lesion in esophagus—CMV
- In all the above cases, endoscopic biopsy is diagnostic.

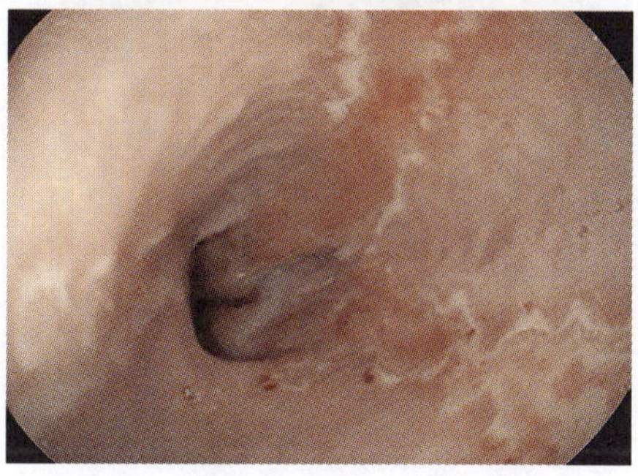

3. Eosinophilic esophagitis
   - Etiology is not clear, but has similarities immunologically to asthma and hence known as "allergic esophagitis".
   - *Clinical features:* Chest pain (post prandial pain) and dysphagia (solid dysphagia more common) and hence it is often confused with gastroesophageal reflux disease (GERD)
   - Eosinophilic esophagitis has a characteristic finding often called the "ringed esophagus" or the "feline esophagus," as the esophageal rings are felt to look like the stripes on a housecat.

   Endoscopy shows multiple esophageal rings, longitudinally oriented furrows are seen, mimicking like a "trachea" also known as trachea like esophagus.

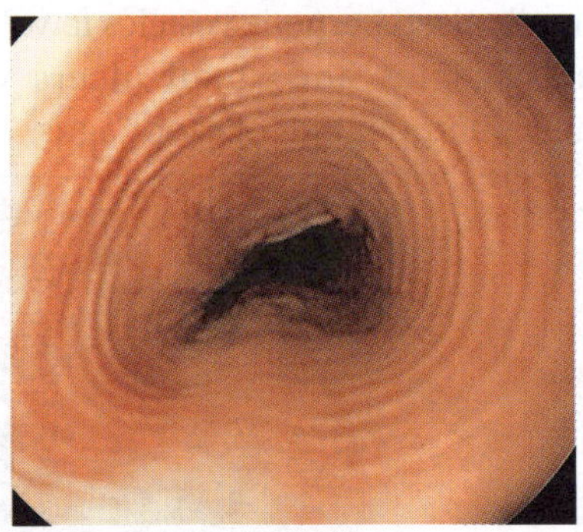

   Ringed trachea-like esophagus in EE:
   - Diagnosis is established by biopsy showing minimum of 15 eosinophils per high powered field, usually at the base of the epithelium.

   *Treatment:*
   - Test for the allergen
   - Give Inhalational or ingestional steroids
   - If dysphagia is not relieved we us, dilatation with rigid dilators: Maloney or Savary dilators.
4. Endoscopy showing this picture in lower esophagus. Your diagnosis is:

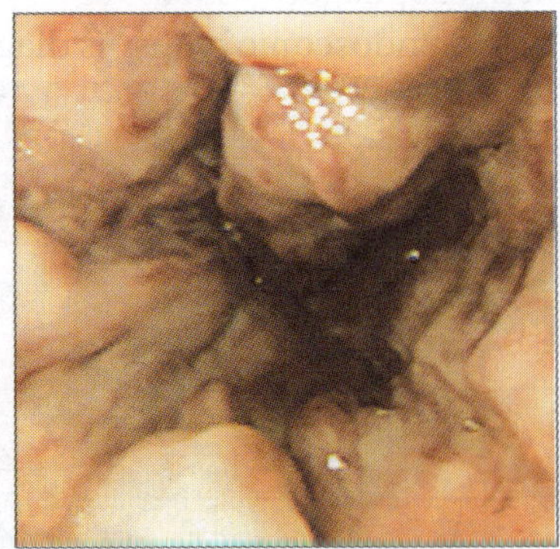

Varices lower end showing dilated columns of veins.

5. Identify the disease.

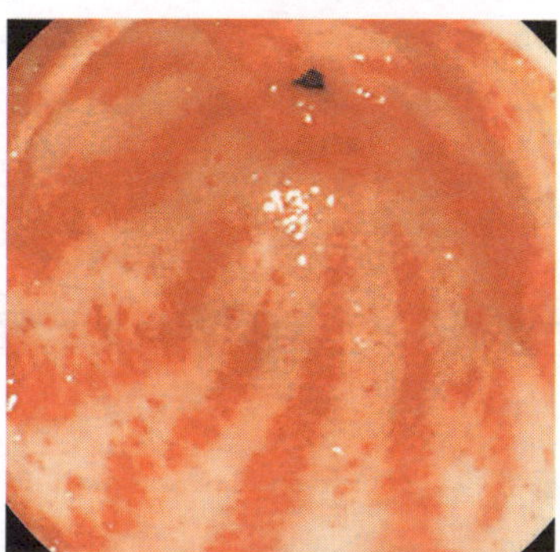

- This is watermelon stomach (gastric antral vascular ectasia)
- Chronic anemia and blood loss seen

6.

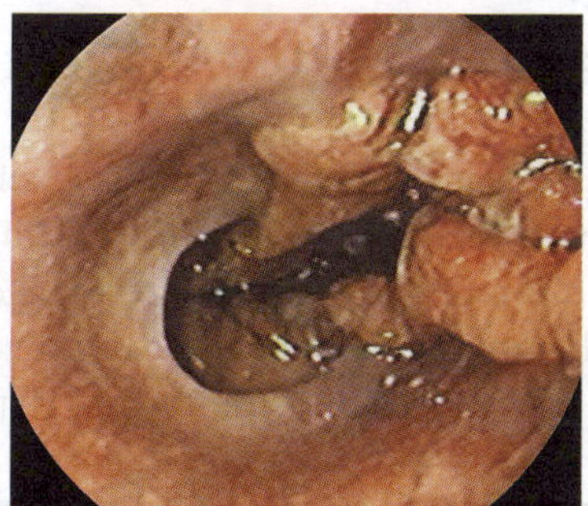

*Source:* Sabiston, 21st edition

Endoscopic view of intestinal-type adenocarcinoma of the gastric cardia.

7.

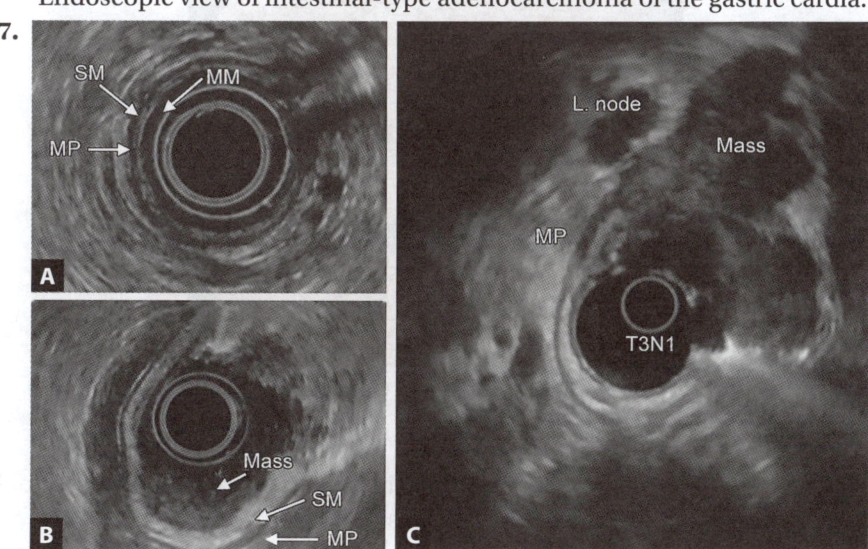


*Source:* Sabiston, 21st edition

Endoscopic ultrasound views of normal stomach (A), T1N0 gastric cancer (B), and T3N1 gastric cancer (C).

**8.**

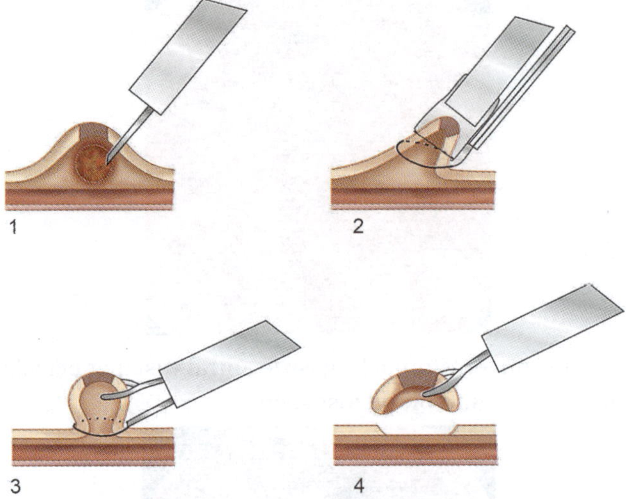


Endoscopic mucosal resection by strip biopsy: Saline is injected into the submucosal layer, and the area is elevated (1). The top of the mound is pulled upward with forceps, and the snare is placed at the base of the lesion (2 and 3). Electrosurgical current is applied through the snare to resect the mucosa, and the lesion is removed (4). (*Source:* Sabiston, 21st edition)

**9.**

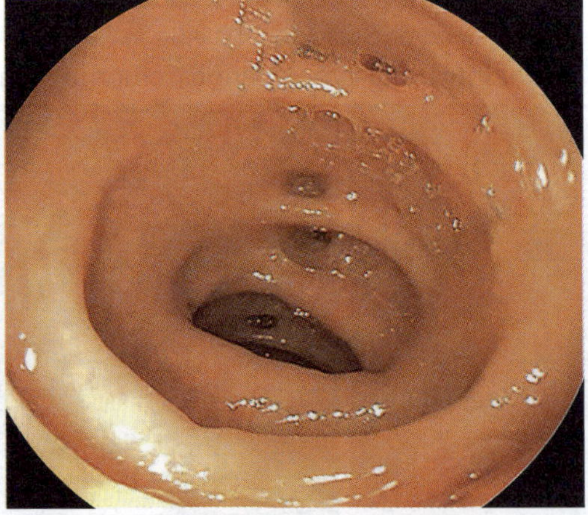

*Source:* Sabiston, 21st edition

Endoscopic view of diverticulosis.

The modified Hinchey classification six is the most commonly used tool to describe the severity of diverticulitis:

*Stage 0:* Mild clinical diverticulitis

*Stage Ia:* Confined pericolic inflammation—phlegmon

*Stage Ib:* Confined pericolic abscess (within sigmoid mesocolon)

*Stage II:* Pelvic, distant intra-abdominal or intraperitoneal abscess

*Stage III:* Generalized purulent peritonitis

*Stage IV:* Fecal peritonitis

10. 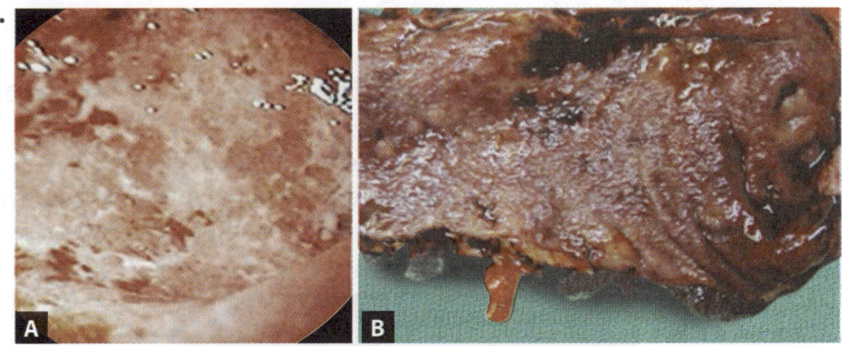

*Source:* Sabiston, 21st edition

(A) Endoscopic view of moderately severe ulcerative colitis. Note the bleeding and ulceration; (B) Macroscopic view of right colon following total proctocolectomy for fulminant ulcerative colitis.

11. 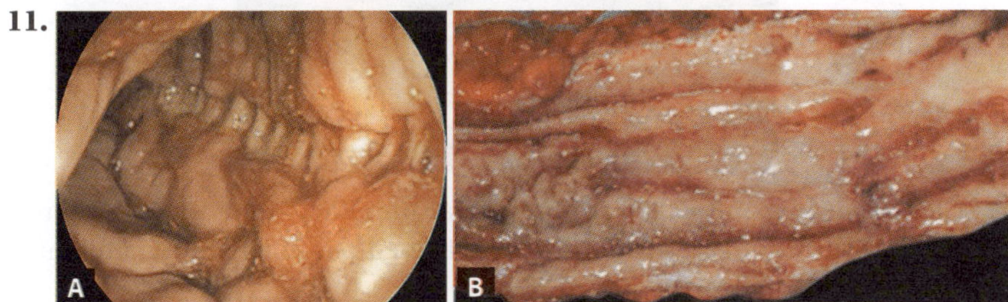

Bear-claw ulcers in Crohn colitis. (A) Endoscopic view; (B) Macroscopic view. (*Source:* Sabiston, 21st edition)

12. 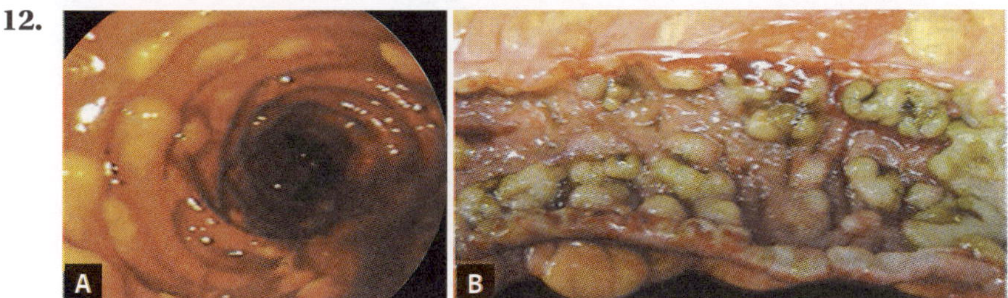

*Source:* Sabiston, 21st edition

(A) Endoscopic view of pseudomembranes associated with *Clostridium difficile*; (B) Pseudomembranes overlying the colon mucosa at the time of colectomy. The patient had active *Clostridium difficile* colitis with coexisting Crohn colitis.

Antibiotic treatment of *Clostridium difficile* infection:

- *First episode (Duration 10 days):*
  - Oral vancomycin 125 mg four times daily OR
  - Fidaxomicin 200 mg twice Daily
- If vancomycin and fidaxomicin are not available—metronidazole 500 mg three times daily can be given for nonsevere disease.
- *First episode—fulminant (hypotension, shock, ileus and megacolon) (at least 10 days, duration should be individualized):*
  - Vancomycin, 500 mg four times daily (oral or by nasogastric tube).
  - *In case of ileus:*
    - Consider adding rectal instillation of vancomycin.
    - I ntravenously administered metronidazole (500 mg every 8 hours) should be administered together with oral or rectal vancomycin.

**13.**

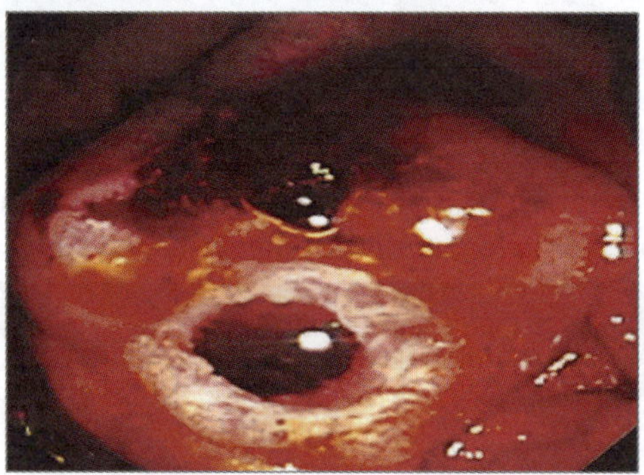

Classic endoscopic view of intraductal papillary mucinous neoplasm (IPMN) showing viscous fluid oozing from a patulous ampulla of Vater. (*Source:* Sabiston, 21st edition)

# CHAPTER 58 Histopathology

## QUESTIONS

### HISTOLOGY IMAGES SPOTTERS AND REVISION POINTS

**Q1. What fine-needle aspiration cytology (FNAC) is showing in given image?**

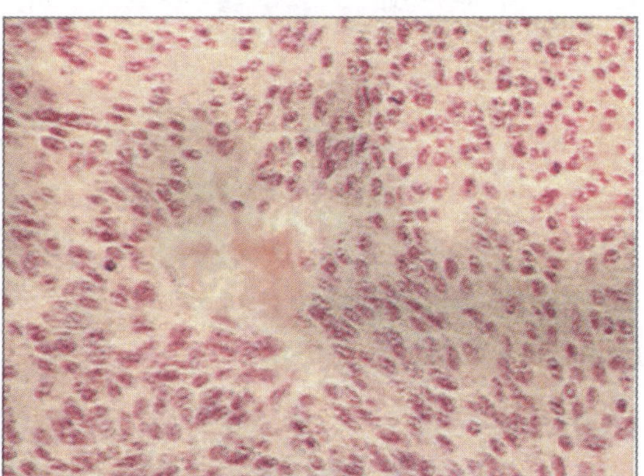

**Q2. Identify the type of carcinoma in thyroid showing the following FNAC findings.**

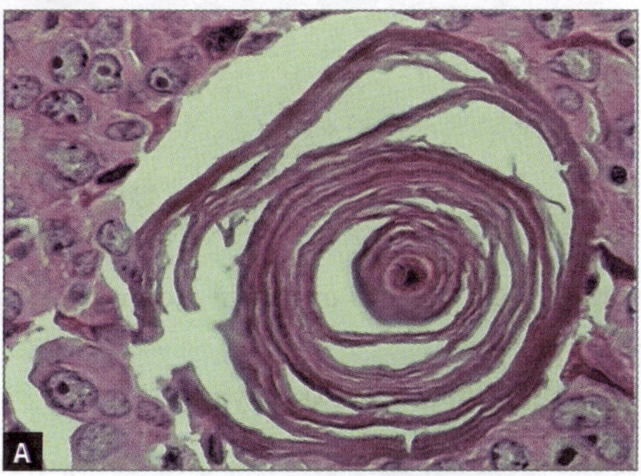


*Source:* Sabiston, 21st edition.

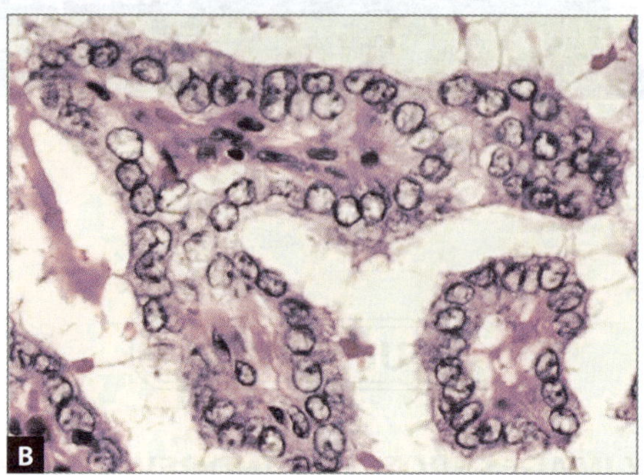

*Source:* Sabiston, 21st edition.

**Q3. Describe Indian file pattern in lobular carcinoma breast.**

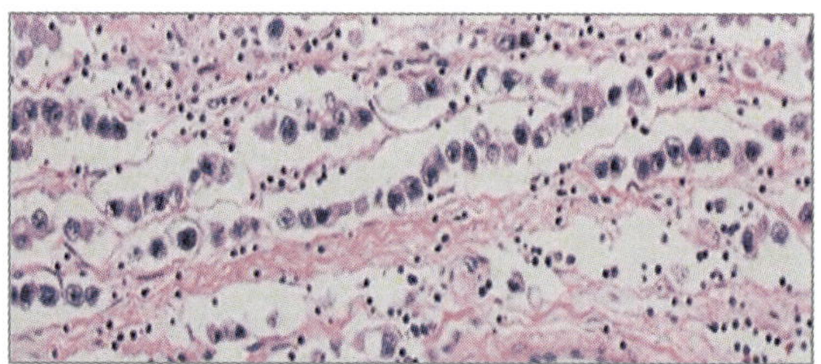

*Source:* Sabiston, 21st edition.

**Q4. Describe Paget's cells.**

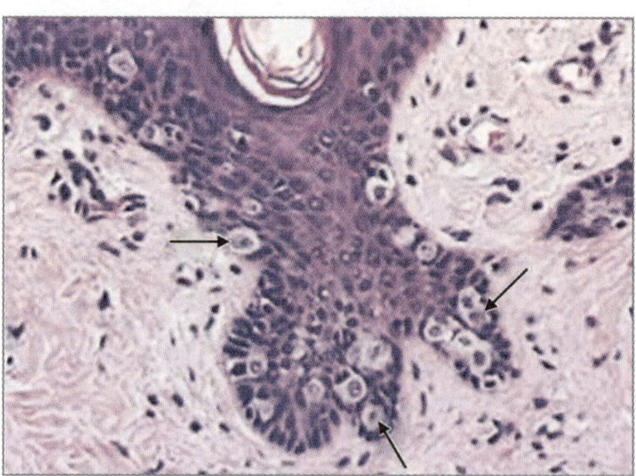

**Q5. Explain histologic section of active ulcerative colitis and Crohn colitis.**

**Q6. Describe malignant intestinal polyps.**

**Q7. Explain the ovarian-like stroma and computed tomography (CT) scan of the tail of the pancreas mucinous cystic neoplasm (MCN).**

**Q8. The following biopsy image from a chronic nonhealing leg venous ulcer—identify the microscopy finding.**

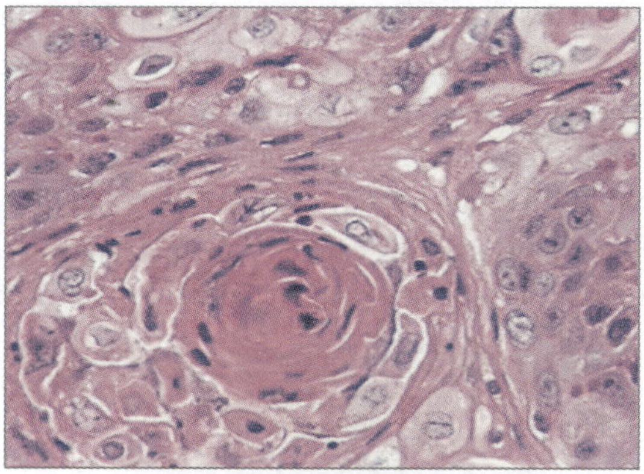

*Source:* Sabiston, 21st edition.

**Q9. Wedge biopsy form the edge of an ulcer shows the following pathological finding. What is your diagnosis?**

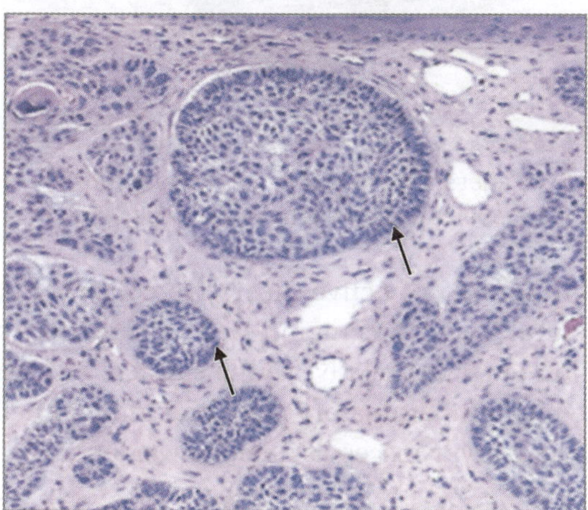

## ANSWERS

**Ans. 1** The FNAC showing amyloid stroma seen in medullary carcinoma of thyroid.

**Ans. 2.** Images A and B shown are—psammoma bodies and orphan Anne empty pale nuclei seen in papillary carcinoma of thyroid.

**Ans. 3** Mammography shows calcification in adjacent tissues (neighboring calcification—unique feature of lobular carcinoma).

**Ans. 4** *Paget's disease:*

- Present as chronic eczematous eruption of the nipple, which may be subtle, but may progress to an ulcerated, weeping lesion.
- Paget's disease is usually associated with extensive ductal carcinoma in situ (DCIS) or may be associated with an invasive cancer.
- Palpable mass may or may not be seen.
- Pathognomonic of this cancer is the presence of large, pale, and vacuolated cells (Paget's cells) in the rete pegs of the epithelium.

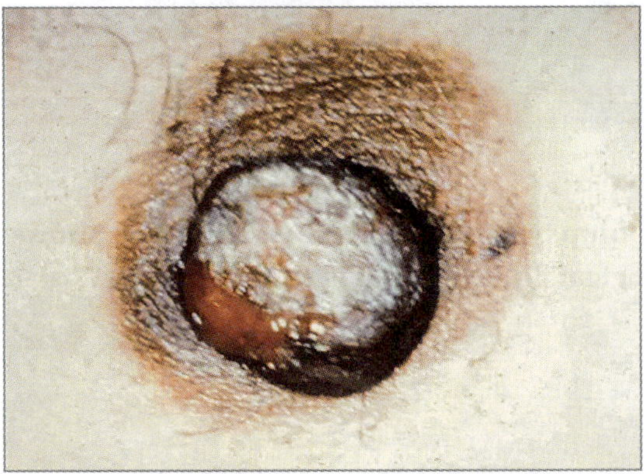

Paget's disease showing nipple erosions.
*Source:* Bailey and Love, 27th edition.

**Ans. 5** Histologic section of active ulcerative colitis. There is glandular architectural distortion manifested by irregular branching and orientation of glands relative to the surface. The lamina propria is expanded with inflammatory cells, and intraepithelial neutrophils are present. A crypt abscess is noted (lower left).

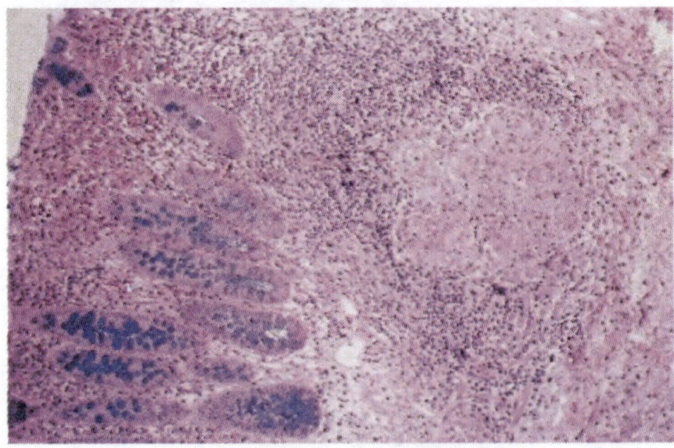

Crohn colitis with noncaseating granuloma.
*Source:* Sabiston 21st edition.

**Ans. 6** One of the important risk factors is the depth of penetration. This can be defined by the Haggitt classification:

- *Level 0:* Carcinoma limited to the mucosa, carcinoma in situ
- *Level 1:* Carcinoma invading into the submucosa, limited to the head of the polyp
- *Level 2:* Carcinoma invading to the level of the neck (junction of the head and stalk)
- *Level 3:* Carcinoma invading any part of the stalk
- *Level 4:* Carcinoma invading into the submucosa of the colon wall, below the level of the stalk, but above the muscularis propria

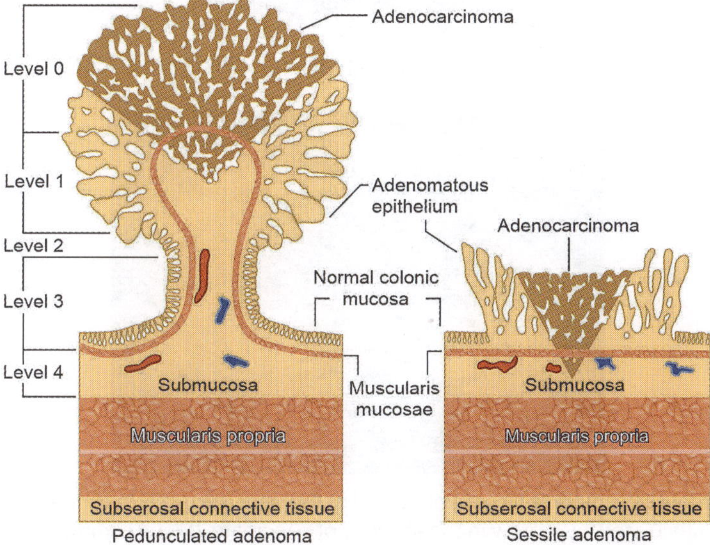


*Source:* Sabiston, 21st edition.

*Haggitt classification:* Anatomic landmarks of pedunculated and sessile adenomas

Recommendations for repeat colonoscopy following endoscopic removal of polyps.

- Small (<10 mm) hyperplastic polyps in rectum or sigmoid 10 years
- *Low risk:* 5–10 years (AGA guidelines) and 10 years (ESGE guidelines)
- One to two small tubular adenomas <10 mm, with low-grade dysplasia
- *High risk:* 3 years

Villous histology or high-grade dysplasia or size ≥10 mm or ≥3 polyps:

- Piecemeal removal of polyp 6 months
- Sessile serrated polyp <10 mm 5 years
- Sessile serrated polyp >10 mm or with dysplasia or traditional serrated adenoma 3 years

**Ans. 7**

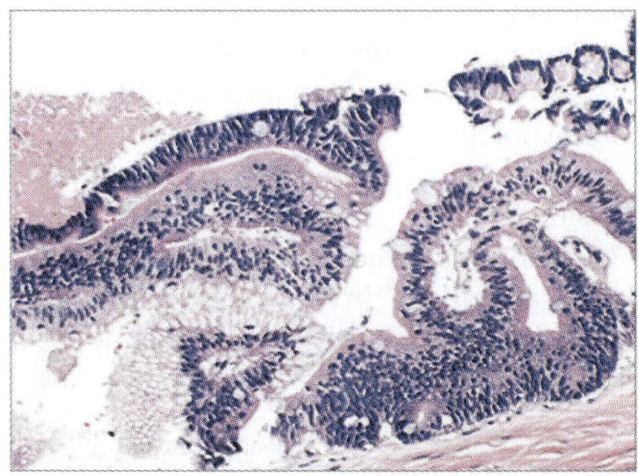

Ovarian-like stroma is a histologic feature often seen in MCNs.

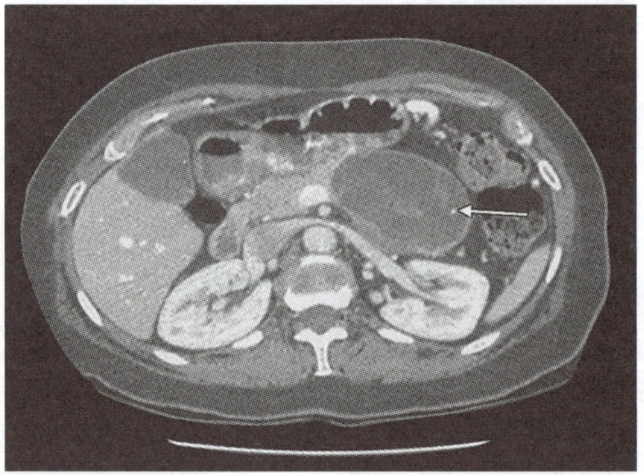

Computed tomography scan of the tail of the pancreas MCN showing a large multiloculated cyst arrow in the absence of pancreatic ductal communication.
*Source:* Sabiston, 21st edition.

**Ans. 8** *Squamous cell cancer:* This is keratin pearl appearance in a squamous cell cancer. Probably a Marjolin's ulcer

**Ans. 9** *Basal cell cancer:*

- The image shows peripheral palisading of nuclei, which is characteristic of basal cell cancer.
- Keratin pearl (onion skin) appearance is typical of squamous cell cancer.

CHAPTER 59

# Instruments

## INSTRUMENTS IMAGES SPOTTERS AND REVISION POINTS

**1.**

Linear stapler

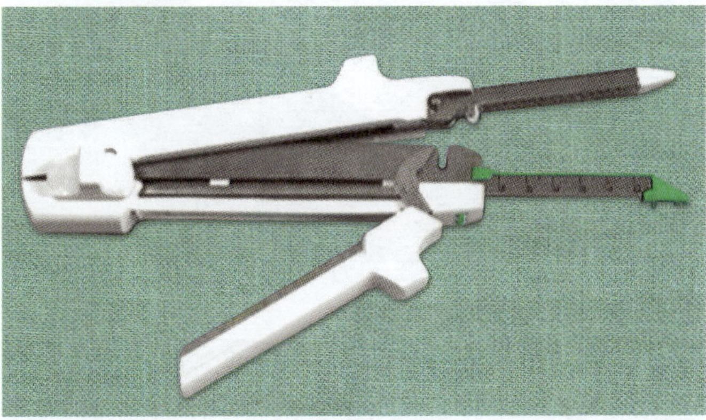

Circular stapler

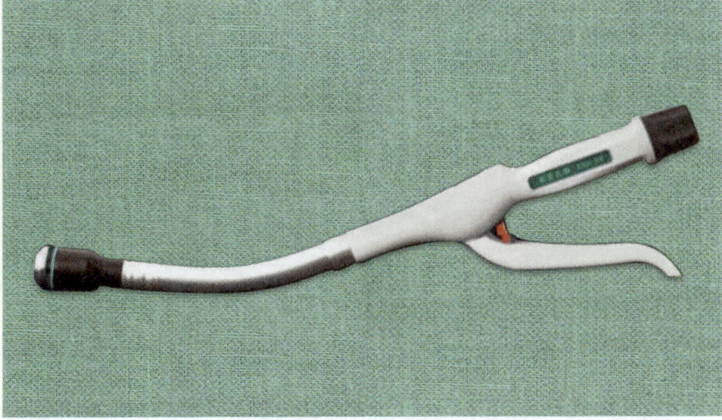

*Staplers:*

- 1st One to use Stapler is - HULTL
- Linear staplers are used for side-to-side anastomosis of bowel as in gastrojejunostomy.

- Circular staplers are used to do end-to-end anastomosis of bowel as in anterior resection, esophagojejunal anastomosis.
- Circular staplers have a separate head (Anvil) which must be introduced into proximal lumen and two ends are anastomosed.
- After stapling integrity of anastomosis is checked by seeing the "doughnut".

**2.**

Corrugated open drain

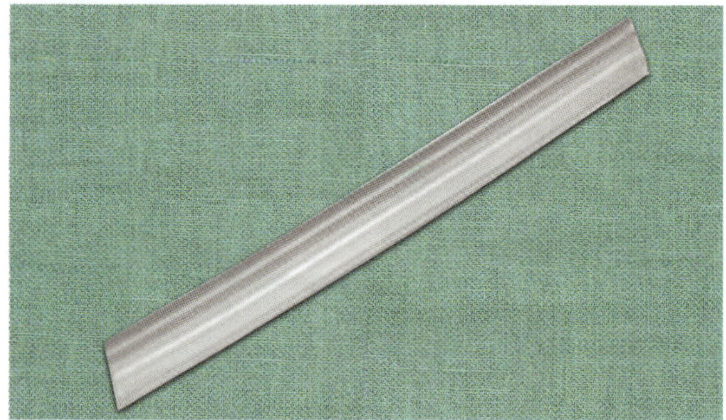

Closed suction drain

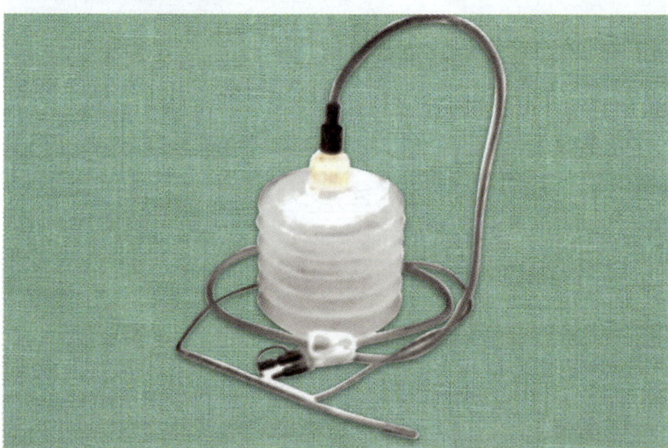

| *Open drains* | *Closed drains* |
|---|---|
| • Include corrugated rubber or plastic drains<br>• Drain fluid collects in a pad or stoma bag<br>• Increased risk of infection seen | • Consists of tubes draining into a bag or bottle<br>• Abdominal drains, ICD drains, suction drains are examples<br>• Infection risk is less |

**3.**

Methods of creating pneumoperitoneum

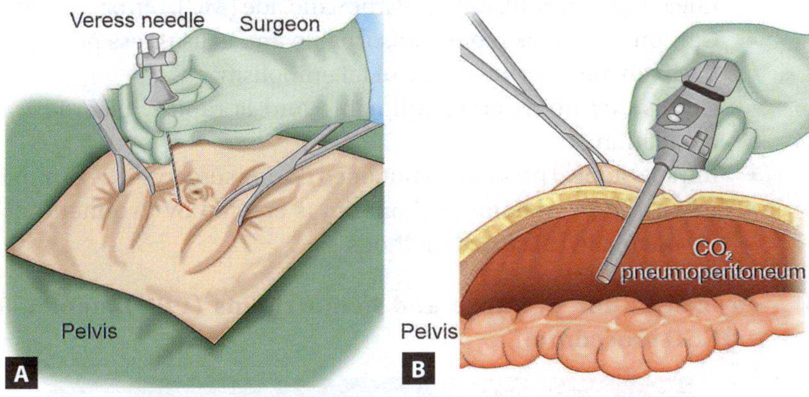


Hasson cannula for open technique

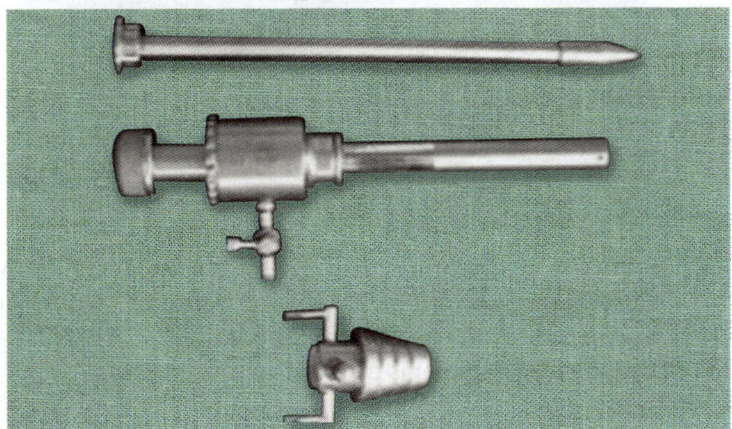

Verres needle for closed method (risk of bowel injury is less as it has safety valve at tip)

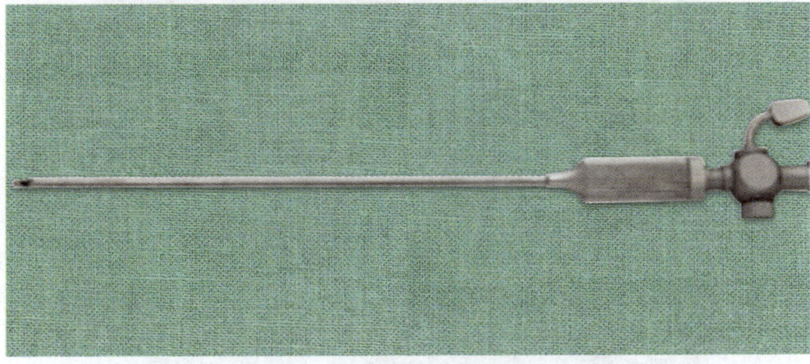

*Laparoscopic surgery*:

- Insufflation of gas in peritoneal cavity and operating via small holes. Gases insufflated are carbon dioxide (MC), nitrogen, and air.
- Carbon dioxide is rapidly absorbable and causes less postoperative pain and less incidence of fat embolism.
- $CO_2$ is 200 times more diffusible and is rapidly cleared from circulation.
- Intraperitoneal pressure maintained during surgery—12–15 mm Hg
- Laparoscopy pneumoperitoneum is created by two methods—(1) open and (2) closed methods.

**4.** **Procedure for prolapse and hemorrhoids (PPH) stapler for LONGO procedure.**

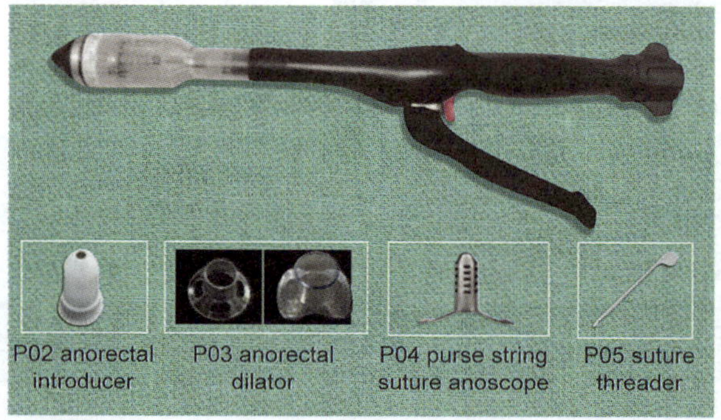


- Minimally invasive proctoscopic hemorrhoidectomy (MIPH) is also known as PPH (LONGO procedure or stapled hemorrhoidopexy).
- Circular cutting stapler is used in this procedure.

**5.**

Hudson brace (NEET SS 2023)

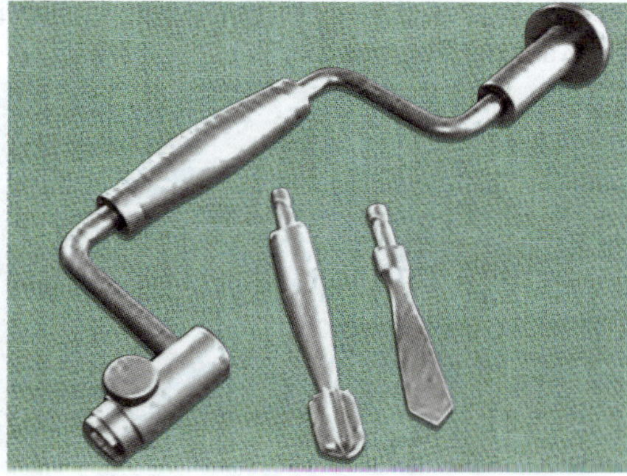

Hudson brace with perforator burr is the bone drills used to drill single or multiple holes in the skull.

**6.**

Lister sinus forceps

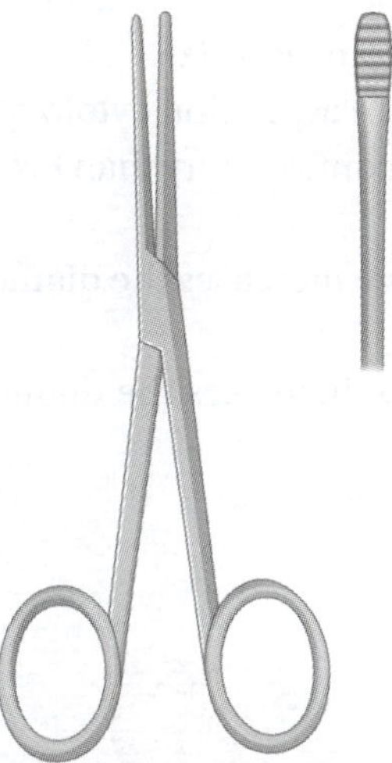

- This is an instrument used in those days for opening the ostia of sinuses in cases of sinusitis. The tip is blunt. The instrument is used by surgeons now to drain abscess.
- This method of drainage of abscess is known as Hilton's method.
- This is used in places with multiple nerves and vessels to avoid injury to them during incision and drainage.
- Specifically used in neck, axilla, and parotid region abscess

**7. Identify the size of this instrument used in taking biopsy from breast.**

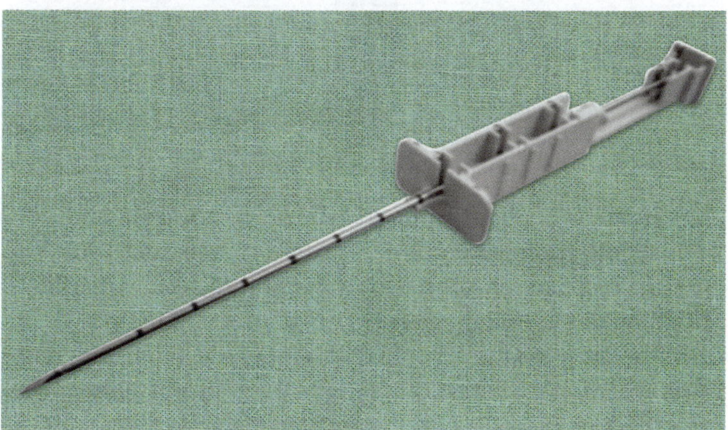

*18-gauge*

- This is tru-cut biopsy needle used to take biopsy from breast.
- Sizes are 18 G and bigger.
- Gauge size number increases the sample taken diameter decreases.
- 22 G is smaller than 18 G size.
- 22 G is fine needle aspiration cytology (FNAC), 18 G is tru-cut.
- Tru-cut is more confirmatory than FNAC and yields more material for study.
- As the French size increases the diameter increases—14 Fr <16 Fr <18 Fr
- As the gauge size increases the diameter decreases—18 G >22 G > 24 G
- 1 French unit = 3 mm size

**8.**

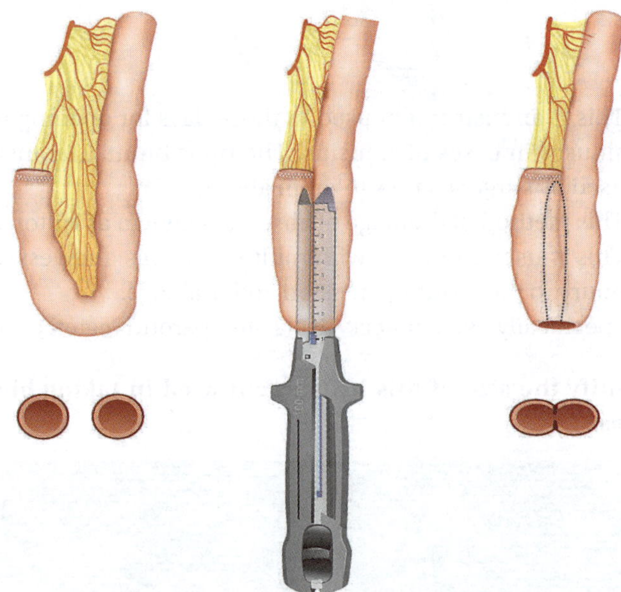

*Source:* Sabiston, 21st edition.

Creation of an ileal J-pouch using a cutting linear stapler. For replacement of the rectum, a reservoir is created from the distal ileum. The stapler joins two limbs of intestine with staples while dividing the intervening wall. The diameter of the pouch is created twice as large as the original diameter of the ileum. The limbs of the J-pouch should be 15 cm in length. Two fires of a linear stapler are required, either a 75- or 100 mm stapler can be used

9.

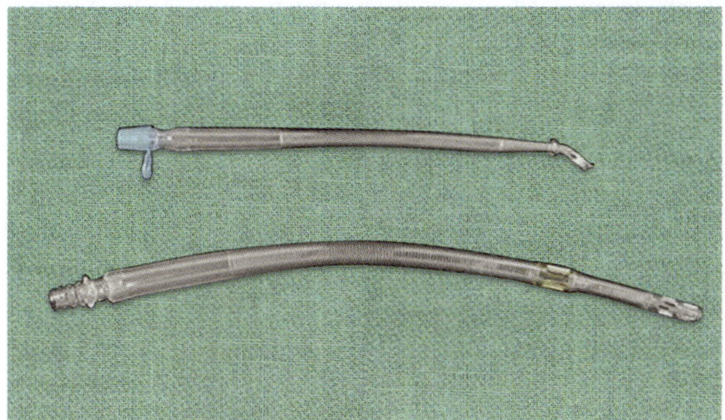

*Source:* Sabiston, 21st edition.

*Aortic cannula (top)*: The specially designed tip is angulated to allow laminar flow of blood into the aortic arch.

*Dual-stage venous cannula (bottom)*: The first stage is the fenestrated basket that usually rests at the level of the hepatic veins and captures all venous return from the inferior vena cava. The second-stage basket is located such that it remains within the right atrium and captures venous return from the superior vena cava, azygos vein, coronary sinus, and direct collateral drainage into the right atrium. The venous drainage is a passive siphon aided by gravity.

10.

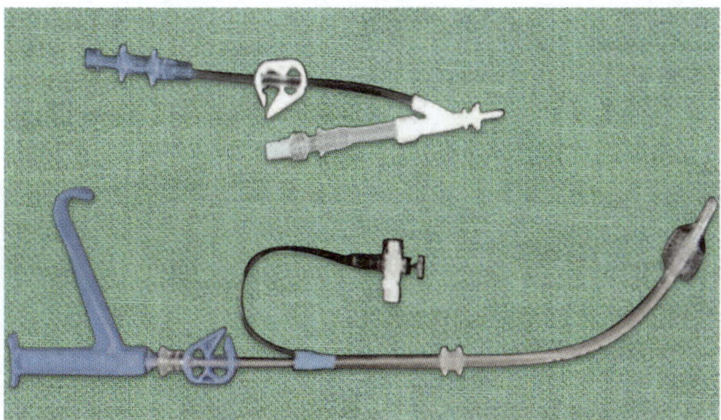

*Source:* Sabiston, 21st edition.

Retrograde cardioplegia cannula (bottom) used to administer cardioplegia solution into the coronary sinus. The self-inflating balloon distends, forming a seal only when cardioplegia solution is administered. Antegrade cardioplegia cannula (top) used to administer cardioplegia solution into the aortic root. The side port functions as a sump.

**11.**

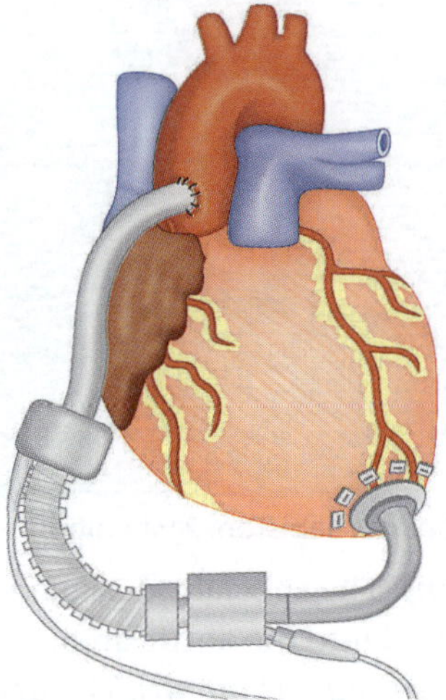

*Source:* Sabiston, 21st edition.

An axial flow left ventricular assist device, which can be used as temporary mechanical support or a bridge to transplantation for a patient in end-stage cardiomyopathy due to coronary artery disease not amenable to bypass surgery. The inflow of blood into the pump is from the apex of the left ventricle. The blood is then pumped into the ascending aorta through specially designed grafts that are incorporated into the pump. The axial flow pumps are less bulky and relatively easy to implant. They have only a single moving part, which is the axial impeller.

**12.**

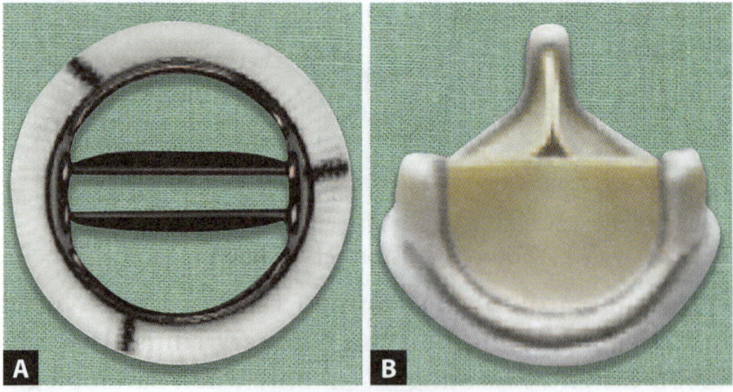


*Source:* Sabiston, 21st edition.

*Prosthetic valves*: Prosthetic heart valves most often implanted are made from (A) synthetic material such as pyrolytic carbon (mechanical valve) or (B) allogeneic biologic tissue such as bovine pericardium (bioprosthetic valve).

**13.**

Hemorrhoid ligator Barron's bander

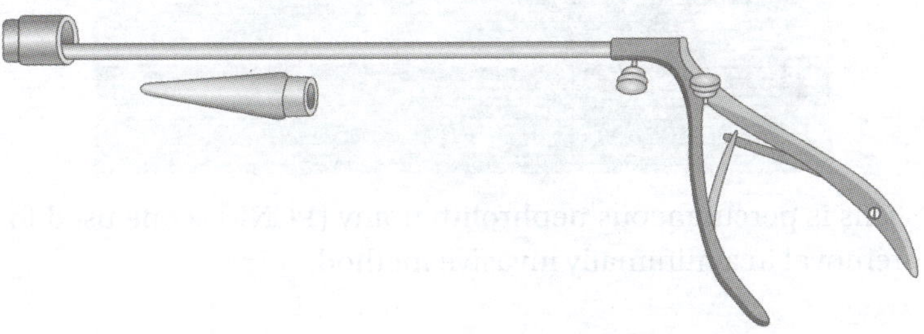

Special hemorrhoid bander for grades 1 and 2 hemorrhoids using rubber band.

**14. Sengstaken–Blakemore tube.**

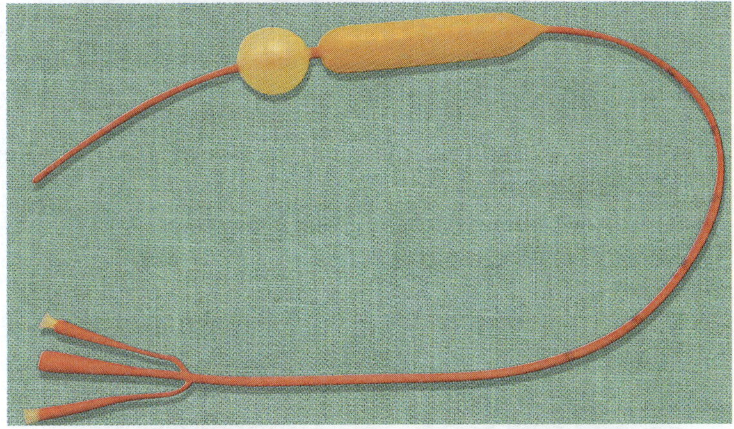

- Modified Sengstaken contains four lumens (old Sengstaken-Blakemore tube contains three tubes)—one for aspiration from stomach, one from esophagus, one for esophageal balloon dilatation, and last one for gastric balloon dilatation.
- The gastric balloon inflated to 250 mL of air and esophageal balloon to a pressure of 40 mm Hg using air
- The potentially lethal complication is accidentally inflating gastric balloon inside the esophagus resulting in perforation of esophagus.
- Balloons should be temporarily deflated after 12 hours to prevent esophageal necrosis.

**15. Identify the use of this instrument.**

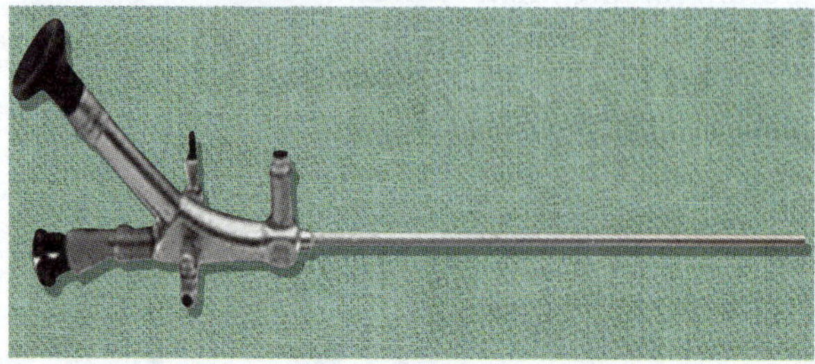

This is percutaneous nephrolithotomy (PCNL) scope used for stone removal in a minimally invasive method.

**16.**

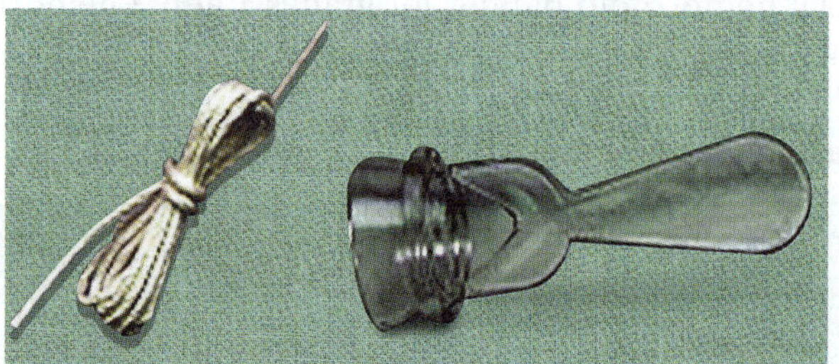

- Plastibell or Hollister device is the device used for sutureless circumcision in infants.
- The device can be safely removed after 7 days.

**17.**

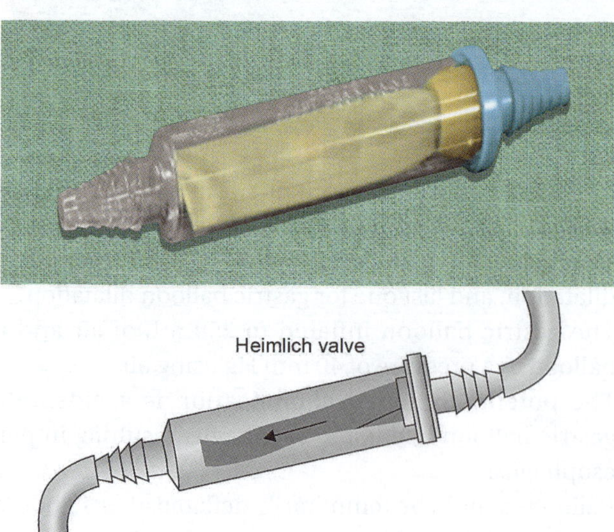

*Heimlich valve*:

- It is a chest drain valve specially designed flutter valve used to replace underwater bottle in chest drainage.
- This valve allows unidirectional flow.
- This will be very helpful in spontaneous pneumothorax, open thoracotomy, and recurrent pleural effusions.

**18. What is the material used in making up these grafts for vascular anastomosis?**

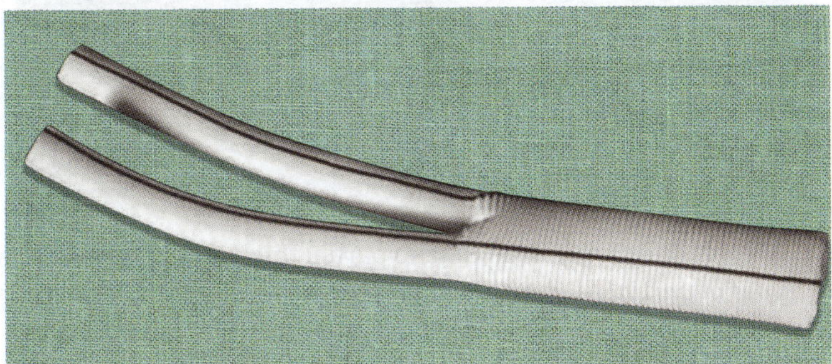

*Dacron*:

- This is a bifurcation graft used to anastomosis aortobifemoral graft.
- Also known as PANT graft

**19.**

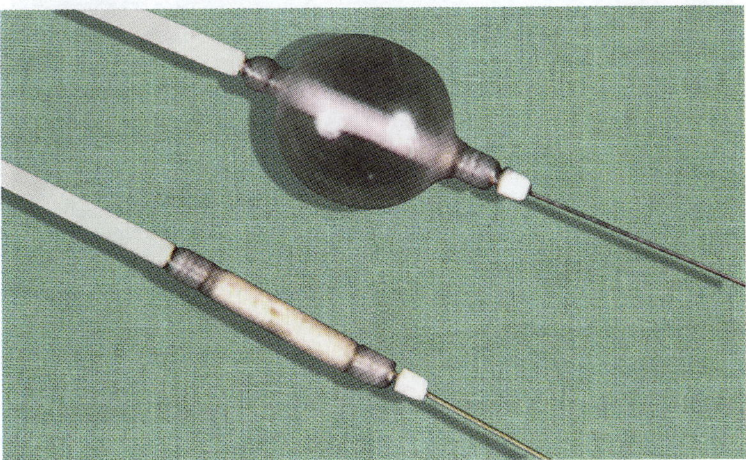

This is known as Fogarty balloon catheter used for percutaneous transluminal angioplasty, stenting and also to remove the emboli.

**20. What is the use of this instrument shown below?**

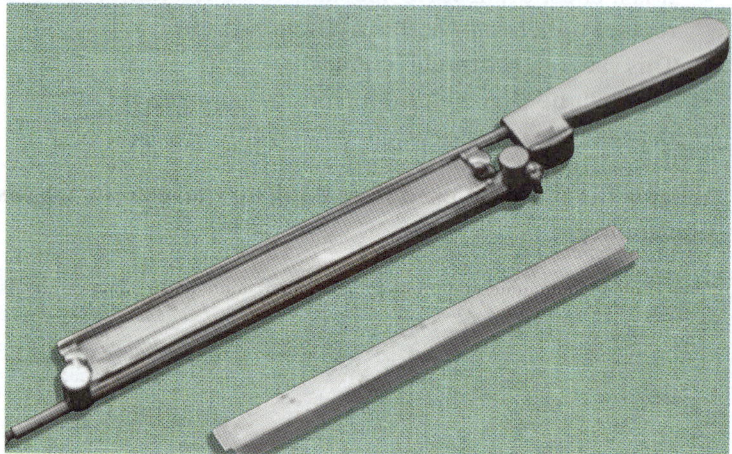

This is humby knife used to take partial thickness grafts.

*Types of partial thickness split grafts:*

- *Thin (Thiersch-Ollier):* 0.006–0.012 inch thickness
- *Intermediate (Blair Brown):* 0.012–0.018 inch thickness
- *Thick (Padgett):* 0.018–0.024 inch thickness

**21. What is the name of the instrument?**

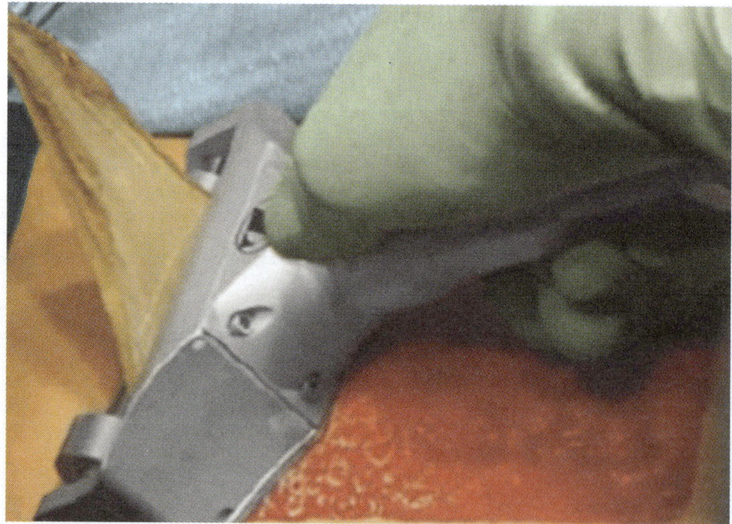

Power dermatome is used to take skin graft.

**22. What is the instrument shown below?**

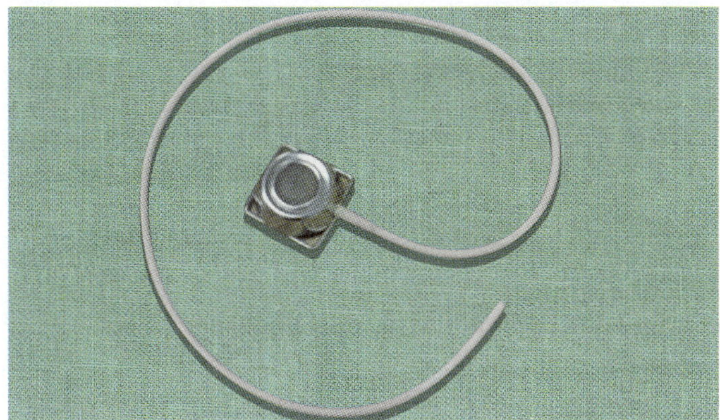

*Chemoport to infuse chemotherapy*:

- It is used to deliver chemotherapy to cancer patients who must undergo treatment frequently.
- Chemotherapy is often toxic, and can damage skin and muscle tissue, and therefore should not be delivered through these tissues.
- Ports provide a solution, delivering drugs quickly, and efficiently through the entire body via the circulatory system.
- Usually chemo port is kept in infraclavicular area.

**23. What is the use of this instrument?**

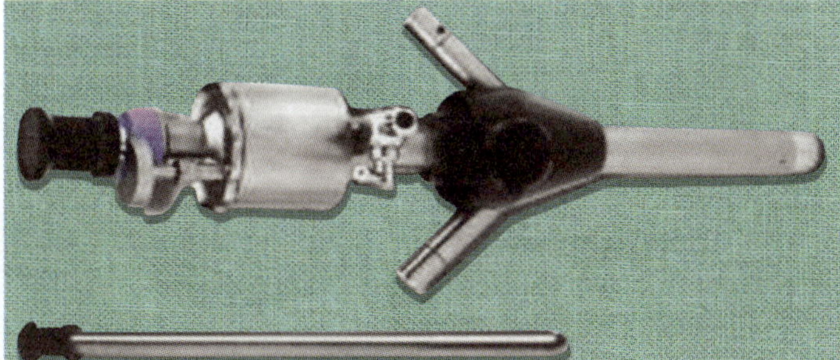

- Hassan cannula used in creating pneumoperitoneum by open method.
- The risk of vascular injury is less with open method but the risk of bowel injury is same or high as compared to closed technique using Veress needle.

**24. What is the name of this catheter?**

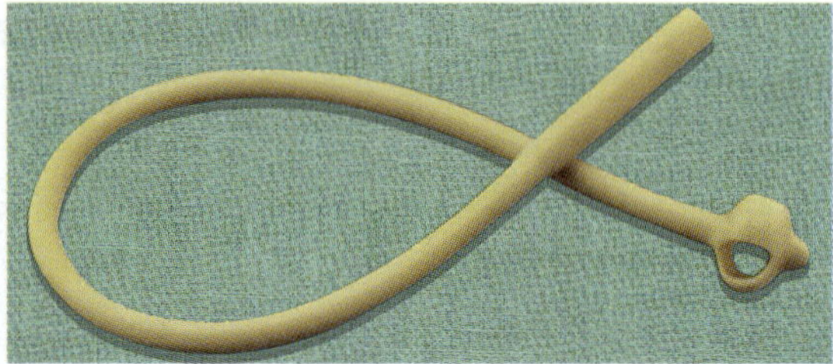

*Malecot's catheter*:

- This is self-retaining Malecot's catheter.
- Used to drain the abscess
- It has capacity to get retained once placed in a cavity.
- It has also been used for feeding purpose.

**25.**

Mayo's venous stripper

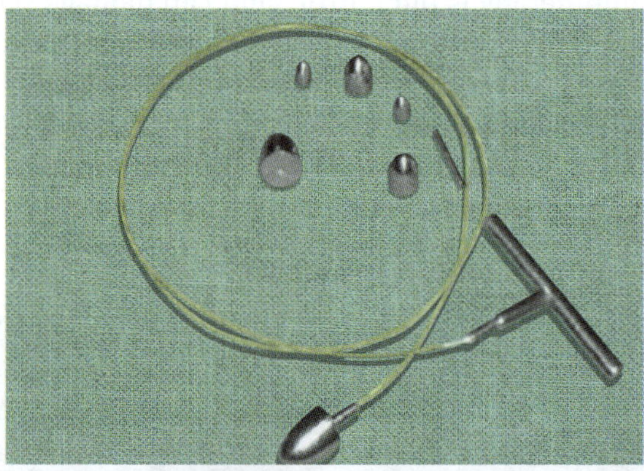

- It is used in stripping of varicose veins.
- The stripping should not be done beyond the midcalf level to prevent injury of saphenous and sural nerves.

**26.**

Gigli saw wire with handle

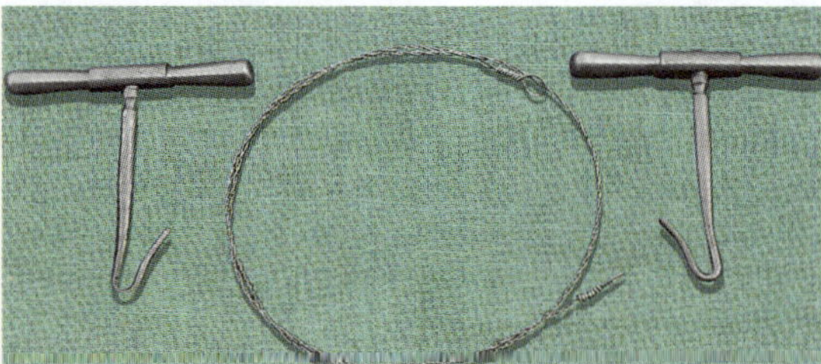

- It is used to cut the bone during below knee or above knee amputations.
- This has to be moved both sides like a saw while cutting. Saline should be poured at the time of cutting.

**27.**

Linear stapler

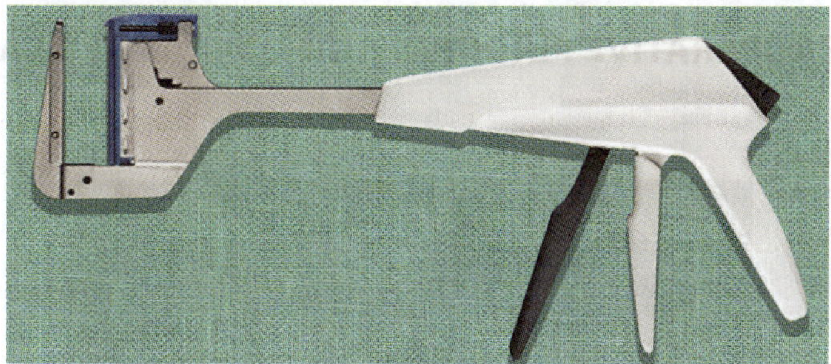

- This is used to insert two rows of evenly spaced staples into the tissues.
- It will not be cutting; it will only staple the tissues.

# 60 CHAPTER Intraoperative Images

## INTRAOPERATIVE FINDINGS AND OPERATIVE IMAGES

**1.**

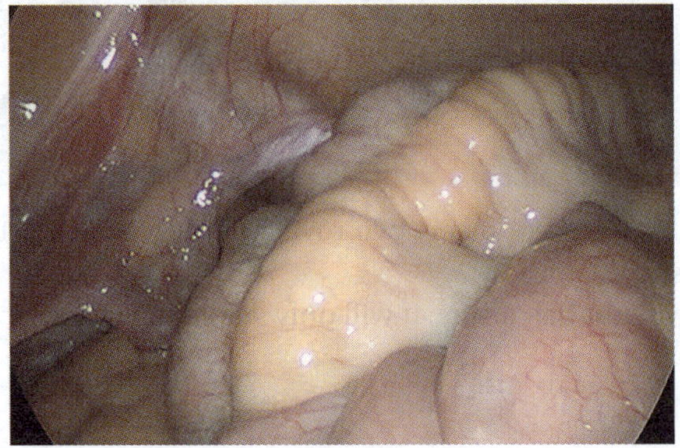

*Source:* Sabiston, 21st edition.

Crohn disease with evidence of creeping fat. Laparoscopic evaluation of extensive fat wrapping caused by the circumferential growth of the mesenteric fat around the bowel wall.

**2.**

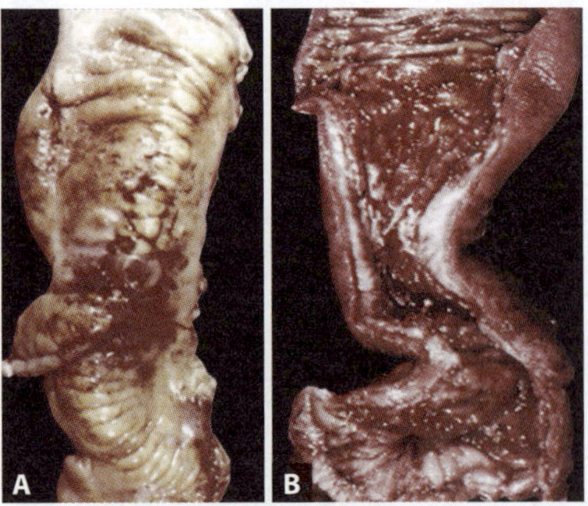


*Source:* Sabiston, 21st edition.

Gross pathologic features of Crohn disease.

(A) Serosal surface demonstrates extensive fat wrapping and inflammation. (B) Resected specimen demonstrates marked fibrosis of the intestinal wall, stricture, and segmental mucosal inflammation.

**3.**

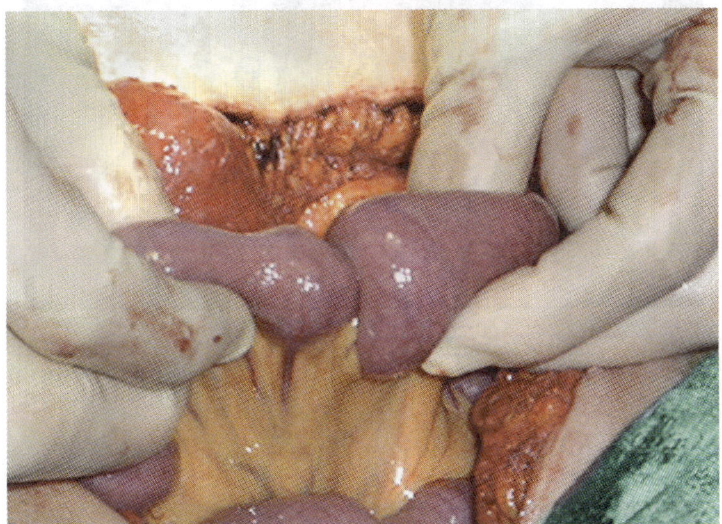

*Source:* Sabiston, 21st edition.

Jejunojenunal intussusception in an adult patient.

**4.**

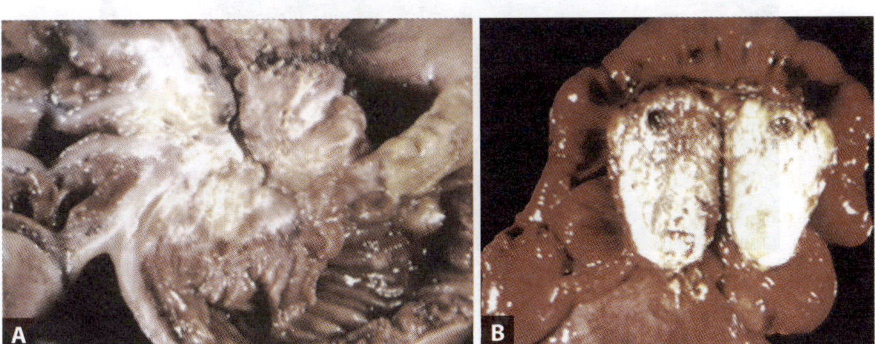


*Source:* Sabiston, 21st edition.

Gross pathologic characteristics of neuroendocrine tumor (NET). (A) NET of the distal ileum demonstrates the intense desmoplastic reaction and fibrosis of the bowel wall. (B) Mesenteric metastases from a NET of the small bowel.

**5.**

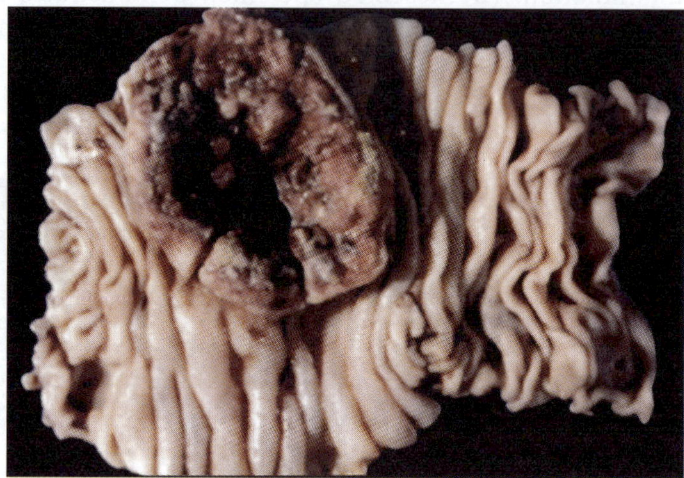

*Source:* Sabiston, 21st edition.

Lymphoma of the small intestine. Small bowel lymphoma is manifested as perforation and peritonitis.

**6.**

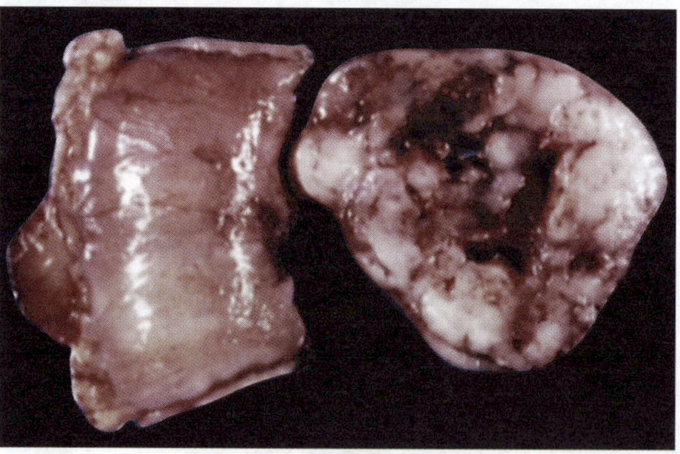

*Source:* Sabiston, 21st edition.

Small intestine gastrointestinal stroma tumor (GIST). Small bowel GIST with hemorrhagic necrosis.

**7.**

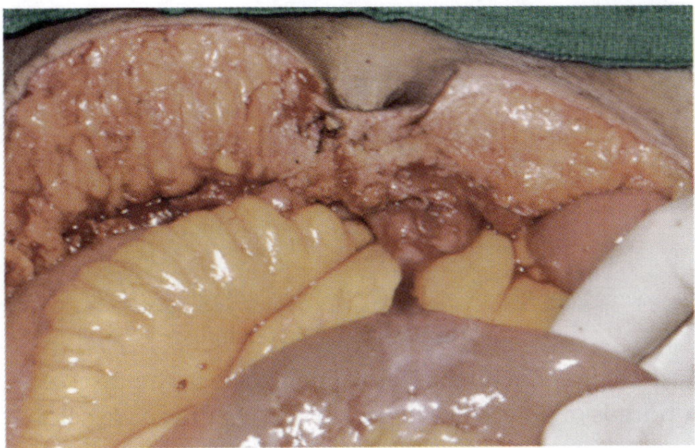

*Source:* Sabiston, 21st edition.

Persistent omphalomesenteric remnant. Omphalomesenteric remnant persisting as a fibrous cord from the ileum to the umbilicus.

**8.**

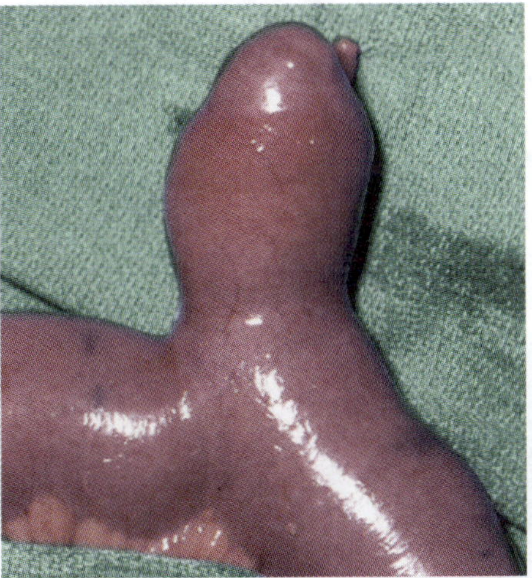

*Source:* Sabiston, 21st edition.

*Meckel diverticulum:* Common presentation of a Meckel diverticulum projecting from the antimesenteric border of the ileum.

**9.**

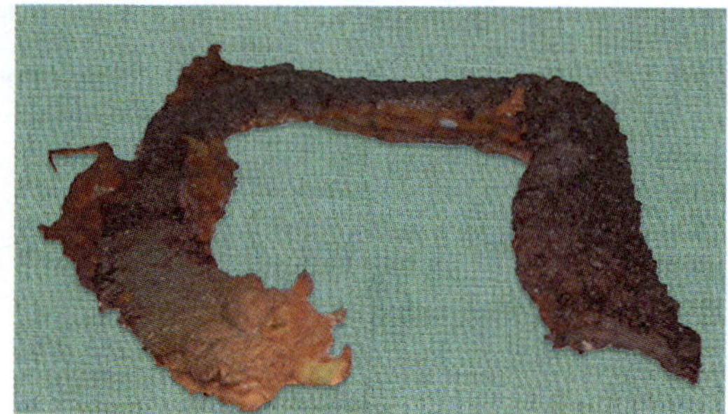

*Source:* Sabiston, 21st edition.

Classical familial adenomatous polyposis in the resected specimen. Hundreds of polyps are well visible along the entire colon.

**10.**

The Spigelman classification is used to grade the severity of and guide the clinical management of duodenal polyposis.

*Criteria:*

| | ***Points*** | | |
|---|---|---|---|
| | ***1*** | ***2*** | ***3*** |
| Polyp number | 1 | 2 | 3 |
| Polyp size (mm) | 1–4 | 5–20 | >20 |
| Histology | Tubular | Tubulovillous | Villous |
| Dysplasia | Mild | Moderate | Severe |

**11.**

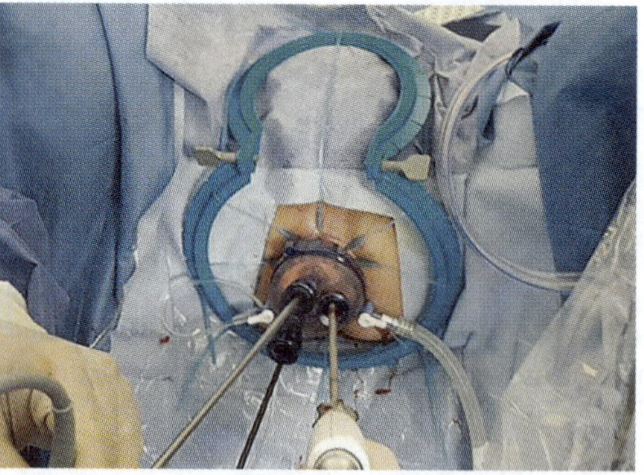

*Source:* Sabiston, 21st edition.

Transanal total mesorectal excision (TME). Transanal laparoscopy for the dissection of the rectum from below.

12.

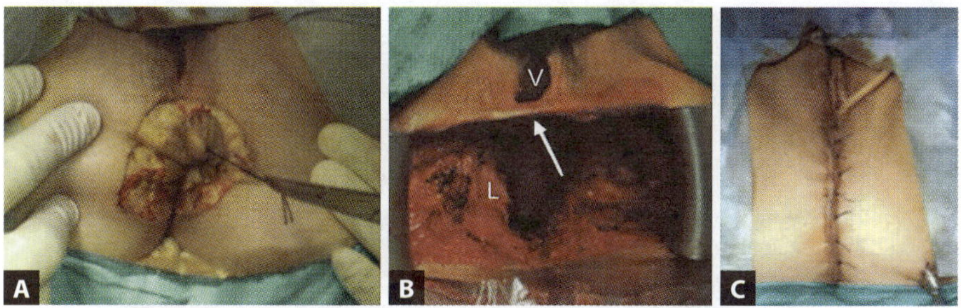


*Source:* Sabiston, 21st edition.

(A) *Perineal incision in miles procedure:* A purse-string suture is placed around the anal canal and the entire anal sphincter excised. (B) Photo of operative field after specimen has been removed. Perineal incision shows large defect in the pelvis (white arrow denotes posterior vaginal wall) (L: levator; V: vagina). (C) Perineal incision following skin closure following miles procedure.

13.

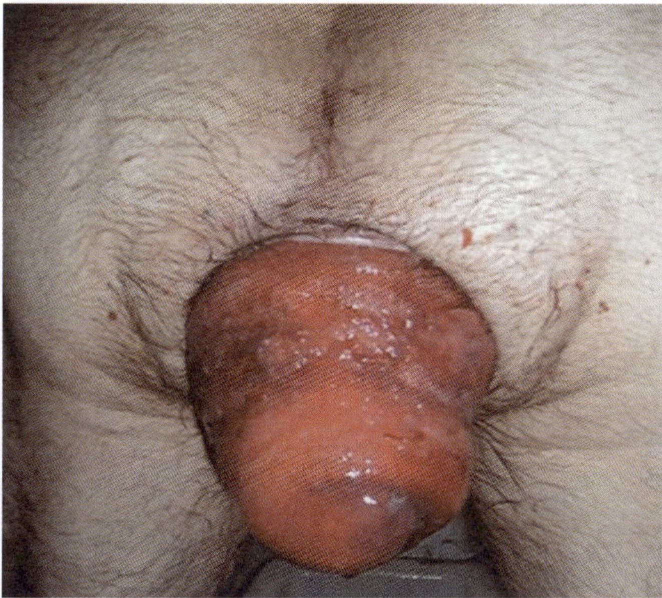

*Source:* Sabiston, 21st edition.

A patient with a huge external rectal prolapse.

**14.**

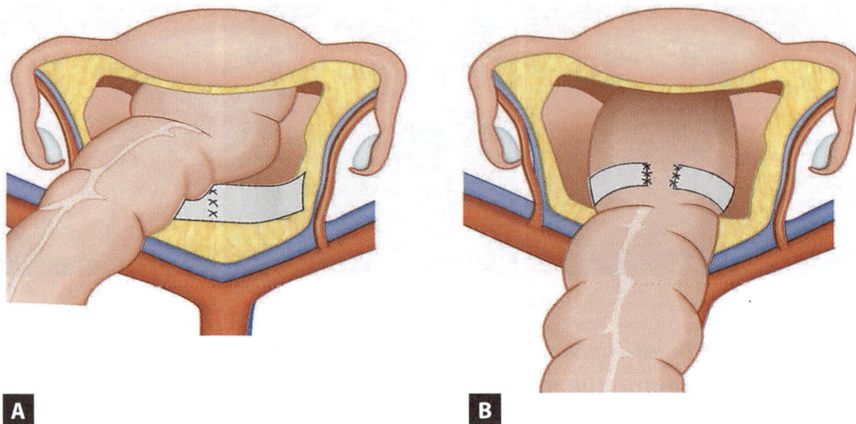

Source: Sabiston, 21st edition.

The posterior mesh rectopexy (modified Ripstein operation). (A) The rectum is mobilized and the mesh is fixed to the presacral fascia. (B) The mesh is fixed to both sides of the rectum.

**15.**

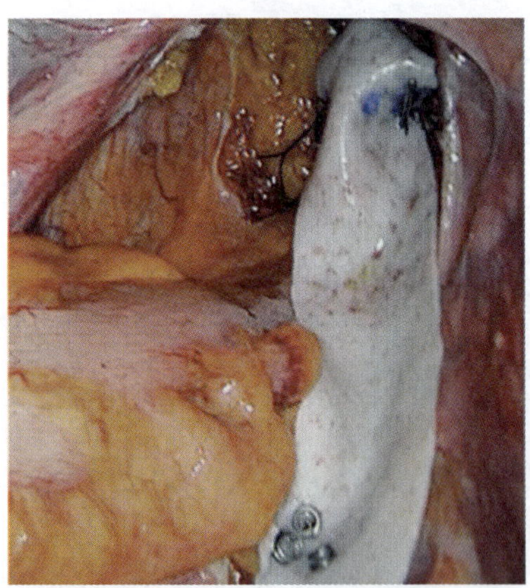

Source: Sabiston, 21st edition.

Ventral mesh rectopexy. The mesh is attached to the anterior rectal wall and the sacral promontory.

16.

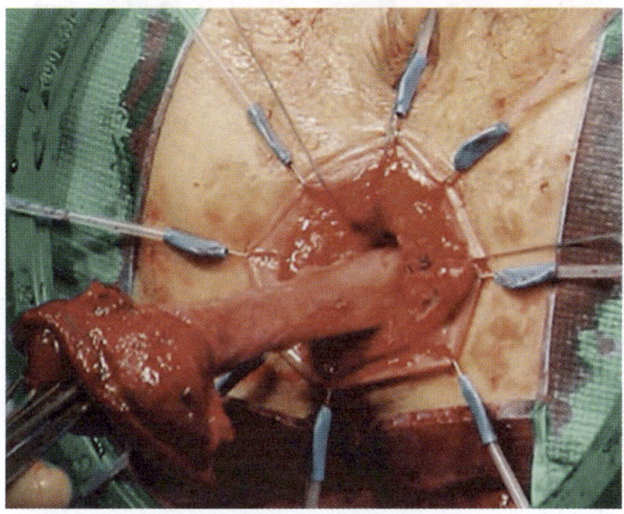

*Source:* Sabiston, 21st edition.

The Altemeier procedure or perineal proctectomy. The redundant rectosigmoid colon is resected through a transperineal approach and a hand-sewn coloanal anastomosis is performed.

17.

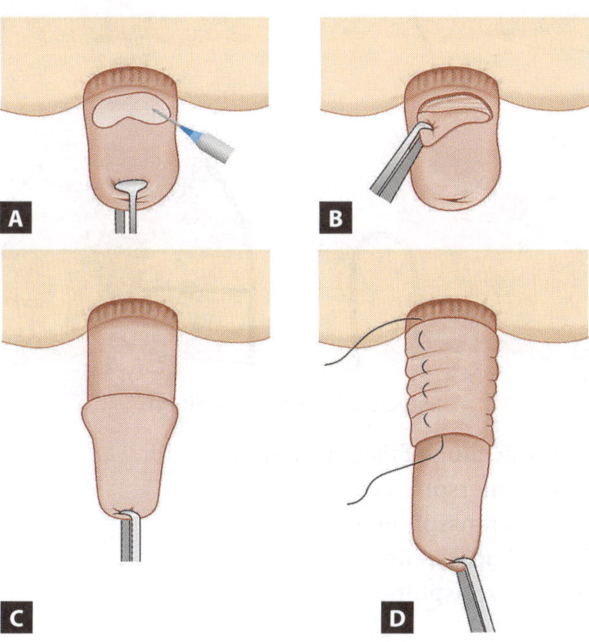


*Source:* Sabiston, 21st edition.

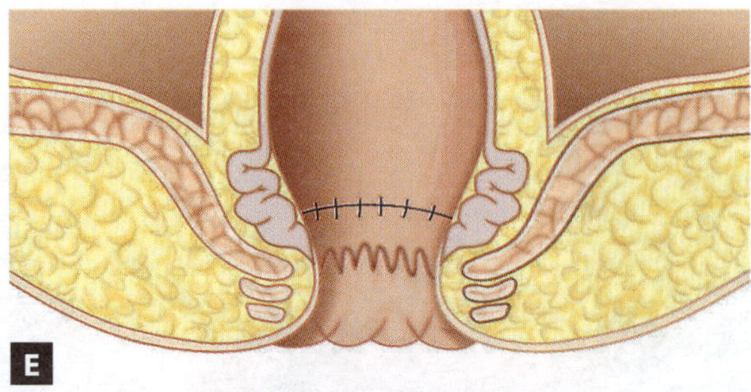


*Source:* Sabiston, 21st edition.

*The Delorme procedure:* The mucosal layer is infiltrated with epinephrine containing solution (A), incised (B), and stripped off the underlying muscularis (C). Plication of the muscularis propria is performed (D). The operation concludes with an anastomosis between the proximal and distal mucosal edges (E).

**18.**

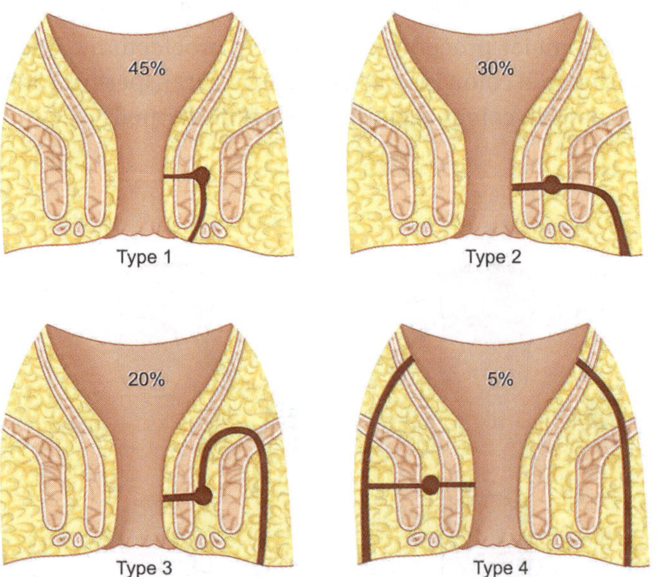


*Source:* Sabiston, 21st edition.

Park classification of fistula-in-ano:
- *Type 1:* Intersphincteric
- *Type 2:* Transsphincteric
- *Type 3:* Suprasphincteric
- *Type 4:* Extrasphincteric

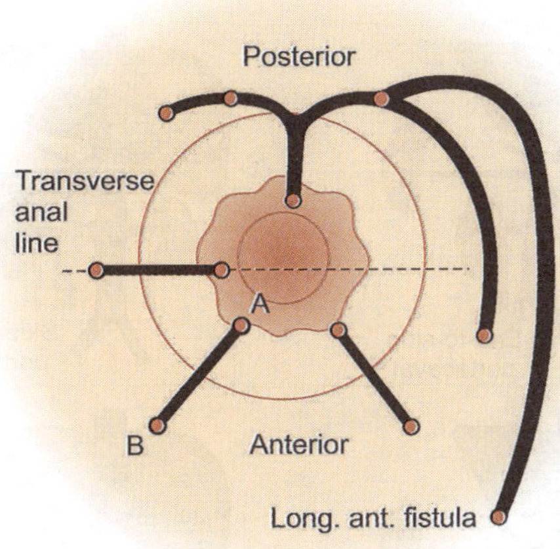


*Source:* Sabiston, 21st edition.

Goodsall rule of fistula-in-ano tracks extension

## 19. Pilonidal sinus.

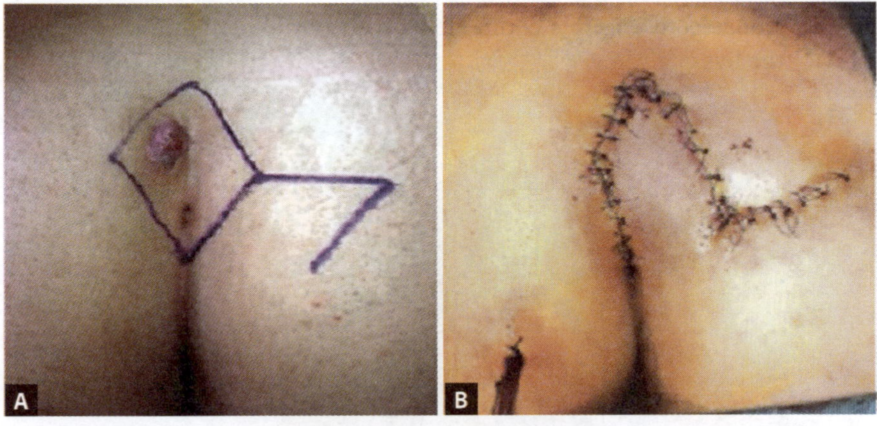


*Source:* Sabiston, 21st edition.

*Limberg flap:* (A) Initial marking of a proposed incision. (B) Completed rotation of the flap.

**20.**

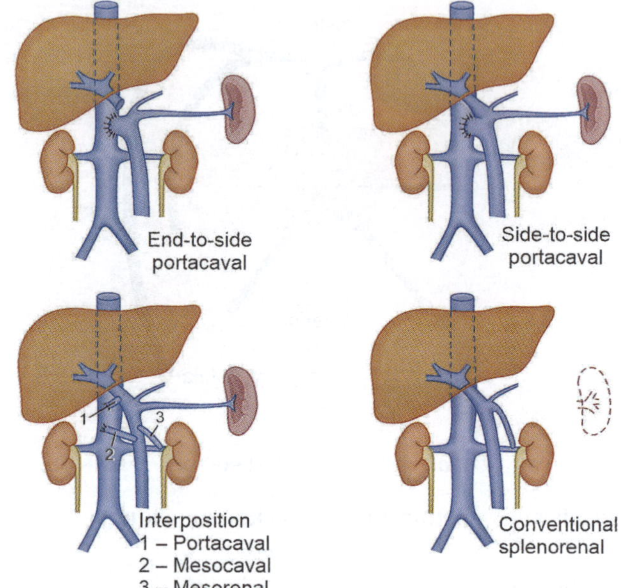


*Source:* Sabiston, 21st edition.

Nonselective shunts completely divert portal blood flow away from the liver.

**21.**

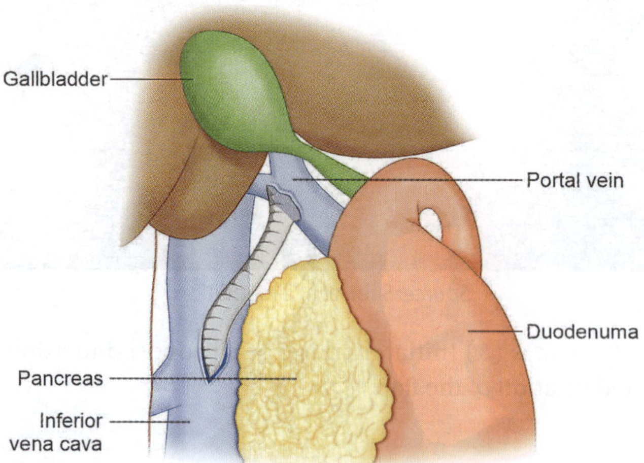


*Source:* Sabiston, 21st edition.

A small-diameter (8–10 mm) interposition portacaval shunt partially decompresses the portal venous system and may preserve hepatic portal perfusion.

**22.**

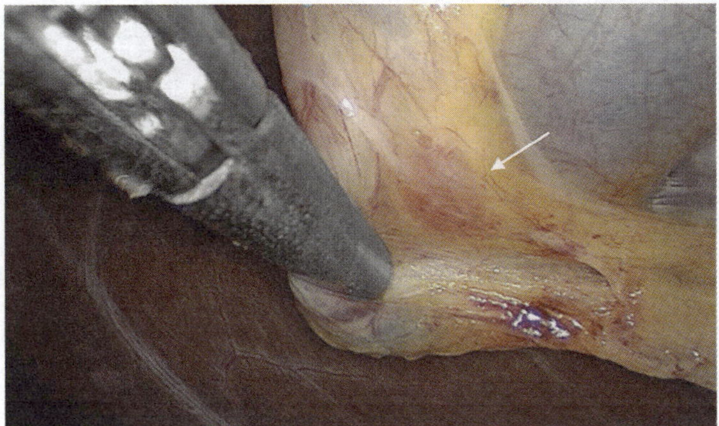

*Source:* Sabiston, 21st edition.

Operative photograph of Calot node. This node (arrow) is useful for identification of the common location of the cystic artery.

**23.**

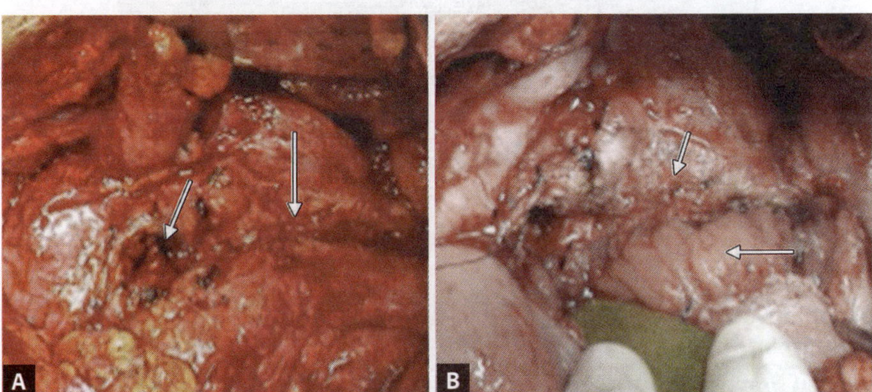


*Source:* Sabiston, 21st edition.

Frey procedure, intraoperative photographs. (A) Significant dilation of the main pancreatic duct at the level of the head (short arrow) and body of the pancreas (long arrow) after the anterior surface of the pancreas has been opened. (B) Side-to-side anastomosis between the pancreatic duct (short arrow) and jejunum (long arrow).

**24.**

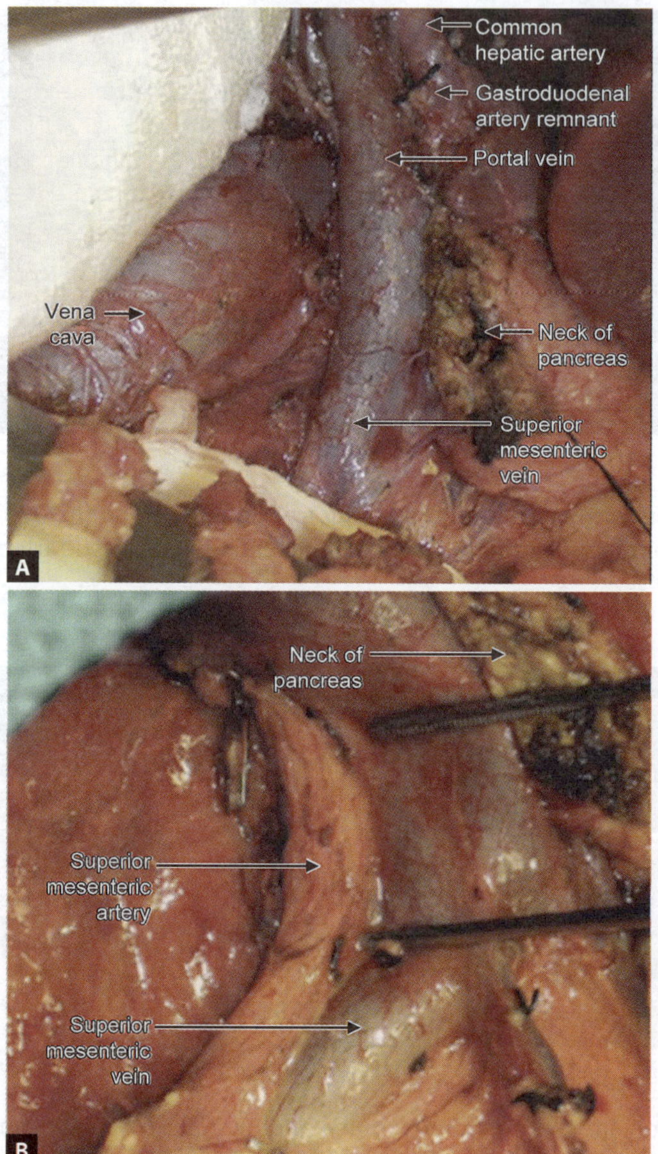


*Source:* Sabiston, 21st edition.

(A) Surgical anatomy after pancreaticoduodenectomy. The superior mesenteric vein (SMV), portal vein, hepatic artery, and vena cava are visualized. Complete lymphatic clearance is noted. (B) Superior mesenteric artery (SMA) dissection illustrating complete clearance of periarterial lymphatic tissue.

**25.**

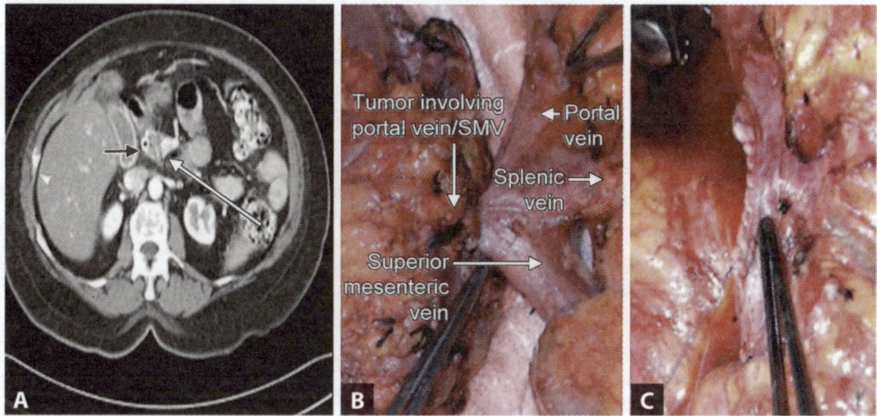


*Source:* Sabiston, 21st edition.

(A) Computed tomography (CT) scan showing pancreatic ductal adenocarcinoma (PDAC) of the pancreatic head with involvement of portal vein–SMV confluence (large arrow). A metal biliary stent is in place (small arrow). (B) Operative image demonstrating tumor involvement of the lateral aspect of the portal vein–SMV confluence. (C) Primary closure of portal vein–SMV confluence after tumor removal with lateral vein resection.

**26.**

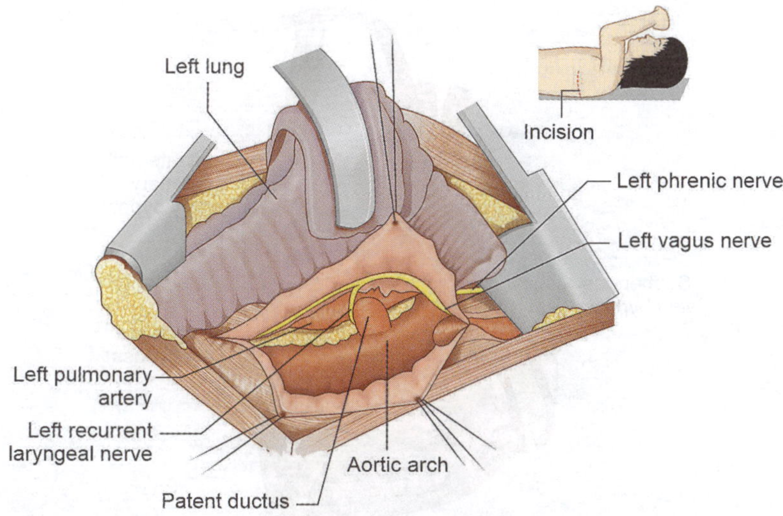


*Source:* Sabiston, 21st edition.

Anatomic relationships of a patent ductus arteriosus exposed from a left thoracotomy [INISS 2023/NEET SS 2022].

**27.**

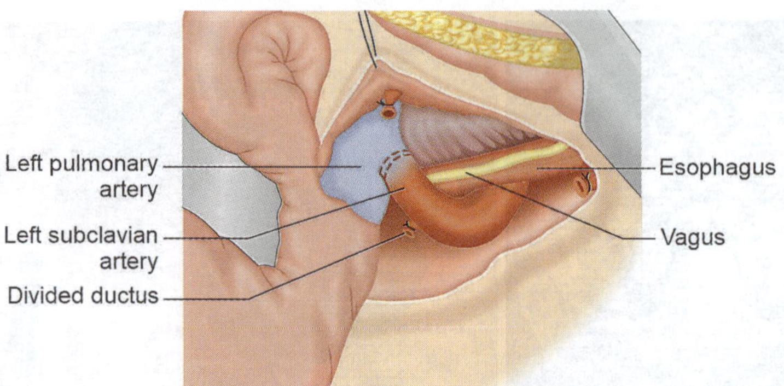


*Source:* Sabiston, 21st edition.

Blalock–Taussig shunt (a: artery).

A connection is made between the first artery that branches off the aorta (called the right subclavian artery) and the right pulmonary artery. Some of the blood traveling through the aorta toward the body will "shunt" through this connection and flow into the pulmonary artery to receive oxygen. However, the child will still have some degree of cyanosis since oxygen-poor (blue) blood from the right atrium and oxygen-rich (red) blood from the left side of the heart mix and flow through the aorta to the body.

**28.**

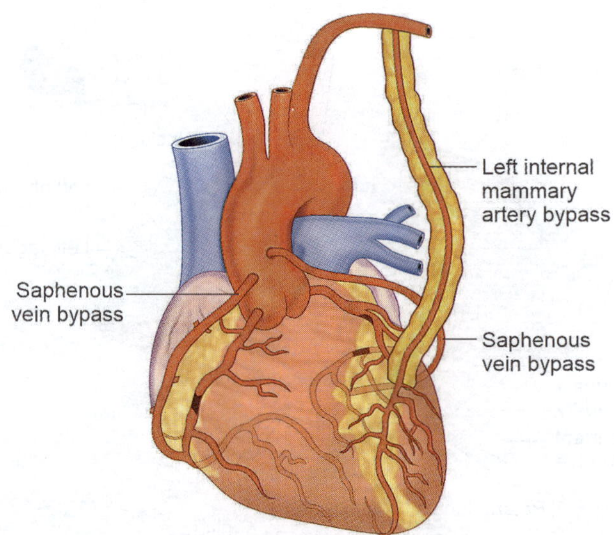


*Source:* Sabiston, 21st edition.

Typical configuration for a three-vessel coronary artery bypass. The left internal mammary artery is anastomosed to the left anterior descending artery. Aortocoronary bypasses are created with reversed saphenous vein to the distal right coronary artery and an obtuse marginal branch of the circumflex coronary artery. The circumflex coronary artery is usually avoided as a target for bypass because its location well inside the atrioventricular groove makes it difficult to visualize.

**29.**

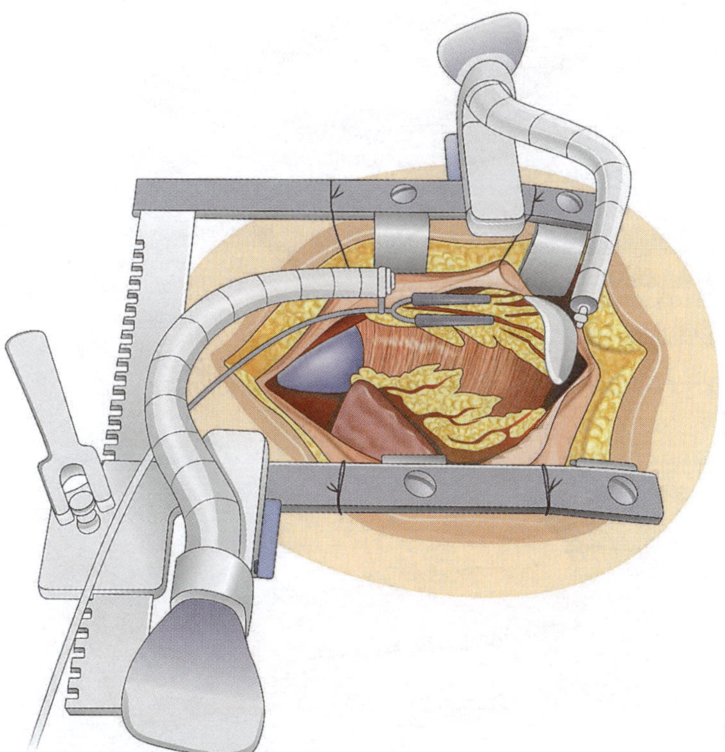

*Source:* Sabiston, 21st edition.

Off-pump coronary artery bypass with vacuum-assisted multi-articulating arms to position and to stabilize the myocardium. This minimizes the movement of the heart, allowing the surgeon to feasibly perform the distal anastomoses. Here, the stabilizer is positioned in preparation for creating a bypass to the left anterior descending artery.

## 30. Lymphedema treatment.

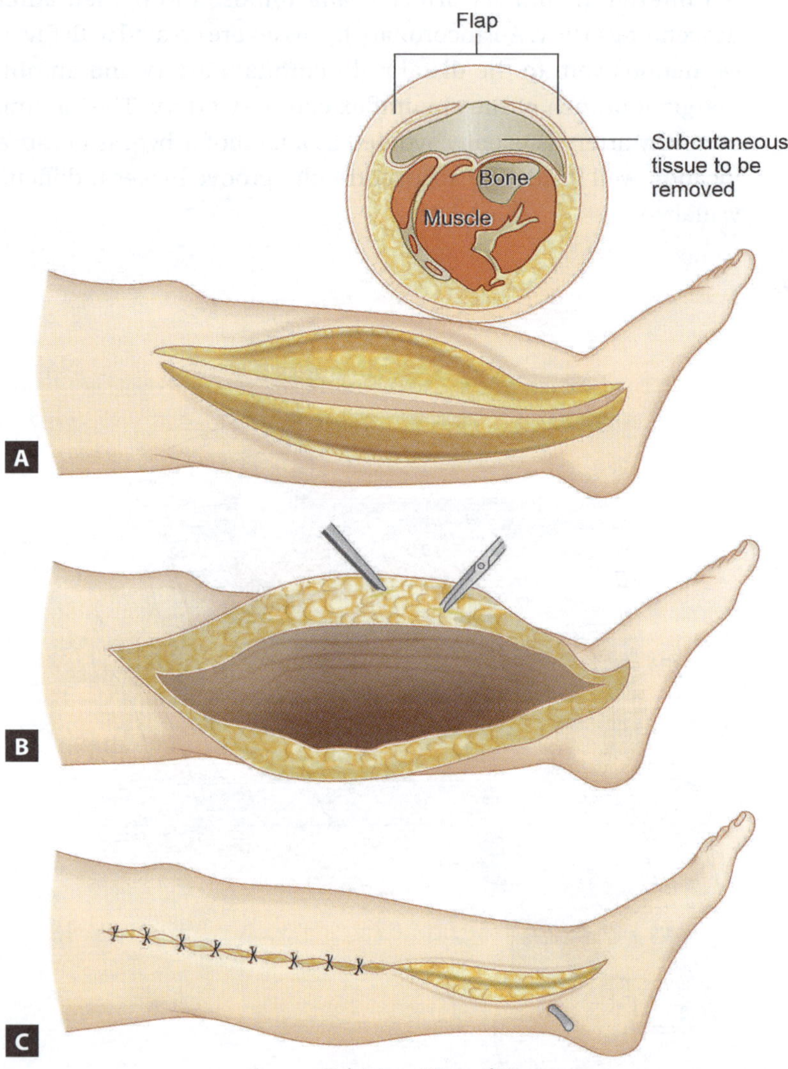


*Source:* Sabiston, 21st edition.

(A to C) Schematic representation of the Kontoleon or Homan procedure. Relatively thick skin flaps are raised anteriorly and posteriorly, and all subcutaneous tissue beneath the flaps and the underlying medial calf deep fascia are removed along with the necessary redundant skin.

**31. Lymphedema treatment.**

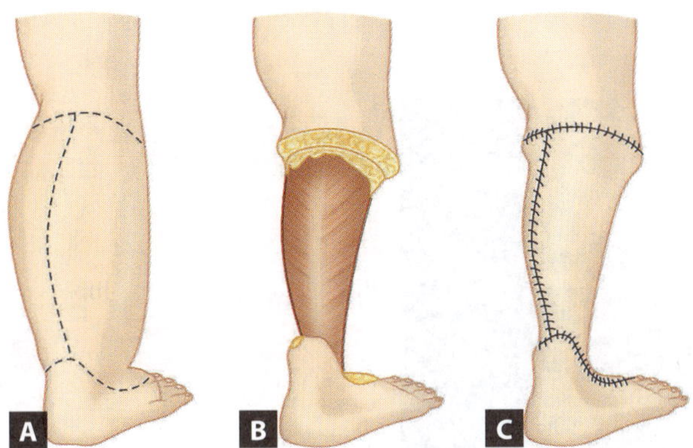


*Source:* Sabiston, 21st edition.

(A to C) Schematic representation of the Charles procedure. It involves complete and circumferential excision of the skin, subcutaneous tissue, and deep fascia of the involved leg and dorsum of the foot. Coverage is provided preferably by full-thickness grafting from the excised skin.

**32.**

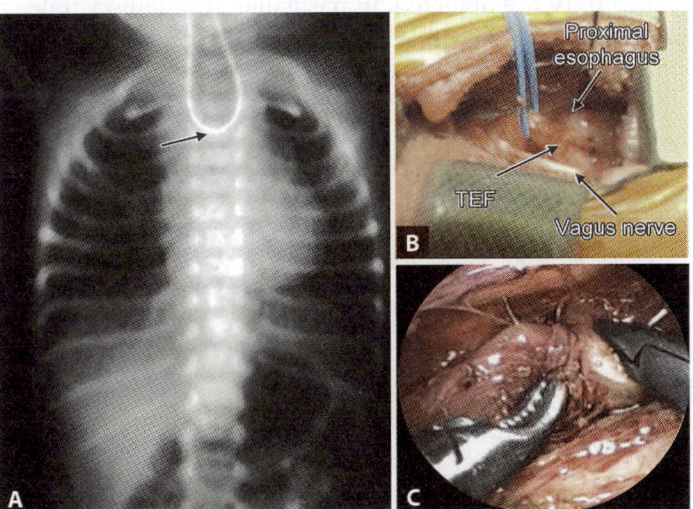


*Source:* Sabiston, 21st edition.

(A) Plain chest radiograph of an infant with proximal esophageal atresia and distal tracheoesophageal fistula (TEF). The distal tip of the orogastric tube is curled up at the level of thoracic inlet (arrow). (B) Distal TEF (arrow) encircled with a blue vessel loop. The proximal blind esophageal pouch is in close proximity (arrow).

(C) Thoracoscopic esophageal anastomosis. Interrupted sutures are placed using intracorporeal technique.

**33.**

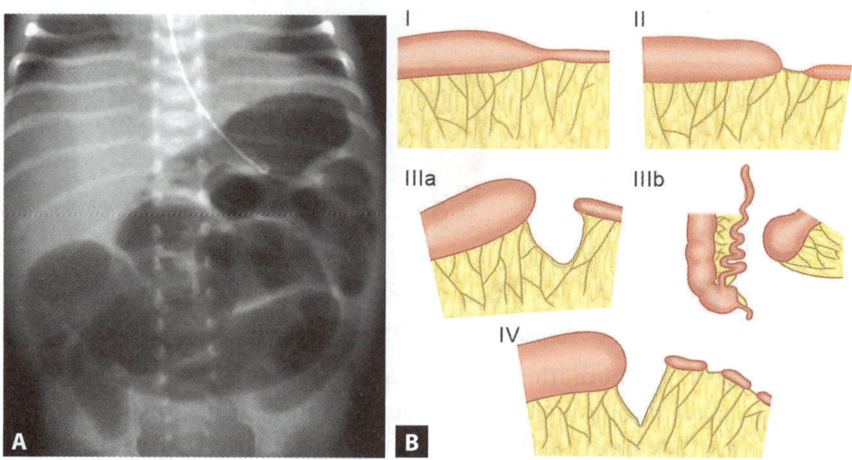


*Source:* Sabiston, 21st edition.

(A) Plain abdominal radiograph shows multiple dilated bowel loops indicating congenital bowel obstruction. (B) Jejunoileal atresia types I to IV are depicted. In particular, IIIb demonstrates an apple peel type of atresia with a large mesenteric gap.

**34.**

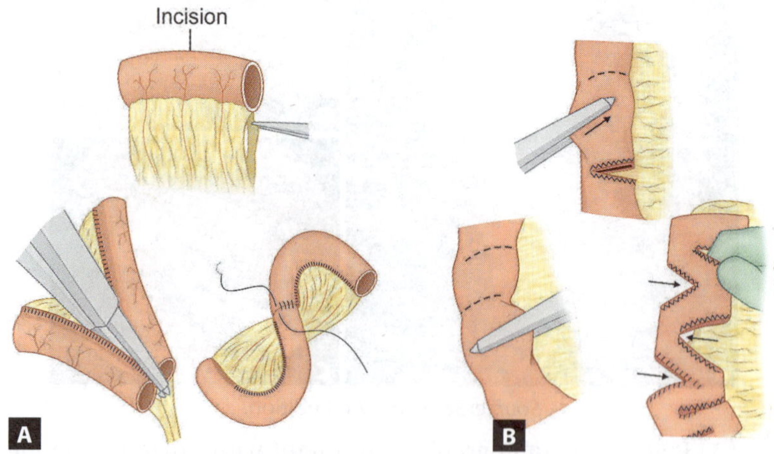


*Source:* Sabiston, 21st edition.

*Bowel-lengthening procedures:* (A) Bianchi technique separates two mesenteric planes. A dilated segment of bowel is stapled longitudinally to create two narrower segments for sequential anastomosis.

(B) Serial transverse enteroplasty (STEP) involves stapling a dilated bowel into V shapes on alternating sides, decreasing width and increasing length.

**35.**

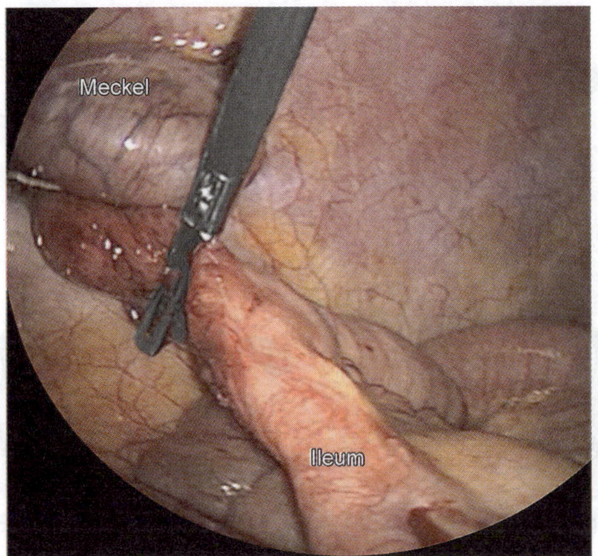


*Source:* Sabiston, 21st edition.

Meckel diverticulectomy performed using an endoscopic stapling device via laparoscopic approach.

Meckel diverticulum is the most common congenital anomaly of the GI tract and occurs in approximately 2% of the population. >70% of symptomatic patients have heterotopic gastric mucosa and another 5% have pancreatic tissue. The rule of 2's is often cited in association with Meckel diverticulum. Aside from its 2% incidence and two types of heterotopic mucosa, it is located within 2 feet of the ileocecal valve, is approximately 2 inches in length, and usually symptomatic by 2 years of age. Meckel diverticulum is caused by a failure of normal regression of the vitelline duct that occurs during weeks 5–7 of gestation. Meckel diverticulum is a true diverticulum containing all intestinal layers.

Bleeding from a Meckel diverticulum may be confirmed by a 99mTc-pertechnetate isotope scan, which detects gastric mucosa.

Segmental ileal resection at the base of the Meckel diverticulum, especially in the case of inflammation or ulceration, with primary end-to-end anastomosis is the gold standard.

Management of incidentally found Meckel diverticulum at the time of laparotomy for unrelated other GI condition has been somewhat controversial, asymptomatic Meckel diverticulum should be left alone.

**36.**

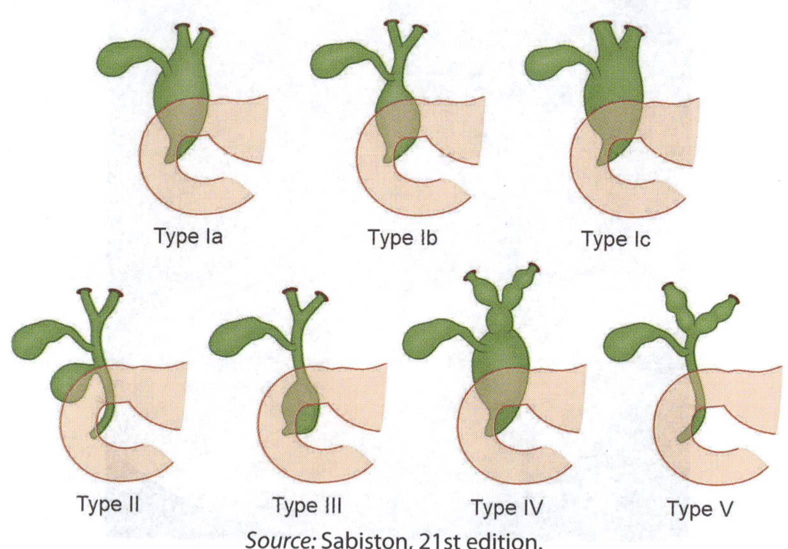


*Source:* Sabiston, 21st edition.

Classification of choledochal cyst.

**37.**

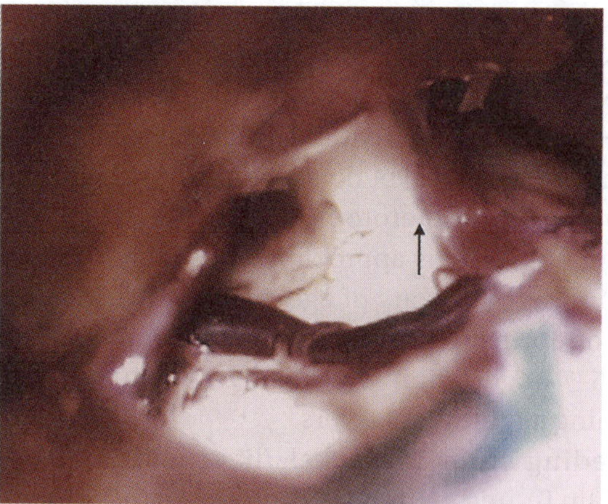

*Source:* Sabiston, 21st edition.

Intraoperative photograph of a patient with typical trigeminal neuralgia. The left trigeminal nerve is compressed superiorly by an arterial branch of the superior cerebellar artery (arrow).

Trigeminal neuralgia is characterized by brief episodes of severe, lancinating pain in one or more of the three divisions of the trigeminal nerve, usually V2 and V3. Patients often describe that it is precipitated by touch or extremes of temperature.

MRI is used to rule out posterior fossa tumors and multiple sclerosis, which can present with related symptoms.

Most patients respond to the oral administration of carbamazepine. Baclofen and gabapentin also have some clinical usefulness in medical treatment.

The most common mechanism is presumed to be related to vascular compression of the fifth cranial nerve as it enters the brainstem.

Microvascular decompression involves a small suboccipital craniotomy for microsurgical exploration of the dorsal root entry zone of the trigeminal nerve on the affected side. The offending vessel, usually the superior cerebellar artery, is then dissected off the nerve, and a barrier (Teflon or polyvinyl alcohol sponge) is placed between the vessel and nerve to prevent continued pulsatile focal compression.

Percutaneous trigeminal rhizotomy techniques generally involve radiofrequency heat lesioning of the trigeminal ganglion, glycerol injection into the spinal fluid of Meckel cave (which causes an osmotic damage preferentially to the smaller pain-carrying nerve fibers), or mechanical trauma to the nerve or ganglion by transient inflation of a No. 4 Fogarty catheter balloon.

**38.**

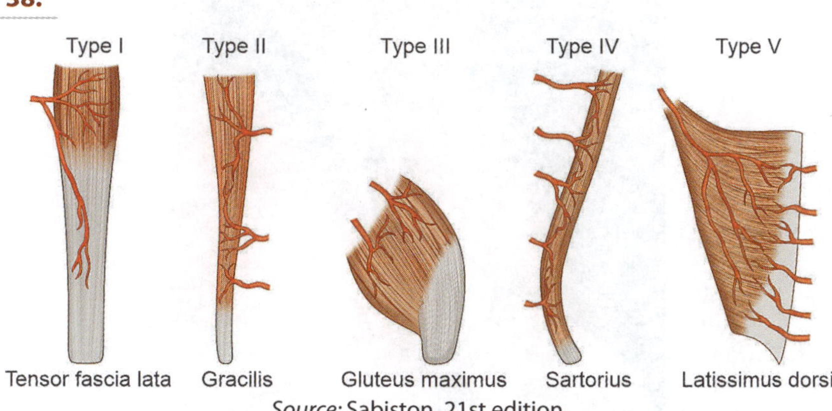


*Source:* Sabiston, 21st edition.

Classification of muscle and musculocutaneous flaps according to their vascular supply:

- Type I, one vascular pedicle
- Type II, dominant pedicle and minor pedicles

- Type III, two dominant pedicles
- Type IV, segmental vascular pedicles
- Type V, one dominant pedicle and secondary segmental pedicles

**39. Name the surgery shown in the surgery.**

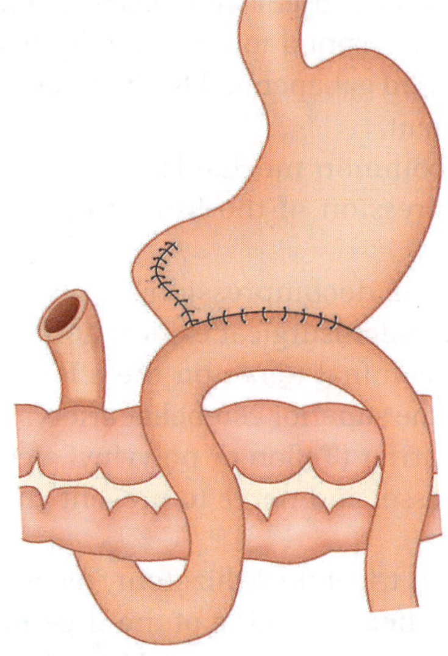

Billroth II reconstruction is gastro jejunal anastomosis.

**40. Name the surgery done for congenital hypertrophic pyloric stenosis.**

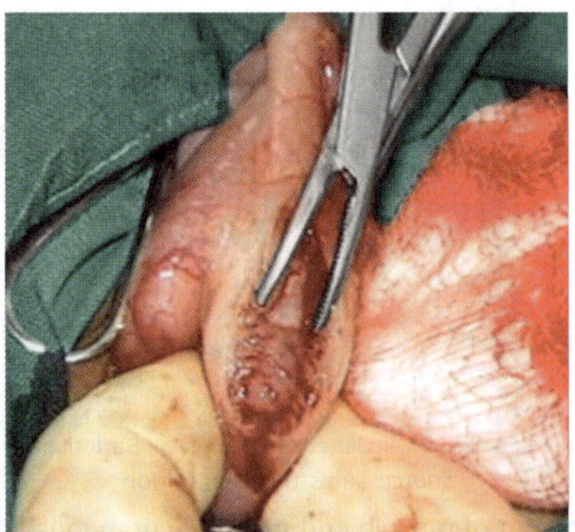

*Source:* Bailey and Love, 27th edition.

*Ramstedt's pyloromyotomy:* Muscle layer is opened until the mucosa bulgcs out.

**41.** ***Identify the disease:*** **Stomach showing cerebriform appearance.**

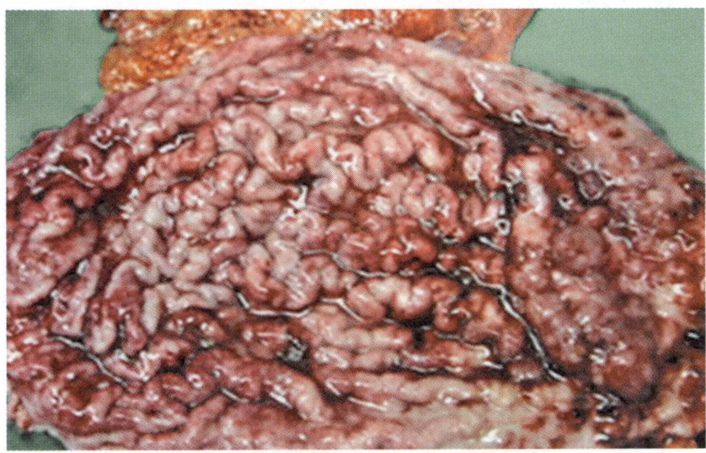

*Source:* Bailey and Love, 27th edition.

*Ménétrier's disease:* Cerebriform pattern of mucosa is Ménétrier's disease.

**42.** **Name of this surgery.**

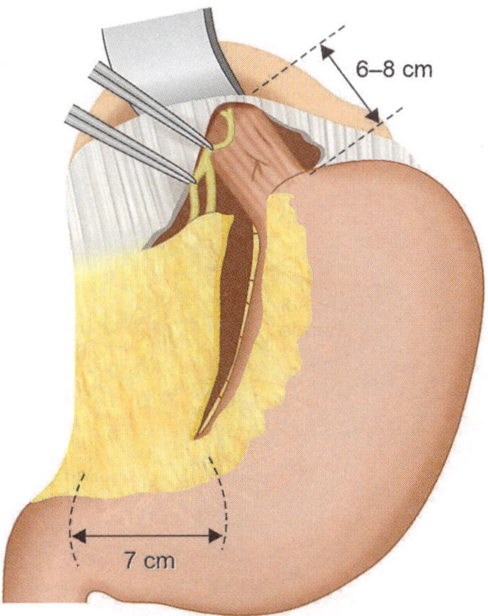


*Source:* Bailey and Love, 27th edition.

*High selective vagotomy (HSV):*

- Nerve of Latarjet is spared in HSV.
- Parietal cell vagotomy is done about 7 cm from pylorus.

**43. Identify the name of surgery.**

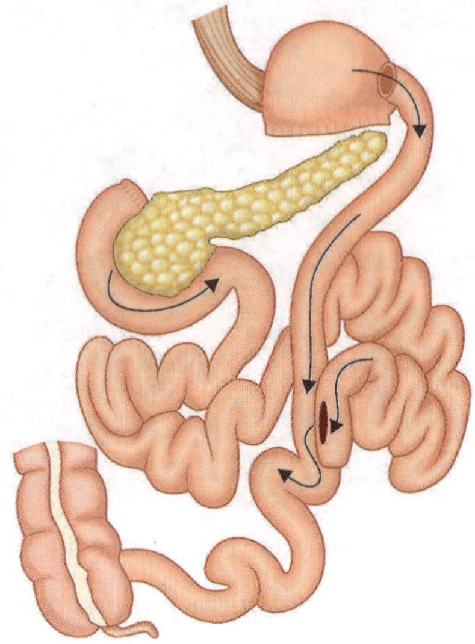

*Source:* Bailey and Love, 27th edition.

Biliopancreatic diversion A type of mostly malabsorptive and partly restrictive bariatric surgery.

**44.**

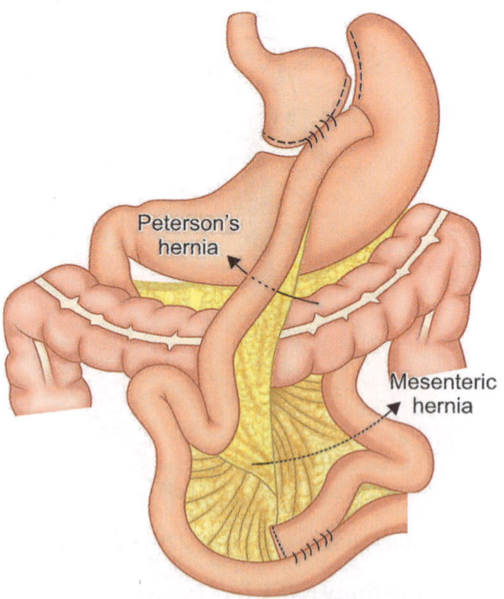


*Source:* Bailey and Love, 27th edition.

Peterson hernia—hernia behind the Roux-en-Y limb

**45.**

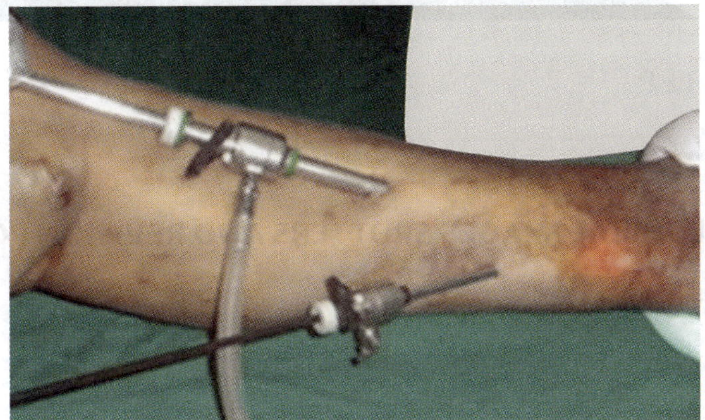

*Source:* Sabiston, 21st edition.

Subfascial endoscopic perforator surgery (SEPS):

# CHAPTER 61 Radiology

## RADIOLOGICAL IMAGES SPOTTERS AND REVISION POINTS

**1. Flail chest**

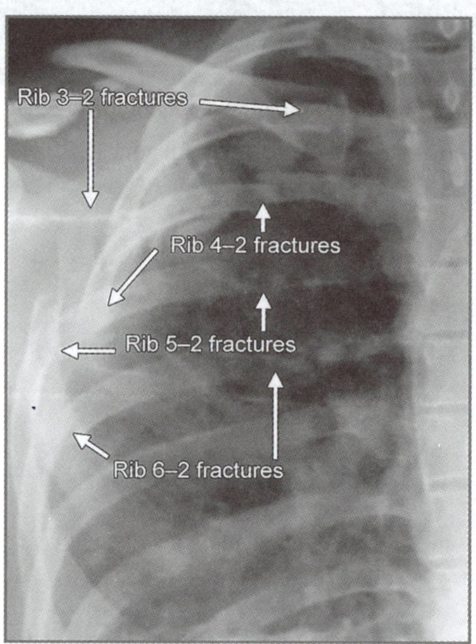


*Source:* Bailey and Love, 28th edition.

- Fracture of three or more ribs
- Paradoxical respiration

**2. A young male met with a road traffic accident and came to the emergency department, he was evaluated and found to have blood pressure (BP)—130/80 mm Hg, pulse rate—88/min, and respiratory rate (RR)—22/min. On auscultation, there was decreased air entry on one side with absent breath sounds. X-ray chest is given here.**

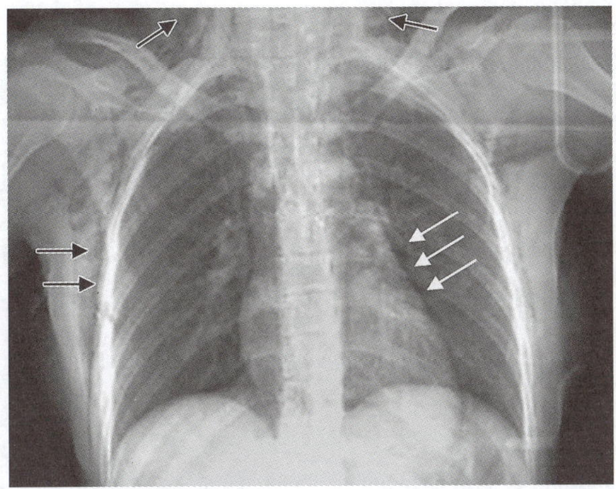

*Source:* Bailey and Love, 28th edition.

*Rupture of esophagus and compressing the pericardium*

- This image shows pneumomediastinum which is a feature of esophageal rupture.
- Decreased air entry implies collection of esophageal contents and pleural effusion on that side.
- Naclerio V sign—Presence of V-shaped gas shadow near cardiophrenic angle on left side in Boerhaave syndrome, esophagus rupture.
- Mackler's triad—Vomiting, chest pain, and subcutaneous emphysema in barotrauma esophagus.

## 3. Pneumothorax

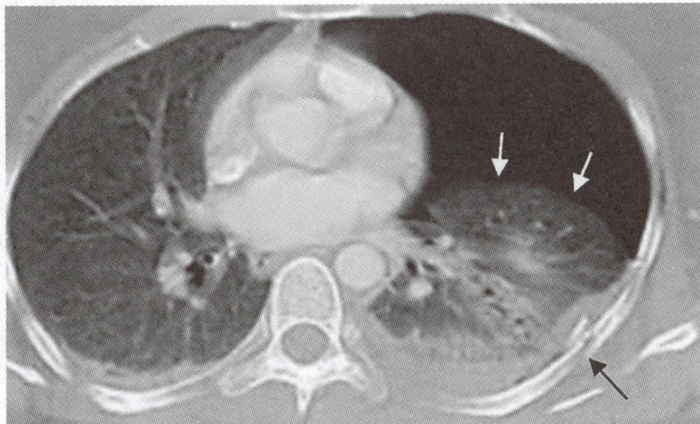

*Source:* Bailey and Love, 28th edition.

- Left thorax shows—air in pleural cavity—with compression of lung.
- Emergency needle thoracocentesis followed by intercostal drainage tube (ICD) must be done.

## 4. Subcutaneous emphysema

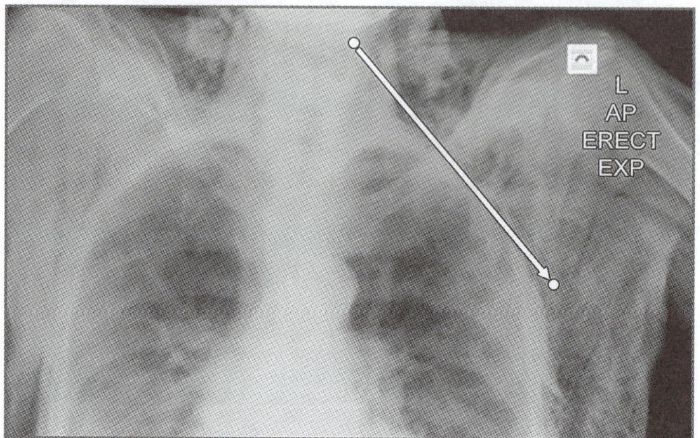


*Source:* Bailey and Love, 28th edition.

The sign we are seeing in this X-ray is "Ginkgo leaf sign".

- The air is outlining the pectoralis major muscle and creating a branching pattern that resembles this Ginkgo leaf veins as shown here.
- This is characteristic sign of subcutaneous emphysema.

## 5. Stafne bone cyst

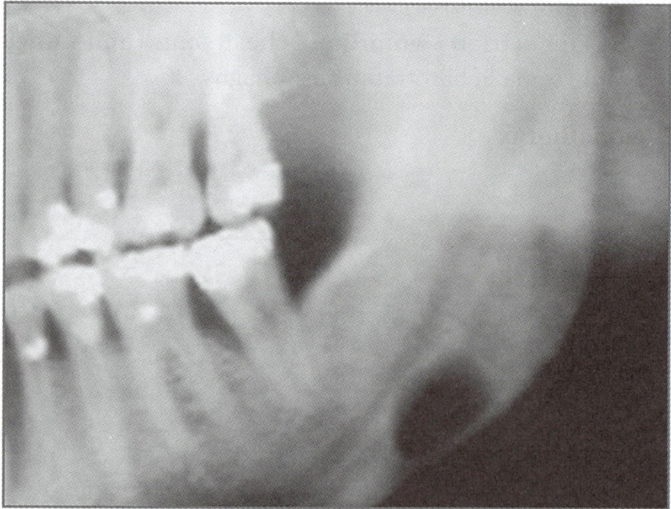

*Source:* Bailey and Love, 28th edition.

*Ectopic salivary tissue*

- Most common site of ectopic salivary tissue—Stafne bone cyst
- Most common site of ectopic salivary gland tumor—Palate

6.

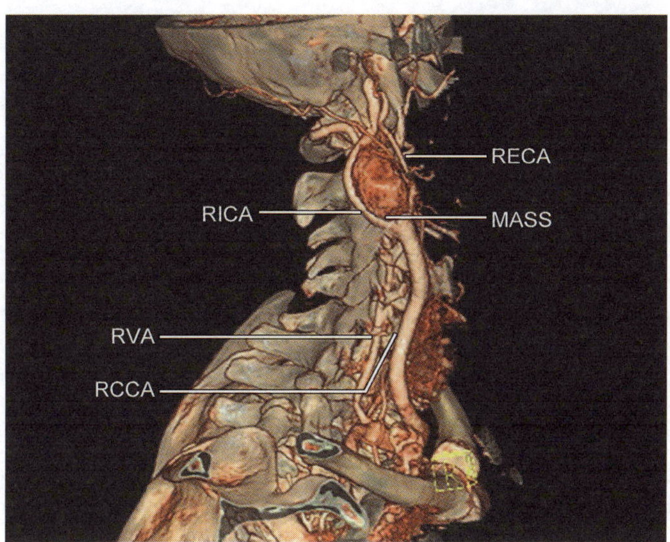


*Source:* Bailey and Love, 28th edition.

Magnetic resonance (MR) angiogram reconstructed showing Lyre sign. (RECA: right external carotid artery; RICA: right internal carotid artery; RVA: right vertebral artery; RCCA: right common carotid artery)

Carotid body tumors arise from chemoreceptor cells (not baroreceptor cells) of carotid body and are stimulated by decrease arterial oxygen tension, e.g., cyanotic heart disease, chronic hypoxia in high altitude inhabitants.

*Lyre sign*

Angiogram finding—splaying of internal and external carotids due to tumor in between biopsy and FNAC are absolutely contraindicated.

*Shamblin classifications, types, and management:*

| ***Types*** | ***Pattern*** | ***Surgical procedure*** |
|---|---|---|
| Type 1 | Localized (25%) | Excision |
| Type 2 | Adherent partially (50%) | Subadventitial dissection (temporary intraluminal shunt may be used) |
| Type 3 | Adherent completely surround internal carotid artery (25%) cases | • En bloc removal of tumor and internal carotid artery (ICA)<br>• En bloc great saphenous vein grafting |

## 7. Bilateral cervical ribs

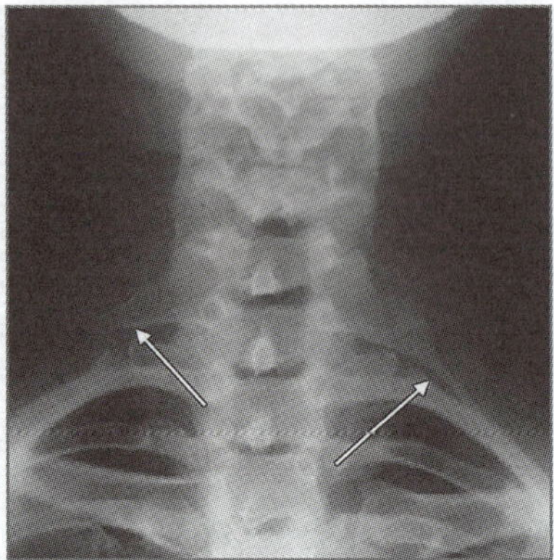

*Source:* Bailey and Love, 28th edition.

*Cervical ribs:* Costal element may develop from anterior part of the transverse process of C7 vertebra. This may develop into cervical rib. Most common in (R) side.

*Symptoms:*

- Neurological symptoms are less common in cervical rib than vascular symptoms.
- If neurological symptoms predominate always rule out disk prolapsed and carpal tunnel syndrome.

*Surgical treatment:*

Excision of cervical rib (extraperiosteal excision)

*Scalenotomy*

## 8. Lyre sign

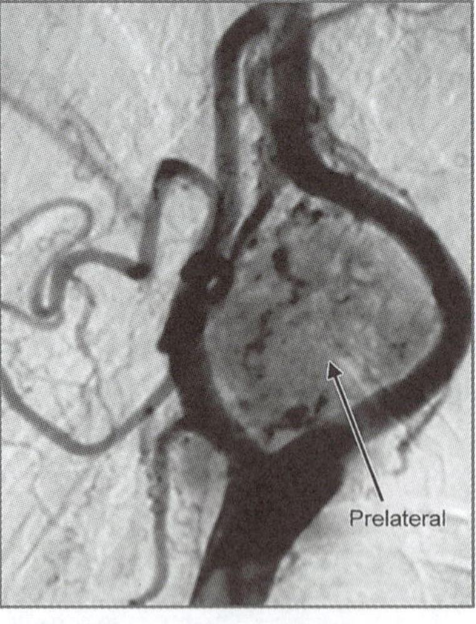


*Source.* Bailey and Love, 28th edition.

- Lyre sign is the splaying of internal carotid artery and external carotid artery.
- It is a typical finding seen in carotid body tumor.

**9. Fistulogram of second branchial remnant.**

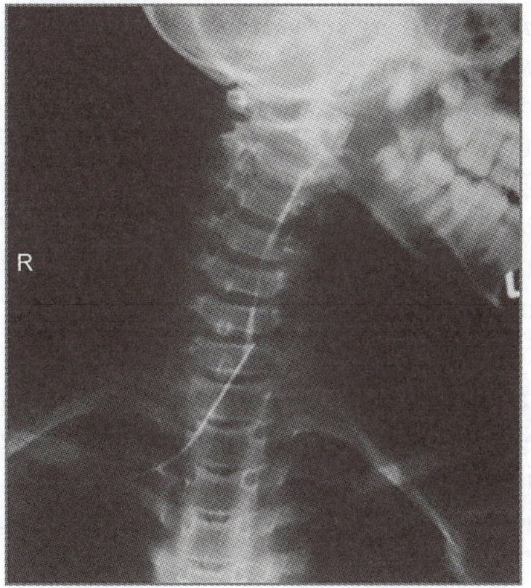


*Source:* Bailey and Love, 28th edition.

- This is a branchial fistula. Inner opening is found in the tonsillar fossa.
- The external opening is found in the lower third of sternocleidomastoid border.

**10.**

Magnetic resonance imaging (MRI) of implanted breast—IOC for cancer breast in implanted women.

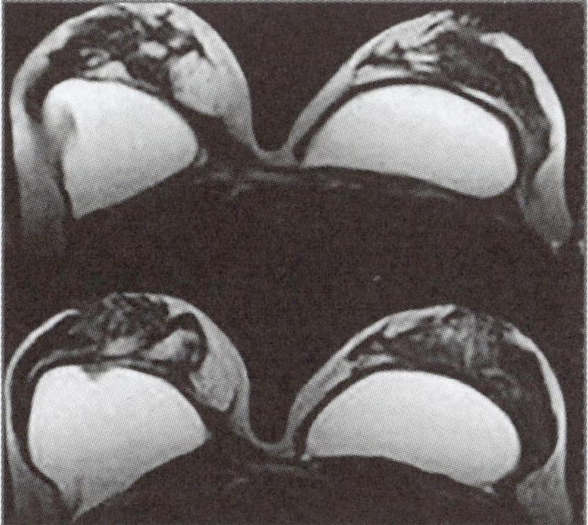

*Source:* Bailey and Love, 28th edition.

*MRI breast indicated in:*

- Distinguishing scar from recurrence in women who had previous breast conservative surgery.
- Gold standard for imaging the breasts of women with implants.
- Evaluating the axilla in both primary breast cancer and recurrence.

*Indications of MRI as screening investigation—American Cancer Society Risk criteria:*

Women at high risk (>20–25% risk) for breast cancer:

- BRCA 1 and BRCA 2 mutation
- First degree relative of BRCA 1, 2
- Radiation therapy to chest at 10–30 years
- Lifetime risk of 20–25% as per risk models
- Li fraumeni and Cowden disease

*Women at moderate risk (15–20%):*

- Personal history of ductal carcinoma in situ, lobular carcinoma in situ, previous breast cancer operated, atypical ductal hyperplasia, or lobular hyperplasia.
- Extremely dense breasts or unevenly dense breasts.

**11.**

Diagnosis of the mammography report in a 30-year-old woman with breast lump felt on self-examination of breast.

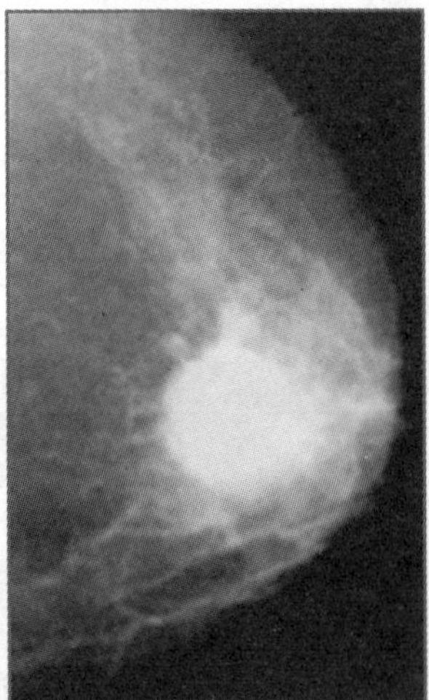

*Source:* Bailey and Love, 28th edition.

*Breast cancer:*

- Mammography shows branching calcification typical of cancer breast.
- Fibroadenoma will have popcorn-type calcification.

**12. What is the investigation done here?**

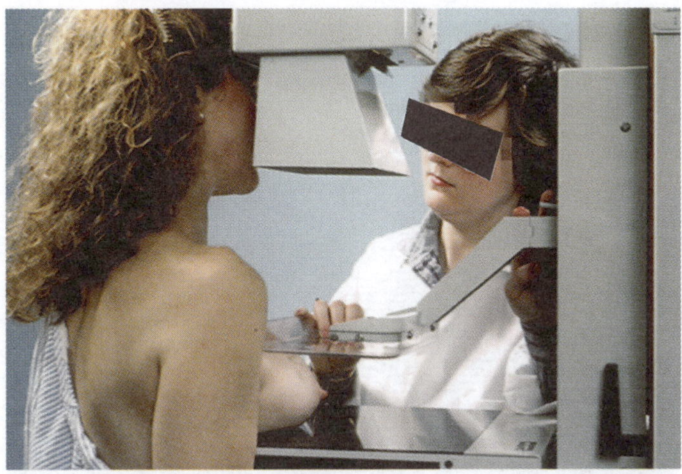

*Source:* Bailey and Love, 28th edition.

*Mammography*

- This is a craniocaudal view of mammography being taken.
- It is a low voltage and high amplitude X-ray.

**13.**

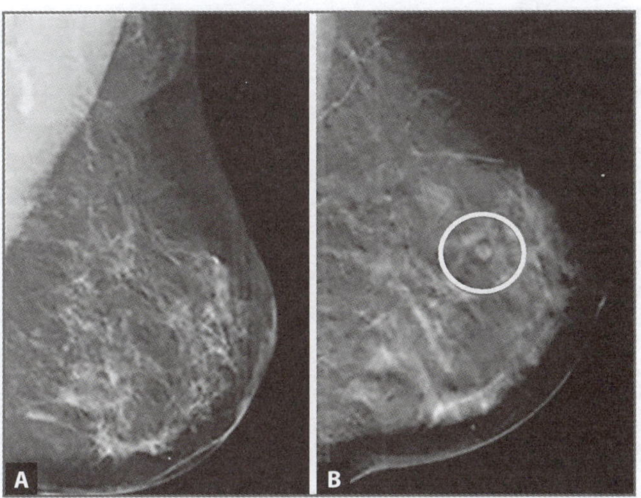


*Source:* Bailey and Love, 28th edition.

*Microcalcification*

- Microcalcification is rounded in Figure B.
- It is a finding more in favor of cancer breast.

## 14. Fibroadenoma

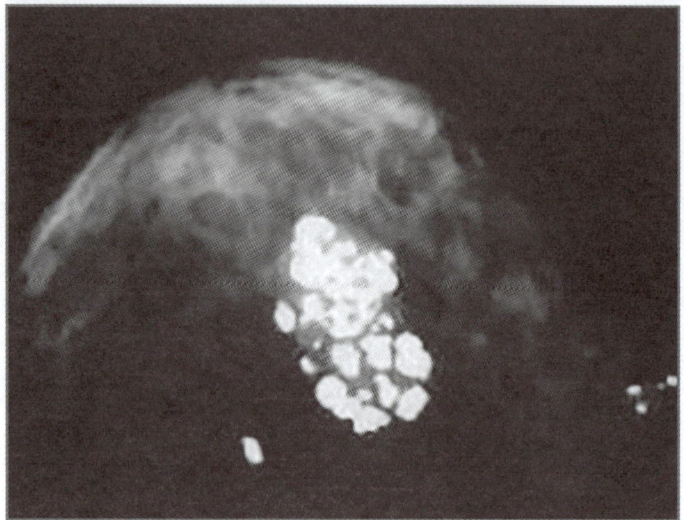

*Source:* Bailey and Love, 28th edition.

- This image shows popcorn calcification—macrocalcification

## 15.

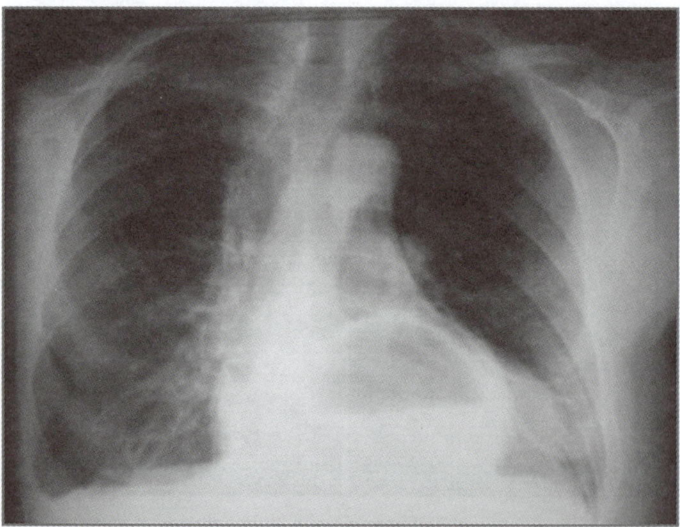

*Source:* Bailey and Love, 28th edition.

- Hiatus hernia type 2 is associated with protrusion of fundus of stomach into the mediastinum.

**16. Identify the barium swallow shown here:**

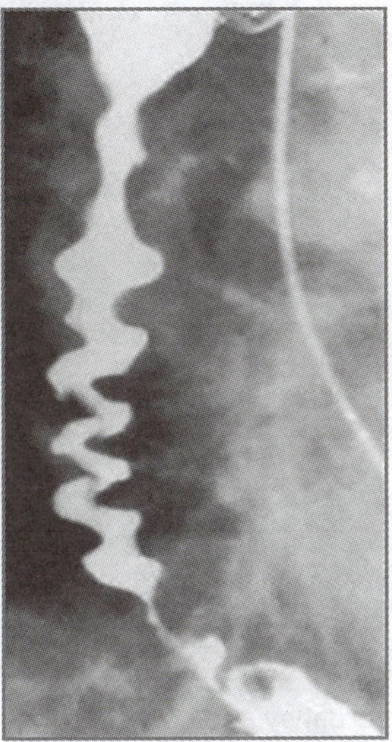

*Source:* Bailey and Love, 28th edition.

Cork screw esophagus in diffuse esophageal spasm

**17. Middle age patient presents with dysphagia for liquids. The barium esophagogram of the patient is shown here. The diagnosis is:**

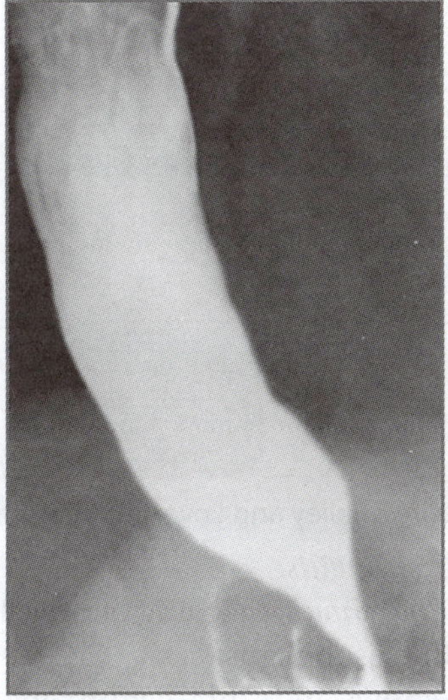

*Source:* Bailey and Love, 28th edition.

Image shows bird-beak appearance of achalasia cardia.

**18. Following image is diagnostic of:**

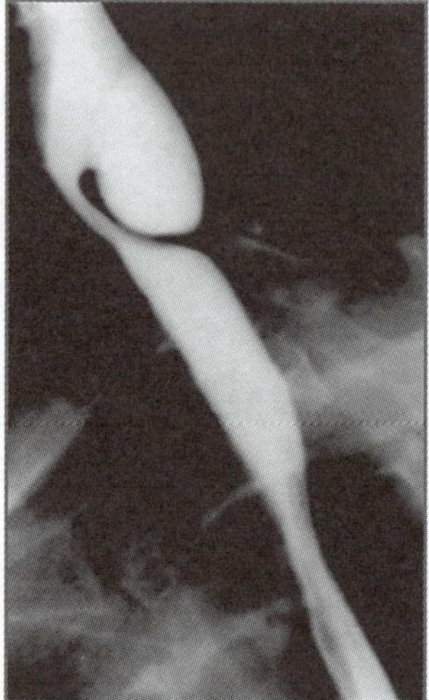

*Source:* Bailey and Love, 28th edition.

- Zenker diverticulum protrudes posteriorly above the cricopharyngeal sphincter through Killian dehiscence.
- IOC for Zenker is barium swallow.

**19. Barium swallow shows—Feline esophagus.**

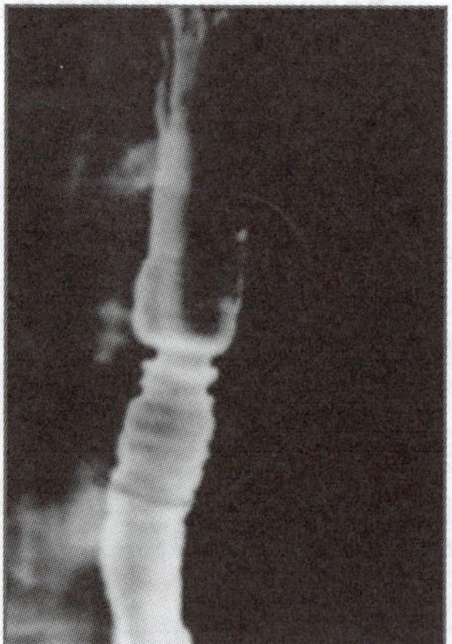

*Source:* Bailey and Love, 28th edition.

*In eosinophilic esophagitis:*

- *Barium swallow shows:* Stacking of rings like "ringed esophagus" known as feline esophagus.
- Endoscopy shows multiple esophageal rings, longitudinally oriented furrows are seen, mimicking like a "Trachea"—also known as trachea like esophagus.

**20.**

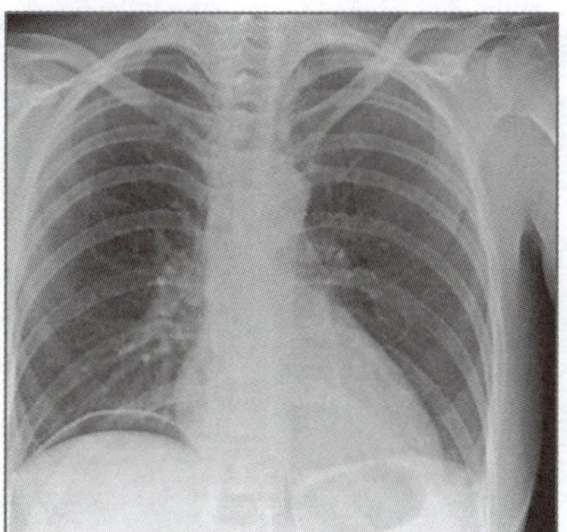

*Source:* Bailey and Love, 28th edition.

*Intestinal perforation*

- Times repeated question—Pneumoperitoneum (air under diaphragm) seen in gastrointestinal tract (GIT) perforations.
- Most common (MC) cause is duodenal ulcer perforation.

*Management of perforation peritonitis:*

- Initial priority—Resuscitation and analgesics. There is no contraindication to give analgesics with fear of masking symptoms of peritonitis.
- Following resuscitation—Principal treatment is surgical by upper midline laparotomy.
- Laparoscopy can be used.
- Most important component in surgery—Thorough peritoneal lavage to remove all fluid and food debris.
- *Options to close are:*
    - Closed the perforated ulcer in transverse direction as in pyloroplasty and then omental patch is kept. Do not tie sutures so tightly.
    - If perforation is difficult to close primarily, we can close the leak with omental patch alone (Modified Graham's patch closure).
    - Gastric ulcers are excised and the edges closed to exclude malignancy.
    - Massive duodenal or gastric ulcers where closure is difficult, we can do distal gastrectomy and do Roux-en-Y reconstruction as procedure of choice.
- All patients are given systemic antibiotics.
- All patients are given gastric antisecretory agents and *Helicobacter pylori* eradication mandatory.

**21. Tell your diagnosis:**

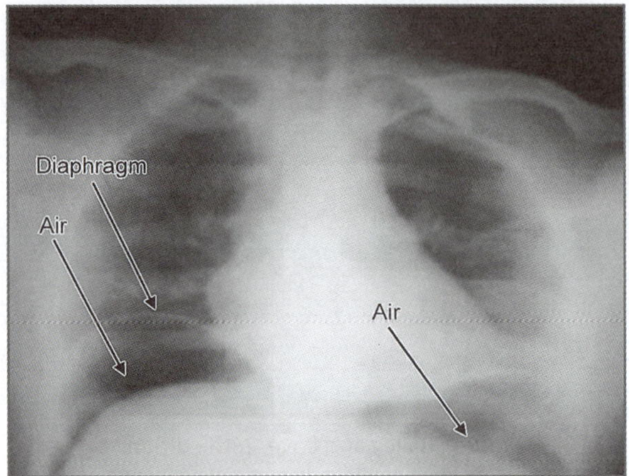


*Source:* Bailey and Love, 28th edition.

*Perforation peritonitis:*

- Air under diaphragm on the right side indicates a hollow viscus perforation.
- The best imaging for hollow viscus perforation is X-ray abdomen erect.
- The minimum amount of air detected on erect X-ray: 1 mL.
- *If patient cannot stand erect due to peritonitis:* Left lateral decubitus X-ray is taken. This image will detect 5–10 mL of air.
- *Chilaiditi's syndrome:* Interposition of colonic shadow between the liver and diaphragm appears like perforation air under diaphragm.

**22. Your diagnosis in this 6-month-old kid.**

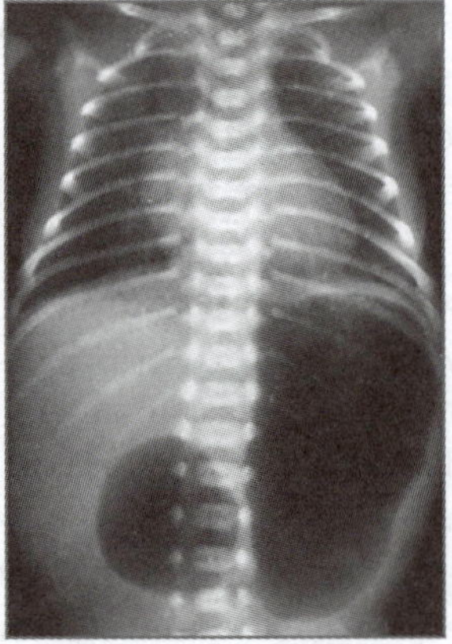

*Source:* Bailey and Love, 28th edition.

*Duodenal atresia*

- Double-bubble appearance shown in X-ray.

**23.**

- Carmen meniscus sign is characterized by lentiform-shaped appearance of inner margin also looking convex in malignant ulcer as shown here.

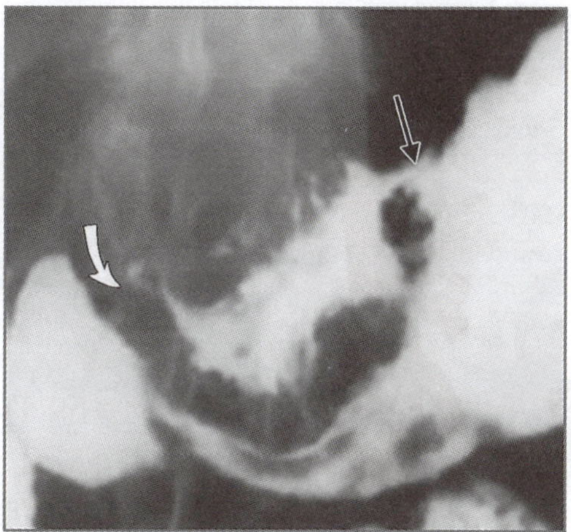

*Source:* Bailey and Love, 28th edition.

- Hampton line is thin radiolucent line at neck of benign gastric ulcer as shown here.

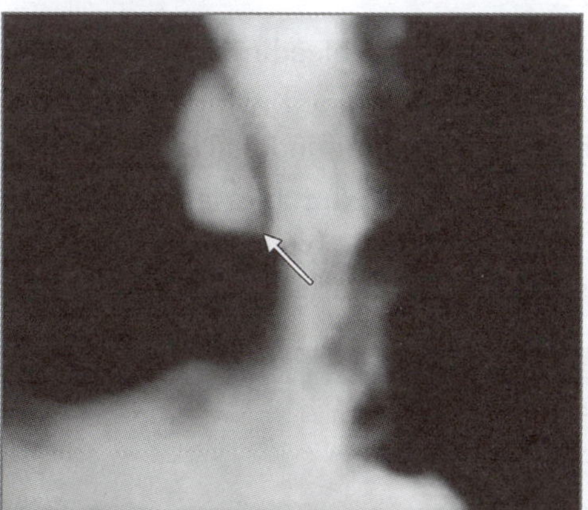

*Source:* Bailey and Love, 28th edition.

**24.**

*Median arcuate ligament syndrome (celiac artery compression syndrome) or Dunbar syndrome:*

- Characterized by a triad of postprandial abdominal pain + weight loss + abdominal bruit.

- Celiac artery arises from aorta at level of T11–L1. Higher origin or lower origin of celiac axis leads to compression.
- Median arcuate ligament that bridges the crura of diaphragm causes compression.
- Diagnosed by dynamic blood flow studies and computed tomography (CT) angiogram.
- Treatment is to release the arcuate ligament by surgery.

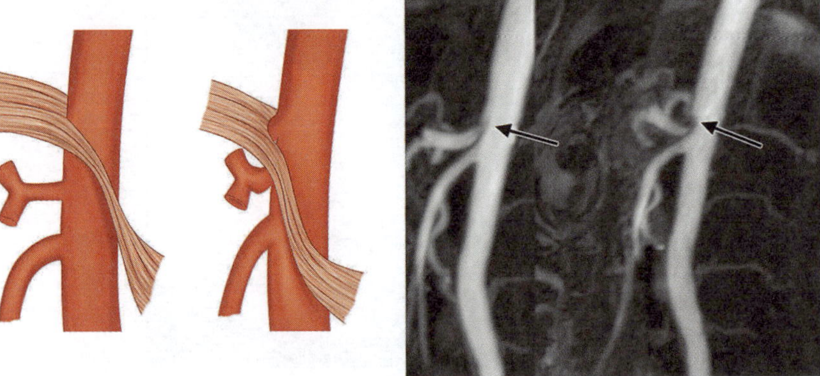

Median arcuate ligament syndrome.
*Source:* Sabiston, 21st edition.

**25.**

Endovascular control of a bleeding duodenal ulcer.

A. An angiogram is obtained, which shows extravasation from a branch off of the gastroduodenal artery.

B. A completion angiogram after glue embolization of the vessel shows resolution of the bleed with preservation of flow through the gastroduodenal artery.

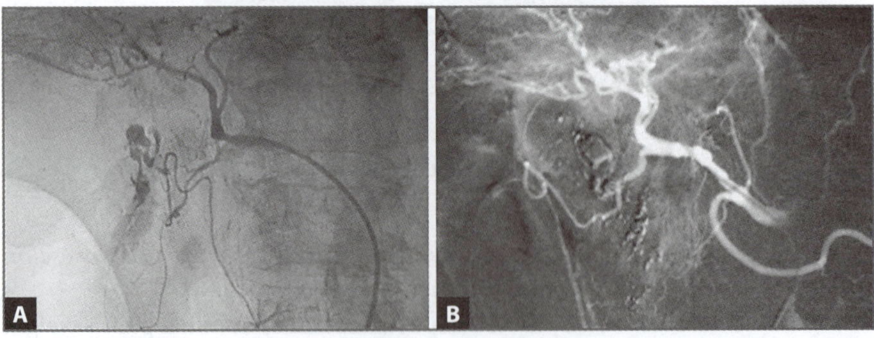


*Source:* Sabiston, 21st edition.

**26.**

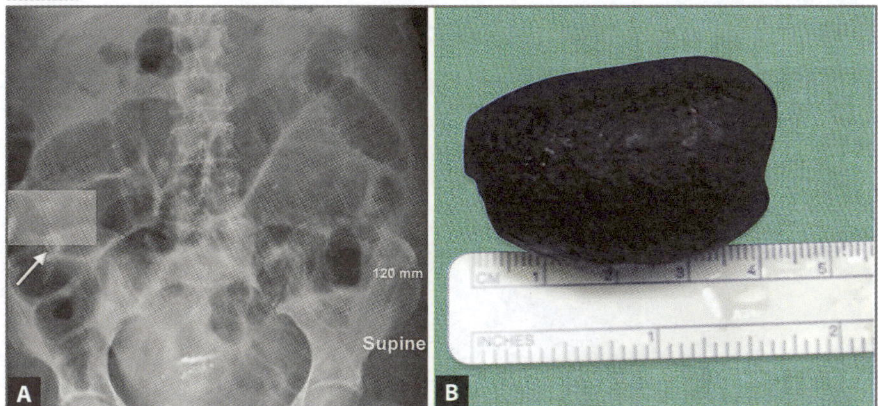


*Source:* Sabiston, 21st edition.

Patient presents with gallstone ileus.

A. Plain abdominal film shows complete bowel obstruction caused by a large radiopaque gallstone (arrow) obstructing the distal ileum.

B. The large gallstone responsible for the obstruction seen in the corresponding plain abdominal film.

**27.**

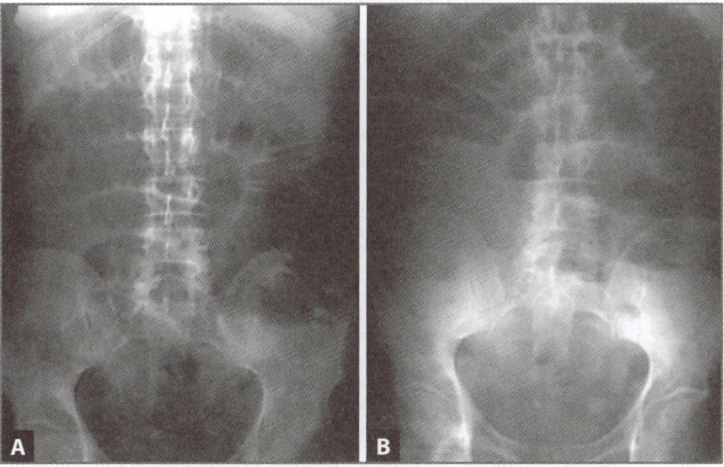


*Source:* Sabiston, 21st edition.

Abdominal radiographs of a patient with a complete small bowel obstruction.

A. Supine film shows dilated loops of small bowel in an orderly arrangement, without evidence of colonic gas.

B. Upright film shows multiple, short air-fluid levels arranged in a stepwise pattern.

**28.**

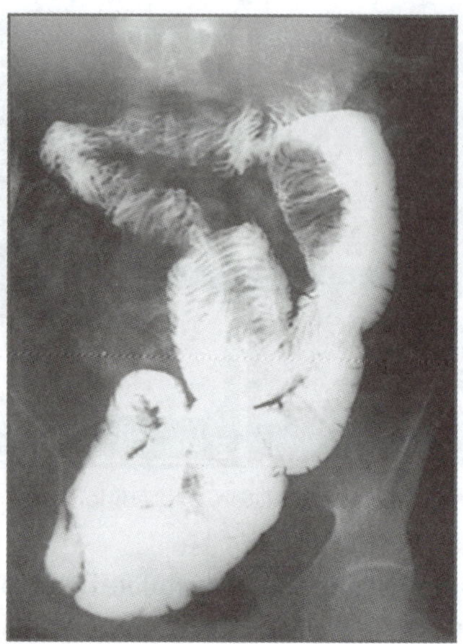

*Source:* Sabiston, 21st edition.

Barium study demonstrates jejunojejunal intussusception.

**29.**

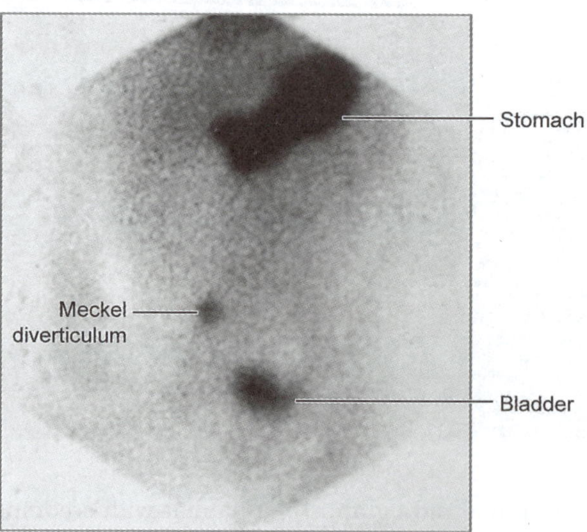


*Source:* Sabiston, 21st edition.

Nuclear imaging of Meckel diverticulum. A 99mTc-pertechnetate scintigram from a child demonstrates a Meckel diverticulum clearly differentiated from the stomach and bladder.

**30.**

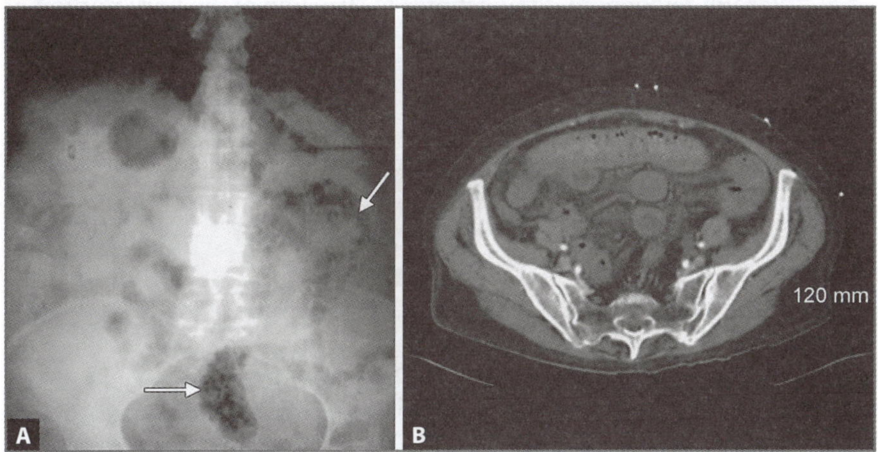


*Source:* Sabiston, 21st edition.

*Pneumatosis intestinalis*

A. Plain abdominal film demonstrates pneumatosis intestinalis (arrows).
B. Computed tomography findings consistent with curvilinear radiolucency appearing as tiny bubbles in the antimesenteric border of the bowel consistent with pneumatosis intestinalis.

**31.**

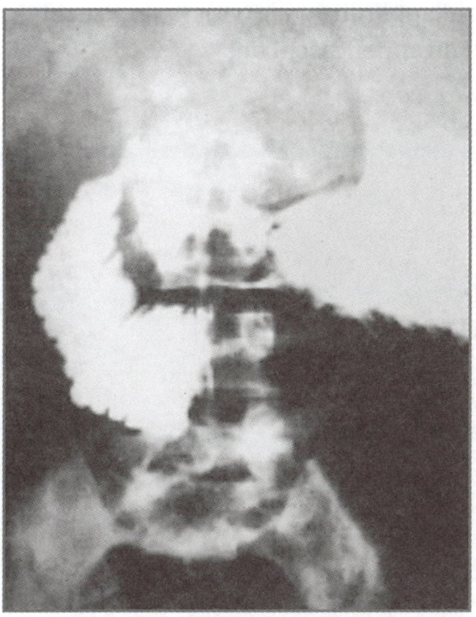

*Source:* Sabiston, 21st edition.

*Superior mesenteric artery (SMA) syndrome*

Barium radiograph demonstrates obstruction of the third portion of the duodenum secondary to superior mesenteric artery compression as a consequence of burn injury.

**32.**

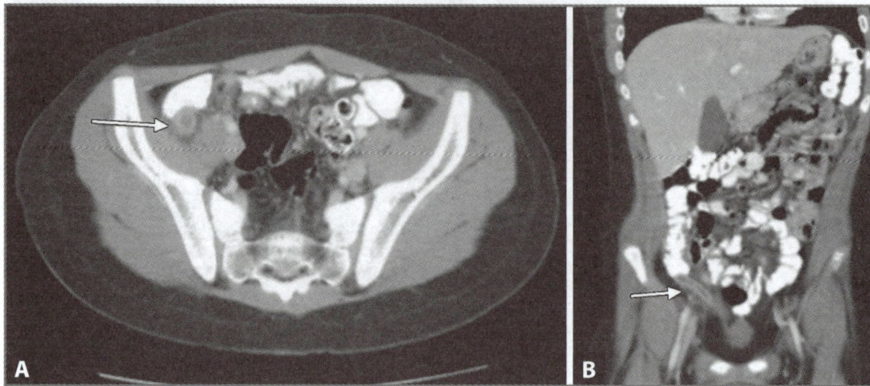


*Source:* Bailey and Love, 28th edition.

Computed tomography scan of the abdomen demonstrates classic findings of acute appendicitis.

A. Sagittal view with arrow demonstrating a thickened, inflamed, and fluid-filled appendix (target sign).

B. Coronal view of same patient. The arrow points to the thickened, elongated appendix with periappendiceal fat stranding and fluid around the appendiceal tip.

*The Alvarado score*

| *Symptoms* | |
|---|---|
| Migration | 1 |
| Anorexia | 1 |
| Nausea | 1 |
| *Signs* | |
| Tenderness in right lower quadrant | 2 |
| Rebound | 1 |
| Elevation of temperature | 1 |
| *Laboratory* | |
| Leukocytosis | 2 |
| Left shift | 1 |
| *Total score* | *10* |

*Source:* Sabiston, 21st edition.

**33.**

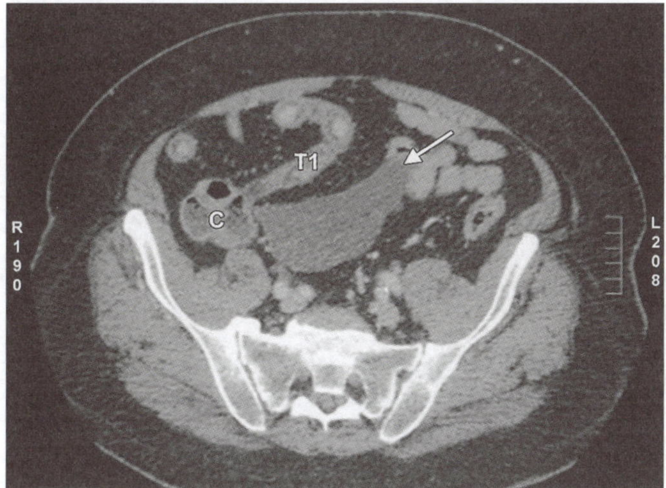


*Source:* Sabiston, 21st edition.

Computed tomography scan of the abdomen in a patient with a benign 10-cm mucocele. The axial image shows a distended fluid-filled mass medial to the appendix (arrow).

**34.**

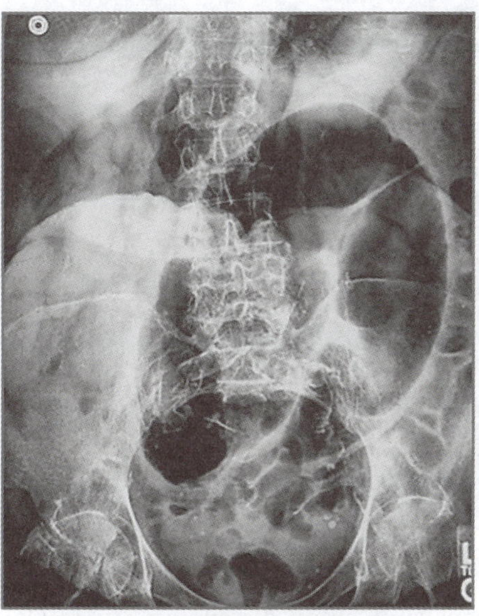

*Source:* Sabiston, 21st edition.

Plain film of sigmoid volvulus. Note bent inner tube appearance.

**35.**

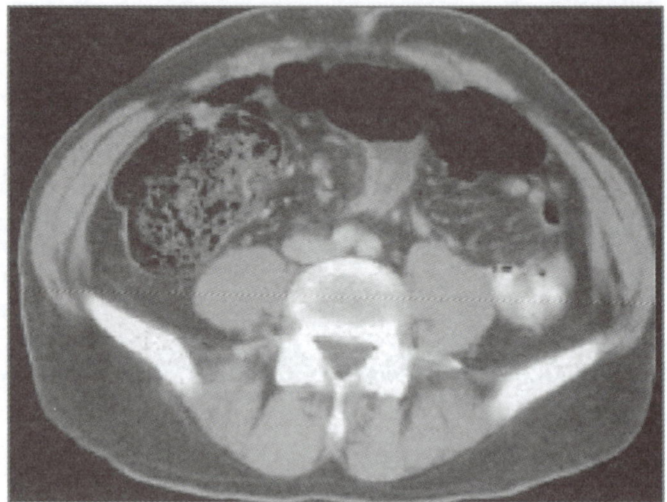

*Source:* Sabiston, 21st edition.

Computed tomography scan of the abdomen in a patient with sigmoid volvulus. Note characteristic whorl in mesentery.

**36.**

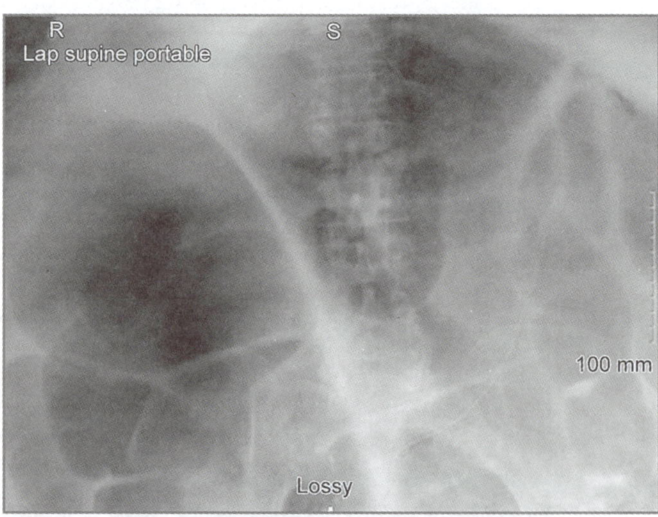


*Source:* Sabiston, 21st edition.

Massive transverse colon distension due to Ogilvie syndrome in a woman with multiple comorbidities including a body mass index of 69, severe pulmonary hypertension, and cardiac disease.

**37.**

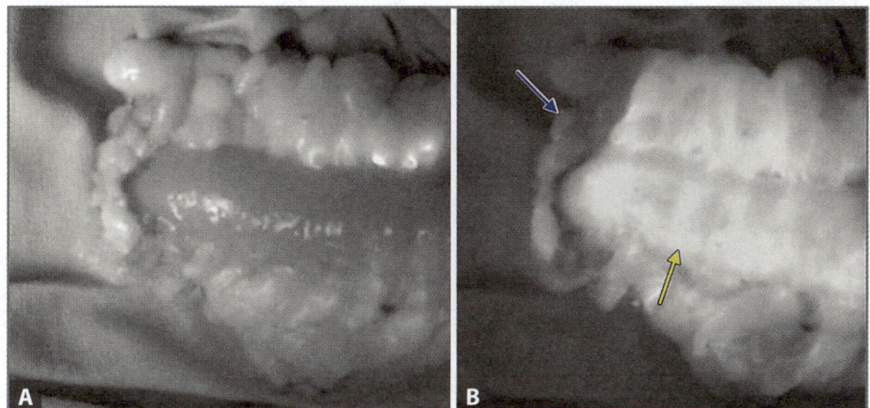


*Source:* Sabiston, 21st edition.

Indocyanine green-based infrared angiography. (A) Colon before injection; (B) Colon after injection: ischemia of resection margin (blue arrow); normal perfusion of colon (yellow arrow).

**38.**

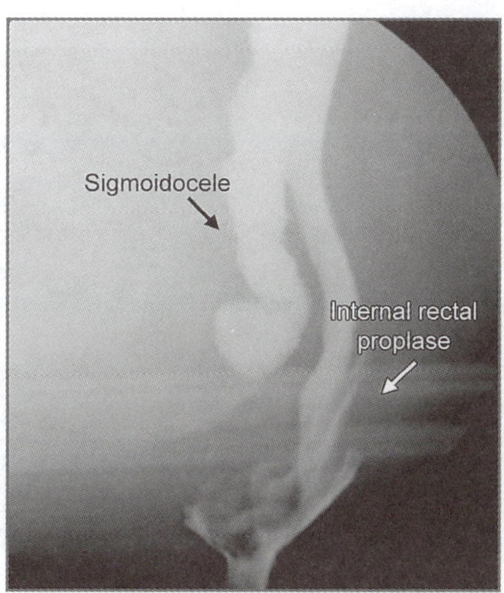


*Source:* Sabiston, 21st edition.

Defecography of a young male patient who presents with internal rectal prolapse (white arrow) and sigmoidocele (black arrow).

**39.**

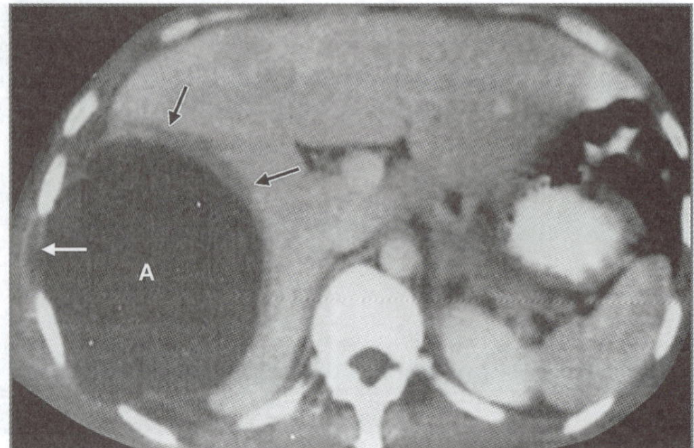


*Source:* Sabiston, 21st edition.

Computed tomography scan of amebic abscess. The lesion is peripherally located and round. The rim is nonenhancing but shows peripheral edema (black arrows).

**40.**

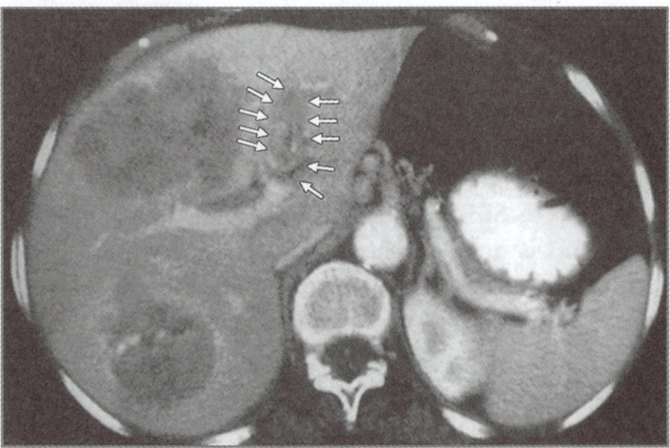

*Source:* Sabiston, 21st edition.

Contrast-enhanced computed tomography scan demonstrating multifocal hepatocellular carcinoma. The left portal vein is invaded and expanded by tumor (arrows).

41.

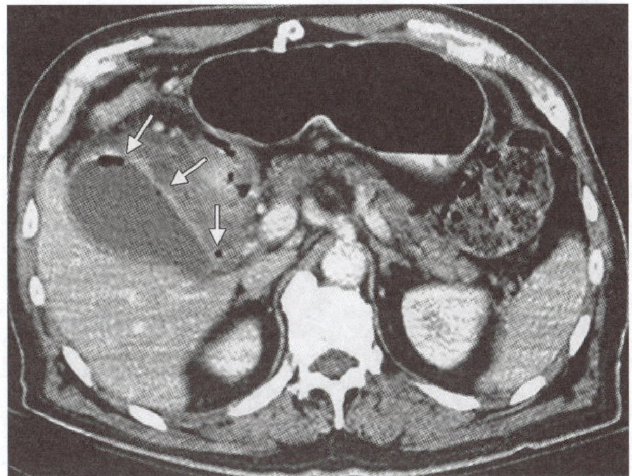

*Source:* Sabiston, 21st edition.

Computed tomography scan of emphysematous cholecystitis. Significant pericholecystic inflammatory changes and air in the gallbladder wall (arrows) are signs of emphysematous cholecystitis.

42.

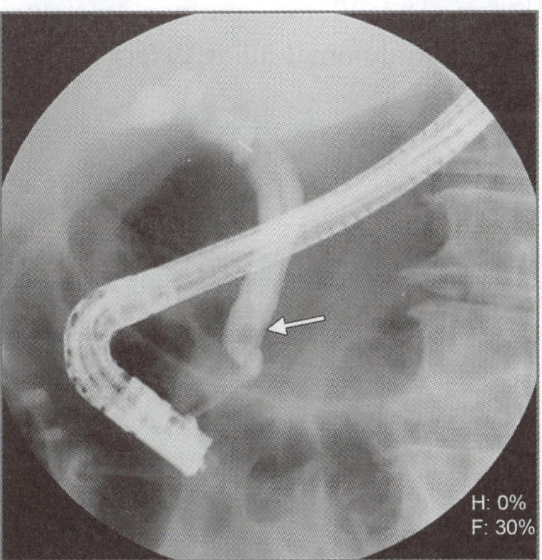


*Source:* Sabiston, 21st edition.

Endoscopic retrograde cholangiopancreatography (ERCP) with choledocholithiasis. With retrograde injection of contrast material, a filling defect noted within the lumen of the common bile duct (arrow) identifies choledocholithiasis. ERCP can also be used to remove the stone through sphincterotomy and balloons or baskets.

**43.**

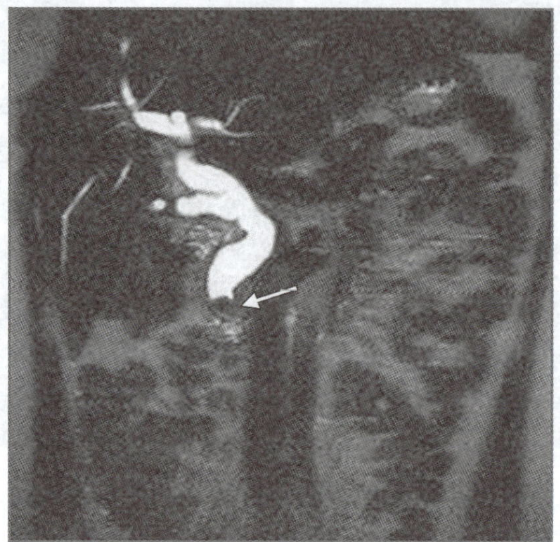

*Source:* Sabiston, 21st edition.

Magnetic resonance cholangiopancreatography with choledocholithiasis. The dilated common bile duct ends abruptly with a convex intraluminal filling defect (arrow) consistent with choledocholithiasis.

**44.**

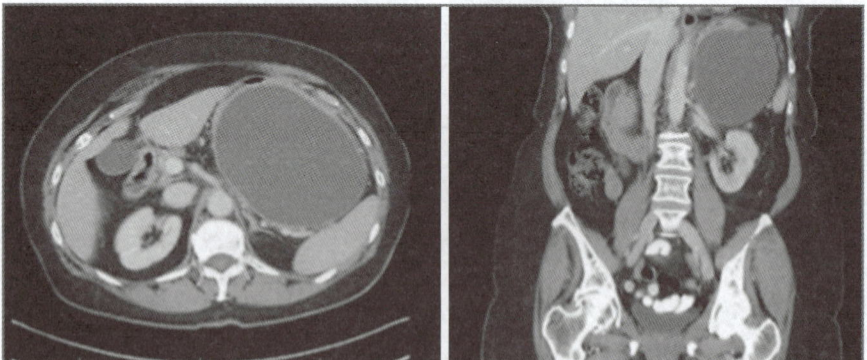

*Source:* Sabiston, 21st edition.

Computed tomography (CT) scans showing a large pseudocyst arising in the tail of the pancreas.

**45.**

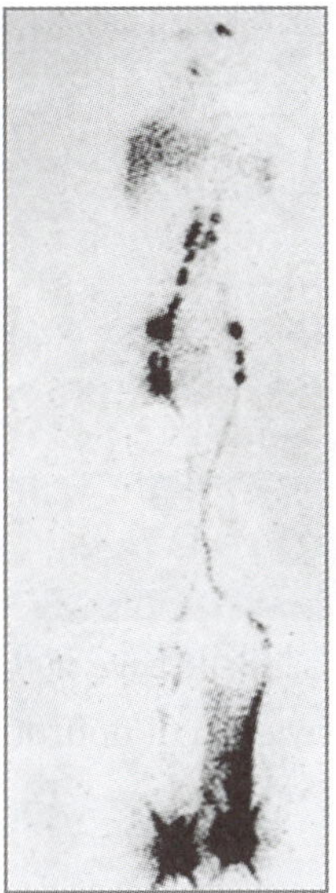

*Source:* Sabiston, 21st edition.

Lymphoscintigraphic pattern in primary lymphedema. Note area of dermal backflow on the left and diminished number of lymph nodes in the groin.

**46.**

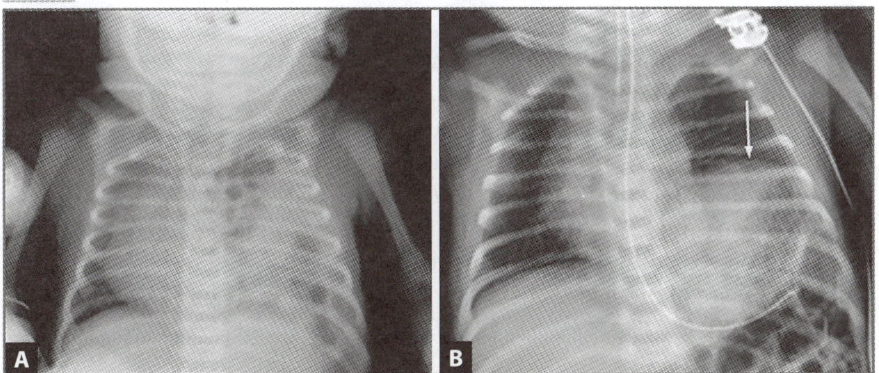


*Source:* Sabiston, 21st edition.

A. Congenital diaphragmatic hernia. Multiple gas-filled bowel loops are located in the left hemithorax, and the mediastinum is shifted to the right.
B. Left diaphragmatic eventration. Hemidiaphragm is elevated (arrow) from phrenic nerve injury-induced paralysis.

**47.**

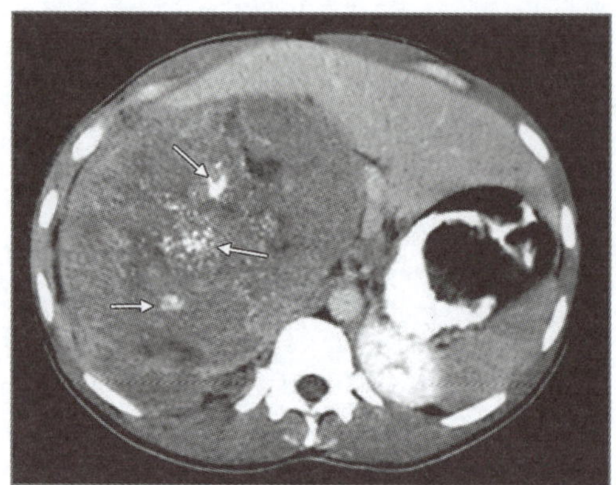

*Source:* Bailey and Love, 28th edition.

Computed tomography scan of neuroblastoma demonstrating areas of calcification (arrows).

*Neuroblastoma*

Malignant tumor arising from neural crest and anywhere along the sympathetic chain.

*Common sites of origin are:*

- *Adrenal medulla:* 38%
- *Sympathetic chain in paravertebral sites of abdomen:* 30%
- *Sympathetic chain in paravertebral sites of chest:* 20%
- Rarely in neck and pelvis

MC tumor diagnosed in infants <1 year age.
MC intra-abdominal malignancy in children.
Sporadic in most cases.
80% cases present before 4 years.
Metastasis is seen in 60–70% cases at the time of diagnosis.
Orbital metastasis presents with ecchymosis.
Paraneoplastic syndromes—Dancing eyes, dancing feet (opsoclonus and myoclonus) watery diarrhea.
MC site of metastasis in older children—Bones (Long bones—MC)

| *Favorable prognosis* | *Unfavorable prognosis* |
|---|---|
| • Age <1 year<br>• Thoracic primary lesion<br>• Well-differentiated tumor<br>• Increased ratio of vanillylmandelic acid (VMA)/ homovanillic acid (HVA)<br>• Normal serum ferritin<br>• Hyperdiploid/triploid<br>• Increased tropomyosin receptor kinase (*Trk*)-A gene | • N MYC amplification<br>• Deletion of 1p<br>• Gain of 17 q<br>• MDR protein+<br>• Overexpressed telomerases<br>• Increased ferritin<br>• Diploid state<br>• Older patients |

The following are the differentiating features between neuroblastoma and Wilm's tumor as they both are common in the same age group and present with mass abdomen:

- *Calcification:* There are specks of calcification visible in neuroblastoma (about 85%) which are generally less common and less prominent in Wilm's tumor (<15%).
- *Intraspinal extension:* Intraspinal extension is seen in neuroblastoma not in Wilm's tumor.
- Aorta and inferior vena cava (IVC) invasion Wilm's tumor invades aorta and IVC. Whereas, neuroblastoma does not invade these structures.
- *Location:* Wilm's tumor and neuroblastoma can be differentiated on location too. CT findings will confirm the intrarenal location of Wilm's whereas neuroblastoma will be seen above the kidney pushing it downward and outward (Drooping lily sign).
- *Crossing midline Wilm's tumors* are typically confined to one side of the abdomen, whereas neuroblastoma usually cross the midline.

**48.**

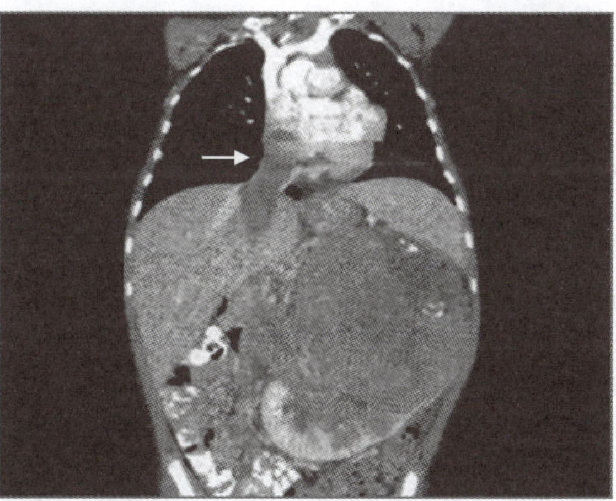

*Source:* Sabiston, 21st edition.

Computed tomography image of Wilm's tumor with a claw sign and a large inferior vena cava tumor thrombus extending to right atrium (arrow).

- *Chromosomal anomalies associated with Wilm's tumor:* 8th and 11th
- Most common age is 1–5 years.
- *Most common and earliest symptom:* Abdominal lump
- *Most common site of distant metastasis:* Lung

- Most common presentation is painless abdominal mass usually discovered by the mother while routinely bathing the baby.
- Other signs and symptoms are abdominal pain, fever, abdominal distention, hematuria anorexia, hypertension, nausea, and vomiting.
- CT scan is used to stage and to diagnose.
- This is a mixed tumor containing epithelium and connective tissue elements arising from embryonic nephrogenic tissue.
- *Triad of:*
  1. Abdominal mass
  2. Pyrexia
  3. Hematuria

*Anomalies associated with Wilm's tumor are:*

- Hemihypertrophy
- Perlman syndrome
- Aniridia
- WAGR syndrome [Wilm's tumor, aniridia, genitourinary anomalies (horseshoe kidney), retardation of intellect]
- Beckwith-Wiedemann syndrome
- Cryptorchidism
- Denys-Drash syndrome
- Hypospadias

*Treatment*

The immediate treatment for unilateral tumors is surgical removal of the affected kidney even if pulmonary metastasis is present.

Wilm's tumor is both chemosensitive and radiosensitive tumor. So, both chemotherapy and radiotherapy play a significant role in its treatment.

(*Note:* Renal cell carcinoma (RCC) is both chemoresistant and radioresistant.)

Combination chemotherapy used in vincristine and actinomycin in localized disease and doxorubicin added for advanced disease.

Radiotherapy is used for advanced disease. The postoperative radiotherapy in Wilm's tumor is started within 10 days of surgery. Delay in starting radiotherapy beyond 10 days leads to tumor cells repopulation and increases the relapse rate.

*Protocols NWTSG—National Wilm's Tumor Study Group*

- Advise surgery first followed by chemotherapy.
- Prechemotherapy based staging International Society of Pediatric Oncology (SIOP).
- Chemotherapy followed by surgery.
- Postchemotherapy based staging system is in SIOP.

- Overall survival is same for both. Both advise chemotherapy first in a bilateral involvement.
- Extension to IVC above set the level of hepatic vein extension set involvement of solitary kidney.

## 49. Staghorn stones

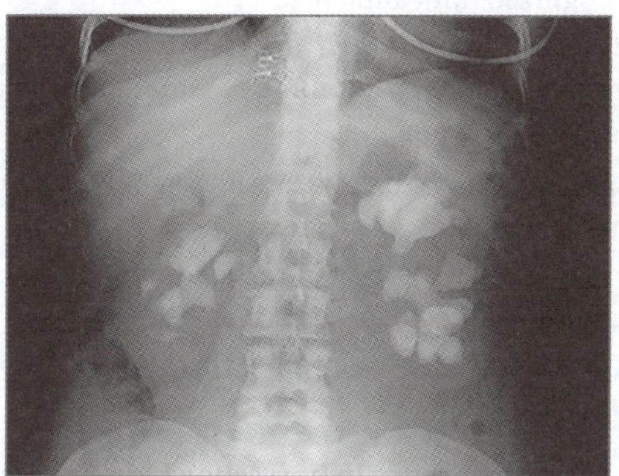

*Source:* Sabiston, 21st edition.

- Usually calcium phosphate, but sometimes is combined with ammonium and magnesium to form the triple phosphate calculus ammonium magnesium phosphate.
- Also known as struvite stone—Smooth and dirty white and solitary.
- Seen in alkaline urine especially with *Proteus* infection, which split urea to ammonia.
- This type of calculus may enlarge to fill all or most of renal collecting system forming a staghorn calculus.

## 50. Ureterocele showing Adder-head appearance in IVP.

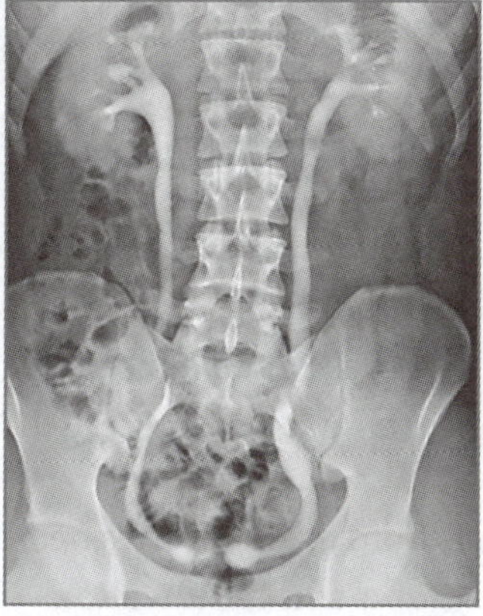

*Source:* Bailey and Love, 28th edition.

- Ureterocele is a ballooning of the distal submucosal ureters into the bladder.
- Ureterocele is thought to result from congenital atresia of the ureteric orifice.
- Although present from childhood the condition is often unrecognized until adult life.
- It may get large enough to obstruct the vesical neck or the contralateral ureters. It is more common in females.
- 10% of cases are bilateral.
- Often associated with duplicate ureters (always involve the ureters draining the upper renal pole).
- The "Adder-head" or "Cobra-head" appearance on excretory urography is noted in ureteroceles.
- Almost always associated with significant hydroureteronephrosis.

## 51. Flower-vase appearance in horseshoe kidney.

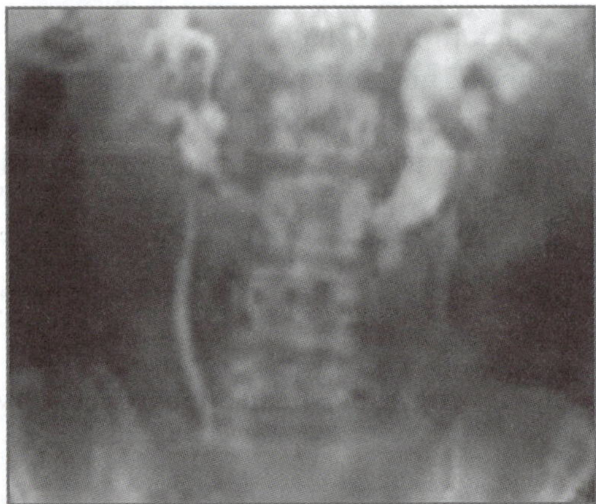

*Source:* Bailey and Love, 28th edition.

- *Most common pole to fuse:* Lower pole.
- *Most common complication:* Urinary infection.
- Fusion seen at L4 vertebra level.
- *IVP shows:* Flower vase appearance.
- *The isthmus is cut only in one surgery:* Abdominal aortic aneurysm surgery.
- Blood supply is from major arteries nearby.
- Pregnancy is not a contraindication—but urinary infection is common for them.

**52. Identify the diagnosis from IVP image here.**

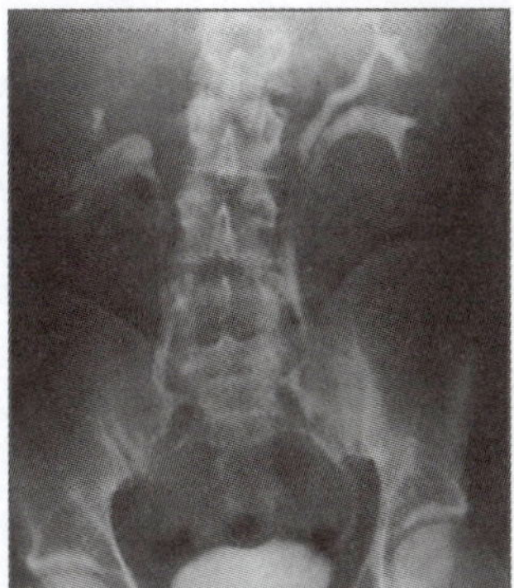

*Source:* Bailey and Love, 28th edition.

*Duplex ureter*

- Ectopic ureters are usually duplicate ureters (in 80% cases) but may also occur in single ureter system.
- MC in females. The classical appearance in IVP is shown below:
- A dilated, obstructed upper moiety ureter, in a completely duplicated system, may produce downward and lateral displacement of the functional lower moiety collecting system, appearing radiographically as the well-known drooping lily sign.

**53.**

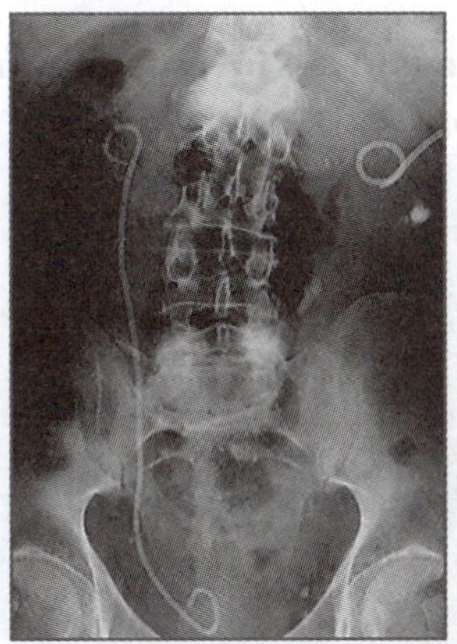

*Source:* Bailey and Love, 28th edition.

*Double J-stent*

- The ureter can be drained into the bladder by the insertion of a pigtail- or J-stent.
- The DJ stent will be straight when kept in guidewire and will become curved once guidewire removed.
- Pig-tailing helps it to be retained.

**54. What is the part of urethra injured on this retrograde urethrogram (RGU)?**

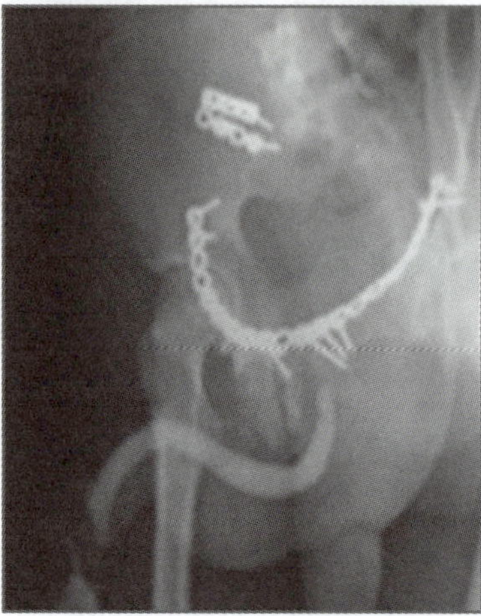

*Source:* Bailey and Love, 28th edition.

- The patient is having fracture pelvis with plate fixations, which is the common cause of urethral injuries.
- RGU shows an abrupt cut-off at level of membranous urethra.
- If per rectal examination done will show—high-lying floating prostate.

**55. Identify the findings in this investigation in a child with obstructive urinary symptoms:**

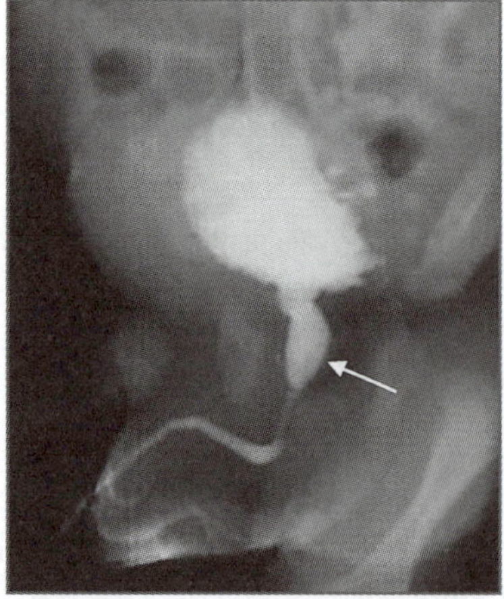

*Source:* Bailey and Love, 28th edition.

- The shown investigation here is micturating cystourethrogram showing posterior urethral valves.

**56. Identify the CT image shown here:**

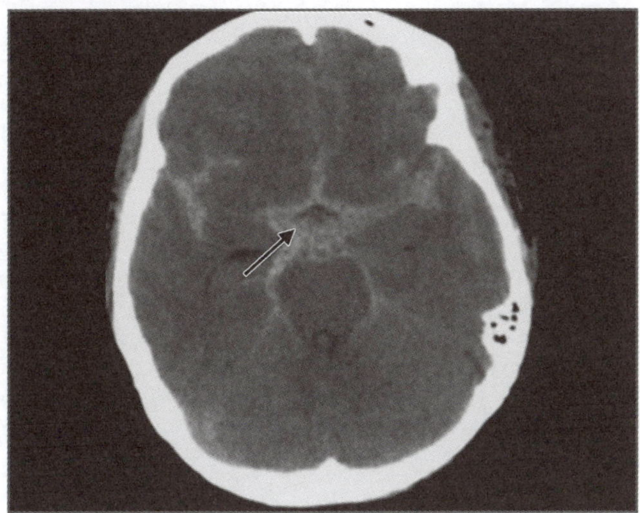

*Source:* Bailey and Love, 28th edition.

*Subarachnoid hemorrhage (SAH):*

- See the first picture which shows hyperdense signal in subarachnoid space due to presence of blood.
- See the second picture which shows isodense signal which is normal.
- CT scan grading of subarachnoid hemorrhage due to berry aneurysm rupture is given by Fisher grading system.

*Fisher grading for appearance of SAH on computed tomography:*

| Grade | CT findings |
|---|---|
| I | No hemorrhage evident |
| II | Diffuse SAH with vertical layers <1 mm thick |
| III | Localized clots and/or vertical layers of SAH >1 mm thick |
| IV | Diffuse or no SAH, but with intracerebral or intraventricular hemorrhage |

# Index

## A

## B

## D

## F

## H

## I

## J



## K



## L

## M

## N

## O

## P

## Q

## R

## S

## T

## U

## X



## Y



## Z